International
Handbook
on Aging

International Handbook on Aging

CONTEMPORARY DEVELOPMENTS and RESEARCH

Edited by Erdman Palmore

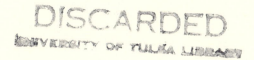

GREENWOOD PRESS

WESTPORT, CONNECTICUT

Library of Congress Cataloging in Publication Data
Main entry under title:

International handbook on aging.

Includes index.
1. Gerontology—Addresses, essays, lectures.
I. Palmore, Erdman Ballagh, 1930–
HQ1061.1535   1980   301.43′5   78-73802
ISBN 0-313-20890-5

Library of Congress Catalog Card Number: 78-73802
ISBN: 0-313-20890-5

First published in 1980

Greenwood Press
A division of Congressional Information Service, Inc.
88 Post Road West, Westport, Connecticut 06881

Printed in the United States of America

10   9   8   7   6   5   4   3   2   1

Dedicated to the gerontologists
around the world
who are helping to make
old age a good age

CONTENTS

TABLES

FOREWORD

Aging has been a major source of curiosity and fear from the time of recorded memory, but only recently has gerontology, the study of aging processes and problems, become a subject of scientific inquiry. The sciences that deal specifically with the understanding of the mechanism of aging and the search for better treatments of the aged physically and mentally, gerontology and geriatrics, have not yet become fashionable. Research in gerontology has been limited and had been carried out under the auspices of a variety of biological and social sciences. The understandable but unfortunate result is that a considerable amount of this work has been published in journals that have nothing in particular to do with gerontology.

The problems of this new interdisciplinary science have been compounded by the pressing need for its development. Within a short period following World War II, the proportion of old people increased in most countries, and while their health and welfare became the concern of most governments, this was not a favorable condition for devoting the resources that are necessary for a better understanding about aging. As a matter of fact, the urgent demands of the increasing population of senior citizens caused a considerable amount of effort to be directed to their immediate needs, and therefore progress in securing basic knowledge was delayed.

This situation started to change in recent years as developments in the field of gerontology took a remarkable leap forward in some countries. These breakthroughs occurred in a variety of disciplines. In some countries, sociology made the greatest progress, while elsewhere welfare delivery or home programs were more successful. In some countries, biology made remarkable advances, and interesting research programs in medicine were initiated. Less dramatic progress or none at all was noted in other countries.

Although gerontologists from around the world meet in congresses and are associated in the International Association of Gerontology, we never have been able to obtain information easily on work in progress in every country, much less to know where to find contacts for organization or research. As president of the IAG, I have received letters from members in various countries, asking, for example, where they could spend a sabbatical year in view of their present knowledge and the kind of work they would like to pursue or the kind of training they would like to acquire.

In this book we have for the first time the accumulated information on the state of gerontology in each of the countries in which some significant work and development is taking place; review of the history of gerontology is included in each case. Passing through the chapters, one can see that the means and motivations for undertaking research and programs have varied in different countries. Similarly the demographics of aging have varied with time and from one country to another. The roles of old people and the status of the aged is depicted as well as the programs for the aged. The research in the various disciplines of gerontology is presented usually with enough information to call a researcher's attention to the most appropriate laboratory or institutions. And finally many authors have presented sources for obtaining further information on aging and the aged in their countries.

This book will be a useful reference for people who already are involved in gerontological studies or who are working with the aged. It is also of great interest for comparative study and is a valuable source of information for those who want to implement programs for the aged while profiting from the experiences of others. The possibility of learning from the person who did the job is always of incomparable value. Whether it is an experiment on a laboratory bench or a plan for home care, the people involved know where the difficulties lie and what progress has been made to overcome them. Such information about the work going on and the persons responsible, when found in one book, contributes to a sharing of ideas and a tightening of connections throughout the world for the benefit of those who are old today and, even more, for all of us who will become old in years to come.

David Danon, President,
International Association of Gerontology

PREFACE

Until recently most gerontology has been limited to the United States and a few West European countries. Consequently most of what we know about aging processes and problems derives from data on whites in Western, capitalist countries. A recent analysis documents that only about 10 percent of bibliographic references in American gerontological journals refer to foreign data and sources. Furthermore most of these were published in the United Kingdom or the United States.

For gerontology to become a truly international science and profession, scholarly inquiry must expand to include studies among all races and ethnic groups and in all major countries around the world. This volume represents a step in that direction. It is an attempt to collect and summarize information on the programs and research in gerontology in most of the countries where substantial work is in progress.

In order to obtain outstanding gerontologists as contributors to this volume, a letter was sent to the head of the main gerontological agency in each country listed in the *International Directory of Gerontological Organizations* inviting each to prepare a chapter on developments in that country. Most agreed, but if a contribution could not be secured from that source, we invited another eminent gerontologist through suggestions from the International Federation on Aging or through personal contacts.

The resulting twenty-eight countries represented in this volume include most of those with substantial organizations, programs, and research on aging. Two notable omissions are Sweden and Australia. The gerontologists who contracted to write chapters for those countries were unable to do so because of other duties, and the urgency of making the rest of this material available precluded reassigning the chapters. We hope to include these and other countries in a future edition. The countries surveyed here include most of the world's largest nations and some of the smallest, among the latter Ireland, Israel, New Zealand, and Uruguay (see table 1). They include highly urbanized countries and some less urbanized ones (such as South Africa and Hungary), and they represent all economic systems: capitalist, socialist, communist. Included are countries with the highest proportion of aged, such as the German Democractic Republic, and some with a low proportion of aged, such as Venezuela; countries with high birthrates, such as Mexico, and some with low birthrates, such as the Federal Republic of Germany; countries with high death rates, such as South Africa, and those with low death rates, such as Israel and Japan.

Yet these nations are not a representative sample of all countries in the world. Gerontology research and programs have developed primarily in countries having two characteristics. The first is a high proportion of aged. The United Nations has defined populations as aged if the nation has over 7 percent aged 65 and over; as mature if 4 to 7 percent are 65 and over; and as young if less than 4 percent are 65 and over. Most of the countries in this volume are classified as aged; there are only three mature countries (Chile, Mexico, and South Africa) and only one young country (Venezuela). The second characteristic is that high proportions of the country are urbanized and industrialized (usually 50 percent or more urban). There is almost no gerontology and there are few programs for the aged among the less developed countries of the world.

It is understandable that the countries with the highest proportion of aged would have the most developed gerontology programs and research. Yet the increase in the proportion of aged has slowed down in the highly developed, industrialized countries, and the less developed nations face the most rapidly rising proportion of aged and all the accompanying problems. Perhaps the less developed nations most need to develop programs for the aged rapidly so that they can anticipate and reduce the problems of aging that the developed countries have experienced.

This volume should be of use to the less developed countries as well as to the researchers, students, program planners, administrators, and others interested in aging around the world. Each section author was asked to include information on unique features of the country; the growth of gerontology; roles and status of the aged; problems of the aged; programs for the aged; research in biomedical, psychological, and social science aspects of the aging; and information sources on aging. Some authors have chosen to emphasize some aspects and deemphasize others. Most authors have emphasized their own disciplines. Some have written lengthy chapters and some short ones; the length is largely dependent on the extent of gerontology and programs in their countries. Some have emphasized positive aspects, and some have been more critical.

The volume also has three useful appendixes; one giving the names and addresses of the major gerontological organizations in each country having one or more such organizations, one describing regional and international organizations in gerontology, and one analyzing the international development of gerontology. Most chapters have bibliographies. In some cases, works have been added to the bibliographies by Greenwood editors.

We hope this volume will contribute to the growth of a truly international science and professional practice in gerontology and thereby improve the quantity and quality of life for the hundreds of millions already aged and the future aged. Perhaps by improving international understanding in a field of pressing common needs, it also will make a small contribution to world peace.

Erdman Palmore

Table 1: DEMOGRAPHIC CHARACTERISTICS OF THE COUNTRIES IN THIS BOOK

Country	1975 Population (Millions)	Percentage 65 and Over	Crude Birthrate (per 1,000)	Crude Death Rate (per 1,000)	Life Expectancy at Birth		Percentage Urban
					Male	Female	
Austria	8	15	12	13	67	75	52
Canada	23	8	15	8	69	76	76
Chile	10	6	28	9	60	66	76
Denmark	5	12	14	10	71	76	67
Federal Republic of Germany	62	14	10	12	68	74	n.a.
Finland	5	10	14	9	67	75	58
France	53	13	15	10	69	76	70
German Democractic Republic	17	16	11	14	69	74	75
Greece	9	11	16	9	70	74	65
Hungary	11	11	18	12	67	73	50
Ireland	3	11	22	11	69	73	52
Israel	3	9	28	7	70	73	82
Italy	56	11	16	10	69	75	n.a.
Japan	111	7	19	7	71	76	72
Mexico	60	4	43	9	63	67	63
Netherlands	14	10	14	8	71	77	77
New Zealand	3	9	21	9	69	75	81
Norway	4	14	14	10	71	78	45
Poland	34	9	18	8	68	75	54
Rumania	21	9	20	9	67	71	43
South Africa	25	4	40	17	50	53	48
Switzerland	6	12	13	9	70	76	55
Union of Soviet Socialist Republics	256	8	18	9	65	74	61
United Kingdom	56	13	13	12	68	74	78
United States of America	214	10	15	9	68	76	74
Uruguay	3	n.a.	21	10	66	72	n.a.
Venezuela	12	2	41	8	66		74
Yugoslavia	21	8	18	8	66	70	34

Source: United Nations *1975 Demographic Yearbook.* Occasional discrepancies between these data and those in the rest of the book are due to different sources or years involved.

International
Handbook
on Aging

AUSTRIA

A. AMANN,

B. DOBERAUER,

W. DOBERAUER,

J. HOERL,

and G. MAJCE

DEVELOPMENT OF GERONTOLOGY

Experimental Gerontology

The beginning of experimental gerontology in Austria goes back to 1450, when Nicolaus de Cusa in Brixen in his treatise *De staticis experimentis* introduced analytics into aging research and by means of measuring and weighing methods tried to assess the functional variations of senescence as compared to youth. Inspired by Nicolaus de Cusa, physicians of the University of Vienna performed a series of experimental gerontological investigations.

The interest in experimental aging research subsided until after World War II when W. Doberauer became interested in this field of work and resumed experimental gerontological research with his collaborators. They carried out their investigations on animals of different ages and dealt chiefly with subjects that are important to clinical geriatrics, among them the influence of age on wound healing (W. Doberauer, 1962a-d, 1963a-c), the growth of benign and malignant tumors and formation of metastasis in relation to age (W. Kovac, A. Lindner, and W. Doberauer, 1966), the difference in water and electrolyte balance in young and old animals (Doberauer, Formaneck, and Wick, 1966a & b) the consequences of radical dehydration, and the age-dependent differences in the course of inflammations (Doberauer and Stoklaska, 1966a & b).

Twenty years ago (1958) Professor Dr. A. Kment, head of the Institute of Physiology, University of Veterinary Medicine, Vienna, introduced experimental gerontology in his institute. Based above all on the ideas of Verzár, Kment and his research team used objective parameters and started to quantify aging as a basic physiologic process; their goal was to explain fundamental aging processes and to identify factors that accelerate or retard it (Kment,

1976; Kment and Hofecker, 1977a & b). The research team includes, besides the head of the institute, Professor Dr. A. Kment (physiology), Professor Dr. G. Hofecker (physiology), Doz. Dipl. Ing., Dr. H. Niedermüller (biochemistry), and Dipl. Ing. Dr. M. Skalicky (physics and mathematics). Other members are two assistant physicians, fifteen laboratory assistants, and ten (at present) candidates for dissertation. The institute is furnished with the most modern physical and chemical laboratories, including a radioisotope laboratory, a biochemical automatic analyzer, an electronic measuring device for biophysical investigations, and a computer. Facilities include laboratories and room for housing fifteen hundred to two thousand experimental rats and a number of larger experimental animals.

The experimental gerontological research of the institute deals essentially with three major overlapping fields: subcellular and molecular aging, aspects of behavioral physiology of aging, and measurements of and influencing of biological age or vitality.

In the subcellular and molecular field, the interest is centered on mitochondria and the macromolecules collagen and DNA. An extended morphometric study on aging changes of heart and liver mitochondria of rat revealed an increase in the number of mitochondria with a decrease of average mitochondria diameter in old rats. The total percentage of mitochondria per volume unit, however, remained unaffected. This change may be interpreted as a compensation of a progressing functional impairment. This applies, however, only to the presenile phase of aging, which probably leads finally to a state of decompensation with an increase in megamitochondria (Kment et al., 1966a, 1966b; Kment and Hofecker, 1977a & b).

Aging of collagen is assessed by the techniques of Verzár (measurement of thermic and chemical denaturation tonicity), as well as with radioisotope examinations of metabolism. The mathematical analysis of results brought new light into structural aging changes of tendon collagen, as well as compartment models of collagen metabolism in young and old animals. The results have revealed the presence of two types of collagen in skin and tendon, have corrected the former ideas about collagen metabolism, and have led to a modification of Verzár's cross-link hypothesis of collagen aging (Niedermüller et al., 1976, 1977a, 1977b; Skalicky et al., 1977; Hofecker, 1975; Hofecker et al., 1972, 1974a, 1974b, 1976, 1977).

DNA investigations deal with restoration processes in this macromolecule. A method has been developed that enables the study of the in vivo kinetics of DNA restoration in rat organs. According to results, restoration capacity decreases with age, and the course in the different age groups shows varying peaks (Niedermüller et al., 1975, 1976; Niedermüller, 1977).

In the complex field of age-related changes, investigations in rats dealt with motor activity and problems of learning, memory, and memory transfer. Motor activity investigated by means of several methods—running wheel, vibrant cage, kinematographic registration, and electronic registration with the Animex® Activity meter—revealted that various forms of motor activity decrease with aging in a different way. For example, purely spontaneous activity remains largely unchanged up to an advanced age, but the reactive activities decrease considerably earlier (Kment, 1963; Hofecker et al., 1974a, 1974b,; Starrach, 1976; Schaffranek, 1976).

Learning tests in the T-labyrinth showed that the learning capacity in approximately 20-month-old rats is largely equivalent to that of young animals. Exploration of the labyrinth is indeed slower in the older animals, but the error rate is lower. Experiments on possibilities of memory transfer in rats revealed that cerebral proteins from animals trained in the labyrinth after subcutaneous injection improved the learning of recipient animals significantly, whereas RNA of trained rats and proteins and RNA of untrained rats showed no measurable effects. The memory transfer was expressed in younger animals by shorter running times and in the old animals by a diminution of error rates (H. Niedermüller, 1976, 1977; E. Niedermüller, 1976).

Verzár's postulate that experimental gerontology should investigate not only fundamental aging processes but also should identify accelerating and inhibiting factors indicates the long-term aim of this research: to explore the possibilities of an intentional influence on aging processes. Such experiments presume the measurability of biological age. Kment compiled a comprehensive aging test program for laboratory rats that took account of the complexity of multicellular aging. It also contained parameters of learning and memory, of motor activity, of skin and aorta elasticity, of tendon collagen, and of tissue respiration. This program was further enlarged, and measuring techniques were improved and combined with electronic data processing. The data compiled by means of this standard test program are at present analyzed by means of multivariate statistical methods in order to obtain standard measures for biological age of laboratory rats (Kment, 1976; Hofecker, 1976). On the basis of these measures, it will be possible to follow the vitality of experimental animals in the course of aging and under the influence of various experimental conditions (Beier et al, 1973).

The influencing of the aging process can have two aims: a prolongation of maximal life span or the longest possible conservation of a high level of vitality within the frame of the genetically determined maximum life span. Kment (1977) underlines that from the sociological standpoint, priority should be given to the conservation of vital capacity within the genetically determined frame. Therefore he postulates that in addition to the investigation of fundamental aging processes, the factors of daily life and their effects on biological age and on vitality should be more closely examined in the animal experiments. Moreover he thinks it necessary to check all approaches toward revitalization that have been found so far by objective, standardized methods of experimental gerontology.

Kment's postulate for objectivation by means of animal experiments sets new measures for the rather ambiguous notion of revitalization, which are also expressed in his definition, inspired by Beier's biophysical vitality model: "revitalization of an organism which has passed the vitality climax is, as has to be objectivated by means of several age parameters, the prolonged maintenance or recovery of a vitality level corresponding to a significantly lower biological age than would accord with the chronological age of the organism" (Kment, 1975). This critical parameter was used in all experiments concerning the influence on aging processes, among others, in the investigation of geriatric drugs, parenterally administered freeze-dried tissue material, running training, and food restriction as well as microclimate (Kment and Hofecker, 1977).

Kment and his collaborators were particularly interested in revitalizing effects. He was the first to carry out comprehensive animal experiments that examined the effects of freeze-dried placenta and testis cells on the aging parameters of rats (Kment, 1963). Statistically significant changes of nearly all parameters toward a younger biological age were observed several months after the last injection. The mechanism of this revitalizing effect is now the object of current investigations.

A recently completed longitudinal study of eleven hundred rats deals with the effects of a restriction of food quantities, a mild regular running training, a combination of both, and the subcutaneous administration of freeze-dried testis cells on a series of aging parameters or vital capacity. The results, which are only partly evaluated, show already that increased exercise, restriction of food uptake, and subcutaneous administration of testis cells are apt to change at least some of the aging parameters of rats in the sense of a revitalization. Testis cells seem to affect the greatest number of parameters and tend to become more pronounced in older age only (Kment et al., 1977). More precise conclusions will be possible after a multivariate analysis of results.

The future experimental gerontologic research program includes a longitudinal study of the influence of environmental stress on the aging and vitality of rats, as well as aspects of molecular and cellular aging and how they are affected by revitalization measures.

In 1976 the Physiologic Institute of the University of Veterinary Medicine in Vienna organized, together with the Austrian Society of Geriatrics, the First Vienna Symposium on Experimental Gerontology. Thirty-eight gerontologists from Europe and overseas surveyed the current problems in experimental gerontology. Such symposia will be held every two years and will encourage experimental gerontology in the spirit of its founder, F. Verzár.

W. Doberauer, who works not only in experimental gerontology but also in clinical geriatrics and social gerontology, founded the Austrian Society of Geriatrics in 1955, was elected president, and still presides over the society. With more than a hundred scientific publications in various fields of gerontology to his credit, Doberauer was elected chairman of the European Executive Committee of the International Association of Gerontology. In 1966 he resigned from this office, since for the term 1966–1969 he was elected president of the association. During this period he became more involved in clinical geriatrics, but there is reason to hope that experimental gerontology will not be neglected in Austria, since A. Kment successfully aroused the interest of his young collaborators and encouraged their work. The continuity of experimental gerontologic research thus seems guaranteed for the next years. This seems particularly important, since without exact experimental gerontologic research, no real progress in clinical geriatrics is possible.

Clinical Geriatrics

Since the foundation of the University of Vienna in 1365, various medical disciplines have investigated the diseases of old age, but no systematic clinical aging research was carried out until this century. When the nursing home for elderly patients in Vienna-Lainz was opened in 1904 with six thousand beds and different specialized units, clinical geriatric research intensified. Shortly after it opened, a physician from New York, I.L. Nascher (1863–1944), visited this home. The good condition of the residents impressed him as much as the low mortality rate did, and he asked the head physician why this institution was so different from other nursing homes. "We treat our residents the same way as the pediatrician treats his children," was the reply, as simple as it was impressive. When Nascher returned to New York, he published in 1909 in the *New York Medical Journal* (90, 358–359) a pragmatic article in which, analogous to the term *pediatrics*, he coined the term *geriatrics* and requested full autonomy for the specialty. Nascher, who worked in New York at Mount Sinai Hospital, had been born in Austria. Thus a man of Austrian origin became the founder of modern geriatrics.

In 1914, the Viennese internist H. Schlesinger issued *The Diseases of Advanced Age*, and in 1937 Müller-Deham wrote *Internal Diseases in Old Age*. The latter later emigrated to the United States and worked at the Goldwater Memorial Hospital in New York; a new edition of his book appeared in 1942 as *Internal Medicine in Old Age*.

During World War II, geriatric research in Austria came to a standstill. It was resumed in 1950 by W. Doberauer and his collaborators, and in 1955 the Austrian Society of Geriatrics was founded. Since then yearly postgraduate courses in geriatrics have been held at Hofgastein where a thousand to two thousand physicians from Austria, Germany, and Switzerland take part. Each year thirty to fifty speakers present and discuss results of their recent research work; the material is published every year by W. Doberauer in *Scriptum Geriatricum*. Up to now nineteen volumes have been issued. In 1969 W. Doberauer (Vienna) published together with A. Hittmayr (Innsbruck), R.

Nissen (Basel), and F. H. Schulz (Berlin) the first *Handbook of Practical Geriatrics* in German (three volumes). This was followed in 1976 by the publication of the *Introduction to Practical Geriatrics* (Bruschke, Doberauer, and Schmidt). Since World War II, more than a thousand scientific publications dealing with geriatric problems have been published, the majority of them in *Scriptum Geriatricum*.

W. Doberauer will soon hand over to one of his colleagues the direction of the geriatric hospitals Baumgarten, St. Rochus, and St. Martin in Vienna, which have sixteen hundred beds. It is hoped that geriatric research in Austria will continue.

Gerosociology

The development of gerosociology was stimulated in Austria by the growing interest of medicine in the social factors conditioning aging processes. Although Charlotte Bühler in the 1920s and early 1930s had designed a psychology of the life span, the main interests of social psychology and sociology, through the influence of the important early works of P. Lazarsfeld, became oriented toward developments during childhood and youth.

After World War II, when W. Doberauer institutionalized courses of specialized geriatric education for physicians, he asked for supplementary sociogerontological background information. The psychiatrists Stransky and Hans Hoff also felt the necessity for a sociological foundation of mental health problems of the elderly in the early 1950s. In response to some of these challenges, Leopold Rosenmayr, who founded the Social Science Research Laboratory at the University of Vienna in 1954, began to extend research activities to the area of aging in 1956 (Rosenmayr, 1975a & b). Rosenmayr had previously studied family and housing problems in the city of Vienna and, in 1956–1957 a study was launched, which Rosenmayr later described in the following terms:

Our projects were designed to fulfill a double purpose: First to meet a request of the City Planning Department to evaluate, sociologically, present housing conditions and in particular to find out to what extent the special type of dwellings built for the aged during the last decade—the "Altersheim-stätten" (self-contained old-age-apartments) —is meeting the requirements of the inhabitants for whom they were specially designed and constructed. Our research was also directed towards gaining a better knowledge of the habits, social relations and special needs of the aged in general, and thus towards the construction of a cumulative and empirically based "sociology of the aged." These two goals can very well be combined because planning housing for the aged should involve a recognition of all their needs. Not merely the utilization of the various parts of the dwelling but also all activities and relationships of the inhabitants have to be studied. [Rosenmayr and Köckeis, 1965b]

This study led to a series of criticisms of city planning and building policies of the city government of Vienna. It emphasized in particular that the local proximity between old and young, which was created by building special homes for the elderly amid large housing units, did not lead to the expected diminishing of the social distance between the age groups. On the other hand, family relations proved to be important, even under conditions of local separation. A stratified random sample of 661 persons 65 and over demonstrated close family cohesion coupled with a remarkable desire for separate dwelling. This led Rosenmayr in 1958 to coin the formula "intimacy at a distance," which he applied not only to family relations but also to ecological aspects, thus expressing specific attitudes characterized by a dialectic between engagement and detachment. Further studies by Rosenmayr and collaborators led to

criticism of mass movements for old-age monocultures (expressing themselves in housing colonies exclusively for persons of higher age)...particularly in view of advertisement campaigns and massive interests of building firms exploiting the romanticisms of leisure worlds. In analogy to housing monocultures, the idea of a uniform role of the elderly from a sociological point of view is equally problematic because, if advocated uncritically, it may lead to a stereotyping of life styles for the elderly. This is particularly out of place in the later years of life where personal maturity should further "individual" instead of "patterned" decisions and solutions. [Rosenmayr and Köckeis, 1965a]

In 1963 *Propositions for a Theory of Aging and the Family* was published by L. Rosenmayr and E. Köckeis, and in 1969 an article by Rosenmayr appeared in René König's *Handbook of Empirical Social Research*. A revised and enlarged edition of the latter article was published in 1976. In the late 1960s— after more than ten years of research—many publications were issued that formed the foundation for the later extended development of sociogerontological studies. Some of these became oft-cited standard publications in German-speaking countries. Some were of particular merit because they contributed to general discussion in social gerontology and therefore are historically of special importance: Rosenmayr's, *Family Relations of the Elderly* (1968) and a further development of this line of research in his "The Family: A Source of Hope for the Elderly?" (1977).

Beginning in 1972 the research activity was considerably extended, which was also expressed by an increase in the number of permanent collaborators (A. Amann, J. Grafinger, J. Hörl, G. Majce). In the same year, the Ludwig Boltzmann Institute for Aging Research was founded, with which gerontologists in Austria had a close cooperation since the beginning. Demographic analyses based on statistical census materials, development and changes of assistance to the elderly, problems of family relations of elderly people who need care, the stress on families due to sick elderly relatives, the cooperation with social services, the theoretical development of social gerontology, and research on the relations between sociology, social policy, and social work are the focus of present activity. Evidence of this is given among others in volume 6/4 of the *Zeitschrift für Gerontologie* (1973) edited by L. Rosenmayr. A strong integration of research and practice, the joint formulation of problems and solutions with people involved in practical welfare work for the elderly, evaluation research, and a new determination of the relation between politics and science are important trends. Consequently a two-volume research report was published in 1974 by L. Rosenmayr and A. Amann, *The Elderly Person in the Structures of Present Society*, and in the same year an extensive explorative case study for problems of home help for the elderly was started; the latter has led in the meantime to a series of publications and another project with practical orientation on evaluation research in home help for elderly people. Also in 1974, G. Majce and J. Hörl published *Forms of Assistance to the Elderly*, a preliminary study for a comprehensive empirical investigation finished by the same authors in 1976, which examined the population that the residents of the homes for elderly people in Vienna came from. In autumn 1976, the institute organized at the university a forum for administrators and decision makers involved in practical work, which aimed at initiating a continuous discussion by eliminating the difficulties of communication between science and policy. In the course of discussions, scientists were made aware of practical aspects and requirements of the topics treated, and an increased understanding and need for scientific social research was created among the people involved in practical work. In cooperation with another research body, a basic work on problems of interdisciplinary assistance for the elderly was carried out (Amann and Velimirovic, 1977), and an extensive publication is being prepared in which the evolution of social gerontology in various countries and the assistance for elderly people which parallels it is examined; this represents the first of its kind in the German-speaking countries.

In 1978 Leopold and Hilde Rosenmayr, together with A. Amann, J. Hörl, and G. Majce, published a book on the elderly in the society (L. and H. Rosenmayr [eds.], 1978) which represents a synopsis of international research in social gerontology, especially on the status of the aged, achievement and old age, social ecology, sexuality and family, social deprivation of the aged, various forms of old age assistance, and demography. Also in 1978, L. Rosenmayr edited a reader dealing with life-phases from philosophical, ethnological, demographic, medical, biological, psychological, psychiatric, and sociological points of view (L. Rosenmayr [ed.], 1978). At present Rosenmayr, Amann, A. Eder, E. Fischer, and Majce, on behalf of the Ministry of Science and Research, are preparing a long-term plan for a research policy on the elderly in Austria.

Two other current projects are worth mentioning: G. Majce is carrying out a family-biographical study of the in-law relations of the elderly, and J. Hörl is investigating the problems of the linkage of familial patterns with bureaucratic organizational patterns of assistance to the elderly.

DEMOGRAPHIC AND SOCIOLOGICAL CHARACTERISTICS OF THE AGED POPULATION

Proportions of Aged

In only one country in the world, the German Democratic Republic, is the proportion of old people higher than in Austria. In 1971, when the last Austrian census was taken, 1,508,408 persons were 60 and more years old. That figure represents 20.2 percent of the Austrian population; 14.2 percent of the Austrians were 65 and over; and 9.8 percent were 70 years and over; 4.7 percent were 75 years and over. This appears, however, to be the peak of this development, at least for this millennium. According to the most recent data available—an interpolation for the year 1977—the percentage of the 60 and over population is 19.8 percent at present (65 and over, 15.3 percent; 70 and over, 10.0 percent); and demographers have made the following prognosis for the rest of the century: in 1981, 14.8 percent of the population will be 65 or older, in 1991 only 13.8 percent and around 2000, the figure will have decreased to 13.4 percent (Ö.St.Z., 1978, pp. 15-16).

The average figures for Austria as a whole are by far exceeded by the figures for the capital of Vienna. As many as 40,400 persons—21.4 percent of the population of Vienna (1,591,000)—were 65 or older in 1977. Persons 70 and above account for 14.1 percent of the total population of Vienna (Magistrat der Stadt Wien [ed.], 1977, p. 32); their number is increasing rapidly and will continue to rise at least up to the end of the 1980s. In 1910 persons 75 and over accounted for 24 percent of the persons 65 years of age; this figure rose to 26 percent in 1934, 33 percent in 1961, and 35 percent in 1971 (Rosenmayr, 1976, p. 278). It would be a mistake to interpret the extremely high percentage of old people in Austria as an indicator of an extremely high average life expectancy in this country. On the contrary, compared to other developed countries Austria must be considered below average. The average male life expectancy at birth was 66.6 years in 1970; thus Austria ranked fourteenth among OECD countries. For females, the position was thirteenth with 73.7 years. The situation is even worse with regard to the remaining life expectancy of the aged: in 1970-72 a 60-year-old man had an average of fifteen more years ahead of him; tied with Belgium, this was the worst result of all the OECD countries. The result with regard to women was 19.1 years, tied with the Federal Republic of Germany for the lowest figure (Scheer, 1977).

We will deal here with only two of the principal causes of the comparatively large aged population of Austria. First, the special sociohistorical situation of Austria must be taken into account. Sixty years ago, it was the nucleus of the

Austro-Hungarian empire, and Vienna, the imperial capital, attracted large numbers of young immigrants from all parts of the empire. Then immigraton figures dropped suddenly, and Austria (especially in the east) began to age very quickly. Second, the birthrate has been very low in Austria, in particular since the late 1960s. As a consequence, in 1975 for the first time, the population of Austria decreased (Ö.St.Z., 1977). (This negative growth occurred only in the eastern part of Austria. The western and the southern parts of the country are characterized by relatively high birth rates.)

Sex Ratio

The enormous surplus of women in Austria results not only from their higher life expectancy (approximately seven years at birth and four years for 60 year olds) but from the influences of two world wars, which were characterized by high death rates for men. Between the census of 1910 and that of 1951, the male population of Austria decreased by 67,000; the female population increased by 353,000 (Gisser, 1976). Until the beginning of the 1990s, the sex ratio of the population above 65 will increase, and there will be nearly twice as many aged women as men. The current (1977) proportion is 172 women for 100 men; a ratio of 193:100 has been forecast for 1990. After 1990 there will be a sudden decrease in the proportion of women, in particular because most of the age groups affected by the wars will be gone.

Marital Status

Unmarried women are by far the largest subgroup among the population above 65. In 1977, 81.4 percent of the men from 65 to 70 but only 41.7 percent of the women of the same age group were married. The percentages for persons from 70 to 75 were 75.6 percent and 30.4 percent respectively; for 75 to 80 year olds, 66.2 percent and 18.9 percent; and only 8 percent of the women above 80 years of age were married, as opposed to half of the men (Ö.St.Z., 1978, pp. 16-17). In 1977, 44.2 percent of the aged population of Austria had been married, 10.2 percent were single, 42.1 percent widowed, and 3.5 percent divorced. If we take the widowed persons as 100 percent, then 83 percent were women (Ö.St.Z., 1977). These patterns are particularly acute in Vienna, which has the following percentages: unmarried women, 49 percent; married women, 17 percent; unmarried men 9 percent; and married men 25 percent (Rosenmayr, 1976).

Household Composition and Family Structure

Although, as is true in most industrialized countries, substantial numbers of the elderly live in households separated from the households of their offspring, a high percentage of old people do live together with their children. A special census, taken in December 1971, on the situation of the elderly in Austria showed that 24 percent of all people 60 and over who were living in private households lived in single-person households. Another 35 percent were aged couples in two-person households (Ö.St.Z., 1972, p. 34). Because of their longer life expectancy and their lower age at marriage, women are more likely to remain in single-person households than men: at the age of 65-75, 10 percent of the men, but not less than 37 percent of the women, live in single-person households, the numbers of those 75 and over being 16 percent and 42 percent, respectively (Ö.St.Z., 1977, p. 27).

The problem of the isolation of women is typically aggravated in the large cities, especially in Vienna. Forty percent of all single-person households are concentrated there. Usually these households consist of unmarried old people, and most of them are old women. In 1971, 111,500 women 65 and over lived in single-person households in the capital of Austria. Nevertheless, a survey in 1974 revealed that nearly 40 percent of those elderly who have grown-up children lived with them in a household.

Table 2: ELDERLY LIVING WITH THEIR GROWN-UP CHILDREN BY AGE AND SEX, 1974

Sex	60-69	70 and over
	percent	percent
Men	31	42
Women	39	38
Total	35	40

Source: Bundesministerium für Wissenschaft und Forschung (ed.), Die gesellschaftliche Reintegration älterer Menschen in Österreich. Vienna-New York: Springer, 1976, p. 48.

In the past 100 years, there has been a marked decline in the portion of single persons. In 1880, for example, 24 out of 100 women aged 60-65 were single, whereas this figure is only 11 today, the figures for men in these years being 20 and 6, respectively (Ö.St.Z., 1977, p. 24,). At the same time, however, fertility has undergone a sharp decrease. Thus the ratio of the elderly to the grown-up children who could care for them has shifted dramatically against the former. Where in 1910, for example, there were three women aged 35-44 for every widowed (or divorced) woman 55 and over, there were only 1.3 in the year 1973. In addition, in contrast to former times, nearly all of those middle-aged women were married and had children, with the consequence that they were not able to fully take care of their aged mothers (H. and L. Rosenmayr, 1978, p. 196).

Nearly 30 percent of the Austrian population aged 60 and over have no living children (Ö.St.Z. 1972, p. 52). But it is only a very small minority of old people who have no relatives (spouse not included) at all, namely 2.6 percent

(Ö.St.Z., 1972, p. 53). About half of this number, however, are married; so, as few as 1.4 percent of the Austrian elderly have neither a spouse nor any other relatives, and one out of every two of them is living in Vienna.

Generally speaking, the elderly have a rich kinship network. A quarter of them have at least three children and other relatives; a further 20 percent have at least two children and other relatives. The elderly inhabitants of the rural small communities have the best kinship networks, whereas the Viennese kinship networks are fairly poor: Only 17 percent of the elderly (60 and over) living in communities with less than 2,000 inhabitants have no living children. The other extreme is represented by the Viennese with 37 percent of this group having no children (Ö.St.Z., 1972, p. 52). A Viennese study from the year 1968 reported that 51 percent of the women 70 and over had no children (IFES, 1968, p. 4).

In addition to the elderly having immediate offspring, a tendency toward an overlapping of generations can be observed. Three percent of the population 60 and over still have living parents, and nearly 12 percent have great-grand-children (Ö.St.Z., 1977). More than two-thirds have brothers or sisters, but only 4 percent of the elderly live in a household with these siblings (Ö.St.Z., 1977).

Employment and Retirement

The official retirement age in Austria is 60 years for women and 65 for men, but a large percentage retire much earlier: 12 percent of men between 50 and 60 are no longer employed, and 52 percent of men between 60 and 65 have already retired. Only 5.4 percent of persons 65 and above are still employed (8.8 percent of the men and 3.3 percent of the women) (Majce and Hörl, 1974); 83.2 percent are pensioners.

A study carried out by the Institute für empirische Sozialforschung of Vienna (IFES) showed that this early dropping out of production in most cases corresponds to the wishes of the persons concerned. Generally those with higher education or professional standing take an interest in continuing to work. The study doubts, rightfully so, "whether the majority of blue and white collar workers under the present alienated conditions of the working world have developed such strong ties to their work that retirement would mean a loss of the contents of their lives" (BMfWF, 1976). In fact 42 percent of the respondents, skilled workers above 50, declared they would retire before reaching the general pensionable age, whereas only 3 percent wanted to continue working beyond that limit. By comparison only 9 percent of those with secondary or postsecondary education planned early retirement, and the same percentage intended to continue their work after reaching the pensionable age. Among self-employed persons, this tendency became even more pro-nounced: 11 percent wanted to retire prematurely, whereas 21 percent intended to go on working beyond age 65 (BMfWF, 1976).

STATUS AND PROBLEMS OF THE AGED

Social Contacts, Isolation, Loneliness

Few data are available on the quality of the social relationships of old people. Counting contact scores yields only a limited indicator of the quality of a relationship. A study of recipients of home-help services in Vienna showed that *high frequency of contact and unfavorable family relationships may very well exist side by side*. The most obvious contact event of old age is the loss of a spouse (BMfWF, 1976). For demographic reasons, women are highly disadvantaged: The probability of their becoming widowed is very high, and the enormous surplus of women in this age group makes it almost impossible for widows to find another partner. A study carried out in Vienna showed that 15 percent of the widowed men over 70 enter a new partnership as compared to only 2 percent of the widows of this age group. Furthermore, half of the widowers but only one out of fifty widows say they hope to find a new partner (IFES, 1968). Another study found that in 1971-73 out of 1,000 widowers aged 60 to 64, 26.7 remarried, whereas only 1.2 out of 1,000 widows of the same age groups took a new spouse (Gisser, 1976, pp. 359, 363).

Regarding intergenerational social contacts, it follows from the differing kinship networks discussed above that in the rural areas there is a substantially greater chance of the elderly living together with their children than in urban areas, particularly in Vienna. "Forty-four percent of the agricultural population, but only 14 percent of the non-agricultural population of Lower Austria [the largest state of Austria], aged 60 and over are household-members of extended families; in Vienna the percentage drops to 11 percent" (H. and L. Rosenmayr, 1978, p. 180).

We should not, however, prematurely interpret household separation of the generations as "isolation" for the elderly. There are two questions to be answered: (1) Is separaton of the households necessarily followed by a loss in family relations? (2) To what degree do the elderly and their children like/dislike their present living arrangements?

In the majority of cases where the elderly live in separate households, the preconditions for maintenance of contact are not abandoned, because the children usually settle rather near their parents' households. A special census in 1975 showed that about half of the population aged 18 to 70 having relatives outside their dwellings can reach their parents in less than half an hour; for another third it takes one-half to two hours. Four-fifths of all grown-up children aged 35 to 70 are able to contact their parents personally (face-to-face) in less than two hours: In Vienna 40 percent of the grown-up children can reach their parents in a half-hour; a further 38 percent report a distance of less than two hours (Ö.St.Z., 1978, pp. 35ff.).

Short distances are reported by the elderly themselves. Not only are there high percentages of intergenerational households, but a survey defining "short distance'' as half an hour's walking distance showed that 45 percent of those people aged 60 to 70 who had grown-up children outside of their own household lived a short distance from them. Another 37 percent could reach their children (or could be reached by their children) by car or public transportation within one hour. The respective percentages for those aged 70 and over were 52 percent ''short distance'' and a further 30 percent ''one hour.'' For only 18 percent of the other elderly does it take more than one hour to reach their children (BMfWF, 1976, p. 48).

Does household separation result in a significant impoverishment of intergenerational family relations? Younger age groups commonly believe that ''the elderly'' suffer primarily from isolation, loneliness, and their children's disinterest in them. Survey research shows, however, that in this regard the opinions and attitudes of the aged population, on the one hand, and of the younger segments, on the other, are grossly at variance. When asked what problems the elderly suffered from the most, the younger people (75 percent of those aged 50 or less) answered most frequently ''being always alone.'' With rising age the percentage who gave this answer dropped. Sixty-seven percent of the people aged 60 to 70 and only 49 percent of those 70 and more answered in this way. A similar discrepancy appeared with a question about the parent-child relation. Thirty-two to 42 percent of those aged 14 to 50 held that one of the most difficult problems of the elderly would be that their children would not care enough for them. But only 27 percent of the elderly 60 to 70 years old and even 15 percent of the 70 and more years old agreed (Fessel and GfK, 1972, p.1).

One may conclude from these findings that a substantial proportion of the elderly are quite satisfied with their relationships to their off-spring. We don't know, however, if this satisfaction is the result of functioning contacts or of the elderly making a resignative adaptation to expectations of a low standard of interaction. The following figures lead to the assumption that both factors are operating, not only as separate effects on different segments of the aged population but also as a mixture on the same people.

Analyzing a special census on the elderly's contacts with relatives and friends, W. Schulz summarizes: ''Attainability is the most essential determining characteristic of a person for the frequency of being met by others. This variable explains the frequency of contacts best. If it is possible to reach the parents within less than half an hour they are met once or more a week by 77.8 percent of the Viennese population. Where the contact can be made in half an hour to two hours, only 49 percent maintain visiting contacts of at least once a week. A distance of two to six hours reduces the weekly meeting to 7 percent'' (W. Schulz, 1978, p. 89).

This pattern also applies to the rural areas, although the elderly living there more frequently have the advantage of living together with their children or in their immediate vicinity. Frequency of contacts radically declines if the children's household is farther off than the neighboring village. Two-thirds to four-fifths of the aged whose children live in the same or in the neighboring village are visited several times a week, and the percentage is reduced to only 4 percent if the distance exceeds the neighboring village (IFES, 1971, II, p.5).

In Austria 16.4 percent of the adults aged 35 to 45 with parents living in a separate household meet them nearly every day, another 30 percent at least once a week. The same figures apply to the children aged 45 to 55 and 55 to 70. One has to add, of course, those who share the household with their parents: 17 percent of the 35 to 45 age group, 11 percent of the 45 to 55 age group, and 2.6 percent of the 55 to 70 age group (Ö.St.Z., 1975, pp. 34 and 37).

Because of the exclusion of the people aged 70 and over from the special census of social contacts, contact frequency from the view of the elderly can be presented here only for the 55- to 70-year-old parents. If one takes only those who have children outside of their household, nearly 25 percent of them meet their children almost every day, another third at least once a week. Only a sixth meet their children as seldom as once a month or even less often (Ö.St.Z., 1978, p. 43). This finding is independent of whether one has a spouse or not, or whether the household is shared with other relatives or not.

Another special census (December 1971) unfortunately does not control for the variable of whether one has children or not in presenting data on visiting/being visited. Due to this failure, the contact frequencies appear more unfavorable than they really are: the childless elderly lower the averages. Daily visits were received—following the cross-tabulations of this (1971) census—by 7.4 percent of the persons 60 and over in Austria. Another 17.8 percent were visited several times a week, and still another 15.9 percent once a week. There were no marked differences that were dependent on community size, age, and household composition (Ö.St.Z., 1972, pp. 80-82).

The survey of the Ministry of Science and Research tried to specify the kinds of contacts. One has to note that this survey generally reported less favorable results, regarding, for example, visiting frequency, than the special censuses presented thus far. It demonstrated that contacts with the children are restricted largely to visits by and with the children, but even these activities are not frequent. As table 3 shows, only 17 percent of those over 50 are frequently visited by their children; 39 percent are never visited. Spending vacations together is the rarest common activity.

For visits to and by friends or relatives, the study showed that 25 percent of the persons 60 and over receive visitors at least several times per week; 14 percent visit other people on the same frequency scale. Fifty percent receive visitors less than once a week, and 8 percent never do. A slight deviation of this pattern occurs with the very old (80 and above). On the one hand, there are more among the very old who receive daily visits, but, on the other hand, there are more who receive no visitors at all, (Ö.St.Z., 1972). Sex differences, if any, are minor.

Table 3: PARTICIPATION OF PARENTS AND CHILDREN IN JOINT ACTIVITIES

	Participation of Children in the Activities of their Parents (N=516)[a]					Participation of Parents in the Activities of their Children (N=1,066)[b]				
	Frequently	Occasionally	Rarely	Never	No Personal Activities	Frequently	Occasionally	Rarely	Never	No Personal Activities
Invitation to the home	17	26	14	22	17	13	20	15	46	4
Going out	5	17	12	37	25	2	10	11	72	4
Weekend trips	7	10	12	31	36	2	11	11	61	13
Vacations	5	8	8	41	38	7	7	6	56	24

Source: Bundesministerium für Wissenschaft und Forschung (ed.). Die gesellschaftliche Reintegration älterer Menschen in Österreich. Vienna-New York: Springer, 1976. p. 49.

a. All respondents older than 50 and having only grown-up children
b. All respondents aged 16 to 49 whose parents are still alive

Neighborhood and extrafamilial contacts, in general, are relatively rare and do not go deeply. The importance of neighbors lies mainly in their being immediately available in emergencies and their offering small-scale assistance (Rosenmayr and Köckeis, 1965a, b).

The question is still open as to whether the aged parents prefer to live alone or in a common household with their children and which arrangement is preferred by the children. As Rosenmayr observed in 1958 when he studied special apartments for the aged in Vienna, old people prefer *intimacy at a distance*; they dislike sharing households, but they do not want to live too far from the younger generation (Rosenmayr, 1959). According to the special census of December 1971, only 7 percent of aged couples living together in the same household and only 10 percent of unmarried aged people wanted to live with their children in the same household (Ö.St.Z., 1972).

From the 1974 survey, however, we know that the wish for shared living in an intergenerational household is more frequently expressed by the elderly than by their children; a quarter of the aged parents but only a tenth of their children would like this arrangement. A similar pattern is true for living in vicinity (see table 4).

Table 4: WISH FOR COMMON HOUSEHOLD/LIVING IN CONTACT VICINITY, 1974

	Wish for Common Household		Wish for Living in Contact Vicinity[a]	
	Parents[b]	*Children*[c]	*Parents*[d]	*Children*[e]
Yes	23%	10%	67%	48%
No	66%	77%	19%	35%
Don't know/not yet considered	11%	13%	14%	17%

Source: IFES, Reintegration älterer Menschen. 2nd report, tables volume. Vienna 1974 (mimeo.), pp. 65, 66, 67, 78, 80.

Notes: a. "Contact vicinity" = not more than half an hour walking distance
   b. Persons 50 and above with children outside household
   c. Persons aged 16-50 with parents outside household
   d. Persons 50 and over whose children's households lie outside "contact vicinity"
   e. Persons aged 16-50, whose parents' households' lie outside "contact vicinity"

Without doubt elderly persons, because of the high probability of bereavement and desolation, run a particularly high risk of loneliness. The percentage of persons feeling lonely rises in proportion to age. Whereas only 3 percent of the 16 to 50 year olds are often lonely, this is the case with 9 percent of the 50 to 60 year olds, 13 percent of the 60 to 70 year olds, and 15 percent of persons older than 70 (BMfWF, 1976). This loneliness occurs particularly among women; 17 percent in the age group above 50 feel "frequently lonely" as opposed to only 1 percent of 50-to-60 year-old men, among whom the percentage does not exceed 10 percent even in the age group of persons above 70. Women seem to feel lonely more often than men not only because they lose their partners more frequently. Controlling for the marital status, we find that among the married women above age 50, loneliness is complained about four times as often as among men: 3.5 percent of the men but 12 percent of the women. This phenomenon is probably due to the sex-role-specific family orientation of women. Whereas the percentage of married men who feel lonely hardly varies depending on children (5 percent of married men without children, 4 percent with children in vicinity, and 3 percent with children not in vicinity), women seem to be affected by the idea that they do not see their children often enough, and thus they develop feelings of loneliness. Only 4 percent of married women above 50 who have no children feel often lonely from the subjective point of view (this percentage of lonely women rises remarkable in case of women with children: 13 percent with children within vicinity and 11 percent with children beyond contact vicinity). The loneliest persons on the whole are not unmarried women without children (19 percent) but married women with children living outside an easily realized contact vicinity (BMfWF, 1976). Therefore loneliness is not so much due to the absence of reference persons but to the knowledge about potentially existing but unrealized opportunities of contact.

Health

In September 1973, a microcensus was taken in Austria on the state of health of the Austrian population. According to this study 21 percent of the 60 to 70 year olds, 18 percent of the 70 to 80 year olds, and 17 percent of those 80 and above did not complain of any physical ailments. Apart from the fact that the typical phenomenon of multimorbidity also occurred in Austria, the most important complaints were circulatory trouble, pains in the joints, muscles, and nerves, and cardiac conditions. In the oldest age group, the following conditions were also frequently reported: sleeping problems (26 percent), fatigue or weakness (28 percent), vertigo (25 percent), deficient vision (25 percent), and walking handicaps (22 percent) (Ö.St.Z., 1977). Between about age 60 and 80, the physicomotoric abilities decrease by one-quarter or one-third on the average, varying according to the type of activity specified. The greatest difficulty seems to be posed by the carrying of shopping bags; this fact should stimulate our considerations of how we could assist such handicapped people in supplying them with consumer goods. American, Danish, and English studies (Shanas, et al., 1968) show similar tendencies, which imply a decrease in physical abilities in high age (see table 5).

Apart from these more objective questions concerning various physical abilities the Austrian microcensus study also undertook to analyze the subjective well-being of the respondents. Generally about 55 percent of the

Table 5: SOMATIC ABILITIES OF PERSONS OVER 60 YEARS OF AGE

Able to Perform the Following without Difficulties	Men				Women			
	60-64	65-74	75+	80+	60-64	65-74	75+	80+
Climb stairs	93%	87%	75%	67%	91%	85%	67%	57%
Carry shopping bags	92	87	71	59	93	83	60	45
Bend over to pick up objects	91	85	70	60	92	85	67	57
Number in 1,000s	186	292	113	48	248	411	219	95

Source: A. Amann and H. Velimirovic, *Beiträge zu einer Strukturanalyse der Altenarbeit* (Vienna, 1977).

respondents said that their state of health was "very good," and only a minority (approximately 10 percent) complained of bad health (Amann, 1975b). Striking differences occurred depending on age, sex, and other considerations. In the age group of the 60 to 64 year olds, two-thirds of the respondents said their state of health was on average very good to good, whereas only about one-third of the persons aged 75 and above responded in that way (Amann, 1975a).

Finances and Housing

The aged population is among the less well-off groups of the population, although old-age and retirement pensions in Austria guarantee a certain standard of living through a special scheme of linking pensions with wages and although the average pension increases lie above the level of increase of the cost of living. On the other hand, the living standard of the working population is improving faster than that of the pensioners, not only because the nominal income growth rate exceeds the growth rate of the pensions, but also because the inflation rate for the goods and services typically consumed by the households of the active population is smaller than that of the typical goods and services used by pensioners (Rosenmayr and Majce, 1978, pp. 234ff.). As a consequence, while the proportion of necessary expenditures (for nutrition, dwelling, heating, and lighting) decreased for the working population (white and blue collar), it increased for the pensioners from 50.0 percent in the year 1966 to 54.1 percent in the year 1975 (Rosenmayr and Majce, 1978, p. 249). A study carried out in Vienna showed that if a percentage of 35 percent of total expenditures being spent on food is considered the poverty line, then 30 percent of the households of pensioners in Vienna must be considered poor (these 30 percent equal 17 percent of the total population of Vienna) (Wiener Kammer für Arbeiter und Angestellte, 1974). Women are the most disadvantaged: "According to the study carried out in Vienna it is mainly unmarried women, an incredibly high percentage of whom are part of the defined poverty group: in 1971 nearly two thirds of women receiving old age pensions (64%) and 78% of the women receiving widows' pensions belonged to this group.

According to a projection based on an IFES-study, 40% of single-person households of pensioners in Vienna fall within this poverty group, and the majority of them are unmarried elderly women'' (BMfWF, 1976).

The picture is not much different with regard to housing. There is an overrepresentation of old people in substandard accommodations. In March 1975, two-thirds of all homes but only 37 percent of the single-person households of persons over 60 years of age had private bathrooms. Thirty-nine percent of these single-person households had no private bath or toilet compared to only 20 percent of all homes in Austria. Considering that old people often have walking difficulties, it is noteworthy that although 40 percent of all apartments in Austria are situated in houses with elevators, only 25 percent of the aged population live in such apartments. A total of 338,000 apartments are located on the fourth floor (third floor according to Austrian terminology) or higher, and as many as 92,000 of these are inhabited by old people (Ö.St.Z., 1977).

Leisure and Cultural Activities

The most popular leisure activity among the aged population of Austria is watching television. According to their own statements, 41 percent of retired men, 42 percent of retired women, and 34 percent of housewives without employment spend "much time" watching television. This is followed by the traditional leisure activities such as walking (BMfWF, 1976).

Cultural and artistic activities and sports are not very popular: During the course of a year, four-fifths of the population over 65 in 1972 had not seen an opera or operetta, nor had they been to a museum, an exhibition, or a concert. The same phenomena were observed for only 54 percent of the 15 to 18 year olds and for 57 percent of the 19 to 25 year olds (Ö.St.Z., 1977). Reading books is not very popular: 48 percent of the men 70 and over and 58 percent of the women of the same age read no books at all (IFES, 1977). Generally books dealing with questions of how to cope with one's existence are read least frequently. Such books accounted for 20 percent of those read by 65- to 70-year-old men but dropped to 8 percent among men above 70; the percentage among women was even lower: 9 percent and 4 percent, respectively (Rosenmayr, 1976). This lower level of book reading among the older population can be explained by the fact that their educational levels are far below the national average (table 6).

Table 6: HIGHEST SCHOOL LEVEL REACHED

Age Group	Primary Level	Secondary Level	Postsecondary Level
25-34	45.8%	50.9%	3.3%
35-64	62.0	35.4	2.7
65 and over	75.8	22.6	1.7

Source: UNESCO, Statistical Yearbook (1974).

Institutionalization

The aged in Austria do not look favorably on old people's homes (Majce, 1978). They have little desire to be admitted to such institutions: only 1.7 percent want to go to a hospital; 1.9 percent to an old people's home (Ö.St.Z., 1972); and even of those 60 and over who consider their state of health "bad and in need of help," only 4.4 percent want to go to an old people's hospital and only 4.2 percent to an old people's home (Ö.St.Z., 1972). This negative attitude is particularly strong in rural areas.

In 1972, a study carried out by Kaufmann and Balog showed that at that time, thirty-two thousand old people (approximately 3.5 percent of the aged population) were living in residential institutions (Kaufmann and Balog, 1974). At least as many persons who need either institutional care or home nursing, are, according to the estimation of IFES, being cared for by their families at home (Gehmacher, 1971).

The causes for transfer to a residential institution are varied. In 1962 in one of the first Austrian studies in this area, Doberauer found that illness (39 percent) and the need for care (28 percent) are named most frequently as causes. These were followed by problems within the family (14 percent) and insufficient living space (12 percent) (Doberauer, 1962d). Hörl and Majce found in a recent study that—at least with regard to old people's homes in Vienna—high age, the need for care, and in particular social isolation appear to be the main components in the complex of factors resulting in transfer to an institution (Hörl and Majce, 1976). The same study showed a tendency toward the opinion that admittance to a residential institution is in many cases equivalent to severing all contacts with the outside world (Hörl and Majce, 1976).

PROGRAMS AND RELATED RESEARCH

In the field of empirical research, two subjects have received particular attention: the analysis of living conditions of old people who are in need and the analysis of possibilities of cooperation and coordination between research and practice. The emphasis of the theoretical considerations lies in the perspective that any approach to an understanding of the role and place of services and care for those in need has to be embedded in a wider and comprehensive approach to an understanding of all social services. From the societal level, the research must be considered within a systemic model of other relevant institutions like those of closed care, the family, the social security system, and basic structures of cultural and social concern. From the level of the interrelationships between the individual and social groups, it has to be considered within a life span and intergenerational framework. Its substantive theoretical dimensions have to be seen in the vast range of differences to be found among individuals of the same chronological age in later life and among individuals who have been commonly classified as "old," "impaired," "helpless," and "on welfare." Systems of help, care, and support must be based upon a recognition that the biological, psychological, and sociological processes of aging continue to differentiate individuals at any chronological point in the life span; we have to stress the understanding that "aging" begins with birth, and that the social determination of the biological aging process demands control at earlier points of time than is usual if we are to reach a better understanding and integration of the aged in any phase of societal development.

Modern work with and help for the aged sees its most important objective as the expansion, improvement, and intensification of the so-called open care for the aged; the priority of domiciliary help systems over forms of intramural aid has been internationally accepted.

An expansion and differentiation of communal institutions can be effectively brought about only if it is based on the findings of empirical research and is accompanied by evaluating research proocesses. This combination of socio-political action and social scientific research not only covers questions of living conditions of the aged population but also methodological questions on the connection between the problems that arise, the methodologies used to analyze the field, and the transfer of knowledge between research and practice.

On Special Needs and Services

Studies dealing with the living conditions of specific groups of the aged population in Austria can be seen conceptually under the following perspectives: one concerned with the theory of needs and socioeconomic allocation, one dealing with systems theory and functionalism, one oriented toward role theory and its criticism, and one concerned with interaction, activity, and exchange theory. Works from the first perspective are the most recent ones and will be the starting point of the discussion.

Needs are conceived of as perceived and socially recognized physical, psychic, economic, or social shortages or deficiencies of an individual or a group of individuals (Amann and Majce, 1976). If for a long period of time (longer than it is socioculturally defined as "normal") such a need cannot be satisfied by the individual himself because of the significantly restricted availability of adequate resources, one has to speak of "neediness." This brings in the essential social dimension of the problem: for the abolishment or relief of a situation of neediness, activities of others are required (Amann and Majce, 1976). This approach, combining theories of needs and interaction, is characteristic of a study carried out in 1974–1975 at the Institute of Sociology at the University of Vienna in cooperation with the Ludwig Boltzmann Institute for Research on Aging.

The subjects were clients of the home-help services for the elderly in Vienna (the home-help services are the most elaborate and highly developed part of the services for the elderly in Vienna). Most of these persons had a number of handicaps and impairments for which they were being given care. The research design was oriented to an exploratory study (using the techniques of case study and life history method) with depth interviews with clients and multiple interviews with several other persons. The latter covered the home helps, the client's relatives and neighbors or friends, as well as respective comparative persons (their relatives and friends) who had been selected by a matched-pair method (Amann et al., 1975; Amann 1975a). Some of the most important results from 271 interview protocols illustrate the special situation of persons receiving home help for the elderly, as well as the specific problems arising in course of the discussion on social disadvantages in old age.

Work with the elderly (especially home-help services) is usually concerned simultaneously with problems arising from insufficient housing conditions, loneliness and lack of contact, deficient physical and/or psychic health, and nonfunctioning family relations. Clients are the physically handicapped due to accidents or sudden illness, persons with shattered identities due to an illness or the death of their partner, the socially isolated, those downtrodden in spirit and soul, the forgetful, those termed psychotic, and finally the very old, who may be referred to as "people at risk."

Events and developments in the personal biography of the individual are of particular importance. Accidents, loss of partner, other traumatic experiences, economic setbacks, personal dilemmas, and so forth exert a decisive influence on behavior and attitudes. There is a strong connection between depressing and shocking experiences during preceding years and a progressive deterioration of health in the present (in the sense of a primary sociogenesis). A bad state of health and negative experiences (such as forced change of domicile because of a terminated lease or rental contract) dominate attitudes and plans for the future. The realization that they cannot change the situation brings resignation. In most cases, these people severely reduce their contacts to a small group of persons (usually their closest relatives) and to a gradual disengagement from their accustomed social environment. Thus arises a situation characterized by dependence on others, comparative helplessness, social isolation, and disintegration (Amann and Velimirovic, 1977; Amann et al., 1975; Amann, 1975b).

Clients of home-help services depend twice as often as average old people do on help for the necessary tasks of daily life. They are characterized by multimorbidity and by a syndrome of relative social deprivation (Amann, 1977). Sensory diseases, cardiovascular diseases, diseases of the joints, and diseases of the digestive organs are among the most common impairments. Low income occurs in connection with poor health, poor living conditions, and social disintegration (few or no social contacts). Because of the long process of getting accustomed to the living situation (perhaps they lived fifty years in the same apartment) and because of the impossibility of altering the situation of their own accord, the reaction is contentment with the poor conditions and a lowering of the aspiration level under the pressure of being forced continuously to adapt downward.

Based on this phenomenon, the study developed a theoretical approach to the syndrome of social deprivation in old age that can be applied to the specific conditions of the situation in which old people have become dependent on help. This approach includes the following dimensions:

1. Deficiencies in the perception and/or opening up of opportunities. The individual's capacity to realize or to effect opportunities in which to change his situation is impaired.
2. Lack of power. The perception of the reality that a change in one's situation cannot be brought about by one's own efforts.
3. Restrictions in exchange. The relative incapability to guarantee reciprocity of behavior, corresponding to the expectations of significant others.
4. Self-alienation. The relative discrepancy between a socially ideal form of existence and the socially real situation an individual is facing.
5. Decay of aspirations. External conditions forcing a downward adaption and the resultant resignation with regard to higher levels of aspiration.

These dimensions apply economically, socially, physically, and psychically; thus theoretical frames of reference become available for economics, physical and social helplessness, and the decay of economic and social aspirations. Two further studies (Amann, 1978; Amann, 1979) have developed a categorial scheme for the analysis of patterns of services, help, and support that complements this approach. This categorial scheme is employing concepts of biographic theory, of social interaction analysis, and of psychoanalysis.

The Importance of the Domicile in High Age and the Change of Domicile

Another study (mainly concerned with a functionalistic approach) dealing with the specific problem of the change of domicile in high age was carried out in 1974 in Graz, a city of 250,000 inhabitants (Falk and Spielhofer, 1975).

A sample of 155 persons aged 71 years and 166 persons aged 66 years was drawn. The primary questions of the study referred to conditions surrounding the change of domicile in old age, the reactions of the persons concerned, plans for the change of domicile, and the dependence of such processes on socioeconomic factors. The group aged 66 was chosen since the period following the average retirement date seems to be of particular importance; the group aged 71 was used for control purposes.

One of the most notable findings of the study was the discovery of a relatively high mobility among the aged; approximately 2 percent of the aged population changed their domicile every year and approximately 25 percent did so during the course of twelve years. Seven percent of the 71 year olds and 8 percent of the 66 year olds intended to change their domicile within five years after the interview to other private dwellings. This result is of great interest since the mobility rate has been lower during the course of life of these older people than for younger cohorts and, besides, the readiness to change dwellings must be considered much lower in Central Europe than in the United States, for example. If the population is divided into persons who actively planned and carried out a change of domicile and persons who reacted mainly to outside forces, the following pattern can be observed: the 71 year olds more frequently (50 percent) changed their domicile as a reaction than the 66 year olds (39 percent). Causes for reactive behavior were listed as follows: forcible eviction, termination of contract, death of the spouse, apartment too expensive, poor state of health, deficiencies in the old apartment, housework too difficult. The following were listed among the causes for preventive or active (as compared to reactive) change: the desire to live near the children, apartment too large or too small, connection (spatial) with friends, the desire to meet more people, better location of the apartment, private ownership of new dwellings. It was also generally found that the persons changing domiciles had a higher standard of living than those who did not change; and within the group of persons changing, the preventive group had a better standard than the reactive group.

The fact that reactive causes for a change of domicile are more common than preventive ones corresponds to the findings of another study carried out at the beginning of the 1970s as a comparison between forty-seven persons (69 to 82 years of age) in private homes and thirty persons (69 to 82 years) in residential institutions (Krammer-Hirsch, 1974). This study also showed a specification of the planning behavior of the elderly depending on social stratification. In the lower class, only 5 percent made plans for the coming year, in the middle class 18 percent, and in the upper class 54 percent. In the lower class, intentions and desires were mainly concerned with basic necessities of everyday living; in the upper class, they dealt more with cultural and social consumption. This study showed, however, that a change of domicile does not depend entirely on social stratum.

The danger of becoming dependent on care with increasing age is increased with substandard housing conditions; a person with a motoric handicap living in a well-equipped apartment on the ground floor is less likely to need help than a person with the same state of health living in an ill-equipped apartment on the fifth floor in a building without an elevator.

Studies on the Relationships between Research and Practice

The starting point for action research or evaluation research is the participation of the research workers in the shaping of social conditions; this means the combination of practical and political action with systematic research. This type of research finally abandons data collecting as the primary task of the research work (which is typical of survey research) for a scheme characterized by three criteria: (1) the research worker does not just enter a situation for a short moment (the interview situation). (2) He takes part in a social process for a longer period of time and helps to stimulate its development. (3) He does not work with isolated individuals in an artificial survey situation, but with groups within their social framework, and he also takes part in the application and evaluation of the results of the research (Haag and Krüger, 1972; Fischer and Amann, 1979).

This rather demanding program is being applied in a research project (which has been going on for two years) within the framework of open help for the aged in Vienna. It is the first step of a process designed to find and test new opportunities for cooperation between research and practice and to study conditions and consequences of the transfer of scientific knowledge within this cooperation. Although methods and theories of accompanying research are well known and widely discussed, there is hardly any international experience available in the field of care for the aged. This research project undertakes to reach the goals set above in the following areas: training for persons to provide aid to the aged, continued education for persons engaged in assisting the aged, the design and development of a uniform professional image, coordination between the various bodies providing aid for the aged, and centralization versus decentralization, among others (Amann, et al., 1977).

One dimension within the framework of aid for the elderly deals with questions on how staff is recruited, motivations and incentives for becoming a social worker or home helper, attitudes toward clients, and expectations and realities with regard to their work. A pilot study carried out in Vienna dealt with these questions and has yielded some interesting results (Achleitner, 1974). Twenty-six social workers (mainly women between 23 and 55 years of age)—civil servants in higher social services positions—were questioned in an exploratory manner. It is particularly striking that even among these experts, we find some of the generally held old-age stereotypes. The daily confrontation with problems and conditions of aging in their daily work has not helped them to achieve a differentiated insight into the situation; it has served only to reinforce the original stereotypes in many cases.

Some respondents explained that being old is a disadvantage in our society. This was the answer given nearly exclusively by workers whose professional approach is individualizing (oriented toward casework as the main method of their work). Furthermore it was found (and this illustrates the general social understanding in many sectors of social work) that the impact of economic factors on the general old-age situation is taken into account only to a limited extent (Achleitner, 1974). Only reform-oriented social workers who consider social work as an agent of social change consider this aspect to be of primary importance. Perspectives of one's own situation as a social worker and the interpretation of social work as an interdependent element of the society rest on a traditional interpretation of society. The family ("the trend toward the nuclear family") is the primary cause of the age problem, say the respondents. "The dissolution of the three-generation family deprives the aged of important functions" is an objectively wrong slogan, says Achleitner (1974). The alleged disappearance of the modified extended family is frequently deplored. The younger ones are often accused of causing the problem situations of the aged. These answers underscore the insufficient sociological training of social workers, which in many cases leads to the adherence to a conservative ideal of the family.

Numerous other reports and publications deal with special questions on the situation of the aged, for example, with the structural prerequisites for an optimal regionalized and decentralized system of care for the aged (Gehmacher, 1971); with questions of coordination and integration between public assistance and aid provided by the family (Rosenmayr, 1975); and with the present situation of aid for the aged in general and with home aid in particular.

THEORETICAL BACKGROUND OF GEROSOCIOLOGICAL RESEARCH

Recent theoretical work in social gerontology aims at a fusion of system theory starting from biological considerations on the one hand and historical perspectives on the individual and social relations and structures. This concept was elaborated for the first time in a paper presented at the Eighth World Congress of Sociology at Toronto (Rosenmayr, 1974) and is summarized here.

Toward a Sociological Definition of Aging

An age status within the age stratification system is determined according to the values and norms of global society. Patterns of problem resolution and the division of labor bring about the societal fixing and evaluation of certain biological ages.

The assignment of a certain status to an age group is the result of the position that society assigns to this age group in the pattern of the division of labor. Individuals and groups are evaluated also according to their position in system elucidation (science, communication, mass media) and decision making in the economic and political subsystems. Social status heavily determines age status.

Furthermore, age statuses and their relative position in society depend on whether and how public means are allocated. This argument is used to show that roles can only follow primary social decisions and developments that entail the allocation of resources. Individuals and groups having close relations with system elucidation or amelioration are particularly highly rewarded. The relatively high position of the elderly in patriarchal, particularly artisanal, societies we have known so far is a function of their position in system elucidation and/or amelioration.

Homeostatic models that intrinsically tend toward balance (and that serve biology adequately) are deemed inadequate to serve as a frame for describing human individuals, populations, and their age structures. Adaptive system models are needed to frame or structure theoretically such problems as relationships between socioeconomic dynamics, culture, values, and age structures. When and if value structures are involved, even a refined model of balance is inadequate. Historical evolution, although to some extent based on them, finally transcends systems processes; they might be called transhomeostatic.

Exchange Theory in Its Application to Aging

A recent study (Rosenmayr, 1976) explores the value of exchange theory for research in the development phases of the life course and for the evaluation of statuses as equilibrium points in the aging process. Special application for gerosociology is required. In order to do this, one has to start with a biological perspective, which interprets life processes as changes between equilibrium states. Rosenmayr starts with biological assumptions and then contrasts them with sociological ones.

The influx of energy and material into a living system is balanced by certain energy and material losses. A ''normally'' functioning living system establishes an equilibrium or balance (homeostasis) between what we might term *assimilation* (gain from the environment) and *yield* (flow to the environment).

In the biological sense, yield means some form of loss or, more neutrally, transfer to the environment. This is contrasted with the sociocultural notion of yield, which includes symbolic creativity, humanitarian action, empathy, and solidarity.

Elaborating a human and social science point of view, Rosenmayr defines individual life time as composed of individually and socially experienced and implemented applied time spans. These spans or units are used for participation and activities in society, its institutions, and its groups, and they lead to certain positions (for example, of information, communication, and control). This perspective avoids a unilateral pessimistic connotation in the notion of ''becoming older,'' which is the result of generalizing biological changes over psychological and social developments and will permit study not only of certain aspects of physical decrease but also those of psychological, social, moral, or cultural increase. These latter aspects are encountered by focusing on the accumulative and reinforcing consequences of actions in units of time that occur in processes of learning, memory, evaluation, and individual and interpersonal experience. To a certain extent, biological aging can be controlled by psychological and sociological forces.

A stage in the life course may be defined as the status or balance point that is the result of the duration and outcome of both psychological, social, and cultural accumulation and build-up on the one hand and deprivation and reduction on the other. The latter may be of a biological as well as of a psychosocial nature (for example, in the case of development under conditions of deprivation). Psychosocial influences are vitalizing only under certain conditions. A status representing a balance between processes of aging constitutes the position in the life span. Such statuses as balance points characterize psychosocial development. They are not as fixed as the chronological ones, and they need frequent revision, structuring, and adaptation to the society and problem studied.

The sociocultural concept of aging implies a notion of a reflexive personality and reflexive human assimilation and yield processes. They are structured by the symbolically elucidated basis of action, and thus they are connected with acts of evaluation of both assimilation and yield and with evaluating balancing: an estimate is made of what one might term gratification and frustration and, in correspondence with the assimilation-yield dyad, a balance of what one receives and what one offers, or perceives to receive and to offer.

Individuals, as they are engaged in assimilation and yield processes, have expectations and strategies concerning these processes and their aims. They have their ideas, values, and norms concerning the amount and type of yield they should offer in relation to their expected, present, or earlier amount of assimilation.

The social environment is considered to be an external milieu that can potentiate and/or encourage adjustments in the assimilation-yield balance. Some societies provide opportunity and encourage people to exhibit diverse ways of yielding. The social work organizations might increasingly encourage that tendency. Elderly people in some cultures have greater opportunity to give to society through participating in the family, educating the young, generating or supporting history, contributing to religion, art, music, or literature, and participating in socially productive tasks. The assimilation-yield model is used to study different life phases in the aging process on the basis of the exchange concept and to determine age statuses.

Rosenmayr has described the limits of exchange theory. He states that the norm of reciprocity cannot be considered as sufficient to allow for the integration of the elderly and argues that the conceptualization and concretization of socially generated and guaranteed life chances is necessary.

The Concept of Cumulative Deprivation

Another theoretical line pursued by the research team of the L. Boltzmann Institute concerns the cumulative deprivation of specific groups of old people, one being elderly women, single, divorced, or widowed *and* living alone. The complexity of causes for cumulative deprivation is an indication of the fact that this seems to be a phenomenon we might term *socially dependent self-infliction* (Rosenmayr, 1975). We can use the term since the causes for some of the deprivations lie in certain actions or omissions that can be said to be the ''fault'' of the individual who ''commits'' them. Even on very low incomes, it should be possible for these persons, for example, to buy a refrigerator for food storage, and a bad state of health is very often due to unreasonable behavior (never consulting a physician, ignoring medical advice, or not following dietary regulations). On the other hand this self-infliction is socially dependent: in the course of the lifelong socialization processes, class-specific attitudes are developed that may be substantial impediments to planned and rational behavior from which the individual might have benefited, given different social encouragement and support.

The social devaluation not only generally reduces the chances of social participation and of access to resources but works as a multiplication of factors in terms of the cumulating disadvantages of the economically weakest and socially most isolated groups of the aged (Rosenmayr, 1975b; Rosenmayr and Majce, 1978). Differences between socioeconomic strata are thus greater among the elderly than among the younger. This is due to greater differences in their initial social situations and to biographically created conditions which led to reduced chances of the deprived of coping with aging processes.

We know from a number of studies that the state of health is substantially worse in the lower socioeconomic classes. On the basis of previous studies on deprivation during earlier phases of life, Rosenmayr emphasizes the difficulty of activating the deprived, be it in their ecological setting, in medical institutions, in clubs of the aged, or day centers. They tend to retreat to the social fringes. Applying this concept of socially dependent self-infliction and the mechanism of cumulative deprivation to the isolated widowed women, Rosenmayr and Majce (1978) show that they practically never go on a vacation; they are often too weak and lack the initiative to leave their usually poor living environment. In cases where help is needed most, it is usually most expensive, most time-consuming, and most difficult to furnish economically, socially, and psychologically. The greater the need in one dimension, the more this need is coupled to other types of deficiencies. The resources of society are being wasted because of the self-inflicted, society-dependent resistance against individual intentions to help and against helpful social actions is not being properly realized.

REFERENCES

Achleitner, W. 1974. Probleme der Kooperation im Dienste der älteren Mitbürger. In L.Rosenmayr and A. Amann, eds., *Der alte Mensch in den Strukturen der Gegenwartsgesellschaft*. Mimeo. Vienna.

Amann, A. 1975a. Grundlagen zur Forschung in der sozialen Gerontologie—Ein methodenkritischer Versuch. Ph.D. diss., Univ. of Vienna.

———. 1975b. Zur Bedürfnis- und Versorgungssituation älterer Menschen. In K. Fellinger, ed., *Altenhilfe—ein kooperatives Problem.* Vienna.

———. 1975c. *Empirisch-theoretische Erkundungen über den Kontext sozialer Benachteiligung im Alter—Einzelfallanalysen zu Problemen der Altenheimhilfe.*

Amann, A.; Fischer, E.; and Friedl, W. 1977. Begleitende Forschung in der Alten- (Heim-) Hilfe. Mimeo. Vienna.

Amann, A., and Majce, G. 1976. Some remarks on the concept of need and health and their treatment in gerontological research. In J.M. Munnichs and J. van den Heuvel, eds., *Dependency or Independency in Old Age.* The Hague: Nijhoff.

Amann, A.; Majce, G.; Pavelka, F.; and Wieser, G. 1975. Zur sozialen und personalen Lage alter, hilfsbedürftig gewordener Menschen in Wien. In Die gesellschaftliche Reintegration älterer Menschen. Mimeo. Vienna: Institut für empirische Sozialforschung.

Amann, A., and Velimirovic, H. 1977. *Beiträge zu einer Strukturanalyse der Altenarbeit. Eurosocial Ocasional Papers* no. 4.

Amann A., and Wieser, G. 1978. Zur Praxis der Altenhilfe im Wohlfahrtsstaat—Am Beispiel der Heimhilfe in Wien. Österreichische Zeitschrift für Soziologie.

Beier, W.; Brehme, K.H.; and Wiegel, D. 1973. *Biophysikalische Aspekte des Alterns multizellularer Systeme.* Leipzig: VEB Thieme.

Bundesministerium für Wissenschaft und Forschung (BMfWF) 1976. Die gesellschaftliche Reintegration älterer Menschen in Österreich. Vienna: Springer.

Deutsch, E. and Doberauer, W. 1966. Kritischer Beitrag zur medikamentösen Beeinflussung des Lipidspiegels im Blut. Paper presented at the Seventh International Congress of Gerontology, Vienna.

Doberauer, W. 1954. Ergebnisse genagelter Schenkelhalsbrüche bei Menschen hohen Alters. *Klinische Medizin* 9:381–390.

———. 1955. Die neurogene Appendizitis bei Menschen hohen Alters. *Klinische Medizin* 5:209–219.

———. 1956a. Aspekte der Altersheilkunde: Sozial-Medizinische Folge der ''Begegnung'' *Klinische Medizin* 10: 2-5.

———. 1956b. Entwicklung und Wandel der Problemstellung in der Lehre vom Altern. *Asklepios Lannach, Stmk.* 3:129–133.

———. 1956c. Hinweise zur Entwicklung und Bedeutung der Geriatrie. *Klinische Medizin* 10:430–446.

———. 1957a. Chirurgische Behandlung Neurogener Enteropathien bei Menschen hohen Alters. Paper presented to the International Symposium on Medical-Social Aspects of Senile Nervous Diseases, Venice.

———. 1957b. Chirurgische Eingriffe am sympathischen Nervensystem alte Menschen. In W. Doberauer, *Alter und Krankheit,* pp. 273–300. Vienna.

———. 1957c. Ernährung im Alter. *Klinische Medizin* 9:102–113.

———. 1957d. Neurogenic appendicopathy. *Journal of Gerontology* 4:398–400.

———. 1958. Altersheilkunde und Altenbefürsorgung. In *Soziale Berufe.* Vienna: Waldheim-Eberle, 8–9.

———. 1959a. Geriatrische Chirurgie. In *Almanach für ärztliche Fortbildung,* pp. 181–193. Munich: J. F. Lehmann.

————. 1959b. Das Verhalten der Fibrinwerte bei radikaloperierten und inoperablen Krebskranken im Alter. In *Geriatrie und Fortbildung*. Gesellschaft z.Forderung wissenschaftlicher Forschung, pp. 49-103. Vienna.

————. 1960–1961. Kleine Chirurgie im Alter. In *Almanach für die ärztliche Fortbildung*, pp. 203–226. Munich: J. F. Lehmann.

————. 1961. Therapeutische Probleme bei alternden Menschen. *Monatskurse für die ärztliche Fortbildung* 5: 358-361. Munich: J. F. Lehmann.

————. 1962a. Beeinflussung von Wundheilungsvorgängen durch das Lebensalter. *Geront. Clin. S.* Karger 4: 112–127.

————. 1962b. Der Einfluss des Lebensalters auf die Granulations—gewebsbildung. In *Scriptum Geriatricum 1962*, pp. 167–197. Vienna, Österreichiscme Gesellschaft für Geriatrie.

————. 1962c. Die Fortbildungskurse für Geriatrie in Bad Hofgastein. In *Geriatrie 62*. Lannoo, Tielt-Den Haag.

————. 1962d. Vom Versorgungshaus zum altersheim und Alterskrankenhaus, In *Der Mensch im Alter*. Frankfurt: Schriftenreihe der Medizinisch-Pharmazeutischen Gesellschaft.

————. 1963a. Zum Einfluss des Lebensalters auf die Heilung künstlicher Hautdefekte. *Klinische Medizin*.

————. 1963b. Greis, Arzt und soziale Hilfen. In *Forbildungskurs f. Sozialarbeiter*. Vienna: Selbstverlag d. Österreichischen Komitees für Sozialarbeit.

————. 1963c. Die Stellung der Geriatrie in der Gesamtmedizin. *Der Deutsche Apotheker*. 12.

————. 1964a. Die Betreuung alter Menschen. 3. Enquete des Österreichischen städtebundes. *Österreichische* Gemeinde-Zeitung. *Verlag für Jugend und Volk* 22.

————. 1964b. Greis und arzt. *Soziale Berufe* 8.

————. 1965. Karzinom und Geriatrie. In *Monatskurse für die ärztliche Fortbildung*. Munich: J. F. Lehmann. 1:22–24.

————. 1968. Wundheilung und Wundheilungskomplikationen im Alter. In *Handbuch der praktischen Geriatrie*. Stuttgart: Ferdinand Enke Verl.

————. 1971. Ist ein Leben zwischen 100 und 120 Jahren lebenswert? *Medical Tribune GmbH., Wiesbaden*.

Doberauer W., and Doberauer, B. 1971. Patofisiologia del envejecer. *Tribuna Medica.* 8:399.

————. 1972. Die zerebrale Dekompensation im Alter. *Ärzliche Praxis*. 34:1847–1850.

Doberauer, W.; Formanek, K.; and Wick, G. 1966a. Auswirkungen einer Entwässerung auf den Wasser- und Elektrolythaushalt bei alten und jungen Ratten. *Zeitschr. f. Alternsforschung* 3–4.

————. 1966b. Unterschiede in der Salurese bei alten und jungen Ratten. *Zeitschr. f. Alternsforschung* 3–4.

Doberauer, W.; Schulz, F.-H.; and Friedel, W. 1957. Über den Fibringehalt des Blutplasmas alter Menschen. *Klinische Medizin* 9:361–367.

Doberauer, W., and Stoklaska, E. 1966a. Alter und experimentelle Entzündung. Paper presented at the Seventh International Congress of Gerontology. Vienna.

————. 1966b. Der einfluss des Lebensalters auf die Ausbildung von Rattenpfotenodemen. *Gerontologia Clinica* 8:5–11.

Doberauer, W., and Twrdy, E. 1971. Spezielle Pharmakotherapie in der Geriatrie. In *Klinisch Pharmakologie und Pharmakotherapie.* Munich, Berlin, and Vienna: Urban und Schwarzenberg.

————. 1972. Klinik und Pharmakotherapie der Nebenwirkungen in der Geriatrie.

Falk, G., and Spielhofer, H. 1975. Räumliche Umwelt und Wohnmobilität älterer Menschen—Ihre Determinanten und Konsequenzen. In Die gesellschaftliche Reintegration älterer Menschen. Mimeo. Vienna: Institut für empirische Sozialforschung.

Fessel and Gfk. 1972. Probleme alter Menschen. Mimeo. Vienna.

Formanek, K; Wick, G.; and Doberauer, W. 1966. Altersbedingte Unterschiede im Wasser- und Elektrolythaushalt nach radikaler Entwässerung. Paper presented to the Seventh International Congress of Gerontology, Vienna.

Gehmacher, E. 1971. Die gesellschaftliche Stellung alter Menschen, ihre Vorstellungen und Wünsche. In *Probleme des Status und der Betreuüng alter Menschen: Schriften zur Sozialarbeit des österr.* Vienna: Komites für Sozialarbeit, pp. 11-20.

Gisser, R. 1976. Demographische Grunddaten der weiblichen Bevölkerung Österreichs. In *Bericht über die Situation der Frau in Österreich. Part 4,* Vienna: Bundeskanzleramt.

Haag, F. and Krüger, H. eds. 1972 *Aktionsforschung.* Munich.

Hofecker, G. 1975. Untersuchungen zur isometrischen Messung und mathematischen Analyse der chemischen Kontraktion und Relaxation von Rattenschwanzsehnen. In *Habilitationsschrift.* Vienna: Eigenverlag Vet. Med. University.

————. 1976. Messungen des biologischen Alters im Tierversuch. *Aktuelle Gerontologie.* 6:103–110.

Hofecker, G.; Kment, A.; and Niedermüller, H. 1974a. Untersuchung über isometrische Spannungsentwicklung und lösliches Kollagen in Dorsaien und ventralen Sehnen des Rattenschwanzes. *Aktuelle Gerontologie* 4:291–295.

————. 1974b. Assessment of activity patterns of one- and two-year-old rats by electronic recording. *Experimental Gerontology* 9:109–114.

————. 1976. Die motorische Aktivität der Ratte als Altersparameter. Abstracts of the Congress of the Hungarian Gerontological Association, Budapest, October.

Hofecker, G.; Niedermüller, H.; Skalicky, M.; and Jahn, J. 1977. Die chemische Kontraktion von Schwanzsehnenfäden der Ratte als Altersparameter: Mathematische Analyse der Kontraction-Relaxation. *Aktuelle Gerontolie* 7:535–542.

Hörl, J., and Majce, G. 1976. Die Rekrutierungspopulation der Wiener Altersheime. Mimeo. Vienna.

Institut für empirische Sozialforschung (IFES), 1968. Betagte Menschen in Wien, part I. Mimeo. Vienna.

————. 1971. Der subjektive und objektive Lebensrahmen in Niederösterreich, vol. 1-2. Mimeo. Vienna.

————. 1975. Die Reintegration älterer Menschen. Mimeo. Vienna.

Kaufmann, A., and Balog, A. 1974. Altershilfeeinrichtungen: Österreich. In *Altenhilfe in Österreich—Eine Dokumentation, zusammengestellt vom Arbeitskreis Altenbetreuüng des Österreichischen Komitees für Sozialarbeitünd des Österreichischen Städtebundes,* pp. 5–65. Vienna: Institut für Stadtforschung.

Kment, A. 1963. Die tierexperimentelle Objektivierung des Revitalisierungseffektes nach Zellinjektionen. In F. Schmid and J. Stein, eds., *Zellforschung und Zellulartherapie.* Berne and Stuttgart; Hans Huber.

————. 1975. Der Revitalisierungsbegriff und seine tierexperimentelle Objektivierung. Proceedings of the Symposium of Gerontology, Lugano, April.

————. 1976. Die Bedeutung der Experimentellen Gerontologie für die klinische Geriatrie. *Aktuelle Gerontologie* 6:93-102.

Kment, A. and Hofecker, G. 1977a. Experimental Gerontological Investigations on the Subject of Vitality and Revitalization. Proceedings of the International Gerontological Symposium, Singapore, February.

————. 1977b. Electron Microscopical Gerontological Studies on Rat Liver Mitochondria. In D. Platt, ed., *Liver and Ageing*. Stuttgart and New York: F. K. Schattauer.

Kment A.; Hofecker, G.; and Niedermüller, H. 1977. Langzeituntersuchung über den Einfluss von Lauftraining, reduziertem Nahrungsangebot, Lauftraining und Nahrungsrestriktion und parenteral verabreichten Testiszellen auf verschiedene Altersparameter der Ratte. *Aktuelle Gerontologie* 7:463–469.

Kment, A.; Leibetseder, J., and Adamiker, D. 1966. Gerontologische Untersuchungen an Rattenlebermitochondrien. Z. Altersforsch 19:241–247.

Kment, A.; Leibetseder, J.; and Burger, H. 1966. Gerontologische Untersuchungen an Rattenherzmitochondrien. *Gerontologia* 12:193–199.

Kovac, W.; Lindner, A.; and Doberauer, W. 1966. Histologische Untersuchungen von Impftumoren bei jungen und alten Ratten. Paper presented at the Seventh International Congress of Gerontology, Vienna.

Krammer-Hirsch, F. 1974. Schichtsspezifische Unterschiede in der Situation alter Menschen in Wien. Master's thesis, University of Vienna.

Majce, G. 1978. ''Geschlossenen'' Altenhilfe—Probleme des Heimunterbringung. In L. Rosenmayr and H. Rosenmayr, eds., *Der alte Mensche in der Gesellschaft*, pp. 261–297. Reinbek bei Hamburg: Rowohlt.

————. 1979. Der alte Mensch und die Familie. In Bundeskauzleramt, ed., *Bevicht öber die Situation der Familie in Österreich* (Familienbevicht 1979), vol. 1: Struktur und Bedentuugswandel der Familie. Vienna. pp. 160–175.

Majce, G., and Hörl, J. 1974. *Formen der altenhilfe—Aufgaben und probleme der offenen und geschlossenen Altenhilfe*. Vienna: Institut für Stadtforschung.

Niedermüller, E., 1976a. Die Auswirkung der Übertragung von Proteinen und Ribonukleinsäuren aus dem Gehirn trainierter und untrainierter Ratten auf das Lernvermögen von jungen Ratten. Phil. diss., University of Vienna.

Niedermüller, H. 1976b. Experimentell gerontologische Gedächtnisuntersuchungen. *Aktuelle Gerontologie* 6:111–121.

————. 1977. Experimentell—gerontologische Untersuchungen zur DNA-Reparaturkapazität von Ratten. In *Habilitationsschrift*. Vienna: Vet. Med. Univ.

Niedermüller, H.; Hofecker, G.; and Kment, A. 1975. Gerontologische Untersuchungen des Nukleinsäurestoffwechsels bei der Ratte. I. Mitteilung: Hemmung der de novo Synthese von Thymidin mit Methotrexat. *Aktuelle Gerontologie* 5:445–451.

————. 1976. Untersuchungen zur Altersabhängigkeit der DNA-Reparaturkapazität in verschiedenen Organen der Ratte. In H. Altmann, ed., *DNA—Repair and late effects*. Eisenstadt; Rötzer.

Niedermüller, H.; Hofecker, G.; and Skalicky, M. 1977. Stoffwechselkitnetik des Kollagens junger und alter Ratten. *Aktuelle Gerontologie* 17.

Niedermüller, H.; Skalicky, M.; and Hofecker, G. 1976. Zelluläre und extrazelluläre Aspekte des Kollagenalterns. Abstracts of the Congress of the Hungarian Gerontological Association, Budapest, October.

Niedermüller, H.; Skalicky, M.; Hofecker, G.; and Kment, A. 1977. Investigations on the Kinetics of Collagen Metabolism in Young and Old Rats. *Experimental Gerontology* 12.

Österreichisches Statistiches Zentralamt (Ö.St.Z.) 1950–1978. *Statistische Handbücher für die Republik Österreich, 1950 to 1978*. Vienna.

——. 1972. Lebensverhältnisse älterer menschen—Ergebnisse des mikrozensus Dezember 1971. Beiträge zur österreichischen statistik, no. 310. Vienna.

——. 1977. Sozialstatistische daten 1977. Vienna.

Rosenmayr, L. 1957a. Altersstruktur und Gesellschaftsform. *Internationales Journal für phophylaktische Medizin und Sozialhygiene* 1:1–5.

——. 1957b. Das Altersproblem vom Standpunkt der Soziologie. In W. Doberauer, ed., *Medizinische und soziale Altersprobleme*, pp. 419–426. Vienna.

——. 1959. Alte Menschen in de Grosstadt—Ergebnisse von soziologischen Forschungen über Wohnverhältnisse. Familienbeziehungen und soziale Schwierigkeiten von alten Leuten in den Wohnungen, Helmstätten und Altersheimen der Stadt Wien. Mimeo. Vienna.

——. 1968. Family relations of the elderly. *Journal of Marriage and the Family* 30.

——. 1974. Elements of an Assimilation-yield Theory: An Exchange Model for Gerontology. Mimeo. Toronto.

——. 1975. Familiäre ünd ausserfamiliäre Betreuung alter Menschen. In K. Fellinger ed., *Altenhilfe—ein kooperatives Problem*. Vienna.

——. 1976. Schwerpunkte der Soziologie des Alters (Gerosoziologie). In L. König, ed., *Familie Alter. Handbuch der empirischen sozialforschung*, 7:218–406. Stuttgart: Enke.

——. 1977. The Family: A Source of Hope for the Elderly? In Ethel Shanas and Marvin B. Sussman, eds., *Family, Bureaucracy, and the Elderly*, pp. 132–157. Durham, N.C.: Duke University Press.

——, ed. 1978. Die menschlichen Lebensalter—Kontinuität und Krisen. Munich: Piper.

——. 1979. Progress and Unresolved Problems in Socio-gerontological Theory. *Aktuelle Gerontologie*, 9, pp. 197–205.

Rosenmayr, L., and Köckeis, E. 1963. Propositions for a theory of aging and the family. *International Social Science Journal* 15.

Rosenmayr, L., and Rosenmayr H., eds. 1978 *Die alte Mensch in der Gesellschaft*. Reinbek bei Hamburg: Rowohlt.

——. 1965a. Housing conditions and family relations of the elderly. In *Patterns of living and housing of the middle-aged and older people*. Proceedings of the Research Conference, Washington, D.C., March 1965.

——. 1965b. *Umwelt und Familie alter Menschen*. Neuwied and Berlin: Luchterhand.

Schaffranek, E. 1976. Experimentell-gerontologische Langzeituntersuchung. über den Einfluss von Nahrungsrestriktion, Lauftraining, sowie Nahrungsrestriktion und Lauftraining, und Testiszellen auf die Spontanaktivität der Ratte. Vet. Med. Diss., Univ. of Vienna.

Scheer, I. 1974. Wie gesund sind wir? Eine internationale Prognose bis 1982. Schriftenreihe der Arbeitsgemeinschaft für Lebensniveauvergleiche: Was heisst gesund leben?

Schulz, F-H., and Doberauer, W. 1958. Hypothyreose und alter. *Aktuelle Geriatrie.* Verlagsbuchandlg. Gesellschaft z. Forderung wissenschaftlicher Forschung. Vienna. pp. 127-131.

————. 1959. Die bedeutung der biomorphose für die geriatrie. *Die medizinische* 2:70–73.

————. 1960b. Regeneration und Alter. *Klinische Medizin* 10:475–482.

————. 1960a. Blut, Blutverlust und Blutersatz im Alter. *Geriatrie und Praxis* 5:125–130.

Schulz, F-H.; Dolega, P.; and Doberauer, W. 1958. Über Fehldiagnosen in der Geriatrie. *Aktuelle Geriatrie,* pp. 67-77.

Schulz, W. 1978. *Sozialkontakte in der Grosstadt.* Vienna: Institut für Stadtforschung.

Shanas, E.; Townsend, P.; Wederburn, D.; Friis, H.; Milhg, P.; and Stehouwer, J. 1968. *Old People in three industrial societies.* London: Atherton.

Skalicky, M.; Niedermüller, H.; and Hofecker, G. 1977. Ein mathematisches Modell der Stoffwechselkinetik des Sehnen- und Hautkollagens der Ratte. *Aktuelle Gerontologie* 7.

Starrach, A. 1976. Longitudinalstudien über das Verhalten der motorischen Aktivität unter dem Einfluss von Nahrungsrestriktion, Lauftraining, Nahrungsrestriktion und Lauftraining und Testiszellen bei der Ratte. Vet. Med. Diss., University of Vienna.

Wick, G.; Formanek, K.; and Doberauer, W. 1966. Abhängigkeit der Wasser- und Elektrolytausscheidung im Harn vom Lebensalter. Paper presented at the Seventh International Congress of Gerontology, Vienna.

Wiener Kammer für Arbeiter und Angestellte. 1974. *Armut in Wien.* Vienna.

Zwerina, R.; Doberauer, W.; and Lachnit, K. S. 1966. Behandlungsergebnisse bei der Verwendung von Dibenzodiazepin an einem geriatrischen Krankengut. Paper presented at the Seventh International Congress on Gerontology, Vienna.

CANADA

GILBERT ROSENBERG
and BERNARD GRAD

DEMOGRAPHY

In 1931, life expectancy at birth in Canada was 60.0 years for males and 62.1 for females. By 1971, it had risen to 69.3 years for males and 76.4 for females. It is predicted that by 1987, the corresponding figures will be 70.2 and 78.6 years. Thus life expectancy is increasing for both sexes, although the gap between males and females is continuing to widen (Clark and Collishaw, 1975). This increased life expectancy has combined with a decrease in natality to increase the proportion of aged persons in our society.

In 1851, persons over 65 years of age accounted for about 3 percent of the total population. By 1971, this percentage had increased to 8 percent (1.7 million persons) and is projected to be 11 percent (3.3 million persons) by the year 2001. By 2031, 20 percent of the population may be over sixty-five years of age.

For the very elderly (85 and over), who are much more likely to need health and social services, the projected increase in absolute numbers is from 142,000 persons in 1971 to 351,000 in 2001 (nearly two and a half times), representing the most rapidly growing segment of the total population (Auerbach and Gerber, 1976). Although the proportion of elderly in Canada is lower than in most other developed countries (see table 1), it appears that this proportion is entering a phase of rapid increase.

For those over 65 years of age, there is an ever-widening numbers gap between the sexes, which is of comparatively recent onset. Until 1951, the proportions of each sex over 65 were nearly the same. Since then, however, the proportion of women over 65 has increased much faster than the corresponding proportion of men. By the year 2001, the proportions will be 9 percent and 13 percent for males and females, respectively.

A consequence of the growing tendency of wives to outlive their husbands is that an increasingly large number of older women are left living alone. Less than 5 percent of people under 55 years of age live alone, but for people older than 55, the proportion living alone increases rapidly, particularly for women. Over 30 percent of women 75 years of age and over live alone; the corresponding percentage for men is 15 percent (Clark and Collishaw, 1975).

Like many other countries, Canada is currently in the midst of an inflationary period accompanied by stagnation (or recession). In this period, governments at all levels have looked at social programs as areas in which fiscal restraints should first be implemented. At such times, those in the older age groups nearing retirement are particularly vulnerable since compulsory retirement becomes a way to dispose of "surplus" labor (Canadian Council on Social Development, 1976).

These developments point to the need for greater knowledge about the elderly so that efforts can be quickly instituted to render this increasing segment of the population as self-sustaining as possible. To this end, information from the whole spectrum of science is required. Our purpose here is to provide a brief history of those who have made a start in taking up the challenge to meet the problems of the aged in Canada.

THE BEGINNINGS OF CANADIAN GERONTOLOGY

The Gerontologic Unit of the Allan Memorial Institute of Psychiatry of McGill University was established in 1944 by Dr. D. Ewen Cameron at a time when there were few such centers in the world and none in Canada. From the outset, the research in this unit was conducted throughout the whole spectrum of human aging. There were biochemical and physiological investigations on experimental animals as well as on humans and clinical studies of normal and pathological behavior. Research was also conducted upon the psychological and sociological aspects of aging, especially upon those concerned with the adaptation of the senescent person to his environment.

The earliest studies conducted in the Gerontologic Unit were concerned with enzyme changes during senescence (Stern et al., 1950, 1951; Birmingham and Grad, 1954), detoxification mechanisms in aged persons (Stern and Askonas, 1945, 1946, 1947), attempts to produce in experimental animals brain changes similar to those seen in senile and presenile conditions (Stern and Reed, 1945; Stern and Elliott, 1949), personality studies in menopausal women (Stern and Prados, 1946), and the mechanism of reactivation in the depressions of old age (Stern and Menzer, 1946).

The studies on enzyme activity showed that the peptidase activity of leukocytes increased during aging and thus suggested one reason why catabolic processes are perhaps more active in the aged.

The detoxification mechanisms in young and old persons were compared by measuring their ability to synthesize hippuric acid before and during the feeding of glycine. Elderly persons showed a reduced ability to synthesize hippuric acid when glycine was not fed. This difference disappeared when glycine was given, thus suggesting some deficiency of the elderly organism to furnish glycine rather than an impairment of the mechanism of conjugation of glycine to benzoic acid to form hippuric acid (Stern et al., 1946; Stern and Askonas, 1947).

Also investigated were biochemical mechanisms possibly operative in the development of certain histological changes in the brains of patients with presenile and senile psychosis. Thus the intravenous administration of 25 percent glucose solution to rabbits resulted in brain changes that corresponded to the initial stages of Alzheimer's fibrillary degeneration encountered in man and in senile and presenile conditions. This finding suggests that the fibrillary changes observed in senile psychosis and Alzheimer's disease may be associated with dehydration.

The first psychosocial investigations conducted by the Gerontologic Unit were largely concerned with the position of the elderly in the family (Stern, 1948) and with their specific emotional problems, such as grief reactions (Stern and Prados, 1951) and reactivation of depressions. The elderly subjects for these investigations were obtained from the Allan Memorial Institute and also from clients referred by special agencies to an Old Age Counselling Centre whose chief psychiatrist, Dr. Karl Stern, was also director of the Gerontologic Unit. These studies led to a deeper understanding of the psychodynamics of the emotional reactions of the elderly. It was also found that the psychotherapeutic approach must be different from that used with younger age groups; directive control of the environment played a far greater role in the therapy of the elderly.

RESEARCH

Thyroid Function

Dr. Karl Stern was succeeded by Dr. Martin Hoffman in 1952 as director of the Gerontologic Unit, and from then until 1955, biomedical studies were concerned mainly with the age changes in thyroid function. Attempts were made to measure the amount of thyroid hormone secreted by young and old rats utilizing two different methods. One involved the use of the antithyroid substance, thiouracil (Grad and Hoffman, 1955), and the other made use of a method involving radioactive iodine (Grad et al., 1956). Both methods revealed that the amount of thyroid hormone produced by the senescent animals is about 20 to 30 percent below that put out by the young. In addition, microscopic examination of the thyroids showed that the older animals presented a picture of lesser activity. The same was found to be true of the pituitary, which controls the rate of thyroid function. Thus the lesser activity of the thyroid gland in the aged rat was caused by its less active pituitary (Hoffman et al., 1954–1955).

Further studies, however, revealed the following surprising results. Despite the lesser production of thyroid hormone by the aged animal, the same amount of thyroid hormones was found circulating in the blood in both age groups. Moreover removal of the thyroid gland from both young and old animals resulted in a quantitatively similar decline in the basal metabolic rate in both groups (Grad, 1953). Further studies clarified this apparent enigma; it was found that a given amount of thyroxine stimulated the tissues of the aged rat to a greater extent than it did those of the younger ones, and toxic effects appeared more readily in the old than in the young. Hence although the older animal produced less thyroid hormone, it could not be considered hypothyroid (Grad, 1969). That is, the aged animal produced less thyroid hormone because its peripheral tissues were more sensitive to the hormone, and therefore less of it was required to maintain the normal metabolic rate. The thyroid gland of the aged animal did not produce less thyroxine because it had undergone senescent changes that made it incapable of producing more. These investigations received a Ciba Foundation Award for 1954–1955 on problems of aging (Hoffman et al., 1954–1955).

Adrenocortical Function

Other investigations conducted during this period were concerned with the possible relationship between the sodium over potassium ratio Na/K in saliva and the adrenocortical function. They were begun by B. Grad soon after he joined the Gerontologic Unit in 1949. Dr. Grad is still employed there and has had a major role in most of the biomedical studies conducted in that unit since 1949. His demonstration that adrenocorticotropic hormone (ACTH) administration caused a fall in the salivary Na/K was the first to show that the anterior pituitary–adrenal cortex axis plays a role in controlling the sodium concentration in saliva. Another finding in this study was that the salivary Na/K had a diurnal variation that paralleled anterior pituitary–adrenocortical function as determined by other criteria (Grad, 1952).

This study was extended to include the investigation of the salivary Na/K in fifty-two male and fifty-six female subjects ranging in age from 5 to 99 years. The results showed no significant change in the Na/K during normal aging nor was there any change in the diurnal variation of this ratio during senescence. The ratio, however, is reliably elevated in elderly schizophrenics and in patients with senile dementia (Kral and Grad, 1960; Grad and Kral, 1961).

Psychological and Neurological Research

In 1953 Dr. James S. Tyhurst, a psychiatrist, commenced extensive studies not only on aging but also on individual reactions to community disasters and catastrophies (Tyhurst, 1950a, b). His studies on aging were concerned with the effect of retirement on the aged. Contrary to the findings of others, he found that retirement did not hasten death. Indeed some evidence showed that the immediate postretirement period is characterized by a lower mortality (Tyhurst, 1956).

In 1955, when Dr. V. A. Kral assumed the directorship of the Gerontologic Unit, studies concerned chiefly with attempts to learn more about the etiology and pathogenesis of senile psychosis were started. As part of a series of investigations on the possible role of stress on the etiology and/or pathogenesis of senile psychosis, two studies compared the stress tolerance of patients with senile psychosis with that of normal subjects of similar age and background. In one of them, the stress applied was blindfolding the subject for half an hour. This was found to be nonstressful to the normal group; it appeared to disturb those in the patients' group. This finding was shown not only in the results of psychological tests taken before and after the stress but also in the greater decline of circulating eosinophils (an index of adrenocortical function) in the patients than in the normal subjects (Azima and Kral, 1960) A result pointing in the same direction was seen in studies in which the stress was a pricking pain produced by heat utilizing the Hardy-Wolff-Goodell dolorimeter. In this case, the senile patients showed a reliably greater fall in the salivary Na/K than did the normal persons. Both stresses are considered mild under normal circumstances, and none of the subjects suffered unduly. An extension of these studies appeared to suggest that the salivary Na/K response to stress might possibly be used as a prognostic indicator of impending mental breakdown in aged individuals who were still nevertheless able to live and function in the community without yet becoming manifestly ill.

Because of the greater reactivity of patients with senile psychosis to stress than that of normal elderly persons, it was decided to investigate in detail the hypothalamo-hypophyseal-adrenocortical system in the two groups of subjects. Adrenocortical function was studied first in normal young and normal elderly persons and then in senile subjects under conditions of rest and following stimulation with ACTH. The rate of removal of an infusion of cortisol, the major corticoid in humans, was also investiagated in senile psychotic patients and in normal subjects.

These studies showed that under resting conditions, adrenal cortical function in the normal elderly subjects was significantly below that of normal young people, at least during the first six hours following awakening in the morning (Grad and Kral, 1967). On the other hand, under the same conditions, there was no significant difference in adrenal cortical function between senile and psychotic patients and normal elderly persons (Grad et al., 1966).

Next, two separate studies were conducted on the responsiveness of the adrenal cortex of normal elderly subjects and of elderly patients with the chronic brain syndrome to forty international units of ACTH. Sixty-two persons were tested in the first study and ninety in the second, with equal numbers of men and women in each study. Patients with senile psychosis (S) were investigated in both studies, while those with psychosis due to cerebral arteriosclerosis (CAS) were studied only in the second. In the first investigation, blood samples were collected four and six hours after ACTH; in the second, the collections were made eight and ten hours after ACTH administration (Kral et al., 1967; Grad et al., 1969).

The first study showed that an elevation of the plasma corticoid (PC) level occurred in normals as well as in arteriosclerotic and senile patients, with the elevation almost identical in both groups at four hours; at six hours, the elevation was higher in the senile patients than in the normals but not significantly so. On the other hand, the second study revealed that the high PC values that the female S patients achieved at four and six hours were more or less maintained at eight and ten hours, while the corresponding values for the normal females declined markedly at these times.

In the males, the PC levels rose markedly in the S patients at eight and ten hours relative to their levels obtained at four and six hours, while in the normals, the values from four to ten hours after ACTH administration remained at about the same level. Thus in both males and females, the S patients had significantly higher PC values eight and ten hours after ACTH injection than the normal controls. Patients with CAS has PC values at the eight and ten hour interval, which were significantly below those of the S patients but significantly above those of the normals (Grad et al., 1969).

These facts, considered together with the finding that the rate of removal of infused cortisol was the same in the S patients as in the normals (Grad, unpublished), suggests that the greater increase in the PC level of the S patients to administered ACTH was not due to deficient mechanisms of removal of cortisol in the S patients but probably to a greater responsiveness of the adrenal cortex of the S patients as compared with the normals. Inasmuch as the anterior pituitary and the hypothalamus are also involved in protecting the organism against stress, differences in the reaction to stress between the two groups of subjects may also exist in either one or both of these organs. Further studies are needed in this area.

The significance of these findings should be assessed in the light of the following facts. Patients with the chronic brain syndrome in mental hospitals number about 100,000 in the United States and about 10,000 in Canada. Many more live in private homes or receive care in residences for the aged. The problem in terms of numbers alone is severe, and it is made more difficult by the fact that modern drug therapy, which has been efficacious in the endogenous psychoses, has been of limited symptomatic value in the organic psychoses. Thus persons who require a great deal of nursing care are a considerable medical and economic problem, which is likely to increase because of the ever-increasing proportion of elderly persons in our society.

Hitherto the etiology and pathogenesis of the organic psychoses were unknown, but the current studies point to the fact that the neuroendocrine response of these persons to stress is maladaptive and that the adrenal cortex at least is overreactive, with the possible involvement of the anterior pituitary and the hypothalamus. Such involvement of the neuroendocrine system is likely to be present decades before the symptoms of the organic psychoses become manifest; therefore, the possibility of early detection of persons with a propensity for this condition arises, as does the control of senile psychoses following institution of proper preventative methods.

An interesting sidelight of these studies was the finding that under resting conditions, adrenocortical function was significantly less in women than in men, but its response to exogenous ACTH was marked by a sharper response to ACTH during the first six hours, with a more marked decline during the next four hours than that of men (Grad et al., 1969).

Stress

Another study conducted involved stimulation of the adrenal cortex by a naturally occurring stress. This study involved the determination of the PC level (as well as symptom presentation) in a group of fifty-four normal and psychotic elderly persons undergoing relocation from one nursing home to another (Kral et al., 1968).

Normal aged men appeared to suffer more from the relocation than normal aged women did, and psychotic aged persons more than psychiatrically normal subjects of similar age. These results were apparent not only from the incidence of the symptom presentation subsequent to the relocation but also from the fact that in the normals the PC level rose in the men after relocation while it tended to decline somewhat in the women. In the psychotics, it rose in both sexes, and more so in the men (Kral et al., 1968).

The results obtained in the relocation study confirmed the findings obtained with the ACTH administration, for the latter showed that by eight and ten hours, the PC levels were higher in men than in women, while in the relocation study the PC level was determined one or two weeks after relocation, which is long after six hours after the stress at which time the women appear more reactive.

In addition to these studies of stress in humans, a series of studies were (and still are) being conducted on the effect of stress in young and old animals (Grad and Kral, 1957). The stress chosen for study was one undergone annually by a large number of people: cold. When young and old animals were exposed to the cold, the mortality was found to be very reliably higher in the old animals than in the young. Thus, exposure of mice to a temperature of 43–46°F killed over 80 percent of the old mice but less than 30 percent of young, when the animals had been adapted to a temperature of 80°F. It was also known that old mice can be made to survive lethal temperatures when accustomed to them gradually, but this adaptation was less effective in the old than in the young. Moreover metabolic studies revealed that when exposed to the cold, the old mice lost more weight and ate less, and their heat production was less markedly stimulated than that of the young. The sugar level in the blood of the old mice did not increase to the same extent as that of the young, and the elderly developed an anemia (the young did not). In short, those mechanisms normally set into motion when a warm-blooded animal is exposed to the cold were not operating as effectively in the old as in the young (Grad and Kral, 1957). These experiments are being conducted at the present time along the lines of a search for the mechanism(s) responsible for the loss of substances that could improve resistance to stress among the elderly.

One process observed during aging is the loss of cells from many tissues and the resulting loss of size and function. This is particularly true of the kidney, whose function in an eighty-year-old man is on the average about half that of a thirty-year-old male. However, cytophotometric measurements of Feulgen-stained nuclei demonstrated that the DNA content of nuclei of proximal tubules of the kidney was the same for young and old rats. The same was found to be true of neurons of the granular layer of the cerebellum and for diploid and tetraploid liver cells. Thus there does not appear to be any loss of DNA from individual nuclei during aging (Enesco, 1967b).

In more recent years, work has also been conducted on the determination of the PC level in individual mice. Work conducted by others in this field had hitherto always employed samples of blood pooled from several animals. This was necessary because the methods of bioassay utilized were not sufficiently sensitive to determine them in individual mice. However, by means of a competitive protein-binding radioassay, the corticosteroids in the blood and urine of individual mice were successfully determined in the Gerontologic Unit laboratory (Grad and Khalid, 1968). A study on the PC level conducted in several hundred young and old mice from two to thirty-three months of age showed that the values were high at two months of age, dropped to a low point at four months, and rose to a second peak by eight months, especially in females. Thereafter there was a gradual decline until old age. Females had significantly higher values than males did.

The importance of being able to assess accurately adrenocortical function in animals was that it permitted the execution of experiments not possible to conduct in persons that yield information complementary to the findings in man. Moreover, it could provide answers to hypotheses within one or two years; in humans, the work would require a lifetime. One such hypothesis is that severe emotional deprivation in early infancy or early childhood produces maladaptive responses to stress in later life, possibly contributing subsequently to a chronic brain syndrome in the human.

Psychosocial

The past several years have been marked by a rapid rate of expansion of investigation in the psychosocial field by the Gerontologic Unit. This was made possible by an expansion of the number of patients of the older age group available to the unit. When the unit was first established, the case material came essentially from the Allan Memorial Institute itself, as well as from the Old Age Counselling Centre. Later the sources of such case material were expanded to include the Jewish General Hospital (where a geriatric clinic was established), the Maimonides Hospital and Home for the Aged, the Douglas Hospital, and the Queen Mary Veteran's Hospital. In addition, the Gerontologic Unit also established contact with many of the Golden Age Clubs in Montreal.

This work led to an extensive revision of existing concepts of the nature of mental ill health in the aged (Kral and Gold, 1961). First of all, the so-called organic psychoses of the aged—senile and arteriosclerotic psychoses—form only a minor part—about 25 percent—of the case material that psychiatrists see in daily practice. However, this group occupies one-third of all beds in psychiatric institutions and one-sixth of all hospital beds in the United States and Canada. Research in this area is therefore vital.

About 25 percent of elderly patients seen in daily practice have affective psychoses, mainly depressions, and these respond favorably to the same type of treatment as used in the younger age group. Nearly half of the aged patients suffer from neurotic conditions that essentially represent their psychological reactions to the biological, psychological, and social facts of growing old. Another practical and important observation relates to the fact that aged subjects frequently react to acute stresses of a physical as well as a psychological nature with acute confusional states that can be mistaken for the acute onset of senile psychosis but have a considerably better prognosis when diagnosed in time and properly treated (Kral, 1961, 1962, 1965).

This advance in our knowledge concerning mental ill health in the aged has significance not only with respect to the kind of therapeutic services to be provided for the aged individual but also with respect to the plans that should be drawn up on a national basis for therapeutic centers and buildings to provide the necessary psychiatric treatment for older citizens.

During this period a series of psychosocial investigations were conducted on the possible role of stress in the development of senile psychosis. Thus stress histories were taken of patients with senile psychoses and compared with those of normal elderly persons of similar age and background. These studies showed no reliable difference in the amount of stress endured by each of the two groups. However, one particular stress occurred with greater frequency in the patients with senile psychosis than it did in the normal elderly persons. There was evidence that severe emotional deprivaton occurred with significantly greater frequency during the childhood of the patients than it did during the same period of the control group. Moreover the patients with senile psychosis appeared to react subsequently to stress in a more exaggerated manner, for example, by falling ill following stresses that did not similarly affect the normal group (Grad, unpublished).

During this period, extensive time was devoted to the study of memory dysfunction so commonly found in aging people. A major advance was the discovery, made by Dr. V. A. Kral, of two types of senescent forgetfulness: a benign type that occurs with equal frequency in both sexes, progresses slowly, and is not significantly correlated with survival time and mortality, and a malignant type that occurs more frequently in women, progresses much faster, and is significantly correlated with an increased death rate and a shortened survival time (Kral, 1962).

These findings were verified on an extensive material comprising nearly seven hundred patients, 60 years and over, suffering from various mental disorders. Patients who presented the malignant type of forgetfulness, the senile amnestic syndrome, had a significantly higher death rate and a significantly shorter survival time than patients of the same age without memory impairment or only the benign type of senescent forgetfulness. A five-year follow-up of this group demonstrated that the type and degree of memory dysfunction was a reliable indicator of the general health and survival of the aged individual. No reliable relationship, however, was found between the senile amnestic syndrome and a specific cause of death (Wigdor and Kral, 1961). This led to the conclusion that the increased death rate of the patients with the senile amnestic syndrome was due to a lower stress resistance than that found in old people who do not show this type of memory impairment.

The following hypothesis emerged from these investigations: the disease process of the amnestic syndrome interferes directly or indirectly with the function of the centrencephalic system (Krall and Muller, 1966b). In this connection previous studies have shown that an important part of the integrative mechanism that enables the organism to withstand stress is localized in the hypothalamus. It would appear, therefore, that the localization of the senile brain disease, either in the hypothalamus or in the area functionally connected with it, may account for the significant correlation between the senile amnestic syndrome and the markedly reduced stress resistance and consequent increased death rate of these patients (Krall et al., 1967).

A study of electroencephalogram findings in patients with far advanced senile dementia demonstrated bilaterally synchronous slow wave discharges similar to those found in patients with hepatic coma, although the state of consciousness in these patients was not impaired to the same extent as in the hepatic group. Rather, their clinical condition was characterized by profound apathy. It was concluded that these discharges represent a dysfunction of a coordinating system involving cortical as well as subcortical structures (Muller and Krall, 1967). These findings seem to be in agreement with those made in the studies on stress resistance of the aged, as well as the studies on senescent memory dysfunction.

Also shown in studies conducted in the Gerontologic Unit was that irreversible strokes occurred significantly less frequently in subjects who on psychiatric examination showed signs of organic brain syndrome due to senile brain disease than those with cerebral arteriosclerosis, although the latter were younger than the former (Kral, 1964).

Another study showed a significant positive correlation between hypertension and high Bender gestalt scores, which are indicative of impaired visual motor coordination or poor perceptual organization. This indicated that hypertension leads to impairment of the visual motor part of gestalt perception and this may be one of the earlier signs of impaired brain function. This confirmed the previous findings that psychological testing can detect organic deficit in clinically well-preserved aged people (people who are able to compensate at least for some of their organic deficits) (Kral and Wigdor, 1963).

Drugs

Several studies were also conducted on the use of certain drugs in geriatric patients. Thus imipramine was found to be a useful, relatively safe adjuvant in the treatment of depressive states in the aged.

The workers of the Gerontologic Unit were the first to test another antidepressant, trimipramine, which was found to be an effective drug for the treatment of geriatric patients suffering from endogenous depressions (Kral et al., 1964).

Similarly thioridazine was found to be suited for the treatment of a variety of mental disorders in the aged (Kral, 1961). When dosage was moderate and controls were applied, serious side effects were lacking. On the other hand, procaine hydrochloride (Novocain) treatment, according to Aslan's method, did not appreciably alter the symptomatology and course of senile and arteriosclerotic brain disease. However, it was found to be temporarily helpful in alleviating depressive symptoms in these patients (Kral et al., 1962).

Studies with an oral androgen administered to patients with senile memory dysfunction demonstrated a significant, although temporary, increase in memory scores, particularly of logical memory. This improvement was attributed to increased alertness and improved concentration rather than to a direct effect of the hormone on the biochemical process underlying memory function itself (Kral and Wigdor, 1959, 1961).

In a series of studies with Dr. H. Lehmann and Dr. T. Ban, methods were developed to assess the changes in the behavior, both verbal and nonverbal, and the mood changes of geriatric mental patients (Lehmann et al., 1968; Silver et al., 1968). These studies led to the standardization of certain psychological and psychophysiological testing methods, which proved useful for the clinical evaluation of the many new psychopharmaceutical drugs being offered by the pharmaceutical industry.

Complementing these studies was another series directed toward the understanding of memory function in biochemical terms and toward developing a treatment for geriatric patients suffering from senile memory impairment. Because preliminary findings by Dr. D.E. Cameron and Dr. L. Solyom appeared to indicate that ribonucleic acid (RNA) improved memory function in senile patients, an extensive series of investigations was begun on the effect of this and other substances on the learning ability in the rat (Cameron and Solyom, 1961; Cameron et al., 1961, 1963a & b, 1964). These studies were based on the premise that RNA may be involved in the encoding and retention of memory traces. Age-dependent failure of the neuronal RNA system may be one of the intrinsic factors of senescent memory dysfunction (Cameron et al., 1966; Beaulieu, 1966; Solyom et al., 1966, 1967; Beaulieu and Solyom, 1966; Enesco, 1967a, 1968). These studies found that RNA administration produced clinical improvement and increased memory scores in patients suffering from senile brain disease and cerebral arteriosclerosis as measured by the Wechsler Memory Scale, the counting test, and the acquisition and retention of the conditioned galvanic skin response (GSR). Intravenous RNA treatment seemed to be more effective than oral administration.

In another study, the activity of the serum ribonuclease was investigated in relation to age and the memory function of aged persons. A significant positive correlation was found between ribonuclease activity and age, but none with memory function, in a group of senile and senescent patients (Sved et al., 1967).

In rats, intact yeast RNA in contradistinction to hydrolyzed RNA facilitated acquisition of bar pressing when injected intraperitoneally. Old and young animals benefited significantly from this treatment (Beaulieu, 1966; Solyom et al., 1967, 1968). To clarify the mechanism of RNA action, studies were conducted on the fate of twelve cc. of $C_2$14C_8RNA administered to mice and sacrificed four hours later (Enesco, 1966). RNA was taken up by the intestine, liver, kidney, pancreas, and spleen but not by the neural tissue of the brain, although it was observed in the choroid plexus and ependyma. Thus the therapeutic effects of RNA treatment do not appear to be explicable on the basis that RNA encodes memory information within the brain. Other studies showed that RNA is not a central stimulant and does not increase the general level of activity. However, RNA injections could have a limited stimulant action in rats brought about by increased levels of circulating nucleotides and xanthine bases resulting from RNA breakdown. At the present time, this hypothesis appears to be the best available to explain the results of the animals experimentation.

The effect on learning of several substances known to increase the endogenous RNA content of central nervous system cells significantly was also explored. Thus both malononitrile dimer (Solyom and Gallay, 1966) and vitamin B_{12} (Enesco, 1968) reliably increase the acquisition of bar-pressing response. On the other hand, chronic administration of vitamin B_{12} did not increase the memory scores of patients suffering from arteriosclerotic and senile brain disease. However, it was found that the ratio of the serum level of vitamin B_{12} to folic acid is changed in cases with memory impairment.

Paralleling these investigations were studies on the use of the conditioning of the eyeblink response and of the GSR. Learning scores derived from conditioning, discrimination, and delayed and trace reflex formation were used in the assessment of senile brain disease (Solyom, 1968a). Conditioning was also used as an investigative tool in the physiopathology of senescence and senility (Solyom and Barik, 1965). Finally, the examination of perseveration in its neurophysiological and psychological aspects, as well as time estimation, in senescent and senile individuals in comparison with that of younger persons was also undertaken (Solyom, 1968).

Current Research

An active research program, led by Dr. B. Grad, continues at the Gerontologic Unit despite the current lack of funds for research on aging. Although Dr. V. A. Kral retired as director of the unit in 1973, he remains associated in an advisory capacity. More recently, research on gerontology and geriatrics has taken strong root in hospitals outside the Allan Memorial Institute, notably the Maimonides Hospital and Home for the Aged under Dr. Gilbert Rosenberg, the Douglas Hospital under Dr. H. F. Muller, and the Montreal hospitals under the wing of the Department of Veterans' Affairs. Here Dr. Blossom Wigdor, Dr. F. W. Lundell, and J.Z. Csank have played prominent roles. Collaboration between these research centers and the Gerontologic Unit remains strong.

The most recent studies conducted in the Gerontologic Unit alone or in collaboration with others have involved the use of Levodopa therapy in elderly patients with Parkinson's disease (Grad, et al., 1974; Wener et al., 1976), biological and psychological predictors of survival in a psychogeriatric population (Muller and Grad, 1974; Muller et al., 1975), and changes in adrenocortical function in elderly people under stress, as, for example, during relocation (Grad, unpublished). Studies on the so-called placebo effect and the doctor-patient relationship in general were also carried out (Grad, 1966, 1967). Some of the recent investigations of the unit have also included the use of experimental animals to elucidate the role of psychological and dietary factors on the resistance to disease (Grad, unpublished).

The Gerontologic Unit of the Allan Memorial Institute of Psychiatry has played a crucial role in Canadian gerontology not only because of the work carried out directly under its aegis but also because it served as a mainspring for development of gerontology throughout the country at a time when the study was in its infancy. Although many other organizations—most notably the Canadian Council on Social Development—have long been active in the field of aging, the unit was the first to focus primarily on the problems of the elderly, particularly from a clinical and research viewpoint.

More recently gerontologic studies are being carried out in other parts of Canada. Basic biological studies are in process under the direction of Dr. S. Goldstein at McMaster University (Goldstein et al., 1969, 1978; Goldstein and Lin, 1972) in Hamliton, Ontario, and under Dr. W. F. Forbes at Waterloo University (Forbes, 1964; Forbes and Ramsbottom, 1969) in Waterloo, Ontario. On the psychological side, many studies have been developed under the direction of Professor D. Schonfield at the University of Calgary (Schonfield, 1966, 1970), Calgary, Alberta. The many centers of activity in the area of social research, planning, and practice are too numerous to mention here. On the clinical side, the teaching of geriatrics has been strengthened by the arrival of several active young geriatricians from England, notably Dr. R. Fisher, who is working at the Sunnybrooke Hospital in Toronto, Ontario, Dr. R. Cape, who is in London, Ontario, and Dr. D. Skelton, who is working at the University of Manitoba and Deerlodge Hospital in Winnipeg, Manitoba. These are in addition to the group of indigenous Canadian physicians who have long labored to include a geriatric input in medical education, as well as a greater awareness of the problems of the elderly in the community as a whole. Most notably these include Dr. J. MacDonell of the Deerlodge Hospital and University of Manitoba, in Winnipeg, Manitoba, Dr. B. Fahrni of the University of British Columbia in Vancouver, British Columbia, Dr. R. Bayne at McMaster University in Hamilton, Ontario, and Dr. C. Paradis at the University of Laval in Quebec City, Quebec. Nonetheless in most parts of the country, the teaching of geriatrics and gerontology represents a very small fragment of health education.

Care of the Elderly

Care of the elderly received a great boost when the Senate of Canada established a special committee in 1963 ''to examine the problem involved in the promotion of the welfare of the aged and aging persons, in order to ensure that in addition to the provision of a sufficient income, there are also developed adequate services and facilities of a positive and preventative kind so that older persons may continue to live healthy and useful lives as members of the Canadian Community and the need for the maximum cooperation of all levels of government in the promotion thereof.''

The final report of the Special Committee of the Senate on Aging, published in 1966 (Croll, 1966), reviewed the status of the elderly in Canada, including their health, housing, and finances. Chaired by Senator David Croll, the committee in the course of three years of meetings gathered and sifted a vast amount of information and made many recommendations. Some of the data and recommendations are now dated but can be clearly recognized as the source of much of what has now become accepted practice in Canada. Others are still as pertinent today as when first reported in 1966, for example, "that home care programs for elderly people be greatly extended for those who are discharged early from hospital or who would otherwise require to be admitted." Home care for the elderly, like day hospitals, is still sadly lacking in most parts of the country.

Senator Croll has continued to demonstrate concern for the welfare of our older citizens. In December 1977 the Senate of Canada established a special investigating committee, under the chairmanship of Senator Croll, to investigate mandatory retirement and other related aspects of retirement and income security for pensioners. Numerous organizations have submitted briefs to this committee including the Canadian Association on Gerontology. It is anticipated that the final report by the Croll committee will have as significant an impact on the welfare of the elderly in Canada as did that of the Committee on Aging in 1966.

CANADIAN ASSOCIATION ON GERONTOLOGY

In 1971, a small group of gerontologists meeting at the Douglas Hospital in Montreal established the Canadian Association on Gerontology, with Dr. W. F. Forbes of the University of Waterloo, Ontario, as its first president. The association has shown steady growth and currently has more than seven hundred members. Meeting annually, it is acting as a catalyst to foster and support the growth of gerontology in many parts of the country. Most of the active gerontologists in Canada are members, and they have made significant contributions to international gerontology by taking part in all of the recent international congresses of gerontology. Most recently several members contributed to the National Consultation on Aging held in Toronto in February 1977 and sponsored by all of the provincial social service departments. That meeting served to confirm that the Canadian Association on Gerontology would be the main professional gerontological organization involved in planning with the federal and provincial governments for future meetings on a national scale dealing with the problems of the elderly.

A sequel to the Consultation of 1977 took place in October 1978 when a National Symposium was held in Ottawa. The symposium was sponsored by the ministers of social affairs of the provincial governments, and the Canadian Association on Gerontology was actively involved in both the organization of the program as well as in participation at the sessions. Themes of the symposium included implications of the demographic changes in the Canadian population over the next twenty-five years, health and care needs of an aging population, concerns and expectations of the old in Canada, cultural and ethnic aspects of aging, and others. The symposium was useful in that it brought together representatives of the federal and provincial governments and the voluntary sector in plenary sessions and workshops. At the symposium, the minister of National Health and Welfare, the Honorable Monique Bégin, announced the establishment of a national Bureau on Aging. The bureau was subsequently established in early 1979. Although this can be taken as a hopeful sign of increasing governmental concern for the elderly, it is too soon to say how significant a role this bureau will play in Canadian gerontology.

The Canadian Association on Gerontology has also been meeting with the Royal College of Physicians and Surgeons of Canada with a view to clarifying the place of geriatric medicine in medical education and in the spectrum of medical specialties in Canada. As a result, it is likely that the Royal College will establish a certificate of special competence in geriatric medecine. The certificate will lead to postgraduate training programs in geriatric medicine with certification being required for physicians involved in the teaching of geriatrics or involved in long-term care to a significant extent.

The College of Family Physicians of Canada has been in existence for about twenty years. Until now, only sporadic efforts have been made to include geriatric medicine in its continuing education activities. In 1977, however, meetings were initiated with the Canadian Association on Gerontology with a view to incorporating geriatric medicine more consciously into the activities of the college at all levels of training and postgraduate education. These steps reflect recognition of the aging of the Canadian population and of the changing medical climate in which Canadian physicians are increasingly working.

Further impetus has been given to the development of geriatric medicine in Canada by the recently published report of a working party of physicians convened by the Department of National Health and Welfare (MacDonell, 1977). This report has charged that "formal curriculum content of geriatrics has been meagre and structured training programs almost nonexistent." It also points out that "a specific body of knowledge relating to normal aging and to Pathological Aging exists and should be a structured component of under-graduate medical curricula."

Recent statements emanating from the 1977 annual meeting of the Canadian Medical Association lending similar support for the teaching of geriatrics serves to round out those principal policy-making bodies involved in the implementation of a geriatric medicine education and training program. Thus, there is widespread support for the growth of geriatrics in Canada.

In February 1979 social gerontology in Canada received a substantial boost when the Social Sciences and Humanities Research Council of Canada announced a program to promote research in the social, economic, and cultural implications of our aging population. Included will be special research grants, post-doctoral awards, and reorientation grants, the latter intended to provide support to researchers with full-time university appointments who wish to orient their research toward aspects of the aging population. The interest generated by the initial announcement suggests that the program *may* have a significant influence on the future course of social gerontology in Canada.

REFERENCES

Auerbach, L., and Gerber, A. 1976. *Implications of the changing age structure of the Canadian population*, 3. Ottawa; Science Council of Canada.

Azima, F. and Kral, V. A. 1960. "Effects of blindfolding on persons during psychologic testing. *Geriatrics* 15:780–792.

Beaulieu, C. 1966. The effect of RNA on experimentally induced memory impairment. *Psychonomic Science* 6:339–340.

Beaulieu, C., and Solyom, L. 1966. The effect of DNA on operant conditioning. *Journal of Psychology* 64:223–226.

Birmingham, M. K., and Grad, B., 1954. Peptidase activity in the thymus of a normal and a leukemic strain of mice during growth and aging. *Cancer Research* 14:352–359.

Cameron, D. E.; Kral, V. A.; Solyom, L; Sved, S.; Wainrib, B.; Beaulieu, C.; and Enesco, H. 1966. RNA and memory. In *Macromolecules and behavior*, ed. J. Gaito, pp. 129–148. New York: Appleton-Century-Crofts.

Cameron, D. E., and Solyom, L. 1961. Effects of ribonucleic acid on memory. *Geriatrics* 16: 74–81.

Cameron, D. E.; Solyom, L.; and Beach, L. 1961. Further studies upon the effects of the administration of ribonucleic acid in aged patients suffering from memory (retention) failure. *Neuro-Psychopharmacology* 2:351–355.

Cameron, D. E.; Solyom, L.; Sved, S.; and Wainrib, B. 1963. Effects of intravenous administration of ribonucleic acid upon failure of memory for recent events in presenile and aged individuals. In *Recent advances in biological psychiatry*, ed. J. Wortis. New York: Plenum.

Cameron, D. E.; Sved, S.; Solyom, L.; Wainrib, B.; and Barik, H. 1963. Effects of ribonucleic acid on memory defect in the aged. *American Journal of Psychiatry* 120:320.

————. 1964. Ribonucleic acid in psychiatric therapy. In *Current psychiatric therapies*, ed. Jules H. Masserman. New York: Grune & Stratton.

Canadian Council on Social Development. 1976. *Fifty-sixth annual report*. Ottawa.

Clark, J. A., and Collishaw, N. E. 1975. Canada's older population. In *Staff papers, long range health planning, health and welfare, Canada*. pp. 1–5. Ottawa.

Croll, D. 1966. *Final report of the Special Committee of the Senate Committee on Aging*. Ottawa, Ontario: Queen's Printer and Controller of Stationery.

Enesco, H. E. 1966. Fate of ^{14}C-RNA injected into mice. *Experimental Cell Research* 42:640–645.

————. 1967a. RNA and memory: a re-evaluation of present data. *Canadian Psychiatric Association Journal* 12:29–34.

————. 1967b. A cytophotometric analysis of DNA content in rat nuclei in aging. *Journal of Gerontology* 22:445–448.

————. 1968. Effect of vitamin B12 on neuronal RNA and on instrumental conditioning in the rat. In *Recent advances in biological psychiatry*, ed. J. Wortis, pp. 134–143. New York: Plenum.

Forbes, W. F. 1964. The role of electron paramagnetic resonance spectro-scopy in aging research. *Gerontologist* 4.

Forbes, W. F., and Hamlin, C. R. 1969. Determinations of -SH and -SS- groups in proteins. II. The age-dependence of -SH and -SS contents in the soluble protein fractions of the eye lens. *Experimental Gerontology* 4:151–158.

Forbes, W. F.; Hamlin, C. R.; and Lerman, S. 1967. Age dependence of -SH and -SS-content in the insoluble fraction (albuminoid) of eye lenses. *Gerontologist* 7.

Forbes, W. F. and Lerman, S. 1966. Effect of radiation and aging on ocular lens proteins. In *Proceedings of the Seventh International Congress of Gerontology.*

Forbes, W. F. and Ramsbottom, J. V. 1967. Concerning the mechanism of radical transfer consistent with the free radical theory of aging. *Gerontologist* 7.

———. 1969. The reactivity of free radicals in the solid phase. In *Proceedings of the Eighth International Congress of Gerontology* 1969, 2.

Forbes, W. F., and Sullivan, P. D. 1966. The effect of radiation on collagen I. Electron-spin resonance spectra of 2537A-irradiated collagen. *Biochemica Biophysica Acta* 120.

Forbes, W. F., and Wang, H. M. 1969. Free radicals derived from tobacco smoke constituents. In *Proceedings of the 8th International Congress of Gerontology*, Washington, D.C.

Goldstein, S., and Littlefield, J. 1969. Effects of insulin on the conversion of glucose $C^{14}O_2$ by normal and diabetic fibroblasts in culture. *Diabetes* 18:545.

Goldstein, S. The biology of aging. 1971a. *New England Journal of Medicine* 285:1120.

Goldstein, S. 1971b. On the pathogenesis of diabetes mellitus and its relationship to biological aging. *Humangenetik* 12:83.

Goldstein, S. 1971c. The role of DNA repair in aging of cultured fibroblasts from xeroderma pigmentosum and normals. *Proceedings of the Society of Experimental Biological Medicine* 137:730

Goldstein, S., and Lin, C. 1972. Rescue of senescent human fibroblasts by hybridization with hamster cells in vitro. *Experimental Cell Research* 70:436.

Goldstein, S.; Littlefield, J.; and Soeldner, J. 1969. Diabetes mellitus and aging. diminished plating efficiency of cultured human fibroblasts. *Proceedings of the National Academy of Science* 64:155.

Goldstein, S.; Moerman, E.J.; Soeldner, J.S.; Gleason, R.E.; and Barnett, D.M. 1978. Chronologic and physiologic age affect replicative life span of fibroblasts from diabetic, prediabetic and normal donors *Science* 199:781-782.

Grad, B. 1952. The influence of ACTH on the sodium and potassium concentration of human mixed saliva. *Journal of Clinical Endocrinology and Metabolism* 12:708–718.

———. 1953. Changes in oxygen consumption and heart rate during growth and aging in rats: Role of the thyroid gland. *American Journal of Physiology* 174:481–486.

———. 1954. Diurnal, age and sex changes in the sodium and potassium of human saliva. *Journal of Gerontology* 9:276–284.

———. 1966. The "laying on of hands": Implications for psychotherapy and the placebo effect. *Corrective Psychiatry and Journal of Social Therapy* 12:192–202.

Grad, B., 1969. The metabolic responsiveness of young and old female rats to thyroxine. *Journal of Gerontology* 24:5–11.

Grad, B., and Hoffman, M. M. 1955. Thyroxine secretion rates and plasma cholesterol levels of young and old rats. *American Journal of Psychology* 182:497.

Grad., B., and Khalid, B. 1968. Plasma corticoid levels in young and old male and female C57B1/6J mice. *Journal of Gerontology* 23:522–528.

Grad, B., and Kral, V. A. 1957. The effect of senescence on resistance to stress. I. Response of young and old mice to cold. *Journal of Gerontology* 12:172–181.

CANADA 57

————. 1961. Adrenal cortical stress effects in senility. II. The response to heat stimulation produced by the Hardy-Wolff-Goodell dolorimeter. *Canadian Psychiatric Association Journal* 6:66–74.

Grad, B.; Kral, V. A.; Berenson, J.; and Kappos, W. J. 1969. The delayed effect of ACTH administration on the plasma corticoid level of normal elderly persons and patients with a chronic brain syndrome. *Journal of the American Geriatrics Society* 17:15–24.

Grad, B.; Kral, V. A.; Payne, R. C.; and Berenson, J. 1966. Adrenal cortical function in the psychoses of later life. *Laval Medical* 37:126–134.

————. 1967. Plasma and urinary corticoids in young and old persons. *Journal of Gerontology* 22:66–71.

Grad, B.; Wener, J.; Rosenberg, G.; and Wener, S. 1974. Effects of Levodopa therapy in patients with Parkinson's disease: Statistical evidence for reduced tolerance to Levodopa in the elderly. *Journal of the American Geriatrics Society* 22:489–494.

Grad, B.; Wilansky, D. L.; and Hoffman, M. M. 1956. Changes in thyroid function during aging. Paper presented to the Ninth Annual Scientific Meeting of the Gerontological Society, Chicago, Illinois, November 8, 1956.

Grauer, H., and Kral, V. A. 1960. The use of imipramine (Tofranil) in psychiatric patients of a geriatric outpatient clinic. *Journal of the Canadian Medical Association* 83:1423–1426.

Kral, V. A. 1961a. The use of thioridazine (Mellaril) in aged people. *Canadian Medical Association Journal* 84:152–154.

————. 1961b. Recent research in prevention of mental disorders at later age levels. In *Recent research looking toward preventive intervention: Proceedings of the Third Institute on Preventive Psychiatry*, ed. R. H. Ojemann.

————. 1962a. Senescent forgetfulness: benign and malignant. *Canadian Medical Association Journal* 86:257–260.

————. 1962b. Stress and mental disorders of the senium. *Medical Services Journal* 8:363–370.

————. 1964. Localized cerebral ischemia: Its incidence in senile and arteriosclerotic psychosis. In *Cerebral Ischemia*, ed. Ernst Simonson and Thomas Hodge McGavack, pp. 146–161., Springfield, Ill.: Charles Thomas.

————. 1965. Neurotic reactions and attitudes of the aging. *Health News*, 10–13.

Kral, V. A., and Gold, S. 1961. Psychiatric findings in a geriatric outpatient clinic. *Canadian Medical Association Journal* 84:588–590.

Kral, V. A., and Grad, B. 1960. Adrenal cortical stress effects in senility. *Canadian Psychiatric Association Journal* 5:8–18.

Kral, V. A.; Grad, B.; and Berenson, J. 1968. Stress reactions resulting from the relocation of an aged population. *Canadian Psychiatric Association Journal* 13:201-209.

Kral, V. A.; Grad, B.; Payne, R. C.; and Berenson, J. 1967. The effect of ACTH on the plasma and urinary corticoids in normal elderly persons and in patients with senile psychosis. *American Journal of Psychiatry* 123:1260–1269.

Kral, V. A.; Cahn, C.; Deutsch M.; Muller, H.; and Solyom, L. 1962. Procaine (Novocain) treatment of patients with senile and arteriosclerotic brain disease. *Canadian Medical Association Journal* 87: 1109–1113.

Kral, V. A.; Lehmann, H. E.; Ban, T. A.; Ast., H.; Barriga, C.; and Lidsky, A. 1964. The effects of trimipramine on geriatric patients. In *Trimipramine, a new antidepressant,* ed. H. E. Lehmann, M. Berthiaume, and T. A. Ban, pp. 69–75.

Kral, V. A., and Muller, H. 1966a. Memory dysfunction: A prognastic indicator in geriatric patients. *Canadian Psychiatric Association Journal* 11:343–349.

―――. 1966b. Centrencephalic dysfunction in senile dementia. In *Excerpta Medical International Congress Series No. 150. Proceedings of the Fourth World Congress of Psychiatry.* Madrid.

Kral, V. A., and Wigdor, B. T. 1959. Androgen effect on senescent memory function. *Geriatrics* 14:450–456.

―――. 1961. Further studies on the androgen effect on senescent memory function. *Canadian Psychiatric Association Journal* 6:345–352.

―――. 1963. Clinical and psychological observations in a group of well-preserved aged people. *Medical Services Journal* 19:1–11.

Lehmann, H. E.; Ban, T. A.; and Kral, V. A. 1968. Psychological tests: Practice effect in geriatric patients. *Geriatrics* 23:160–163.

MacDonell, J.A. *Medical education in geriatrics: Report of a working party convened by the Health Standards and Consultants Directorate, Health Programs Branch, Department of National Health and Welfare, Ottawa, Canada.* 1977.

Muller, H. F., and Grad, B. 1974. Clinical-psychological, electroencephalographic and adrenocortical relationships in elderly psychiatric patients. *Journal of Gerontology* 29:28–38.

Muller, H. F.; Grad, B.; and Engelsmann, F. 1975a. Biological and psychological predictors of survival in a psychogeriatric population. *Journal of Gerontology* 30:47–53.

―――. 1975b. Five year follow-up of geriatric EEG's. *Electroencephalography and Clinical Neurophysiology* 38:108.

Muller, H. F. and Kral, V. A., 1967. The electroencephalogram in advanced senile dementia. *Journal of the American Geriatrics Society* 15:415–426.

Schonfield, A. E. D. 1966. Coding and translation processes in older age groups. *Gerontologist* 6:30.

―――. 1967. Geronting: Reflections on successful aging. *Gerontologist* 7:270–273.

―――. 1969a. Age and remembering. In *Proceedings of seminars, Duke University Council on Aging and Human Development, Durham, Duke University,* ed. F. Jeffers, p. 88.

―――. 1969b. In search of early memories. In *Proceedings of the 8th International Congress of Gerontology,* Washington, D.C..

―――. 1970. Family life education study: The later adult years. *Gerontologist* 10:115–118.

Silver, D.; Lehmann, H. E.; Kral, V. A.; and Ban, T. A. 1968. Experimental geriatrics: Selection and prediction of therapeutic responsiveness in geriatric patients. *Canadian Psychiatric Association Journal* 561–563.

Solyom, L. 1968a. Trace reflex formation in senescence and senility. *Recent Advances in Biological Psychiatry* 10:294–301.

―――. 1968b. Perseveración: El aspecto neurofisiólogico. *Revista de Psicologia General y aplicada* 23:23-43.

Solyom, L., and Barik, H. C. 1965. Conditioning in senescence and senility. *Journal of Gerontology* 20:483–488.

Solyom, L.; Beaulieu, C.; and Enesco, H. E. 1966. The effect of RNA on the operant conditioned behavior of white rats. *Psychonomic Science* 6:341–342.

Solyom, L.; Enesco, H.; and Beaulieu, C. 1967. The effect of RNA on learning and activity in young and old rats. *Journal of Gerontology* 22:1–7.

————. 1968. The effect of RNA, uric acid and caffein on conditioning and activity in rats. *Journal of Psychiatric Research* 6:175–183.

Solyom, L., and Gallay, H.M. 1966. Effect of malononitrile dimer on operant and classical conditioning of aged white rats. *International Journal of Neuropsychiatry* 2:577–584.

Stern, K. 1948. Observations in an old age counselling center. *Journal of Gerontology* 3:48–60.

Stern, K., and Askonas, B. A. 1947. Glycine-creatinine metabolism in its relationship to aging. *Journal of Gerontology* 2:296–302.

Stern, K.; Birmingham, M. K.; Cullen, A. M.; and Richer, R. 1950. Peptidase activity in the blood consituents of young and old people. In *Proceedings of the Canadian Physiological Society, Fourteenth Annual Meeting*, p. 42.

————. 1951. Peptidase activity in leukocytes, erythrocytes and plasma of young adult and senile subjects. *Journal of Clinical Investigation* 30:84–89.

Stern, K., and Elliott, K. A. C. 1949. Experimental observations on the so-called senile changes of intra-cellular neurofibrils. *American Journal of Psychiatry* 106:190–194.

Stern, K.; Hinds, E. G.; and Askonas, B. A. 1945. Aging and detoxification. *American Journal of Psychiatry* 102:325–329.

Stern, K., and Menzer, D. 1946. The mechanism of reactivation in depressions of the old age group. *Psychiatric Quarterly* 20:56–73.

Stern, K., and Prados, M. 1946. Personality studies in menopausal women. *American Journal of Psychiatry* 103:358–368.

Stern, K., and Reed, G. E. 1945. Presenile dementia (Alzheimer's disease): Its pathogenesis and classification. *American Journal of Psychiatry* 102:191–197.

Stern, K.; Tyhurst, J. S.; and Askonas, B. A. 1946. Notes on hippuric acid synthesis in senility. *American Journal of the Medical Sciences* 212:302–305.

Stern, K.; Williams, G. M.; and Prados, M. 1951. Grief reactions in later life. *American Journal of Psychiatry* 108:289–294.

Sved, S.; Kral, V. A.; Enesco, H. E.; Solyom, L.; Wigdor, B. T.; and Mauer, S. M. 1967. Memory and serum ribonuclease activity in the aged. *Journal of the American Geriatrics Society* 15: 629–639.

Tyhurst, J. S. 1950a. Behavior under stress. Defence Research Board Symposium, paper no. 19. Ottawa.

————. 1950b. Experiences with individual reactions on field survey. *Chemical Corps. Medical Division Reports* 237:23–25.

————. 1956. Retirement: A study of transition. *Association for Research in Nervous and Mental Disease*, 34.

Wener, J.; Rosenberg, G.; Grad, B.; and Wener, S. 1976. Cardiovascular effects of Levodopa therapy in young and old patients with Parkinson's disease. *Journal of the American Geriatrics Society* 24:185–188.

Wigdor, B. T., and Kral, V. A. 1961. Senescent memory function as an indicator of the general preservation of the aging human organism. *Proceedings of the Third World Congress of Psychiatry* 1:682–686.

CHILE

JOSÉ FROIMOVICH

The development of gerontology in the Republic of Chile can be discussed in terms of the three main institutions devoted to policy formulation and programs and research on aging: the National Committee for the Aged, the Chilean Society of Gerontology, and the Laboratory of Experimental Medicine.

NATIONAL COMMITTEE FOR THE AGED

By Supreme Decree Number 364, 1975, of the Ministry of Health, the National Committee for the Aged was instituted, taking over its functions on October 31, 1975. The essence of the decree follows:

This Committee will have the following as its fundamental aims:

1. To study and propose a national policy regarding the problem of old age, upon which to develop programs and actions.

2. To elaborate and propose an integral action program to attend the needs of old people in the country, according to the resources available.

3. To promote scientific and technical research concerning the problem of the aged and to propose the proper corrective and/or preventive measures.

4. To study preventive actions for the situations causing invalidity and indigence in old people.

5. To devise and propose recovery and rehabilitation measures permitting [the aged] to subsist by themselves or to undertake tasks that are compatible with their limitations.

6. To study the coordination of measures required to orient and get the best possible profit of the resources provided for the assistance of old people, both in public and private areas.

7. To suggest the systems and structures adequate for the surveillance, coordination, and fulfillment of the approved policies and programs.

8. To study the possibility of training personnel to work with senescent people.

9. To stimulate the carrying out of community education programs on senescence.

10. To stimulate the creation of special job sources for the aged.

11. To devise organization systems that permit the gathering of aged people to live in a common, economic, and true-to-their resources manner.

This Committee will be formed by the following persons:

1. The President of the National Council for the Protection of the Aged, who presides;

2. A representative from the Ministry of Health;
3. A representative from the Ministry of Internal Affairs;
4. A representative from the Secretary of State;
5. A representative from the Ministry of Education;
6. A representative from the National Health Service;
7. The Directing Doctor in the Geriatrics Center of Santiago;
8. A representative from the Chilean Society of Gerontology.

To the effect of fulfilling in an efficacious and opportune way the aims and functions of this Committee, information and antecedents may be required from any public service of the State Administration.

The Superior Chiefs of these Services shall supervise the remittance of the required antecedents and reports and also facilitate the attendance of their depending personnel when solicited by the Committee.

Considering the multisectorial nature of the matter to be attacked, the work is approached from the following sectors, each one of them constituting a working subcommittee: demography and family, social medicine and health, education and social mobilization, housing policy, social organization, social security and labor policy, census on institutions and resources, and law.

National Policy for the Aged

Old-age problems are not exclusively health ones; they involve many aspects of national life. Thus a thorough and accurate analysis shall provide useful approaches filling the heterogenous needs of this group of the population.

Perhaps because of the complexity of the problem, there has not been a policy established favoring old people, nor has any sector of national life identified the problem as its own; each one considers the root of it to be in some other part of the national interest. The health sector believes it is essentially social in character; the social sector judges that it is up to health or to education; and education conceives the problem as a labor and economic one. Thus everybody fails to reach the bottom of the problem. Because of this refusal of any one area to take over responsibility, it is necessary to determine in which field of the national affairs a national policy for the aged would be established. Once the question of responsibility has been cleared up, the corresponding sector or sectors must be committed to study the problem and give solutions.

The National Committee for the Aged thinks of the problem as being a socioeconomic one; hence its prime concern would correspond to the field of social security, which covers almost all areas pertaining to old age. Social security, in its modern and integral concept, is the branch of the socioeconomic policy of a country by means of which the community protects its members, providing socially sufficient conditions of life, work, and health, which improve productivity and common well-being and promote progress. The concept goes much further than the usual idea that social security is the same as social prevention. This distinction is made because of its particular importance for this work, since many things concerning the economic aspects of social security have been discussed only briefly, because their study and resolution correspond to other branches of the state.

However, it is recognized that everything in this chapter, from a strictly social viewpoint, will be closely and intensely related to economic problems and social prevention, which mechanisms are the primal root and source of every measure in behalf of old people, although as you will see, there are programs and actions addressed to different areas. Thus I want to state clearly that everything presented here lies within the framework of social security in its widest sense, and is addressed to a whole spectrum of possibilities of a social character, and that maybe it will become a complement or an aid to the resolutions about economic systems of prevention, under study by the government. Summarizing, no pronouncement is made concerning economic matters, which are considered as belonging to social prevention, but only those social aspects useful to support the well-being of old people in the country are discussed.

The general aim is to help all the old people to enjoy the maximum spiritual and material well-being, to be able to become useful and valued in their community, and to become integrated with the rest of society, with their aid, respect, and acceptance.

A national policy for the aged must be grounded on the following general bases. Every national policy for economic and social develpment must consider the situation of the aged. In other words, every policy in favor of the aged must be included within the general national policies of economic and social development, except for what is specific to and characteristic of old people. Finally, the basic social programs, or any other kind of program formulated by the government, must be elaborated for integrated groups of different ages, including old people.

All means should be used to strengthen the nuclear family, so that it can attend to the problems and needs of its aged. Once that source has been exhausted, the community must be helped to take care of those over 65. Society must understand the nature of aging as a natural process taking into account consequences of old age in the individual, family, community, and society. The aging of the population also affects the basic social orders and institutions, which must adapt to its new role and accept responsibilities for caring for the aged.

Study and research aimed at determining the role of people over 65 in society must be developed. The policies, plans, programs, and actions regarding the aged must be ample. They should not be aimed exclusively to those over 65, nor only to those less valuable, helpless, or ill. In other words, we must try to include all those over 65. And to succeed in that, action should be take to help people before they reach that age.

The special needs of any human being at any stage of life are related to the prior and future phases of his growth and development, and this fact provides a fundamental orientation to the links between generations in family, community, and society. Also, we must help everyone over 65, whatever his social class, instruction, race, religion, or dwelling place may be; all those factors must be left aside.

A permanent system or structure of investigation, planning, direction, coordination, and evaluation of activities for and favoring the aged must be established. Into that system or structure, the voluntary organizations favoring old people should be guided.

Age discrimination must be eliminated. The right of old people to have services, facilities, and an environment favorable to their capability of participating in society and contributing to it, as well as their right to have protection and security compatible with the level and quality of the life the rest of the population enjoys, should be recognized.

Contact between the national government and international organizations must be sought in order to develop common policies and plans for international solidarity regarding the problems of old age. Some proposals for policy in various areas follow.

Policy on Social Action

Given the importance of eliminating the main problem of old age—loneliness—and given that the Supreme Government lends particular attention to community organization, the government should promote, encourage, and improve social integration within the group of those over 65. Thus the required legislative and other modifications should be introduced to reach that goal.

The actual and effective participation of old people in functional and community organizations must be achieved in the process of development and in the local, communal, and regional spheres. In this way, the creative and experienced contribution of the aged will be directed, and expression and representation will be given to their common interests. The communal administration should especially consider the organizations of old people and/or their incorporation into the community organizations.

A major goal would be for elderly people to live with their families as long as possible, through the development of a range of supporting services and resources. To achieve this, we must strengthen the family and create a feeling of family responsibility among its members.

Local centers to provide assistance for old people in all those aspects in which they may need it must be created.

The carrying out of all the actions must be decentralized, but at the same time they must be coordinated, planned, and evaluated by some national institution.

The volunteering groups assisting old people must be structured and guided in such a way that their labor can be coordinated in a useful and efficacious form.

Educational Policy

Direct action for the aged should include the following:

1. To reinforce at the corresponding levels the concept of permanent education, on the assumption that human beings are capable of learning throughout their lives. They must have access to the different levels of instruction, education, and training.
2. To provide information and orientation for old people regarding work or daily occupation, be it professional, technical, or any other kind. It is important to learn about aging and to understand the psychological changes that accompany it.

To support and help old people in general, the professional and technical information to assist old people in all the spheres involved in the problem must be provided. Therefore, the necessary schools must be opened. The culture, knowledge, and experience of old people must reach future generations. Children, youth, and the community in general should be helped to respect, understand, and assist old people as a way to bring about changes and behavioral attitudes favoring their dignity. Research on gerontological matters needs to be promoted. And humanist principles need to be introduced in education in order to make the individual the center of society. People should be helped to respect each other, including those who are in their last stage of life, because they are members of society, and not because they produce material goods.

Health Policy

An adequate health level for old people should be promoted. They need the attention of general services, be it public, private, or mixed, in their protectional, recovering, rehabilitative, and developmental fields. Particular interest needs to be given to the formation of some research and educational assistance centers, where the peculiar pathologies of old age can be investigated. A new concept of progressive attention in health matters must be applied, properly satisfying the special needs of old people.

The training of geriatricians must be sought, giving geriatrics the character of specialization. Thus new clinical and technical rules will be formulated in order to keep geriatric medical technology at a high level.

Other policies include emphasizing the importance of mental health problems in old people; putting an end to the problem of malnutrition in old people (that is caused not only by economic circumstances but also by loneliness); promoting health maintenance programs for old people, particularly before their retirement; implementing a system of domiciliary health assistance for old people so that they can remain as long as possible with their families; seeking health surveillance for those over 65, with periodic examinations; coordinating or integrating health services for old people and social services; and organizing special assistance programs of opthalmology, odontology, and otology.

Labor Policy

One aim is to encourage people over 65 to continue working on a full- or part-time basis, while keeping their physical and mental abilities properly evaluated. This program should be independent of their right to retirement pensions and general labor policies.

Training in a new job should be promoted for those already retired or retiring. To do this, private enterprise must be motivated. In addition, special labor facilities reserved for those over 65 should be created, permitting them to develop an efficacious, adequate, worthy, and fairly waged job. Finally organizations of workers should be encouraged to give particular consideration to the problems of their aged members.

Social Prevention Policy

The loan regimes of the social prevention system, considered in the social security statute, should comprise and refer specifically to the aged and their own problems, providing them the required assistance.

To get the social security institutions to take care of the essentially social problems—and not only the economic ones—of their affiliates, a social service assisting the incapacitated population must be established. Its aims should be to create and maintain asylums, homes, and similar places for old people; to organize domiciliary assistance for the retired; and to elaborate periodical projects and plans of action. The institution does not have to do the work itself, but it must promote, assist, and encourage the creation of such services by particular institutions, taking direct action only subsidiarily.

Justice Policy

Old people's rights and obligations and their consideration within the context of the whole nation must be kept. No legislation that would contribute to the lessening of their personal dignity must be enacted.

Some of the fundamental and processual rulings that deal with situations applicable to the elderly need improving; for example, rules on guardianships and administration of goods and food. Furthermore, old people need to be advised of their rights so they can use the courts of justice fully. To help them, a specialized legal assistance for elderly persons should be established, both for suing and for the defense of their rights.

Dwelling and Furnishings Policy

Dwelling

Support from all sectors of the nation should be sought so that the aged individual can continue to live with his closest relatives. Only secondarily, and in cases of qualified need, the building of special homes for aged individuals will be promoted, conceived in the general idea of progressively satisfying their needs according to their physical and mental conditions.

The furnishing of special homes for old people must take into account the keeping of indispensable belongings and the provision of assisting services that they could not reach easily by themselves (such as food, laundry, and the barbershop). Special homes for old individuals or couples should be built within the community, not in isolated areas. In the designs, the special architectural needs of old people must be taken into account.

Urbanism

Plans and urban designs will adapt to and suit the requirements of elderly people who are crippled, permitting them to use benches, street crossings, gardens, parks, special stairs, pavements, and means of transportation.

Entertainment and Culture Policy

The adequate backing of facilities and possibilities in matters of recreation for elderly people should be sought. As a group, they have the longest periods of spare time to spend in these activities.

All those over 65 should be encouraged to transmit their experience and knowledge to the new generations. Perhaps they can do so through recreation center programs.

Above all, the cultural abilities of every old individual should be developed and improved through appropriate facilities and opportunities.

Institutional Policy

Bases must be founded for an institutional system that is efficacious in serving old people. Perhaps it could be a specialized organization of a technical character and with possibilities of directly relating to the highest level. Or a relationship could be established with an existing organization capable of carrying out the following functions:

1. Elaboration of the policy and plans for the old people from a multisectoral viewpoint.

2. Maintenance of a system of demographic, economic, social, and similar information regarding those over 65.

3. Advisement and coordination of the sectorial and institutional policies, plans, and actions, including those coming from all spheres concerned with assisting the old.

4. Carrying out of investigations to increase the knowledge of these problems.

5. Attention to the needy old individuals who are in specially designed institutions.

6. Surveillance of public or private institutions whose function is to assist the old.

7. Constant evaluation of the application of policies and plans addressed to elderly people.

Fulfilling these goals is a long-term task. The first stage will attend to the formation of an intersectorial social coordination bureau, whose main functions would be to coordinate the design of specific programs of action according to the national policy, the choice of integrated decisions on interrelated matters, the study of rationalization in the assignment of resources, and the integrated evaluation of progess. The National Committee for the Aged will continue to operate as an assistant committee for the Supreme Government, being linked to it through the Ministry of Internal Affairs.

CHILEAN SOCIETY OF GERONTOLOGY

Founded on March 16, 1961, the Chilean Society of Gerontology includes professionals from the main medical specialties among its members: neurologists, psychiatrists, surgeons, opthalmologists, otolaryngologysts, dieticians, cardiologists, neumologists, pharmacologists, and others. It is officially affiliated with the International Association of Gerontology. Its members are concerned with the scientific problems of gerontology in the Republic of Chile, and they are currently submitting reports on their research to the various international congresses on their specialty.

Some people believe that gerontologists or geriatricians are doctors who prolong the life of human beings. In reality, their most important present medical task is not to prolong indefinitely the life span of people but to make it possible for them to live the number of years that certain immutable genetic laws have determined for them. If a thousand female mice are controlled from their birth until the last one has died, the average life of female mice, which goes from a year to a year and a half, will be determined; in male mice it is about two and a half years; in rabbits, three years; in horses, twenty-five years, and so on. Investigators of all historical ages have agreed that according to genetic laws, humans should live at least 120 years, though this has very seldom occurred. In countries referred to as underdeveloped, most people, according to the statistics of the World Health Organization, have an average life span of 30 years. In many industrialized nations—among them, Holland, Sweden, Switzerland, Norway, the United States, and Denmark—the figure rises to 75 or 80 years. Among the many theories that are advanced for this difference, two main factors have been pointed out: social ones and human ones.

Social Factors

Individuals protect themselves better against the contingencies to which they are continually being exposed if they have a high level of instruction, education, and social evolution. No Englishman, Dutchman, or American would dream of applying to himself a cobweb to heal a wound or a frogskin ointment, risking tetanus, Staphylococcus, and Streptococcus.

In the so-called developed countries, most human beings are protected from before their birth. The mother is taught about proper nutrition to ensure a healthy baby. Usually social laws guarantee her rest, salary, and preventive attention during her pregnancy. Labor usually takes place in specialized hospitals, under the best obstetrical conditions. While the post partum mother rests and is medically cared for, her offspring is cared for by qualified pediatric personnel who give constant attention. The child is usually vaccinated against diseases, such as the measles and whooping cough. In this way he is prevented from falling into the group of precocious child mortality, which currently constitutes a major threat in countries without adequate preventive means or knowledge.

Scientific and technological advances in health matters have made it possible to determine in early pregnancy any pathological abnormalities that might be present. This knowledge permits medical personnel to anticipate any emergency that may appear during labor, birth, and immediately after. Modern equipment manipulated and interpreted by medical personnel specialized in their subject constitutes one of the most profitable contributions to maternity hospitals, since it diminishes the danger of a high-risk labor both for the mother and the offspring.

As the child continues to grow, he is well cared for, well fed, and well dressed; he usually goes to school, obligatory in these countries, and often to college. His youth and adulthood develop under adequate conditions of protection. Most of these countries have child labor laws. His parents usually earn wages that are high enough to permit the family to live comfortably. Many children have regular preventive medical attention, and immediate emergency attention is generally available.

Health is protected in other ways. Sewerage systems prevent infection. Factory workers are usually protected on the job; they often are required to wear special clothing, and the work site usually has good light and ventilation. Work in mines is done under permanent environmental control to prevent fire damp blasts; dampness regulators, goggles, and masks protect workers from the flashing fragments. This social factor has almost completely eradicated a number of diseases, and this accomplishment has much to do with the progress of those countries.

Countries in which the average life is short—30 years or so—evidence an economic and cultural misery. Tuberculosis, hunger, disease, and poor medical attention make the figures of child mortality increase, sometimes up to 100 percent. People earn insufficient salaries and wages, and they are engaged in a constant struggle against hunger. Their working conditions are poor and their medical prevention and treatment inadequate.

Human Factors

Personal habits have a major importance in the prolongation of life. The great increase in the practice of physical exercise has an obvious effect on cardiovascular, respiratory, and modern-day stress relief. By 1980 in West Germany, for example, more than 50 percent of the population will be exercising regularly.

A cheese- and milk-rich diet provides methyl, a radical that has an antiatherosclerotic action on hepatic cells. The use of fish with a high content of polyunsaturated fats prevents the cholesterol synthesis and its subsequent deposits on the walls of the blood vessels. The consumption of citrus fruits, rich in vitamin C, improves the permeability of the capillary endothelium, the passage of foods and oxygen to the cells, and the complete recollection of metabolic residues that would otherwise deposit themselves at a cellular level, impairing the cellular functions. An abundant intake of greens provides minerals and facilitates digestion. Mental relaxation can help prevent cerebral hemorrhages and cardiac infarcts.

But the progress of civilization has its Achilles heel, and this is now restricting the longevity of those living in the most developed countries. Those living in Denmark, Norway, Holland, Switzerland, Sweden, and the United States now face arteriosclerosis with its sequel of cardiac infarcts and cerebral hemorrhages. They have an excessive consumption of foods rich in saturated fats, such as butter, eggs, and ham, sometimes reaching 40 percent of daily meals. In these countries arteriosclerosis may involve all the population older than seven years, and the question is in what proportion they have it rather than whether they have it.

The cell is the most wonderful machine of nature when it is undamaged, rested, and fed; but it can be impaired, made ill, and even destroyed by poisons that are becoming more common everyday: pollution, nervous stress (which is harmful to brain cells' integrity), tobacco, and alcohol. The increase in the incidence of cancer, pulmonary emphysema, and cardiac infarcts is becoming a serious problem in these countries, which, having attained the best social conditions, now face new problems that prevent residents from reaching the 120 years that nature offers.

The intervention of gerontologists to extend life will be required when mankind has reached the 120-years barrier; the genetic laws have to be neutralized.

LABORATORY OF EXPERIMENTAL MEDICINE

Founded and directed since 1939 by Dr. José Froimovich, the laboratory's work has been developed in two fields of action: studies on the early diagnosis of cancer and senescence-related problems.

Early Diagnosis of Cancer

The experimental induction of cancer has been approached. In particular, distillates of tobacco, maté, and fuel oil have been applied at various temperatures to the necks and ears of mice and rabbits, Neoplastic processes have been produced in all cases.

Clinically, a number of chemical, enzymatic, and hormonal elements, whose presence in human beings presenting neoplastic formations varies, have been studied. Some positive results have permitted the diagnosis of neoplasia in human beings whose diagnosis was uncertain.

Problems Related to Senescence

This work covers thirty-eight years of research started in 1939 at the Laboratory of Experimental Medicine by an enthusiastic group of professors, physicians, and scientists. The goal has been to show, with adequate documentation, that with certain therapeutics, the deterioration curve in a percentage of old people becomes stabilized toward the horizontal; in another percentage it has a positive slope; and finally, in a third group, fortunately small, the involution follows its general trend, although to a lower rate. The research development can be laid out in six stages.

First Stage: Production and Retrogression of Old Age in Animals

Several experiments on inducing artificial aging in laboratory animals (rabbits, mice, dogs, cats, and rats) were carried out. Among the methods employed were the extirpation of sexual gonads and the administration by way of the usual foods of a number of products classed as atherosclerosis-favoring incidence (for example, cholesterol, egg yolk, dried bovine marrow, cysteine, and cystine).

Once the typical symptoms of atherosclerosis produced old age, the retrogression from such changes was attempted through methods already used by earlier researchers, such as Brown-Sequad in 1889, and continued with various results by Voronoff, Alexandrescu, Pettinari, Steinach, Bogomoletz, Bardach, Perotti, and others. They worked with transplantation of sexual gonads (testicles and ovaries), ligation of the different ducts, innoculation of antibodies produced by extracts of connective tissue, and so forth. We wished to have evidence that aging, or some of its characteristic traits, can be produced experimentally and that these typical symptoms of aging can be reversed. We were successful in both aspects. The development of these researches is summarized and published in *Arteriosclerosis—Experimental and Clinical Study* (1952).

Second Stage: Human Chemical Constants

Over ten years and with the collaboration of ten chemists, the levels and quantities of various human biochemical constants were studied in the laboratory. Fifty thousand chemical tests were carried out to determine the changes occurring in human blood and tissues during development at the successive stages of childhood, adulthood, and old age. The results were analyzed in groups of both sexes and classed by age in five-year goups (1–5, 6–10, 11–15, and so on, until 96–); there were twenty groups in total. In each group, various factors were assessed and compared, including the fluctuation of seventy-four mineral, hormonal, enzymatic, and vitaminic factors, such as total nitrogen, phosphorated lipids, blood pH, ascorbic acid oxidized, and reduced and total glutation.

The aim was to show whether aging produced significant changes in the chemical elements of blood and tissues, either by the action of aging or because these variations cause aging, and to try to relate those changes and the characteristics of the tissues to certain ages. Because at the level of the external aspects and biological functions, evident changes with age take place, the same must occur inside the organism. Perhaps it was possible to find some variation that could be measured in numbers, which would represent the biological and functional age of the individual.

Significant fluctuations were found: some elements or structures decreased with advancing age, such as hormones, vitamins A, C, and E, the total blood phosphorus, hemoglobin, iron, red cells, gastric ferments, various enzymes, audiometry, logo-audiometry, and aminoacids. etc. Others increased, including total lipids, free cholesterol, triglycerides, and beta lipoproteins.

Third Stage: Histology and Weight of Viscera

One thousand and fifty-four autopsies carried out in Chilean hospitals provided the opportunity of careful study of the macroscopic and microscopic characteristics of the viscera of human beings from childhood to old age, in groups of five years, from 1 to 100 years. It could be established that with increasing age, the number of cells decrease in the various organs, a large proportion of the remaining cells work with diminished ability due to deposition of residuals or to structural decay, and only a fraction of the cells still function properly. The weight of the following organs decreases with advanced age: liver, encephalon, lungs, kidneys, and spleen. However, the heart weight increases. The highly significant results of the research in the second and third stages were published in 1955 in *Geriatrics, Gerontology and Old Age*.

Fourth Stage: Lipotropism

The aim was to study the importance of hepatic functions in activation, transformation, and neutralization of a number of structures playing a major role in the genesis of atherosclerosis and aging, such as enzymes, steroids, provitamins, hormones, hydrogen carriers, and reducers, etc., and their importance in the defense of hepatic cell integrity by means of the lipotropic elements, or its perturbation by the antilipotropic elements. The results of this work are published in *Lipotropism and Aging* (1958, 1961).

Fifth Stage: Human Therapeutics

With a great deal of experimental findings and laboratory tests, obtained after so many years of research, the application in human beings of a treatment for old age, or for some of its manifestations, was initiated in 1955. The work was carried out with the collaboration of 150 senescent subjects over 65 years of age (100 men and 50 women), residing at the Old People Hospice of Santiago, Chile. They were put under a medical treatment of administering them a chemical, Formula F-G-F 60, containing the decreased or altered elements assessed in the second stage. This stage lasted from 1955 through 1957. Its aims, possibilities, and results were presented in a medical session on June 20, 1957.

Sixth Stage: Human Therapeutics with Accurate Control of Results

With the wide laboratory and clinical experience and positive results obtained in the preceding stage, a new process of research was initiated in 1959. One hundred sixty-two aged persons from the Old People Hospice of Santiago were selected (131 men, average age: 74 years old; 31 women, average age: 75.3 years old). None showed serious manifest illness, and all could answer questions, obey therapeutic instructions, and express the effects of treatment. Their limbs were sound so they could undergo physical treatment. The had good visual ability and transparence of ocular media permitting the study of normality or arteriosclerosis of the blood vessels in the bottom of the eye. They were thus healthy old individuals.

Methods were developed in three years in three steps: (1) clinical, instrumental, and laboratory examination of the patients, (2) therapeutics, and (3) control of results. The examination of the patients was carried out with the collaboration of sixty-two professionals in various specialties and with the most complete and accurate methods provided by modern research. Subjective estimations were avoided. The methods employed were intended to measure quantitatively and qualitatively the results of examinations, make comparisons among them, and keep them in the form of printed documents. They included electrocardiograms, electroencephalograms, testicles biopsies, prostate gland biopsies, skin biopsies, vagina biopsies, humerus and thorax radiographies, audiograms, sight tests, blood cholesterol tests, tonometries, and hemograms capable of being analyzed and controlled or used as study and informative material. Almost all the ninety-two tests carried out for each individual before and after treatment were made by the same professionals.

The tests enabled us to search for the actual biological conditions of the Chilean aged. Until then, no figures on the state of aged human beings or their normality or disturbances had been available. A specialist asked an opinion usually had no accurate data. Nobody showed interest in research on the aged because there was no expectation of success or evident goal. The assumption was that no treatment existed for old age.

For three years Formula F-G-F 60 was supplied to the aged subjects, thus providing them those humoral, glandular, structural, and other substances undergoing diminution or other changes with increasing age, and those able to stimulate the depressed organic functions. Because of several hormonal considerations, a male formula and a female formula were prepared. These two formulas gathered the required elements in a given proportion, which was obtained after studying the individual requirements and lack of each of the components.

The results in general were positive, and in some cases very positive, in the physical, sexual, and mental spheres.

1. Hearing: Improvement of 74 percent in men, 93 percent in women.
2. Electrocardiogram: Improvement of 55 percent in men, 37 percent in women.
3. Osseous density: Improvement of 86 percent in men, 83 percent in women.
4. Electroencephalogram: Improvement of 48 percent in men, 57 percent in women.
5. Testicle biopsy: Improvement of 50 percent per cell increase.
6. Skin biopsy: Improvement of 25 percent in men, 21 percent in women.
7. Opthalmology: Improvement of 61 percent in men, 100 percent in women.
8. Vaginal biopsy and frotis: Improvement of 100 percent.
9. Intellectual quotient: 22 percent improvement in men, 18 percent in women.
10. Breathing amplitude: Improvement of 56cc per breath in men and women.
11. Number of breaths: Improvement of four breaths per minute in men, three in women.
12. Twenty-five meter race: Improvement of 4.1 seconds in men, 12.9 in women.
13. Oscillometry: Improvement in both groups.
14. Dynamometry: Improvement in both groups.
15. Lipidogram, glucadogram, and proteingram: Improvement in both groups.
16. Total lipids: Improvement in both groups.
17. Cholesterol esters: Improvement in both groups.
18. Pulse: Improvement of three beats per minute in men, four in women.

Similar improvement results were observed in hemograms, hemoglobin, androgens, estrogens, 17-ketosteroids, uremy, 17-hydroxycorticosteroids, tonometry, logo-audiometry, and so on.

Although the medical treatment has been suspended, the same group of subjects has been kept under control, and comparisons of average mortality, physical, sexual, and psychical conditions have been made with another group of a hundred aged persons of similar ages and way of life, also residents at the hospice.

After the two broad periods of clinical investigation and their previous stages were ended, the conclusion was that there are a number of elements that decrease or change with increasing age and are related to aging symptoms; that there exists a method to supply such elements in a given formula; and that the results and works of investigation are the widest carried out so far in this field.

Film: *For a Better Tomorrow*

A film, *For a Better Tomorrow*, has been prepared, showing as many details as possible, on the results obtained with the administration of Formula F-G-F 60. Originally it was six hours long, but it has been shortened to just over two hours; it is filmed in color and narrated in English and Spanish. The film shows gerontologists and scientists for the first time the possibility of reversing the unmistakable manifestations of old age. These experiences perpare the way for other scientific centers to undertake more sophisticated research.

A panoramic view of this works, together with statistical pictures and photographs of most of the old patients before and after the therapy, has been published in the *Integral Treatise of Gerontology* (1973).

REFERENCES

Froimovich, J. 1950. *Focal infection: Its medical and odontological aspects.* Santiago: Editora Nacional Gabriela Mistral Ltda.

———. 1952. *Arteriosclerosis: Clinical and experimental study.* Santiago: Editora Nacional Gabriela Mistral Ltda.

———. 1955a. *Geriatrics, gerontology and old age.* Santiago: Editora Nacional Gabriela Mistral Ltda.

———. 1955b. *Lipotropism and old age: Clinical and experimental study.* Santiago: Editora Nacional Gabriela Mistral Ltda.

———. 1966, 1971. *Medical and clinical aspects of old age.* Santiago: Editora Nacional Gabriela Mistral Ltda.

———. 1973. *Integral treatise on gerontology.* 7 vols. Santiago: Gabriela Mistral Ltda.

———. 1976. *To live all the life.* Santiago: Editora Nacional Gabriela Mistral Ltda.

———. 1979. *For a better tomorrow.* Santiago: Editora Nacional Gabriela Mistral Ltda.

———. In press. *Fight against old age: Treatments.* Santiago: Editora Nacional Gabriela Mistral Ltda.

DENMARK

BENT FRIJS-MADSEN

The population of Denmark totals 5 million people. About 23 percent of the population live in rural areas. This distribution results from a continuous migration from rural to urban areas.

Denmark is the oldest kingdom of Europe. Since 1849, the country has had a parliamentary constitution. Taxes are levied by the central and local governments alike. The public revenue is provided through taxation of personal income and capital, land taxes, and excise and customs duties. The public expenditure amounts to 50 percent of the total national income. The largest expense on the national budgets in recent years has been the cost of social services and education, followed by public health and national defense. Old-age and invalidity pensions account for the largest group of social services expense.

Scarcely half of the total Danish population are gainfully employed. Of married women, about half work in their own home only; the rest are gainfully employed. Because Denmark has no natural resources of any substantial importance, its production capacity is chiefly dependent on highly qualified manpower and on agricultural land. The largest of gainfully employed persons, 28 percent, work in manufacturing industry, 23 percent in commerce and services, 11 percent in agriculture (in 1930, it was 29 percent), 22 percent in public administration and the professions, 9 percent in building and construction, and 7 percent in transport.

GROWTH OF GERONTOLOGY

During the last thirty years, there has been an increasing interest in gerontology. Dr. Torben Geill, former physician in chief of De Gamles By, Copenhagen, has had an enormous influence and been an inspiration. He was the first president of the Danish Gerontological Society, founded in 1956. In 1963, he was president of the International Association of Gerontology and the president of the Sixth International Congess of Gerontology held in Copenhagen.

The Danish National Institute of Social Research, founded in 1958, has performed and published the results of many valuable social studies of the aged.

The increasing number of departments of geriatric medicine throughout the country and their cooperation with local social authorities have contributed to a better understanding of the disabled and sick elderly and their problems. Also several gerontopsychiatric units have been started. Since 1973, geriatrics (long-term medicine) has been an official subspeciality of internal medicine with its own educational program. Today in Denmark about forty persons specialize in internal medicine combined with long-term medicine.

Scientific meetings, research courses, and Nordic congresses have contributed to many different gerontological research programs.

DEMOGRAPHY

There has been an absolute as well as a relative increase in the population aged over 65. In January 1975 there were 650,000 persons over 65 years of age out of a total number of 5 million inhabitants. That is 13 percent compared with 5 or 6 percent two hundred years ago. In Denmark the change in composition of the population related to age shows the same tendency as in most of the countries in Western Europe. The rise in the number of the elderly is caused by an increase in the group of those over 75 years of age, while the age group 65 to 74 shows a decrease in percentage (table 7).

Table 7: PERCENTAGE DISTRIBUTION BY AGE OF THE ELDERLY, 1976-2001

Age	1976	1986	2001
65–74 years	63	58	55
75 years and over	37	42	45

Source: Danmarks Statistik. 1976. Statistical Yearbook (Copenhagen), Matthiessen, P.C.: personal communication.

The annual increase in population amounts to 0.6 percent, because of a low birthrate. If this tendency remains constant during the coming years, we will have about 125,000 persons fewer in the group of young people. Per 100 persons in the age group between 20 and 65 years in 1976, there were 53 younger persons and children (0–19 years of age). In the year of 2001, the number may only be 43 children and young persons. Thus if the political background permits it, additional public funds may be transferred to the aged.

The average expected life span at the beginning of the century was 50 years for men and 53 years for women. In the year 1973–1974, the figures were 71 for men and 77 for women. The causes of deaths among men and women beyond 70 years of age in 1974 were dominated by the following diseases—malignant neoplasms, ischemic heart disease, and cerebrovascular disease—which accounted for 66 percent of the total causes of deaths.

In January 1975, Denmark contained 2.5 million men and about the same number of women. Fifty-seven percent of those over 65 were women, and 63 percent were women in the age group over 90 years. Their marital status is shown in table 8.

Table 8: PERCENTAGE DISTRIBUTION OF MARITAL STATUS OF THE POPULATION OVER 65 YEARS OF AGE BY SEX

	Unmarried	Married	Widowed	Divorced
Men	8	69	19	4
Women	13	37	45	5

Source: Danmarks Statistik. 1976. *Statistical Yearbook* (Copenhagen).

ROLES, STATUS, AND PROBLEMS OF THE AGED

Between April and June 1962, the Danish National Institute of Social Research carried out an investigation through interviews of a representative nationwide sample comprising about 3,700 elderly people of 62 years of age and over. The following information about the way of living of the elderly people is partly taken from this investigation, which parallels an investigation of old people in England and the United States (Shanas et al., 1968).

Income

The aged in Denmark form a heterogeneous group as to composition and size of income. Only one-fourth do not have income other than their old-age pension. Single women seem to be worse off than single men and couples. Incomes are lowest in the countryside and lower for the aged living with children than for those living alone or with nonrelatives.

The aged as a group, especially single women, show many characteristics of a low-income group. This consumption pattern seems to be explained by traditional patterns of spending and not only by low income. Size of income, on the other hand, exhibits a significant influence on the size and distribution of consumption and expenditures, as might be expected. The daily necessities of food and dwelling make up a notably greater share of the budget of the aged than is the case for the wage-earning population. While wage-earning households in 1963 spent only about one-third of their income on these items, single aged persons spent a little more than half and aged married couples a little less than half their income. This corresponds to the fact that the aged spent an essentially smaller share of their income on durable goods, transport, holidays, leisure, and other more luxurious items, whereas the expenditures for footwear, clothing, washing, cleaning, personal care, nursing, and other consumer goods are on the same level for the two population groups. The two population groups also pay almost the same part of their income in personal taxes.

Employment and Retirement of Aged Men

Men were in active employment at a slightly higher age in 1960 than in 1955. Similarly slightly more of those aged 65 years and over belonged to the labor force in 1960. This might mainly be due to a better employment situation in 1960. If these analyses were repeated in 1976, the results would probably show a decrease of employment of all the aged because of the adverse economic situation and the increasing unemployment rate in Denmark.

The interviews in 1962 showed that about 50 percent of all men age 62 and over are actively employed. The number decreases with increasing age but still amounts to about 15 percent of men age 80 and over. Married men in all age groups have a higher percentage of activity than unmarried and previously married men, perhaps because the married men have a larger burden of support and are in better health.

The length of the working week decreases with increasing age for the actively employed. About half of those 75 years and over who are still employed work fewer than thirty hours a week; this is so for only one-fourth of the 65–66 year olds. About one-fifth of the actives of 75 years and over are employed only seasonally or occasionally, against about one-tenth of the 65–66 year olds. The reduced working hours of the oldest actives in employment might point to the fact that retirement takes place gradually, but it may also be a consequence of the fact that the persons who are already occupied only a few hours per week or work seasonally retire latest.

The self-employed aged continue in active employment longer than wage earners, apart from the farm workers. At the age of 75 years, about 30 percent of the self-employed aged and 50 percent of the farm workers are still working, against only 10 percent of the urban employees. Among the professions and higher-paid self-employed are found the highest percentages of actives within the self-employed; about one-third are still active at the age of 80 years and over. The retirement of wage-earners is concentrated in a fairly small number of years from the age of 65 to 72, while the retirement of the self-employed is spread over more years.

In the interview, retired men were asked why they had retired. Half of those 75 years and over gave poor health or "work too tiring" as the reason.

Forty-one percent of those between 62 and 66 years who feel that they have bad health are still employed. This might indicate that working until the national pensionable age—67 years for men and 62 years for single women—may be a problem for some people. Recently legislation has made it possible to obtain pensions earlier (55 years for men and 50 years for single women).

The Family and the Household

The majority of the aged in Denmark have live children as well as live siblings. About 18 percent of the elderly surveyed were childless, and about the same percentage did not have siblings. The mean was 2.54 children and 2.70 siblings per respondent. About 18 percent of the aged belonged to a family with only one generation living, and 2 percent had neither live siblings nor live children. More than half of the aged had a live family spanning three generations, and in 19 percent of the cases, the subjects had live children, grandchildren, and greatgrandchildren.

Typically the aged in Denmark live apart from, but in the vicinity of, at least one child. About 80 percent of those who were married lived with their spouse only, and 16 percent lived with one of their children, in most cases an unmarried child. Among those not married (in most cases widowed persons), about 60 percent lived alone, and 20 percent lived with one of their children. Relatively few lived with a married child. There are very few three-generation households in Denmark—only 2 percent. This seems to have been the case also before Denmark became industrialized.

Physical nearness is important for the maintenance of contact and frequency of contact with children, although it by no means implies close contacts. In Denmark most elderly people live apart from their children, but a fairly large proportion live near at least one of them. Elderly people in Denmark do not live any nearer to one of their daughters than to one of their sons. The larger number of children an elderly person has, the greater was the chance that he or she lived near at least one of them.

For a long time, the theory that dissolvement of ties between generations takes place primarily in highly urbanized areas has been accepted. Social isolation has often been called a typical aspect of the life of the urban dweller. Comparisons between the interviewed elderly in urban and rural areas can be used as a fruitful point of departure. It was found that the chance that all children live at a distance of about thirty minutes or more from their parents is much higher in rural areas than in large cities. How these conditions affect the contact between generations also appeared from the interview. The chance that an older person who has only one child, and who does not live with that child, has seen the child during the past week is nearly twice as high in Copenhagen (72 percent) as in the rural areas (41 percent). In spite of the fact that the aged in rural areas have better resources for family contact than do their contemporaries in Copenhagen, these sources are used less frequently.

Nutrition

Though very few persons in Denmark suffer from malnutrition or hypovitaminoses, the aged here (like elsewhere) are in constant danger of lack of certain important vitamins, minerals, and other food ingredients. The problem is low energy intake combined with great intake of empty calories. Investigations have shown that 60 percent of elderly patients in a department for limb surgery had an intake of vitamin B_{12} and folic acid below the norms stated in the recommended dietary allowances (Helms, 1977; Hessov, 1977; Hessov and

Elsborg, 1977). The average daily protein intake seemed to be low, apparently because of an intake of sweets and drinks of doubtful nutritional value.

PROGRAMS FOR THE AGED

Social Services

A large number of various types of social services for the aged have gradually been developed. Rules for these services are now compiled and laid down in the Social Assistance Act of June 19, 1974. The basic aim of this act is that the aged shall, as far as possible, be given the opportunity to remain in their homes as long as they wish. Persons who can no longer look after themselves in their own homes, can be admitted to a center for old people (nursing home or sheltered accommodation).

Home Help

According to the Social Assistance Act, local councils are responsible for providing a home-help service in their area so that practical assistance can be given in the aged person's home by trained home helpers. Thus the home-help service aims at meeting a demand for assistance to carry out normal domestic tasks in the client's own home. The home help is given free of charge to persons whose incomes do not exceed the ordinary old-age pension. Otherwise an amount will be charged based on the economic conditions of the recipient. If a home is in need of the help but the local social welfare committee cannot provide it, the committee can instead make a contribution toward the expenses for domestic help engaged by the family itself.

Other practical measures for elderly people in their own homes include meals on wheels (often from a nursing home), laundry services, and chiropody, services that can be extremely important to the aged. Home nursing is provided at the request of a doctor; it is free of charge for the recipient.

Aids

The infirm elderly can obtain financial support for aids, including special garments, that are necessary for the person to carry out a job, that will substantially relieve the affliction, or that will facilitate the daily routine at home. The support is given regardless of the recipient's economic situation. In cases where the applicant has to bear part of the cost but has no means, the social welfare committee can grant financial support. Normally aids and repairs to aids will not be paid for if the cost in the individual case is less than D.Kr. 150 (petty cost limit). On the other hand, for all other aids for which the cost exceeds the petty cost limit, the support will be given without expense to the recipient. An updated list of the aids for which support is granted is published by the Directorate of Social Services.

Centers for aids have been or are about to be established in all counties. These centers are responsible for informing the local authorities (municipalities) of technical aids, giving personal guidance, demonstrating and adjusting the aids. Their work is partly for groups who have contact with handicapped persons and partly for the handicapped individual who is referred to the aids center by the local authority. The aids center is assumed to be in charge of delivery to the local authority of technical aids, either from a depot or by a supplier. Moreover it is assumed that aids not currently in use will be kept in the depot.

Some of the aids supplied include orthopedic and other artificial limbs; bandages; special chairs; seats; cushions; beds, toilet, and bathroom facilities; hearing aids; electrical lamps connected to door bells; and indoor and outdoor wheelchairs.

Telephones

As a condition for granting financial support for a telephone, a person must have a permanent infirmity, due to illness or old age, that prevents the applicant from leaving home unassisted. At the assessment of the need it will be taken into consideration whether relatives living at home can give the necessary assistance.

If the person concerned does not already have a phone, one will be installed at the request of the social welfare committee. Support can be granted for the payment of subscription fees but not for the payment of telephone calls. In many areas telephone links have been established, and each member of the telephone link is called every day.

Dwellings

The social welfare committee can grant the necessary support to arrange a more suitable dwelling for disabled persons or persons suffering from a permanent disease or being infirm due to old age.

Support is considered necessary if the arrangement, after a judgment in each individual case of the housing arrangement and the applicant's affliction or handicap, is deemed to relieve or essentially diminish housing disadvantages connected with the applicant's stay at home. Support can be granted no matter whether the recipient is a flat dweller, has an owner-occupied flat, is a houseowner, or lives permanently with relatives or others.

Support for dwelling arrangements comprises financial assistance for alterations to and arrangement of already existing dwellings. Thus, according to the provisions of the act, support for the acquisition of a self-contained flat cannot be granted; however, it will be possible to obtain support for a small extension to a room or the like if this is deemed expedient.

In connection with the building of a self-contained dwelling, disabled persons or persons suffering from a permanent disease or being inform due to old age can apply to special services for support aimed at relieving their handicap. Often only minor alterations are necessary, such as removing door-steps, putting up banisters, adding handles, changing toilet facilities, and the like.

If the applicant lives in his or her own house and if the arrangement involves a considerable expense, which results in an improvement of the building and an increase of its value, the support will be granted in the form of an interest-free loan. No payment is required, but the loan will be due for payment in case of change of ownership. In such cases a mortgage deed should be drawn up and registered.

For elderly people who cannot look after themselves in their own homes, pensioners' dwellings have been built. They can be situated in a group of special blocks or scattered among the ordinary housing. This measure merely aims at meeting the pensioners' demand for a more appropriate dwelling.

Another type of dwelling for pensioners who are able to look after themselves is the service flat. These flats are grouped in large blocks in which there are collective arrangements—for example, a restaurant. This form of dwelling also meets a certain demand for practical assistance in the home.

Day Care

The local authority shall provide for admission to a day-care home for persons whose condition requires permanent supervision and care that cannot be given in their own homes during the daytime. Otherwise these persons will remain in their homes, because relatives or other persons can look after them the rest of the time.

Moreover the local authority ensures that day-care centers are established in their area for the welfare provisions that can best be carried out at a center. Day-care centers are intended for physically and psychically impaired persons in need of special welfare provisions.

Welfare

Welfare centers are intended for elderly people in need of activating work that they cannot be given through other welfare work.

Examples are club activities, education, lectures, study group work, occupational therapy, and gymnastics intended for pensioners. Welfare work of this nature can be carried out at day-care centers reserved for persons in need of special welfare work.

The local authority is responsible for starting or supporting welfare work for old-age pensioners. It decides whether the welfare work shall be started by the local authority itself or, supported by the local authority, be left to associations, organizations, or other private groups. Support can be granted to welfare work that allows the pensioner to remain in his or her own home or allows pensioners to remain active.

Visiting arrangements for pensioners who cannot or who can only with difficulty move outside their homes are an example of welfare work that aims at keeping the pensioner in his or her own home as long as possible. These arrangements enable the visitor to observe whether there is a need for other remedial measures—for example, home help, aids, changes in the particular dwelling, or assistance in the form of delivery of meals. Welfare work of this nature also comprises a number of practical remedial measures for pensioners living in their own homes—for example meals on wheels, laundry services, and chiropody.

Local authorities can, at their own expense, start or support other measures for pensioners that cannot be regarded as direct nursing home prevention or activating measures. Some examples are excursions, holiday trips, including trips abroad, film shows, visits to theaters, and other entertainment.

Support can also be given to old-age pensioners to meet the cost of season tickets for public transport. Private means of transport of pensioners who for reasons of health cannot use public transport will be granted after an assessment of the need in each case.

Homes and Institutions for the Aged

Persons who cannot manage on their own in their own dwellings but whose condition does not necessitate admission to a nursing or day-care home can move into sheltered accommodation specially designed for persons with permanent afflictions. In addition to meeting the demands offered by service flats, it is assumed that sheltered accommodation will generally meet the pensioners' demand for easy access to assistance from a call center.

The local authority makes provision for persons who cannot look after themselves at home because of their state of health to be admitted to a nursing home. Within this category are a variety of homes that can meet a number of the pensioners' demands, such as the demand for a suitable dwelling, the demand for assistance with domestic tasks, and the demand for nursing.

Social legislation does not contain guidelines as to the form of care to be given at nursing homes. Within the group of old people's homes and nursing homes are institutions with a widely differing number of staff members per pensioner. This difference must presumably be taken as an expression of the assistance differing considerably from home to home, both with regard to quantity and quality. However, in all cases nursing homes, as well as the traditional old people's homes, differ from sheltered accommodation in that residents in the latter can come and go at will.

In 1977, there were about fourteen hundred nursing and old-age homes with a total of fifty thousand residents and a staff of about fifteen thousand. The standard of the average Danish nursing home is rather high. Most are relatively modern, and each resident has his or her own room. In most of the institutions built within the last ten years, each resident also has his or her own bathroom.

Departments of Geriatric Medicine and Medical Long-term Treatment Units

In the early 1960s, geriatric hospitals were established by several local authorities. After some years, it became evident to many that it would be an advantage if disabled and ill old persons were treated and rehabilitated in close connection with the general hospitals.

In 1970 a working group appointed by the National Health Service proposed that so-called long-term units should be established in the hospitals. Today about twenty units of this sort have been built in connection with regional hospitals and large general hospitals throughout the country. The medical heads of the units are specialists in internal medicine with geriatrics or long-term treatment as a subspeciality. The object is to reactivate and rehabilitate medical patients, most of them elderly persons, with a view to a discharge to their homes or to the lightest possible kind of an institution. The patients are admitted from the acute units, as well as directly from their homes, on the reference of a general medical practitioner. The evaluation of the fitness of the patients for treatment in a medical long-term unit is made by the chief consultant of the unit in accordance with the directions applying to the other units of the hospital. The geriatric unit has the assistance of consultants from the acute hospital units, and it is possible to transfer a patient from the medical long-term treatment unit to the other special units according to the general rules of transfer. Some of the medical long-term treatment units or geriatric units have their own staff of physiotherapists and occupational therapists, and others have the necessary assistance for rehabilitation by the specialized medical rehabilitation units. Day hospital facilities are valuable parts of the units, and it is considered important to have the closest possible cooperation with local social authorities, often with conferences once a week. The specialists in long-term treatment take part in the evaluation of the elderly persons who want to move from their homes to some institution.

RESEARCH

In Denmark gerontological research is carried out in many different places; we have no gerontological institute or center. For many years De Gamles By in

Copenhagen was the center of clinical research, until 1966 under the leadership of chief physician Torben Geill. Earlier this institution had its own departments of pathology and clinical chemistry, but in 1976 the function of the institution was changed from a geriatric hospital to a nursing home. Basic biological research is carried out at the University of Arhus (under the leadership of Professor A. Viidik, Institute of Anatomy) and at the University of Copenhagen (under the leadership of Professor P. Ebbesen, Department of Tumor Virus Research, Institute of Medical Microbiology). The research projects of the Arhus group have been focused on age changes in the extracellular matrix of connective tissues and various factors (pregnancy, trauma, changes in hormonal balances) that can change this process or can be altered by it.

The Copenhagen group has focused its interest on cell biology, studying local and general factors of importance for the increase in skin susceptibility to carcinogens observed with aging. In the Department of Prosthetic Dentistry, Royal Dental College, studies of the age changes in the human oral mucosa are carried out (by Professor N. Brill and coworkers). Among other research projects, the Glostrup Population Study, started in 1964 by P. From Hansen and coworkers, must be mentioned. From this survey many different works have been published. Groups of psychologists are conducting gerontopsychological studies, and the Danish National Institute of Social Research is the center of the social and economic studies among the aged. In many of the clinical geriatric departments all over the country, clinical research programs are carried out. An epidemiological World Health Organization project is carried out in cooperation with the Neurological Department, Frederiksberg Hospital, and the Danish Institute of Clinical Epidemiology. It deals with the control of stroke in the community. Seventeen research teams in Europe, Asia, and Africa are collecting data concerning stroke patients (Marquardsen, 1976).

Communication and the exchange of information related to gerontology are established by the scientific societies, the Danish Society of Long-term Medicine, and the Danish Gerontological Society. There still exists no Danish or Scandinavian gerontological journal, but the Nordic Gerontological Society has a monthly newsletter, *NGF Aktuelt*.

REFERENCES

Danmarks Statistik: *Statistical Yearbook* 1976. Copenhagen. 80:19.
Eriksen, M. and From Hansen, P., 1976. Investigation of the 70 year-old population in Glostrup. *Ugeskrift for læger*, 1976, 138. 76-76.
From Hansen, P. and Hagerup, L. 1968. Population surveys. The epidemiological method and techniques of examination. *Ugeskrift for læger* 130: 1139.

Fürstnow-Sørensen, B. 1973. Care of the old, 4th rev. ed. Copenhagen: Ministries of Labour and Social Affairs, International Relations Division.

Helms, P. 1977. Investigation of diet in a nursing home. *Ugeskrift for læger* 139:815-821.

Hessov, I. 1977. Investigation of the nutrition among elderly patients in a department for limb surgery. *Ugeskrift for læger* 139:825-827.

Hessov, I. and Elsborg, L. 1977. Folic acid and vitamin B12 in the diet of elderly patients in a surgical department. *Ugeskrift for læger* 139:825–827.

Marquardsen. J. 1976. An epidemiologic study of stroke in a Danish urban community. In *Stroke*, ed. Gillingham et al., Edinbourgh.

Matthiessen, P.C., personal communication.

National Health Service, 1970. *Long stay treatment in rehabilitation in hospitals.* Copenhagen.

Østergaard, F. 1977. Social services for the aged in Denmark. Paper prepared for the EEC Working Party on Problems in National and Social Care of the Elderly, Luxembourg, May 10th-14th, 1977.

Shanas, E.; Townsend, P.; Wedderburn, D.; Friis, H.; Milhøj, P.; and Stehouwer, J. 1968. *Old people in three industrial societies.* New York: Atherton Press.

FEDERAL REPUBLIC OF GERMANY
(West Germany)

BARBARA FÜLGRAFF*

INTRODUCTION

Social developments in highly industrialized countries have given gerontology a bifurcated focus: on the one hand the field seeks to understand aging as a phenomenon of society and social change, exploring the demography of aging and the influence of older people on the economic, social and political structure, institutions, and functions of society, while, on the other hand, it seeks to understand the way in which time-related biological and psychological changes and environmental and cultural factors influence the development of personality and the behavior of older adults, their roles and statuses. Thus, gerontology comprises and combines knowledge and methods of several scientific disciplines.

The range and complexity of the field render it difficult to organize a systematic review of research activities within the limited space of an article. Therefore, a few main topics have been selected, largely on the basis of research publications and projects undertaken by West German investigators.

At the outset, this section will give a brief summary of the situation, scope, and institutions in the field of social gerontology in West Germany. Attention will then be drawn to some background facts about the West German elderly population to improve understanding of the research issues to be presented in the third part of the article. The choice of topics reflects the prevailing research structure which, in turn, is dependent on social, economic, and political precedents. A critical analysis of these precedents is not intended within the frame of this publication. To conclude, we shall discuss tendencies or changes in research stategies, as well as in social policy, and describe some of the research gaps.

*Source: Copyright 1978 by the Gerontological Society. Reprinted by permission from *Gerontologist*, Vol. 18, 1, Feb. 1978.

THE DEVELOPMENT OF GERONTOLOGY

As in most European countries and the United States, sociological, economic, and political aspects of aging engaged the attention of scientists rather late in the course of gathering knowledge on the aging process. Biological change and medical problems determined research in its initial periods. According to the German tradition, social problems of aging, up to the 1940s, were mainly viewed from the philosopher's viewpoint; empirical research was scarce. Thus, the concept of expansion and restriction during the life cycle, obvious as it seemed to be in everyday experience, could govern scientific thought for a long time.

Only after World War II, and with considerable delay compared to other European countries, were social gerontological research problems raised. Cooperation between adjacent fields was instituted only as recently as 1967, when the German Sociological Society was refounded and organized in three sections; medical, psychological, and sociological. The Society resumed prewar attempts to extend the scope of research on aging to social problems. It is now trying to respond to the urgent demands of translating research results into sociopolitical or educational action, opening its doors to the practitioners in politics and social work.

It was the urgency of practical problems that gave rise to empirical research: The increasing number of older people, their need for adequate income, housing, and health services, and the socioeconomic and psychosocial problems of the older population in a rapidly developing society, with its influence on social change and on social and bureaucratic structures. The "practical" focus on needs of the elderly, important as it was for the initiation of research, for a long time impeded systematic and basic research on theoretical or hypothetical grounds (Rosenmayr, 1969). It is only recently that social gerontologists are giving higher priorities to developing new or testing formulated theories on aging (Eichelberger, 1972; Lehr, 1972b; Thomae, 1975b).

Research inventories (Karsten, 1965; Riegel, 1968; Lehr, 1971), formulation of research gaps (SOFI, 1972; Thomae, 1972a; Karsten, 1973; Blume, 1974) and institutionalization of social gerontology (v. Bila, 1974; Hinschutzer, 1974a) all have supported Rosenmayr's observation. Hinschutzer, in her documentation of ongoing and completed research, lists a total of 230 projects (1973/1974), 125 of which were being carried out by universities or affiliated groups, with the remainder undertaken by public or private institutions. Main areas of interest were job and retirement, housing, and social-psychological problems such as adaptation and adjustment to old age, social contact or neglect, and pathological developments in aging. The documentation, moreover, indicates a rather varied range of research interest, such as income maintenance, and social security, mental health and services for the aged, policy and social planning, leisure, education, and training. What is lacking, however, is a systematic endeavor to fill in knowledge gaps.

Research is very much based on individuals' interests or obvious pressing needs. Basic research, i.e. testing of hypotheses, research into the aging process, or investigation of needs, and social statistics to be transformed into indicators comprise only a small portion of ongoing research (25 projects). Although the number of listed projects seems to be quite impressive, it has to be measured against the background of research activities in other countries. Lehr (1972a), in her comprehensive analysis of the "Psychology of Aging," publishes about one thousand titles, one-fourth of which are written by German authors—and almost 40 percent of these are published in connection with the research program of the Bonn University. Of these 254 German publications, 5 percent were published before 1950, 18 percent betwen 1950 and 1960, 19 percent between 1961 and 1965, and 57 percent later than 1965. Empirical research results were not available before the end of the 1960s. Our main source of information on psychological and sociopsychological problems of aging remains the longitudinal study conducted at the Psychological Institute, Bonn University (Lehr, 1972a; Thomae et al., 1973), and for social and sociopolitical research the studies of the Institute for Social Research and Social Policy, Cologne (Blume, 1974).

The universities in general and affiliated groups or institutions carry a major burden of research in social gerontology, despite the fact that there is not a single academic position ascribed to that field. Research and training are conducted and realized solely by interested scholars of various disciplines. The 1974 inventory (v. Bila) lists ten university institutes which offer courses in psychology or sociology of aging. A supposedly incomplete "information" from the German Center of Aging (Deutsches Zentrum fur Altersfragen e. V. Berlin) lists 13 institutes which offered courses during the winter-semester 1974/1975 and 16 for the semester 1975/1976.

All these university activities are carried out with very little financial support. Only recently public financing by the Department of Youth, Family, and Health, the Department of Labor and Social Order, or some State governments has increased. Foundations such as the German Research Association (Deutsche Forschungsgemeinschaft), the Fritz-Thyssen Foundation and the Volkswagen Foundation, are gradually moving their funds into this field of aging (Wirtschafts und Sozialwissenschaftliches Institut des Deutshen Gewerklacking). The same holds true for activities of other public or private institutions, which are starting to show interest in investigation in the field of aging (Wirtschafts und Sozialwissenschaftliches Institut des Deutschen Gewerkschaftsbunds, Dusseldorf; Institut fur Altenwohnbau e.V. Cologne; Stadtebauinstitut, Nuremberg; Max-Planck-Gesellschaft fur Bildungsforschung, Berlin; etc.). Endeavors to coordinate research activities, to set up an information and documentation center, and to shape research strategies finally in 1974 led to the establishing of the German Center of Aging (Deutsches Zentrum fur Altersfragen e.V.) in Berlin, which is setting up its organization and starting its first activities in documentation and information.

DEMOGRAPHY

A brief overview will acquaint the reader with some background facts about the aging population, i.e., those 65 and over, in West Germany.

The total number of elderly inhabitants in West Germany lies just below eight million, with three million men and five million women. The percentage of the older population has risen from about 5 percent in 1900 to 14 percent in 1975, bringing Germany into the top group of all the industrialized countries. The percentage of older women has always been considerably higher than that of older men: in 1975, 16.6 percent of all women and 11.4 percent of all men were beyond the age of 65. The average life expectancy at birth of women has risen to 74 years, that of men to 68. The tendency shows that probably no further rise is to be expected for either sex. New diseases arising from environmental or occupational conditions are expected to take their toll. It is expected that the difference in life expectancy between men and women will decrease. One might speculate that changing styles of life, growing participation in the labor force, and resulting stress from work account for these statistical data.

The majority of the older women are widowed or divorced (about 60 percent) compared to only one-fifth of the older male population. The gap is widening with increasing age.

Unlike in other countries (Great Britain or the United States), the percentage of the older population is rather stable among different parts of the country. We observe slightly higher percentages in rural areas, largely as a result of heavy migration of the younger population. The same fact may account for higher percentages in central urban areas with older housing. Mobility among the older population seems to be low. Studies indicate that there is much dissatisfaction among the older population with accommodations and furnishings, especially in rented flats, but little inclination to leave familiar neighborhoods (Dittrich, 1972; DIVO, 1974; Dringenberg, 1975b). Housing policy, therefore, should give priority to improving and restoring urban living quarters wherever possible and financially feasible (Dringenberg, 1975a; Friedrich-Wussow, 1975). In rural areas and in small cities, more than 50 percent of the older population live in their own homes, not all of which, of course, are furnished according to the living standards of the 1970s. Only 4-5 percent of the older population live in old age institutions of various kinds. Current research suggests no significant increase in institutionalized elderly (DIVO, 1974; Bierhoff and Schmitz-Scherzer, 1974). The number of well-off pensioners moving to fancy "senior homes" in the south or at the shore is, as yet, statistically and socially insignificant.

The elderly population depends mainly on old age security benefits (87 percent of the men and 71 percent of the women); 18 percent of the elderly men are in the labor force mainly as self-employed or white collar workers in contrast to 6 percent of the elderly women.

In 1973 flexible retirement was initiated, permitting men to choose the date of retirement between the ages of 63 and 67 and women between 58 and 62, with appropriate adjustments of the old age pension and amount of additional allowable earnings. Recent information indicates that, following this measure, the average retirement age has gone down. Specific studies on the influence of social status, type of work, health, or other factors are still needed.

Although West Germany is considered a state with a relatively progressive and just system of old age pensions, including mandated annual cost-of-living adjustments in the pension rate which is aimed at 60–75 percent of last income, and a solid network of additional benefits from social welfare, poverty is still not totally overcome. We lack reliable knowledge to depict sources, distribution, and effects of poverty. Demographic data, based normally on different income sources without identifying them, are not at all reliable as socially or politically usable information. What are needed are surveys of large samples to investigate not only the extent and distribution of needs and inequalities but also the various causes for poverty's existence.

Geissler (1975) describes poverty as the "new social question." He reveals that about two million households—9 percent of the West German population—are living on a net income below the poverty rate, which is defined as the minimum income below which persons are entitled to social welfare allowances. Among retirees, this reaches 14.5 percent. Among them, the percentage of former manual or unskilled workers is still considerably higher than that of any other occupational group. Highly disadvantaged groups among the older population, moreover, are those persons who have not been able to pay into social security long enough, mainly as a result of war or postwar occupational mobility.

Still more difficult is the financial situation of widowed women. The West German system of old age security, progressive as it is is in many respects, tends to perpetuate existing inequalities of social status and to enlarge them during later years (Fulgraff, 1976a). This at least holds true for the present generation of the elderly, which is still heavily influenced by social and political adversities of the last half-century. Social policy for the aged will have to distinguish problems of transitory nature which need immediate and temporary solutions from those of persisting character which can only be solved by changes in social and individual factors from a preventive perspective.

RESEARCH

Aging and Social Policy

It is now accepted and commonplace in the community of sociologists that the treatment accorded the aged as expressed in social policy and social services sheds some light on the underlying beliefs, sentiments, and values of a society, although we do not know enough about the nature of the correlation. Basic research into the sociological and economic sources of political decisions or priorities is still grievously lacking. Such conditions as occupational retirement (Behr, 1973; Naegele, 1975; Pillardy, 1973; Thomae, 1976), reduced income (SOFI, 1972; WSI, 1975), economic dependencies (Schenda, 1972), subordination to the younger generation (Rosenmayr and Rosenmayr, 1974) or social control, loss of status and influence (Schenda, 1972; Tews, 1975), restrictions of participation (Bungard, 1975; Olbrich, 1974; Renner, 1969; Schmitz-Scherzer et al., 1975; Urban, 1973) have been investigated, yet we can only speculate about their influence on individual ideas, organizational postures, institutional attitudes, operational realities, or practical and necessary decisions concerning the status of the aged in society.

The idea of an explicit policy on aging is equally new and controversial. Changes in the age structure, accompanied by rapid changes in other sectors of society that influence the relative status of the aged, have set the stage. The late 1960s saw a shift of policy objectives in favor of marginal social groups. Whether the elderly are properly labeled a problem group remains a matter of controversy (Blume, 1968; Landwehrmann, 1975; Schenda, 1972; Sieber, 1975; Lehr, 1975a).

More than ever before, however, political groups are paying attention to research results or initiating opinion research. There appears to be greater awareness of the responsibility to make choices about issues which involve the aged as a special category of people.

Policy for the aged, hitherto, has been considered part of social policy as a whole and, therefore, has profited from the general shift in objectives from support and aid to prevention and rehabilitation (Achinger, 1975; Blume, 1968; Fulgraff, 1976b). Objectives of social policy are oriented toward the general goals to improve economic, physical, mental, and social prerequisites for security, recognition, participation, activity. These are codified in the latest amendments to the Federal Social Welfare Act (Bundessozialhilfegesetz) of 1974.

Responsibility for achieving these goals lies primarily with government and private organizations of social welfare (Red Cross, the churches, workers' welfare organizations, etc.), which are, to a large extent, publicly financed. Responsibility extends to guaranteeing sufficient income and providing facilities and services. Participation and activity, however, call for self-responsibility on the part of the aged for which most of them are not sufficiently prepared or trained. Socially and individually desirable development has to exclude a number of factors which diminish the effects of generally positive tendencies. Declining work-life expectancy (Bracker, 1974; Blume, 1972; Klauder et al., 1971; Lehr, 1975a), increasing bureaucratization of retirement practices (Naegele, 1975; SOFI, 1972; Stopp, 1971), economic recession and the concomitant notion of the older persons' being less productive, on the one hand and uncompensated inflation (Geissler, 1975; WSI, 1975) on the other accompanied by a serious loss of social influence and power (Bellebaum and Braun, 1974; Blume, 1968; Eichelberger, 1972; Tews, 1975), which is not balanced by the gross voting power of the elderly (Schenda, 1972; Sieber, 1975), are all working as social obstacles against the development of self-reliance. The individual dimension of obstacles is characterized by unreliable or missing information about rights, provisions, and services (incomplete information through the various organizations or the local authorities, insufficient advice, etc.) (Schenda, 1972; Haag, 1972) and resentment of the aged to the connotation of "welfare."

Practical results of social policy in behalf of the aged as a special group can be observed with respect to financial and social needs. First, measures have been taken to redistribute the gains from economic growth in order to provide a greater share for more elderly people. In 1973, social security coverage was extended to new groups of the population (self-employed, farmers, housewives), worktime became more flexible, unemployment insurance as distinguished from early retirement pay has improved, private pension claims have been secured, and old age assistance (welfare) is employed in cases of "exceptional needs" and as a "help for a living" (Federal Social Welfare Act). Social welfare payments increased by 50 percent from 1967 to 1971; yet, we have no reliable data on how much the share of the elderly population amounted to.

Social needs are responded to by considering the social context within which they occur. Such needs as response and relatedness, social contacts and social esteem are seen as being as important as material subsistence (Behrends, 1972; Bellebaum and Braun, 1974; Fulgraff, 1976a). This tendency shows in an increased offer of "open" services (Blume, 1968; Haag, 1972; Hartwieg, 1972), improved facilities for learning and training (see below), restructuring of living quarters (Dieck, 1973, 1975), and in the great emphasis put on leisure and time-budgeting (Schmitz-Scherzer, 1975b). Motivating the elderly to become active has become the major concern of physicians, nursing personnel, social workers, educators, and administrators. It seems necessary to further discuss the concept critically (Fisseni, 1975) and go into further investigation of the underlying social, political, economic, and individual factors which may dilute or strengthen what seems to be a policy to encourage activity.

Housing

As a research topic in its own right, housing has caught attention only recently, but with growing interest. Since Tartler's basic and comprehensive considerations (1961), theoretical as well as empirical research had been more or less incidental. Most of the more general surveys of the living conditions among the older population (Bracker, 1974; Deininger, 1970; Rosenmayr,

1969; Tismer et al., 1975) covered housing problems only marginally or with a limited perspective. Existing attempts to systematize empirical research either dealt with the problem of housing as one variable to describe personal developments (Lehr, 1972a) or concentrated on the problems of institutionalization (Gores, 1971; Tews, 1975). In recent publications the individual and social meaning of housing has been discussed under such rubrics as the ecology of aging (WSI, 1975), space and mobility (Kuhn et al., 1975), contact and communication (Schmitz-Scherzer et al., 1975), and activity and independence. Social research to verify these hypothesized correlations is still scarce (Dittrich, 1972; Dringenberg, 1975a, b).

The specific post-war situation of the Federal Republic with a large proportion of housing accommodations being destroyed or requiring basic renovation accounts for the fact that problems or needs of specific groups, for a long time, fell behind the general demand. Nevertheless, the specific concern of the older population was already included in the first home-building act of 1950 and improved upon in subsequent amendments.

Public subsidies worked effectively from the middle of the 1960s. Publicly subsidized housing has to meet relatively strict standards as to location, size, rent, equipment, quality, and accompanying services (Dringenberg, 1975b). Plans provide that by 1985, 4-5 percent of the aged population over 60 shall live in homes specifically designed for the elderly (Grofphans, 1974; Hugues, 1973), a doubling of such accommodations within the next ten years.

The basic facts about present housing conditions can be summarized as follows. Most of the aged population in West Germany (96 percent) lives in "normal" homes, while only 4 percent (with regional variances between 2 and 8 percent) inhabits special units such as old age homes or nursing homes (Dittrich, 1972). Demand probably will not increase (Reimann and Reimann, 1974) provided that adequate measures are taken and sufficient means provided to improve residential housing and that general living conditions do not change drastically. The older population, however, is severely disadvantaged compared to other age groups. They live significantly more often in the older, ill-equipped homes (Friedrich-Wussow, 1975), predominantly in the cities. Nevertheless, only a few of them are inclined to move into more modern accommodations. Research indicates that "satisfaction" even with poor homes results from such variables as adjustment to neighborhoods, personal contacts, individual reminiscences, health-related immobility, or financial limitations (Dittrich, 1972; Dringenberg, 1975b).

Attitudes toward housing are highly dependent on the need to feel financially, emotionally, and socially secure as well as the need to feel independent and self-supporting (Dittrich, 1972; Hinschutzer, 1974b)—partly contradictory individual concepts. Attitudes are, moreover, shaped by individual living experiences with family or relatives (Rosenmayr and Rosenmayr, 1974; Tartler, 1961), by general social values such as role prescriptions and aspirations in old age (Schneider, 1970, 1974) or perception of one's power and competence to change the situation.

Major alternative solutions to housing problems seem to be to maintain and improve independent living arrangements in unplanned settings which undoubtedly are the norm for older persons and correspond with the majority of needs. The alternative program of planned congregate arrangements, though of growing interest to part of the older population, will probably remain of secondary importance. It will, however, become of utmost importance to set priorities to assist the more disadvantaged groups among the elderly who are the prospective inhabitants of comfortable yet moderately priced accommodations.

Problems of Older Employees

Among the various fields that deal with aging problems the situation of the aging employee is of the utmost concern not only to social researchers but also to various social groups. It is in this context that most financial and research capacity has been invested. Several Federal and State Departments have inaugurated hearings, and employers' associations and the unions (WSI, 1975)—from contrasting political positions—have surveyed the situation of older employees in order to obtain solid "facts" to be used in the ongoing power struggle to gain social and political influence. The concept of "humanizing work," originating from social-liberal thought, has since become a weapon for economic controversies beyond the immediate interests of labor. The concept, contrary to its basic intentions, turns against the needs and interests of workers by concentrating on productivity as a major justification. It does this by misusing the supposed diminished productivity of older workers as striking evidence of the dehumanized work situation, thus creating a "problem group." Applying an economic perspective, political groups are fighting in fact a political battle in which the beneficiaries turn out to be the victims. Older workers are not in themselves a "problem group," although it can be argued that a variety of economic, social, social-psychological, and other factors work against them (Landwehrmann, 1975).

In such a political landscape it is not surprising to observe that opinions on older employees vacillate between "stereotypes and facts." Even research results are not total proof against manipulative interpretation, whether intentional or not. According to Lehr (1975a) the deficit-model of aging, though convincingly refuted through the numerous publications especially those from the Bonn longitudinal study (Lehr, 1972a; Thomae et al., 1973), still haunts the scientific literature on aging. In an analysis of recent studies on the situation of older women, and of older industrial workers to improve the "quality of worklife" (MAGS), the interpretation "bias" which is partly the result of methodological ambiguity and partly that of unidimensional perspective is revealed. The author concludes that researchers "seem to be unable—for reasons of prejudice and stereotyped beliefs—to objectively investigate the opportunities and limitations in employing older workers in accordance with their achieving abilities and readiness."

What are the facts? Older employees—for reasons of statistical comparison usually defined as the groups beyond the age of 44—are by no means a homogeneous group (Blume, 1972). Different working conditions, depending on the degree of mechnization or automatization, the degree of physical or mental strain, or the power structure affect older persons differently (Naegele, 1975; Shaefer, 1975; Schmidt, 1974a, b). Studies suggest investigating problems of older employees with regard to the variety of causes and effects.

Computations from the Institute of Labor Market and Occupation Research (Klauder et al., 1971) assert that 5 ½ million (60 percent) blue- and (40 percent) white-collar workers are between the ages of 45 and 65, i.e., 30 percent of all dependently employed. Two million of them are women. One million eight hundred thousand employees, i.e., 12.5 percent, are physically or mentally handicapped, a third of whom are severely disabled due to war injuries or accidents. Among the older workers, almost 50 percent suffer from handicaps of various degrees. The study predicts that in 1980 every third employee will belong to the group of "older employees." The increase will be heavier among the age group of 50–55, while for those between 55 and 65 a light decrease is expected. Klauder et al. (1971) conclude that in terms of quantity the problems of older workers will become even more severe, while structural aspects such as labor market and unemployment show a slight retreat. This 1971 conclusion seems already outdated. Recent data from the institute indicate that economic developments of the middle 1970s continue the trend of unemployment of the elderly. Not only does their percentage remain higher than that of any other age group, but unemployment lasts longer. Moreover, older employees suffer from such deprivations as structural de-qualification with resulting adaptation problems, from transfer to less productive workplaces with resulting income reduction, and early retirement with resulting loss of social status (WSI, 1975). Reasons given for dismissals normally do not include the older workers' qualification or productivity but shift the responsibility to rationalization processes, a shortage of orders, or shutdowns. Analyses, however, assert that the stereotype of the older worker comes in handy as long as the labor market situation is tight. Correlation between the average length of unemployment, mean number of openings, and the age of the unemployed ascertains that age is of less importance for the duration of unemployment than the actual number of openings (MAGS, 1974). To alter the structural deficits for the older employees Viebahn (1971) suggests improving regional balance of work-places and regional mobility, without considering that mobility is inhibited systematically (Schmitz-Scherzer et al., 1975; Stingl, 1972). How many of these observations reflect the stereotyped image of the older employee? Again the Bonn longitudinal study (Lehr, 1972a; Thomae et al., 1973) gives evidence how seldom research as yet has become the source and basis for political decisions. General decrease of capabilities and productivity with increasing age is anything but normal (Thomae and Lehr, 1973). High productivity can be maintained into upper age groups, provided that working conditions have been "human" during most of the worklife (Lehr et al., 1970; Naegele, 1975), and provided that the demands are accommodated to the capacities and qualifications of the worker, not vice versa. Over- as well as under-demand equally produce dissatisfaction and reduce activity. Measures of productivity are not at all independent of the context within which productivity is required. Observed differences, to some extent, measure generational instead of age differences, younger workers being better trained and educated. Older workers tend to work with older and less efficient machines, tools, or equipment, while the younger are chosen to run more modern working places (Lehr et al., 1970).

To summarize the reliable findings: the deficit model of aging has been modified and partly rejected through solid research. As an explanatory tool to analyze the situation of older employees, it is not only unqualified but deceiving. It can be used as a welcome device to disguise underlying social and political forces. The WSI study (1975), a comprehensive analysis of statistical and survey data on living conditions of the elderly, concludes: "The extensive division of labor, i.e., the division of work processes into monotonous and repetitive parts and the increasing interchangeability of manpower to realize short-term productivity and to minimize costs lead to physical and psychic damage as well as to waste of qualifications and potentials on the older workers' part. The results prove equally adverse for the individual workers as for economic progress. In any case, high consecutive social costs will have to be encountered for health damages, early disablement, incomplete use of available qualifications, and rapidly increasing foreign labor."

Social Behavior and Social Contact

The scope and variety of topics within this area of research do not allow for detailed report of results. We shall have to limit the presentation of data to a large-scale selection of objectives.

Research on social behavior and contact—including leisure, activity, social relations, family, and problems of institutionalization—has been mostly developed to test hypotheses of activity or engagement (Lehr, 1972a). In sociological perspective, role theory in its various versions has contributed to analysis (Narr, 1976). It is widely acknowledged that the aging process, besides—but not independent of—economic conditions, is shaped predominantly by the amount and intensity of social relations and contacts in old age. It is, moreover, generally agreed that communication problems have accompanied the aging process throughout the centuries, while the nature and quality of problems have changed. It is no longer—at least, not primarily—economic deprivation that accounts for segregation of older persons, but a new kind of social devaluation caused by changes in the family structure, housing patterns, occupational mobility modernization, and other factors. Social communication patterns, therefore, have been studied within the context of life-span developments (Thomae, 1976), including variables such as social status and position, occupation, education, life-styles, as well as sex, size, and nature of community, or familial status (Tismer et al., 1975; Lehr, 1972a; Olbrich, 1974; Renner, 1969; Schneider, 1974). Results indicate that "successful aging" as a subjective rating correlates significantly with a high degree of continuity of contact and activity, regardless of other social or psychological variables, continuity being the key variable to test hypotheses of engagement or disengagement.

There are, needless to say, considerable differences in the amount of objective participation opportunities and, hence, of possibilities to reach a subjectively tolerable degree of satisfaction with old age. Isolation seems to be highly dependent on marital status or death of spouse, since withdrawal from public or political stages into intimate social relationships has been indicative for postwar and post-Nazi adult generations.

The bulk of disadvantageous conditions, however, weighs heavily on older women (SOFI, 1972). Since their average life expectancy is higher than those of men and since, on the average, they have little if any claim on old age insurance in their own right and depend on less than two-thirds of their late husband's benefits, older widowed women rank considerably high among social welfare recipients. Economic pressure is one of the sources for their increased isolation. Another source can be found in the traditional role distribution which confines women mainly to intrafamilial roles, thus limiting their role repertoire and their contacts in later life. Although reliable evidence for a direct correlation between economic reproduction and isolation on the one hand and traditional role sets on the other has not been ascertained, we can conclude that the female unmarried or widowed older person has a considerably lower social and economic status than other groups of the older population and that she experiences stronger limitations of communication, increase of conflict potential, and mental encumbrance.

These general findings are supplemented by some specific aspects of contact and social behavior. It can safely be maintained that scope and frequency of social contact does not serve as a sufficiently differentiating indicator for integration or isolation of older persons (Urban, 1973). The quality of and the individual needs for contact must be taken into account. Lehr (1972a) summarizes research in this field: it would be wrong to assume general social or emotional dependency of the older population. Although such conceptions govern public consciousness, whether derived from stereotyping or undue generalization of individual observations, empirical data, systematically gathered, do not support such a picture.

Marital relations between older persons have not been sufficiently investigated (Tews, 1975). Changes in the structure and quality of marital roles after retirement recently came into focus while planning preretirement programs. It is only the aspect of sexual relations in later years that has been studied in greater detail (Tummers, 1976). Findings indicate a shift in social norm perception of sexuality between the generations. Prejudice and rigidity of judging has decreased in the younger age groups compared to the older. Attitudes toward sexuality—and sexual activity also in later years—seem much more liberal. On the other hand, adverse attitudes, already higher among older respondents, intensify with age, regardless of social status or education. Highly restrictive sexual norms are expressed primarily by women of 65 or more. Sexual activity does not automatically decline with age or changing health; it is not dependent on social status or even on loss of spouse (in the case of male respondents), unless normative or moral attitudes—often combined with religious or clerical commitments—against sexuality prevail. Sexual relations in older marriages seem to be an important factor to produce a satisfying and positive perspective on aging.

Another significant factor is found in family relations. Most important reference groups for older persons are their spouses, their children, and grandchildren. Every fifth older person is in daily contact with members of the family, and more than 50 percent meet with the family at least once a week (Tismer et al., 1975). One quarter of the older men and 40 percent of older women would like to intensify their regular contact with children. These findings vary with age, familial status, education, income, and self-perception of respondents. Older persons—both male and female—who are in close contact with their families report considerably less feelings of uselessness or loneliness. From the older persons' point of view, the most desirable family situation has been described by "inner closeness and distance of space" (Tartler, 1961; Rosenmayr, 1969). The patterns of interaction within the families are structured primarily by the roles of grandparents (Tews and Schwagler, 1973). Older persons, to some extent, also take over more responsibility in household duties or contribute to income. These patterns prevail in low income families with mothers of younger children working or in rural households (SOFI, 1972). Frequent contacts, thus, can serve as an indicator for close emotional bonds as well as for urgent material pressure. Close contacts, therefore, can mean emotional fulfillment, continuity of lifestyles, or practical aid, as well as moral obligation or economic need.

Contacts with other groups of people rank considerably behind those with the family. About one-fourth of the older persons meet regularly with friends or neighbors (Tismer et al., 1975). The amount of extra-familial contacts is widely independent of age or of sex (while again dependent on marital status).

It correlates, however, closely with variables such as education, former occupation, type of community, or with personality. Lack of contact or isolation are not primarily the result of aging but reflect a specific life pattern. Again, feelings of loneliness, depression, or pessimistic outlook correlate with frequency of broader contacts, although direct causal relationships can still be doubted.

Old age is widely and traditionally associated with leisure and spare time. Being free of external scheduling can be perceived as a burden, i.e., an urge to develop new habits for which working life has not provided adequate models or as a chance for change, innovation, or creativity (Kehler, 1974; Recktenwald, 1973). Older people often identify their forthcoming retirement life as "free." Research findings indicate that they see themselves predominantly as free from previous tasks or pressure, without, however, being able to develop a life concept that is based on freedom for different enterprise. Most retirees plan to quantitatively augment their hitherto prevailing leisure behavior.

Surprisingly enough, systematic research on leisure behavior and attitudes is only of recent date, though aspects of leisure have been covered under various other findings in gerontological research. The most comprehensive collection of information has been gathered in connection with the Bonn longitudinal study (Schmitz-Scherzer, 1973, 1975d). Older people generally dispose of the same variety of leisure activities as any other age group (Becker, 1974). Chronological age operates as a "reducing variable" (Schmitz-Scherzer, 1973), but hardly influences the content of leisure. Sex, however, accounts for different patterns of behavior. The same is true for material status, health and its psychological correlates, socioeconomic status, and education. More than in almost any other area of aging, social status—measured by education, income, and occupation—determines leisure behavior. Moreover, continuity and constancy of leisure behavior are frequently observed (Schmitz-Scherzer, 1975d). Changes occur from more active forms of behavior toward passive forms, although it is not clear if the observed shift from physical activity to more contemplative activities indicates withdrawal or continuity of a pre-existing pattern.

The function of mass media use can possibly promote a new type of of social integration (Rudinger in Schmitz-Scherzer, ed., 1973). Among the leisure activities of older people, those organized around the family or the house rank highest. Outdoor activities are limited largely to going for a walk or gardening. Traveling becomes increasingly important; less so cultural or educational activities. According to these priorities (or neglected aspects) studies were directed toward investigating the role of family and leisure behavior (Lehr, 1973a), the effects of institutionalization and of the structure and ideology of old age home (Becker, 1974), the correlation between physical activity and positive self-perception (Sokoll et al., 1974), toward investigating into housing and ecological conditions (Grofphans, 1974; Becker, 1974), or social planning (Kuhn and Plagemann, 1974) and continued education (Fulgraff, 1972). Summarizing the data, Schmitz-Scherzer found "a complex pattern of determinants of everyday activities," and he concludes that "the most relevant variables are situational, social, economic, and psychological, while chronological age is of little significance for the explanation of findings." Although a general theoretical model of aging to integrate results is not at hand the data "clearly demonstrate the ability (of older persons) to react adequately and actively to changes in their surroundings" (Schmitz-Scherzer, in Thomae, 1976).

Learning and Education

Learning, traditionally, was not conceived of as a constituent element of an adult's role. Human life was segmented into a period of learning and acquisition, a period of utilization and production, and a period of "wisdom" and contemplation. Learning was confined to childhood and adolescence. The ideology held that biological developments accounted for such a distribution, while underlying economic requirements or aspects of political power and social privilege were screened (Fulgraff, 1972; Brandenburg, 1974a; Verres-Muckel, 1974; Kallmeyer et al., 1976; Tews, 1976). Even when the necessity for continuing education and lifelong learning became obvious (Polemann, 1972; Breloer, 1973; Schenda, 1974; Schneider, 1976), social distribution of opportunities to learn extended only into the utilization period aimed toward improving productive qualities (Kallmeyer et al., 1976; Tews, 1976) but did not carry through to later years. Educational investments into old age were considered fultile. Old age remained the domain of welfare.

It is only recently that the debate was transferred from the field of welfare to education (Vath, 1973; Sitzmann, 1976; Schneider, 1976). Educational programs for older adults, again, were for a long time and even now are tainted by disengagement theory.

Older people themselves not unexpectedly display the same ambiguous attitude: learning and education, in their view, may be of value for the middle years to further occupational career patterns but do not offer a perspective for the later years. While three-quarters of the older population (55 and over) consider continuing education as important or even very important, only every tenth person has participated in any kind of educational activity during the last five years (Leben im Alter, 1977). The difference between attitude and activity is greatest in the oldest age groups, in the less educated and low income groups, and among those groups of older respondents which were rated as less active, poorly integrated, introverted, and pessimistic in their outlook. The social pattern, again, shows up significantly.

Research contributions to learning in later years were offered from various disciplines. Developmental psychology (Lehr and Thomae, 1969) destroyed the legend of a general decline of learning ability, presenting discriminating research results on patterns of learning (Lehr, 1972a; Lowe, 1972), the learning process (Olbrich and Schuster, 1976), abilities of perception and thinking (Skawran, 1971), of accumulation and retrieval or information processing (Rudinger, 1971; Olbrich and Schuster, 1976) and other variables. These indicate that the observable alterations in learning ability with aging are more of a qualitative than of quantitative nature. Learning ability can be developed or trained like many physical abilities, but it needs favorable conditions.

Sociological research accompanied the scouting process and revealed some of the factors adverse to developing learning ability (Tews, 1975, 1976). Correlations between learning ability and motivation, on the one hand, and previous learning history, socialization (Bauer, 1972), education (Leben im Alter, 1977), social status of family, work-life experiences (Fulgraff, 1971; Lehr, 1972a; Huther, 1976), political and social participation (Kehler, 1974), and additional variables, on the other, were tested and reported with the result that the development of learning ability is, by far, more a question of socio-economic prerequisites or prejudice than an individual achievement. Motivation to learn can be built up and encouraged or be suppressed during a lifelong socialization process. Chances to learn are socially allotted.

These results, in turn, initiated new reflection and thinking about the structure and content of education for the middle and later years to put off the detected limits (Alrichs et al., 1973; Brandenburg, 1974b; Tews, 1976). It was in the field of education and through institutions of adult education that old age problems received a new quality of interest. Educational concepts for the later years, over a long period of time oriented toward adjustment (Ruprecht, 1972; Sitzmann, 1971, 1976), shifted to such new objectives like individual and social development or fulfillment (Autorenkollektiv Hannover, 1973; Reck-tenwald, 1973; Kehler, 1974) to activation and participation. But not only were the concepts revised, the learning processes themselves were restructured according to research results (Breloer, 1974; Recktenwald, 1973; Kallmeyer et al., 1976; Fulgraff et al., 1976) integrating aspects of group dynamics (Goeken, 1975) and interaction processes (Radebold et al., 1973), organiza-tion of learning experience (Breloer, 1974), and environmental and psycho-dynamic factors. Moreover, the institutional limits were overthrown, addres-sing older persons in their own environment such as old age homes (Meyer-Dettum, 1976) or clubs (Fluck, 1977). Education has become an important lever to alter social policy perspective on aging problems: concern for the elderly originated with the welfare organizations, but the remedy is seen in the context of continuing education.

"Timely thought and action," "planning," and "preparation for retire-ment" mark the change in public (Deutsche Gesellschaft fur Personalfuhrung, 1975; Evangelische Akademie Bad Boll, 1975) and scientific thinking (Blume, 1971; Schubert and Stormer, 1974; Kallmeyer, 1975, Kuhne and

Krug, 1976). Researchers went to the public recommending an increase and broadening of pre-retirement education by collaboration between industry and the educational institutions (Blume, 1971) and used the mass media to stimulate these developments (Stosberg, 1972). There is no other single area of concern—and debate—in aging that produced a comparable amount of publication activity during the last few years.

Such developments, necessary as they are, tend to have some unexpected effects: there is a growing danger to overshoot the mark and expect education to become the panacea for all problems. To encourage learning activities requires continual rethinking and accompanying evaluation of measures lest concepts like preparation for retirement settle in as a ritual of education or of "progressive" social policy substituting for necessary endeavor during earlier years (Schenda, 1972). In the long run it is to be hoped that retirement planning will envisage not only a single program a few years before the entry into the third age but will develop into a life-accompanying sequence of courses and concepts to humanize work, improve health requirements and services, consolidate financial positions of older persons, and prepare for the individual and social ramifications of role change.

CONCLUSIONS

The foregoing review, fragmentary as it is, testifies to the broad scope and significance of research in gerontology in West Germany. Some of the research underway and more of the previous investigations are entirely theoretical; much was and is increasingly oriented to immediate problems and action. Relevance and significance of research increasingly is measured in terms of applicability. This not only holds true for the observed emphasis on learning but also for a growing interest in shaping policy decisions.

While research, for a long time, fell largely within the purview of traditional disciplines, interdisciplinary approaches are gaining in importance.

The prevailing themes of research and policy for our immediate future indicate a change in outlook on aging problems. This change is marked by shifts from such concepts as welfare to prevention, from adjustment to activation or intervention, from "sealed fate" to planning and preparation, and from individual liability to social and public responsibility.

A realistic perspective, however, does not give rise to unlimited optimism. There are still grievous knowledge gaps. Practical or political consequences remain even more fragmentary and unsystematic. Concepts need time and involvement on the parts of researchers and politicians to become strategies. There is still great need for balanced financial and institutional support over the entire field. Comparative studies among other countries have been stimulating and informative and point to the need to join in cross-national and cross-cultural research. And this, in turn, emphasized the importance of a large-scale extension and improvement of research capacity.

REFERENCES

Journals with Regular or Occasional Contributions to Social Gerontology

Aktuelle Gerontologie, Organ der Deutschen Gesellschaft für Gerontologie und der Österreichischen Gesellschaft für Geriatrie, Stuttgart (seit 1971).

Altenhilfe. Beispiele—Informationen—Meinungen, hrsg. vom Deutschen Zentralinstitut für soziale Fragen, Berlint (seit 1974) Forts. der Informationen zur Altenhilfe in den Blättern der Wohlfahrtspflege.

Aktiver Lebensabend, Die europäische Monatszeitschrift der älteren Generation, hrsg. vonder Lebensabendbewegung e.V., Kassel (seit 1961).

Das Altenheim, Organ der gemeinnützigen und privaten Alten-und Pflegeheime, Hannover (seit 1962).

Archiv für Wissenschaft und Praxis der sozialen Arbeit, Franfurt (seit 1970).

Blätter der Wohlfahrtspflege, Monatszeitschrift der öffentlichen und freien Wohlfahrtspflege, hrsg. vom Landeswohlfahrtswerk für Baden-Württemberg, Stuttgart (seit 1960).

Caritas, Zeitschrift für Caritasarbeit und Caritaswissenschaft, hrsg. vom Deutschen Caritasverband, Freiburg (seit 1899).

DPWV-Nachrichten, hrsg. vom Vorstand des Deutschen paritätischen Wohlfahrtsverbandes, Frankfurt (seit 1950).

Deutsches Rotes Kreuz, hrsg. vom Präsidium des Deutschen Roten Kreuzes, Bonn (seit 1951).

Informationen aus dem Bereich der Altenhilfe, Beilage zu den BdW., bearb. von G. Haag, (1960-1973), Forst. als Altenhilfe (s.dort).

Die Innere Mission, Zeitschrift des Diakonischen Werkes, Innere Mission und Hilfswerk der ev. Kirche in Deutschland, Stuttgart (seit 1910).

Nachrichtendienst des Deutschen Vereins für öffentliche und private Füsorge, Frankfurt (seit 1967).

Neues Beginnen, hrsg. von der Arbeiterwohlfahrt, Bundesverband e. V., Bon (seit 1950); nach 1971 weitergeführt als: Theorie und Praxis der sozialen Arbeit.

Presse- und Informationsdienst, hrsg. vom Kuratorium Deutsch Altenhilfe, Köln (seit 1968).

Sorge für alte Menschen, modern und wirksam, hrsg. vom Deutschen Zentralinstitut für soziale Fragen, Berlin (seit 1970).

Theorie und Praxis der sozialen Arbeit, Bonn (seit 1970).

Zeitschrift für Gerontologie, Europäische Zeitschrift für Altersmedizin und interdisziplinäre Alternsforschung, Darmstadt (seit 1971) (1968-1970 unter demselben Titel erschienen als *Organ der Deutschen Gesellschaft für Gerontologie und der Österreichischen Gesellschaft für Geriatrie.*

The Research Situation in Social Gerontology

Bibliographies, Inventories

Bila, H. von. Gerontologie. *Bestandsaufnahme zur Situation der Alternsforschung in der Bundesrepublic Deutschland.* Göttingen: Vandenhoeck & Ruprecht, 1974.

Deutsches Zentrum für Altersfragen e.V. *Bibliographien.*(Gerontologie/Lebensverhältnisse Älterer/Wohnen Älterer/Suicid und Suicidversuch im Alter/Offene und halboffene Altenhilfe/Vorbereitung auf das Alter) Berline 1976.

Hinschützer, U. *Gerontologische Dokumentation. Soziogerontologische Forschung und Wohnforschung*, Institut für Altenwohnbau, Köln 1974.

Articles

Bergener, M. Interdisziplinäre Aspekte der Geropsychiatrie. *Aktuelle Gerontologie*, 1973, *3*, 439-450.

Blume, O. Ergebnisse der Altenforschung sowie Lückenanalyse and Vorschläge. Gutachten für das Bundesministerium für Jugend, Familie und Gesundheit, Bonn, 1974. (unpubl.)

Erlemeier, N., Multidisziplinäre Alternsforschung. *Ztschr. f. Gerontologie*, 1971, *4*, 217-226.

Institut für Sozialforschung und Gesellschaftspolitik e.V.,Tätigkeitsbericht 1973-74, Köln, (memeo.)

Karsten, A. Probleme der Alternsforschung. *Psychologische Rundschau*, 1965, *16*, 1-27.

Karsten, A. Erkenntnisse und Forschüngslücken in der Gerontologie. *Anpassung oder Integration? Zur gesellschaftlichen Situation älterer Menschen.* Politische Akadedie Eicholz (Ed.), 1973.

Lehr, U. Psycho-gerontologische Forschung in Deutschland. Rückblick und Ausblick. *Ztschr. f. Gerontologie*, 1971, *4*, 1-7.

Lehr, U. Alter und Leistungsgesellschaft—zum gegenwärtigen Stand der interdisziplinären Diskussion in der Gerontologie. *Bergedorfer Gesprächskreis*, 1973, *43*, 68-77. (a)

Lehr, U. Gerontologie—ein Modell interdisziplinärer Forschung und Lehre? *Aktuelle Gerontologie*, 1973, *3*, 391-397. (b)

Riegel, K.F. Ergebnisse und Probleme der psychologischen Altenforschung. *Vita Humana*, 1958, *1*, 52-64; 111-127, reprinted in: Thomae, H., & Lehr, U., (Eds.), *Altern*, 1968, 142-170.

Soziologisches Forschungsinst. Göttingen (SOFI), Die Soziale Problematik des Alterns,Göttingen, 1972. (mimeo.)

Thomae, H. Forschungsdesiderate auf dem Gebiet der sozialen Gerontologie. *Aktuelle Gerontologie*, 1972, *2*, 561-572.

General Introductions, Overviews

Statistical Data, Surveys

Andert, E. Statistische Informationen zur Situation der alten Menschen in der Bundesrepublik. *Diakonie*, 1975, *1*, 56-60.

Bracker, M. Die Situation der alten Menschen in der BDR. Eine sozioökonomische Analyse, Dipl.Arb., Univ. Regensburg, 1974. (unpubl.)

Deininger, D. Statistische Ergebnisse über die Lage der älteten Menschen. Störmer, A. (Ed.), 1970, 186-203.

EMNID, *Lebensbedingungen und Bedürfnisse alter Menschen, Bielefeld, 1974.*

GeiBler, H. Neue soziale Frage. Zahlen—Daten—Fakten. o.O., 1975. (mimeo.)

Geißler, H. Zur Situation der älteren Frau in der Bundesrepublik Deutschland. *Jahrb.des deutschen Caritasverbandes*, Freiburg: Deutscher Caritasverband, 1976.

Menges, W., Häring, D., & Herrnbrodt, U. Die Prozesse des Alterns in der europäischen Bevölkerung, soziale und ökonomische Folgen. Univ. Frankfurt: Soziographisches Inst., 1970. (mimeo.)

Ministerium für Soziales, Gesundheit und Sport des Landes Rheinland-Pfalz. *Daten und Fakten. Zur Situation der älteren Frau in der Bundesrepublik Deutschland, o.O. 1974.*

Statistisches Bundesamt (Ed.) *Die älteren Mitbürger und ihre Lebensverhältnisse, 1971.* Stuttgart: Kolhammer, 1972.

Statistisches Bundesamt (Ed.) Ältere Mitbürger. Volkszählung vom 27. Mai 1970. Stuttgart: Kolhammer, 1974.

Statistisches Bundesamt (Ed.) Zur Situation der älteren Menschen. *Wirtschaft und Statistik*, 1965, *10*, 670-674.

Wirtschafts- und Sozialwissenschaftliches Institut des Deutschen Gewerkschaftsbundes GmbH (WSI) (Ed.) *Die Lebenslage älterer Menschen in der Bundesrepublik Deutschland, Köln: Bund Verl., 1975.*

Empirical Research (Basic Studies and Analyses)

Arbeitsgruppe Alternsforschung, Altern—psychologisch gesehen. Braunschweig: Westermann, 1971.

Becker, K.F. *Emanzipation des Alters.* Gütersloh: Mohn, 1975.

Bleuel, H.P. *Alte Menschen in Deutschland.* München: Hanser, 1972, DTV (paper), 1975 (2nd ed. rev.)

Boetticher, K.W. *Aktiv im Alter* Düsseldorf; Econ. 1975.

Fülgraff, B. Alternssoziologie. *Archiv für die Wissenschaft und Praxis der sozialen Arbeit*, 1971, *2*, 120-132.

Gores, P. Die sozialen Verhaltensweisen alter Menschen, Phil. Diss., Univ. Köln, 1971.

Henke-Bernd, H. Das dritte Alter. *Theorie und Praxis der sozialen Arbeit*, 1976, *27*, 57-66.

Konrad Adenauer-Stiftung/Politische Akademie Eichholz (Ed.), *Anpassung oder Integration? Zur gesellschaftlichen Situation älterer Menschen*, Bonn: Eichholz, 1973.

Leben im Alter. Kommunikations- und Konsumverhalten. Ed. by Stern. Gruner und Jahr AG & Co., Hamburg, 1977.

Lehr, U. *Psychologie des Alterns.* Heidelberg: Quelle & Meyer, 1972.

Narr, H. *Soziale Probleme des Alters.* Stuttgart: Kolhammer, 1976.

Reimann, H., & H. Reimann. (Eds.) *Das Alter*, München: Goldmann, 1974.

Rosenmayr, L. Soziologie des Alters, König, R. (Ed.), *Handbuch der empirischen Soziologie*, vol. II. Stuttgart: Enke, 1969.

Rosenmayr, L., & Rosenmayr, H. Alte Menschen in Arbeitswelt und Familie. Bellebaum, A., H. Braun (Eds.), *Reader soziale Probleme, I: Empirische Befunde.* Frankfurt/New York: Herder & Herder, 1974.

Schenda, R. *Das Elend der alten Leute.* Düsseldorf; Patmos, 1972.

Schmelzer, H. & Tebert, W. *Alter und Gesellschaft.* Bonn: Eichholz, 1969.

Schneider, H.-D. *Sozialpsychologische Aspekte des Alterns.* Frankfurt: Fischer, 1974.

Schoeller, J., *Das Alter in der industriellen Gesellschaft*. Köln: Bachem, 1971.

Schreiber, T., & Blume, O. *Erhaltung der Selbständigkeit älterer Menschen.* Schriftenreihe des Bundesministeriums für Familie, Juger und Gesundheit, vol. 33. Stuttgart: Kohlhammer, 1976.

Sieber, G. *Die Altersrevolution*. Zürich/Köln: Benzinger, 1972, (2nd ed.) (paper). Reinbeck: Rowohlt, 1975.

Specht, K.G. (Ed.) *Neue Aufgaben in Familie und Beruf*. Stein/Nürnberg: Laetare, 1975.

Schubert, R. (Ed.) Herz und Atmungsorgane im Alter, Psychologie und Soziologie in der Gerontologie, *Veröff. der Dt. Ges. f. Gerontologie*, Bd. 1. Darmstadt: Steinkopf, 1968.

Schubert, R. (Ed.) Flexibilität der Altersgrenze, *Veröff der Dt. Ges. F. Gerontologie*, Bd. 2. Darmstadt: Steinkopff, 1969 (a)

Schubert, R. (Ed.) Aktuelle Probleme der Geriatrie, Geropsychologie, Gerosoziologie und Altenfürsorge. *Veröff. Dt. Ges. f. Gerontologie*, Bd. 3. Darmstadt: Steinkopff, 1969.

Störmer, A. Geroprophylaxe, Infektions- und Herzkrankheiten, Rehabilitation und Sozialstatus im Alter. *Veröff. der Dt. Ges. f. Gerontologie*, Bd. 4. Darmstadt: Steinkopff, 1970.

Tartler, R. *Das Alter in der modernen Gesellschaft*. Stuttgart: Enke. 1961.

Tews, H.P. *Soziologie des Alterns* (2nd ed.) Heidelberg: Quelle + Meyer, 1975.

Tismer, K.G., Lange, U., Erlemeier, N., & Tismer-Puschner, *Psychosoziale Aspekte der Situation älterer Menschen, Schriftenreihe des Bundesministeriums für Jugend, Familie und Gesundheit*, Bd. 28. Stuttgart: Kohlhammer, 1975.

Thomae, H. Angleitner, A., Grombach, H., & Schmitz-Scherzer, R. Determinanten und Varianten des Altersprozesses. Ein Bericht über die Bonner gerontologische Längsschnittstudie. *Aktuelle Gerontologie*, 1973, *3*, 359-377.

Thomae, H. (Ed.) *Patterns of Aging. Findings from the Bonn Longitudinal Study*. Basel/München: Karger, 1976.

Contributions to Theory

Eichelberger, H.W. Relative Deprivation im höheren Lebensalter. Phil. Diss., Univ. Freiberg, 1972.

Thomae, H. Die Bedeutung einer kognitiven Persönlichkeitstheorie für die Theorie des Alterns. *Ztschr. f. Gerontologie*, 1971, *4*, 8-18.

Thomae, H. Vergleichende Psychologie der Lebensalter. *Ztschr. f. Gerontologie*, 1974, *7*, 313-322.

Thomae, H. Psychologische Intervention im höheren Alterein neuer Ansatz in der Gerontologie. *Ztschr. f. Gerontologie*, 1975, *8*, 473-475. (a)

Thomae, H. Die Theorie der Entwicklungsaufgaben und die Altershteorie. *Ztschr. f. Gerontolgie*, 1975, *8*, 125-137. (b)

Special Problems

Social Policy

Achinger, H. Altenhilfe. *Nachrictendienst des Deutschen Vereins für öffentl. und priv. Fürsorge*, 1975, *55*, 268–278.

Behnreds, H. Der alte Mensch im Mittelpunkt. Gedanken über Menschen und Einrichtungen in der Altenhilfe. *Innere Mission*, 1972, *62*, 39-46.

Bellebaum, A., & Braun, H. (Eds.) *Reader Soziale Probleme*, vol. II: *Initiativen und Ma Bnahmen*. Frankfurt/New York: Herder & Herder, 1974.

Blume, O. *Möglichkeiten und Grenzen der Altenhilfe*. Tübingen: Mohr, 1968.

Dick, E. *Methoden der Analyse und Planung in der kommunalen Altenhilfe* (KGST-Gutachten). Göttingen: Stiftung VW, 1974.

Elzholz, G. *Altenhilfe als Gegenstand rationaler Infrastrukturplanung*. Hamburg: Weltarchiv, 1970.

Fülgraff, B. Offene Hilfen Für Alte und Pflegebedürftige. Blohmke, M., v. Ferber, C., Kisker, K.P., & Schaefer H. (Eds.), *Hdb. der Sozialmedizin*, Bd. III, Stuttgart: Enke, 1976.

Haag, G. Zur Bedeutung ambulanter Dienste in der Altenhilfe. *Blätter der Wohlfahrtspflege*, 1976, *6*, 132-138. (a)

Haag, G. Offene Hilfen in Beziehunge zur Alten- und Behindertenwohnungen. *Innere Mission*, 1972, *62*, 178-187. (b)

Haag, G. Möglichkeiten der Kooperation zwischen offener und stationärer Altenhilfe. *Das Altenheim*, 1974, *13*, 27-33.

Hartwieg, W. Offene Altenhilfe als Teil moderner Sozialarbeit. *Nachrichtendienst des Dt. Vereins f. öffentl. und priv. Fürsorge*, 1972, *52*, 207-211.

Inst. fur Sozialforschung und Gesellschaftspolitik, Köln and Inst. für Altenwohnbau, Köln, Auswertung verfügbarer Statistiken für die Altenhilfepolitik in Deutschland, Gutachten für das Bundesministerium für Jugend, Familie und Gesundheit, Bonn. 1974. (unpubl.)

Mayer, F. Hilfe für ältere Menschen als Aufgabe der Sozialarbeit. *Blätter der Wohlfahrtsplflege*, 1972, *119*, 297-99.

Offene soziale Dienste in der Altenhilfe. *Caritas-Korrespondenz*, 1974, *8/9*, 5-8.

Orbens, H. Erfahrungen bei Aufbau einer kommunalen Altenhilfe in einer süddeutschen Mittelstadt. *Ztschr. f. Gerontologie*, 1974, *7*, 304-311.

Paazig, M. Altenhilfe in der Bundesrepublik Deutschland und in West-Berlin, Frankfurt, 1971. (mimeo.)

Paazig, M. *Lebenshilfen für alte Menschen,* (4th ed. rev.) Frankfurt: Deutscher Verein für öffentl. und priv. Fürsorge, 1975.

Rustemeyer, J. Bedeutung und Funktion der offenen Altenhilfe. *Blätter der Wohlfahrtspflege* 1972, *119*, 138-142.

Housing

Dieck, M. Wohnen alter Menschen—Situationsanalyse und wohnungspolitische Schlufolgerungen. *Ztschr. f. Gerontologie*, 1973, *6*, 325-329.

Dieck, M. Wohnen alter Menschen—Wissenslücken und Forschungsdesiderate. *Ztschr. f. Gerontologie*, 1975, *8*, 381-382.

Dittrich, G. (Ed.) *Wohnen alter Menschen*. Stuttgart: DVA, 1972.

DIVO-Inmar GmbH. Die Wohnwünsche der Bundesbürger. Gutachten für das Bundesministerium des Inneren, Bonn 1974. (unpubl.)

Dringenberg, R. Neuere Aspekte der Wohnforschung. Ansätze und Ergebnisse einer Untersuchung des Wohnbedarfs älterer Menschen. *Ztschr. f. Gerontologie*, 1975, *8*, 383-399. (a)

Dringenberg, R. Altenwohnungen—Konzeptionen, Realitäten und Befragten-meinungen. *Ztschr. f. Gerontologie*, 1975, *8*, 400-412. (b)

Friedrich-Wussow, M. Wohnen alter Menschen aus der Sicht der Altenpläne. *Ztschr. f. Gerontologie*, 1975, *8*, 413-432.

Gro Bhans, H. Altengerechtes Wohnen—Wohnungen für alter Menschen. *Ztschr. f. Gerontologie*, 1974, *7*, 258-275.

Haag, G. Zur Wohnraumsituation alter Menschen. Eine Befragung von Besuchern von Altenclubs. *Blätter der Wohlfahrtsplfege*, 1971, *118*, 263-266.

Hinschützer, U. Soziogerontologische Forschungsergebnisse und ihre Umsetzung in Konzepte zur Veränderug der Wohnsituation älterer Menschen. *Ztschr. f. praktische Psychologie*, 1974, *13*, 211-217.

Hugues, T. Die altengerechte Wohnung. Diss. Ing., Univ. München, 1973.

Kiesau, G. Wer alt ist, soll nicht schlechter wohnen. Ergebnisse und Empfehlunger einer Studie des WSI. *Neue Heimat*, 1975, *1*, 13-24.

Schalhorn, K. *Wohnungen für alte Menschen. Altenheime, Wohnstifte, Seniorenezen-tren*. München: Callwey, 1973.

Problems of Institutionalization

Anthes, J. Zur Organisation des Altenheims. Ergebnisse einer Inhaltsanalyse der Hausordnungen von Altenheimen in Nordrhein-Westfalen und Bayern, *Ztschr. f. Gerontologie*, 1975, *8*, 433-450.

Bierhoff, H.W. & Schmitz-Scherzer, R. Die Einstellung alter Menschen zum Alten-heim. *Ztschr. f. Gerontologie*, 1974, *7*, 334-343.

Dittmer, C. Über den Zusammenhang von sozialem Vorurteil und Entmündigung alter Menschen, untersucht am Beispiel von Altenheimordnungen. Dipl. Arb., Univ. Gie Ben, 1975.

Englbrecht, R. Zur soziologischen Problematik der Heimsituation im Alter. Dipl. Arb., Univ. München, 1974.

Fisseni, H.J. Zur Situation von Frauen in Altersheimen: Ergebnisse einer Tageslauf-analyse. *Akteuelle Gerontologie*, 1974, *4*, 29-32. (a)

Fisseni, H.J. Psychologische Auswirkungen von Dauer des Heimaufenthaltes und sozialer Schicht. *Aktuelle Gerontologie*, 1974, *4*, 33-38. (b)

Fisseni, H.J. Anpassung an das Leben im Altersheim. *Aktuelle Gerontologie*, 1974, *4*, 711-715. (c)

Fisseni, H.J. Untersuchungen zum Leben im Altersheim. *Ztschr. f. Gerontologie*, 1974, *7*, 335-375. (d)

Gössling, S. Der alte Mensch im Heim. *Aktuelle Gerontologie*, 1973, *3*, 511-514.

Gössling, S., Knopp, A. *Handkommentar zum Heimgesetz*. Hannover: Vincentz, 1976.

Jansen, W. Die Vorbereitung auf das Altenheim. *Aktuelle Gerontologie*, 1971, *1*, 285-289.

Lehr, U. Institutionalisierung älterer Menschen als psychologisches Problem—Ergebnisse der empirischen Forschung. Schubert, R. (Ed.), 1968, 344-352.

Lohmann, S. *Die Lebenssituation älterer Menschen in der geschlossenen Alters-fürsorge*. Hannover: Vincentz, 1970.

Noam, E. *Im Altenheim leben, Kleinere Schriften*, Nr. 29, Frankfurt: Dt. Verein für öffentl. und priv. Fürsorge, 1971.

Rudinger, G. Psychologische Auswirkungen von Dauer des Heimaufenthaltes und sozialer Schicht. *Aktuelle Gerontologie*, 1974, *4*, 33-38.

Spauwen-Micka, E. Anpassung an das Heim. *Aktuelle Gerontologie*, 1974, *4*, 705-709.

Störmer, A. Heimversorgung der alten Menschen in gesunden und kranken Tagen, Schubert, R. (ed.), 1968, 326-333.

Job and Retirement

Behr, v., M. Beruf und Berufsaufgabe—Probleme der Pensionierung. Dipl. Arb., Univ. München, 1973. (unpubl.)

Blume, O. Problematik von Aussagen über ältere Arbeitnehmer im Betrieb. *Aktuelle Gerontologie*, 1972, *2*, 103-110.

Fehm, K. Elemente einer systematischen Altersökonomie. Das Altenproblem in Wirschaftstheorie und Politik. Diss. rer. pol., Erlangen, 1972.

Fülgraff, B. Substitute für Arbeit im Alter? *Aktuelle Gerontologie*, 1972, *2*, 455-459.

Klauder, W., Kühlewind, G., & Schnur P. Zu den Beschäftigungstendenzen älterer Arbeitnehmer Modellrechnung nach Wirtschaftszweigen bis 1980. *Arbeitsmarkt und Berufsforschung*, 1971, *4*, 1-13.

Landwehrmann, F. Älterer Arbeitnehmer—eine gemachte Problemgruppe. *Ztschr. f. Gerontologie*, 1975, *8*, 255-257.

Ledig, P.K. Die produktive Beschäftigung älterer Angestellter und Arbeiter, Denkschrift, 1971. (mimeo.)

Lehr, U. Der ältere Mensch im Arbeitsproze b-Stereotypen und Tatsachen. *Ztschr. f. Gerontologie*, 1975, *8*, 306-314.

Lehr, U., Dreher, G., & Schmitz-Scherzer, R. Der ältere Arbeitnehmer im Betrieb. *Handbuch der Psychologie*, 9, (2nd ed.). Göttingen, 1970, 778-827.

Ministerium für Arbeit, Gesundheit und Soziales des Landes Nordrhein-Westfalen (MAGS), *Der Ältere in der industriellen*. Arbeitswelt: Düsseldorf, 1974.

Naegele, G. Die Problematik älterer Arbeitnehmer aus sozialpolitischer Sicht. *Ztschr. f. Gerontologie*, 1975, *8*, 238-252.

Paul, H.A. Unfallgefährdung älterer Arbeitnehmer. *Ztschr. f. Gerontologie*, 1975, *8*, 266-276.

Pillardy, E. *Arbeit und Alter*. Stuttgart: Enke, 1973.

Pohl, H -J. *Ältere Arbeitnehmer. Ursachen und Folgen ihner beruflichen Abwertung*. Campus Paperbacks, Frankfurt, 1976.

Schäfer, H. Sozialmedizinische Probleme des alternden Menschen im Beruf. *Aktuelle Gerontologie*, 1974, *2*, 71-76.

Schaefer, H. Sozialer Kontakt—ein Risiko des älteren Arbeitnehmers, *Ztschr. f. Gerontologie*, 1975, *8*, 258-265.

Schmidt, H. Das Problem der beruflichen Anpassung von älteren Arbeitnehmern im Bereich hoch technischer Arbeitsplätze. in der industriellen Produktion. *Aktuelle Gerotonlogie*, 1974, *4*, 21-28. (a)

Schmidt, H. Der ältere Arbeitnehmer am automatisierten Arbeitsplatz. *Aktuelle Gerontologie*, 1974, 791-780. (b)

Stingl, J. Der alternde Mensch und der Arbeitsmarkt. *Aktuelle Gerontologie*, 1972, *2*, 83-88.

Stopp, K. *Arbeitnehmer im Übergang vom Arbeitsleben in den Ruhestand.* Kübel-Stiftung, Bensheim-Auerback, 1971.

Thomae, H. Zur Problematik des älteren Arbeitnehmers. *Ztschr. f. Gerontologie* 1972, *5*, 147-158. (a)

Thomae, H. Veränderungen der beruflichen Leistungsfahigkeit in psychologischer Sicht. *Aktuelle Gerontologie*, 1972, *2*, 89-96. (b)

Thomae, H., & Lehr, U. *Beruflich Leistungsfähigkeit im mittleren und höheren Erwachsenenalter.* Göttingen: Schwartz, 1973.

Viebahn, W. Stellung und Einstellung des alten Menschen zur Arbeit und Arbeitslosigkeit. *Aktuelle Gerontologie*, 1971, *1*, 487-493.

Weltz, F. Erwerbsbereitschaft der Frauen. *Mitt. aus der Arbeitsmarkt-und Berufsforschung, 1971, No. 2.*

Social Behavior and Social Contacts

Bierhoff, W.W. & Bierhoff-Alfermann, D. Zur Veränderung der Einstellung zur jungen Generation bei älteren Menschen. *Aktuelle Gerontologie*, 1975, *5*, 281-290.

Bungard, W. *Isolation und Einsamkeit im Alter. Eine sozialpsychologische Studie.* Köln: Hanstein, 1975.

Erlemeier, N. & Angleiter, A. Unterschungen zur "Rigidität" im höheren Alter. *Ztschr. f. Gerontologie*, 1971, *4*, 194-207.

Fissoni, H.J. Sinn and Unsinn von Aktivierung im Alter. *Das Altenheim*, 1975, *14*, 243-250.

Kühn, D. Plagemann, K., & Schmitz-Scherzer, R. Ökologische Determinanten der Mobilität —ein Beitrag zum Problem der Anpassung. *Aktuelle Gerontologie*, 1975, *5*, 47-50.

Lehr, U. Psychologische Voraussetzungen und Hindernisse bei der Aktivierung älterer Menschen. *Das Altenheim*, 1973, 95-100.

Lehr, U. Der ältere Mensch in der Familie. *Aktuelle Gerontologie*, 1975, *5*, 539-550.

Merker, H. *Generationsgegnsätze. Eine empirische Erkundungsstudie über die Einstellung Erwachsener zur Jugend.* Darmstadt: Thesen Verl. 1973. (a)

Merker, H. Jugend und Erziehung im Erleben alterer Menschen, Ztschr. f. Gerontologie, 1973, *6*, 296-306. (b)

Olbrich E. Veränderung der Sozialkontakte und Anpassungsprobleme im Alter. *Aktuelle Gerontologie*, 1974, *4*, 767-770.

Olbrich, E., & H. J. Fisseni. Konstanz und Veränderung der Rollenstruktur im Alter. Lehr, U., & Weinert, F.E. (Eds.), *Entwicklung und Persönlichkeit.* Stuttgart: Kohlhammer, 1975.

Renner, M.M.Th. Strukturen sozialer Teilhabe im hohen Lebensalter. Phil. Diss., Univ. Bonn, 1969.

Schmitz-Scherzer, R. Konstanz und Variabilität im Alltagsverhalten Älterer—eine Langsschnittanalyse über 5 Jahre. *Ztschr. f. Gerontologie*, 1975, *8*, 113-114.

Schmitz-Scherzer, R., & Kühn, D. Zur Situation der 50-65 jährigen Menschen in Braunschweig. Gutachten für das Bundesministerium für Jugend, Familie und Gesundheit, Bonn, 1976. (unpubl.)

Schmitz-Scherzer, R., Kühn, D., Plagemann, K., & Schick, J. Untersuchungen zur Mobilität im höheren Alter. *Aktuelle Gerontologie*, 1975, *5*, 351-364.

Schneider, H.D. *Soziale Rollen im Erwachsenenalter*. Frankfurt: Thesen Verl., 1970.

Schneider, H.P., Einflu bfaktoren auf die Anpassung im Erwachsenenalter, *Aktuelle Gerontologie*, 1975, *5*, 217-228.

Sokoll, U., Bentz, K., & Schmidt, J. Selbsteinschätzung sporttreibender Männer im Alter. *Ztschr. f. Gerontologie*, 1974, *7*, 255-257.

Tausch, A. Die Auswirkung allgemeiner Sozialkontakte sowie gezielter Kontakte in Form psychologisch hilfreicher Gespräche mit alten Menschen. *Aktuelle Gerontologie*, 1974, *4*, 647-656.

Tews, H.P., & Schwägler, G. Großeltern—ein vernachlässigtes Problem gerontologischer und familiensoziologischer Forschung. *Ztschr. f. Gerontologie*, 1973, *6*, 284-295.

Thomae, H., Anpassungsprobleme im höheren Alter—aus psychologischer Sicth. *Aktuelle Gerontologie*, 1974, *4*, 647-656.

Tümmers, H. *Sexualität im Alter*, Köln: Böhlau, 1976.

Urban, U. Isolation und Einsamkeit der alten Menschen—eine Literaturubersicht. Dipl. Arb., Univ. Koln, 1973.

Leisure

Becker, F.K. Freizeit und Alter. *Ztschr. f. Gerontologie*, 1974, *7*, 235-244.

Kühn, D., & Plagemann, K. Probleme der Altersfreizeit in der kommunalen Sozialplanung. *Ztschr. f. Gerontologie*, 1974, *7*, 288-303.

Schmitz-Scherzer, R. *Freizeit im Alter*. Düsseldorf: Schwann, 1973.(a)

Schmitz-Scherzer, R. (Ed.) *Freizeit—eine problemorienterte Textsammlung*. Frankfurt: Akad. Verl. Ges., 1973. (b)

Schmitz-Scherzer, R. Veränderungen des Freizeitverhaltens. *Aktuelle Gerontologie*, 1975, *5*, 103-106. (a)

Schmitz-Scherzer, R. *Alter und Freizeit*. Stuttgart: Kohlhammer, 1975. (b)

Learning and Education

Abele, M. Aspekte zur Bildung und Weiterbildung von älteren Menschen. *Blätter der Wohlfahrtspflege*, 1973, *120*, 295-298.

Ahlrichs, G., et. al. Chancen und Möglichkeiten einer Weiterbildung älterer Menschen. Hannover, Pädag. Hochsch., 1973. (mimeo.)

Autorenkollektiv Hannover. Überlegungen zur Didaktik einer Bildungsarbeit mit älteren Menschen. *Hess. Blätter f. Volksbildung*, 1973, *4*, 348-361.'

Bauer, A. Soziale und psychische Voraussetzungen des Lernens im höheren Lebensalter. *Hess. Blätter f. Volksbildung*, 1972, *3*, 257-268.

Bechtler, H., & Radebold, H. Ein Trainingsmodell im Arbeitsfeld der sozialen Gerontologie, *Aktuelle Gerontologie*, 1973, *3*, 663-666.

Beer, U. *Altern und Bildung*. Braunschweig: Westermann, 1976.

Brandenburg, A. *Der Lernerfolg im Erwachsenenalter*. Göttingen: Schwartz, 1974.(a)

Brandenburg, A. Alter und Lernleistung. *Bestimmungsgründe des Lernverhaltens Erwachsener*. *Hess. Blätter f. Volksbildung*, 1974, *4*, 277-292.(b)

Breloer, G. Lebensproblematik als Organisationsprinzipder Altenbildung. *Erwachsenenbildung*, 1974, *3*, 104-111.

Breloer, G. Altenbildung als ein Studiengebiet der Erwachsenenpädagogik. *VHS im Westen*, 1973, *25*, 120-124. (a)

Breloer, G. Zur Vermittlungsproblematik der Altensforschung-Aufgaben der Erwachsenenbildung. *Aktuelle Gerontologie*, 1973, *3*, 685-695. (b)

Fluck, B. *Weiterbildung im Alter*, Weinheim: Beltz, 1977.

Fülgraff, B. Lernen in der zweiten Lebenshälfte. Überlegungen in lebenslanger Sozialisation. *Hess. Blätter f. Volksbildung*, 1972, *3*, 249-256.

Fulgraff, B. Learning about old age. Models for adult education, Paper presented at the 10th Intern. Congress of Gerontology, Jerusalem, 1975. (unpubl.)

Fülgraff, B. Der problem- und teilnehmeorientierte Ansatz in der Altenbildung. Vortrag auf dem Kongress der Deutschen Gesellschaft für Gerontologie, Berlin, 1976.

Goeken, A. (Ed.) *Gruppenarbeit mit älteren Menschen. Ein Werkbuch (3rd rev. ed.)*. Freiburg: Lambertus, 1975.

Haag, G. Vom Tätigsein im Alter—Forderungen an Wirtschaft und Sozialarbeit. *Ztschr. f. Gerontologie*, 1974, *7*, 245-254.

Heemskerk, J.J. Gedächtnis und Lernleistungen im höheren Erwachsenenalter. *Aktuelle Gerontologie*, 1974, *4*, 9-20.

Hubrich, H.U. Der alternde Mensch in der modernen Gesellschaft—auch ein pädagogisches Problem. *Aktuelle Gerontologie*, 1972 *2*, 473-480.

Hüther, J. Gegen Vorurteile über berufsrelevante Lernfähigkeiten im Erwachsenenalter. *Ztschr. f. Gerontologie*, 1976, *9*, 36-39.

Kallmeyer, G., Breloer, G., Ebel, M., Fülgraff, B., Recktenwald, H., & Pilwousek, I. *Lernen im Alter. Analysen und Modelle zur Weiterbildung*. Grafenau: Lexika Verl., 1976.

Kehler, J. Wozu Weiterbildung für Ältere und über das Älterwerden? *Hess. Blätter f. Volksbildung* 1974. *3*, 233-241.

Lehr, U. Probleme der Weiterbildung im Erwachsenenalter und Alter. *Aktuelle Gerontologie*, 1972, *2*, 713-720.

Lehr, U. & Thomae, H. *Studien zum Lernproblem Erwachsener, Gutachten f. den Dt. Bildungsrat*, Bonn, 1969.

Löwe, H. *Lernpsychologie. Einführung in die Lernpsychologie des Erwachsenenalters*, Berlin (Ost): VEB Deutscher Verlag der Wissenschaften, 1972.

Meyer-Dettum, B. Erwachsenenbildung im Altersheim, Dip. Arbeit, Univ. Oldenburg, 1976.

Oesterreich, K. Bildung für ältere Menschen, *Ztschr. f. Gerontologie*, 1975, *8*, 145-153.

Olbrich, E., & Schuster, M. Lernen im Erwachsenenalterein theoretischer Beitrag, *Ztschr. f. Gerontologie*, 1976, *9*, 3-17.

Petzold, H. & Bubolz, E. (Eds.) *Bildungsarbeit mit alten Menschen*. Stuttgart: Klett, 1976.

Pina, J. Erfordernisse und Möglichkeiten der Aus- und Weiterbildung im Bereich der Altenarbeit—dargestellt am Beispiel der Grobstadt Berlin. *Aktuelle Gerontologie*, 1973, *2*, 659-662.

Polemann, O. Education permanente für die ältere Generation. *Hess. Blätter f. Volksbildung*, 1972, *22*, 269-275.

Radebold, H., Aus-und Fortbildung in Geriatrie/Gerontologie—Bilanz und Erfordernisse. *Aktuelle Gerontologie*, 1973, *3*, 651-653, 677-683.

Radebold, H., Bechtler, H., & Pina, I., *Psychosoziale Arbeit mit älteren Menschen*. Freiburg: Lambertus, 1973.

Recktenwald, H. Didaktische Probeme einer Weiterbildung der älteren Generation. *Hess. Blätter f. Volksbildung*, 1972, *3*, 269-275.

Recktenwald, H. Autonomes und kompetentes Verhalten. Lernziel einer Weterbildung älterer Menschen. *Anpassung oder Integration?* Bonn: Eichholz, 1973.

Rudinger, G. Determinanten der intellektuellen Leistung im höheren Alter. Phil. Diss., Bonn, 1971.

Ruprecht, H. *Lernen für das Älterwerden*. Heidelberg; Quelle + Meyer, 1972.

Ruprecht, H. Das Problem der Altenbildung in der Erwachsenenbildung. *Erwachsenbildung*, 1974, *3*, 99-103.

Schenda, R. Education permanente in Richtung auf das Alter. Prinzipien einer sozialgeragogischen Bildung der Jüngeren, Göttingen, 1974. (unpubl.)

Schmitz-Scherzer, R. Einige Aspekte zur Lernfahig Keit im Alter als Voraussetzung für die Bildungsarbeit mit alten Menschen, *Aktuelle Gerontologie*, 1975, *5*, 439-443.

Schmitz-Scherzer, R. Lernen im Alter. *Ztschr. f. Gerontologie*, 1976, *1*, 1-2.

Schneider, H.D. *Bildung für das dritte Lebensalter. Der vergessene Bildungnotstand*. Zürich: Brenzinger, 1976.

Sitzmann, G.-H. (Ed.) *Lernen für das Alter*, Diessen: Huber, 1970.

Sitzmann, G.-H. Zur Situation und Aufgabe der Altenbildung. *Das Forum*, 1971, *11*, 17-39.

Sitzmann, G.-H. Weiterbildung im dritten Lebensalter. *Ztschr. f. Gerontologie* 1976, *9*, 40-57.

Skawran, P.R. *Die Intelligenz des älteren Menschen*. Stuttgart: Enke, 1971.

Sterzenbach, A. Geistige Arbeit mit älteren Menschen. *Blätter der Wohlfahrspflege*, 1971, *118*, 169-171.

Stiefvater, A., Bildungsarbeit in der älteren Generation. *Erwachsenenbildung*, 1974, *20*, 111-114.

Stosberg, M. Die Massenmedien im Prozess der Rehabilitierung alter Menschen. *Aktuelle Gerontologie*, 1972, *9*, 553-562.

Tews, H.P., Grenzen der Altenbildung. *Ztschr. f. Gerontologie*, 1976, *9*, 58-72.

Tietgens, H. Bildungsmöglichkeiten für ältere Menschen. *Innere Mission*, 1971, *61*, 10-16; repr. in: Becker, K.F. (Ed.), *Alter-doch dabei*. Stuttgart: Klotz, 1973.

Vath, R. *Das Altern lernen*. Hannover: Schroedel, 1973.

Verres-Muckel, M. *Lernprobleme Erwachsener*. Stuttgart: Kohlhammer, 1974.

Preparation for Retirement

Becker, F.K. *Älter—doch dabei! Ruhestand in der Leistungsgelleschaft zwischen Krise und Möglichkeiten*, (2nd rev. ed.). Stuttgart: Klotz, 1973.

Blume, O. Vorbereitung auf das Alter aus gesellschaftspolitischer Sicht. *Aktuelle Gerontologie*, 1971, *1*, 267-271.

Deutsche Gesellschaft für Personalfuhrung; Institut Mensch und Arbeit (Ed.), *Die dritte Lebensrunde. Gut Vorbereiten, besser gestalten.* München: Verl. Mensch und Arbeit, 1975.

Dreher, G. Auseinandersetzungen mit dem bevorstehenden Austritt aus dem Berufsleben. Eine Untersuchung bei Arbeitern und Angestellten in der Stahlindustrie. Störmer, A. (Ed.), 1970, *8*, 118-124.

Evangelische Akademie Bad Boll: Lernziel Ruhestand. *Der ältere Arbeitnehmer, aktuelle Gespräche*, 1975, *23*, Sonderheft 1.

Fuchs, E. Die Vorbereitung auf das Alter als Aufgabe der Gemeindearbeit. *Die Mitarbeit*, 1975, *24* 264-271.

Fülgraff, B., et al., *Bildungsurlaub "Vorbereitung auf Ruhestand und Alter", eine Dokumentation.* Arbeitsberichte der Kreisvolkshochschule Osnabrück e.V., Osnabrück, 1976.

Kallmeyer, G. *Planung des dritten Lebensalters. Kursmodell für einen Bildungsurlaub.*

Kuhlenkamp, D., et. al., *Didaktische Modelle für ben Bildungsurlaub.* Grafenau: Lexika, 1975

Kuhne, B., & Krug, B. (Eds.) *Vorbereitung auf das Alter. Veranstaltungsangebot— Literatur.* Deutsches Zentrum für Altersfragen e.V., Berlin, 1976.

Pauls, A.H. Sozialmedizinische Gesichtspunkte bei der Vorbereitung auf das Alter. *Aktuelle Gerontologie*, 1971, *1*, 272-277.

Radebold, H. Vorbereitung auf das Altern und Hilfe im Alter. Das Berliner Modell "Informationen für Senioren." *Ztschr. f. Gerontologie*, 1976, *9*, 73-80.

Schneider, H.D. Wie wirksam sind Vorbereitungskurse auf den Ruhestand? *Ztschr. f. Gerontologie*, 1975, *8*, 288-294.

Schneider, W. (Ed.) *Vorbereitung auf Ruhestand und Alter im Bildungsurlaub.* Arbeitsberichte der Kreisvolkshochschule Osnabrück, Osnabrück, 1974.

Schubert, R., & Störmer, A. (Eds.) *Vorbereitung auf das Alter.* München: Banaschewski, 1974.

Sitzmann, G. Die Organisation der Vorbereitung auf das Alter als pädagogisches Problem. *Aktuelle Gerontologie*, 1973, *3*, 695-713.

Sitzmann, G. *Kuratorium Deutsche Altenhilfe, Bundesministerium für Jugend, Familie und Gesundheit.* Vorbereitung auf das Alter, Köln: KDA, 1975.

Störmer, A. Vorbereitung auf das Alter als Problem der Gerohygiene. *Aktuelle Gerontologie*, 1971, *1*, 243-246.

Winter, J. Vorbereitung auf Ruhestand und Alter in der Schweiz. *Ztschr. f. Gerontologie*, 1976, *9*, 81-90.

FINLAND

LEIF SOURANDER*

THE AGED POPULATION

Eleven percent of the total population in Finland—about 500,000 persons—is 65 or over. Finland is to a great extent an agricultural society, but industrialization and urbanization have developed rapidly. The social security system includes national pensions, health insurance, and a well-developed social welfare system. Attitudes toward the aged have changed since World War II. With the development of social security, the responsibility for the welfare of the aged has moved from family, relatives, and private organization to state and community. There is a rapid increase in the number of services for the aged, including domiciliary help, advice, geriatric care, and housing projects. Larger towns have well-developed services for the aged, but in rural regions and small towns, the services are still often limited and unsatisfactory. The problem of the single disabled old person is, despite services, a great problem for both medical and social authorities.

RESEARCH

Societas Gerontologica Fennica

Gerontological research was initiated in Finland by the Societas Gerontologica Fennica (SGF), the national gerontological society founded in 1948; it is a private, voluntary, nonprofit organization. The most active member of the society was the late professor Eeva Jalavisto, who was president from 1952 to 1964. Professor Jalavisto did much for gerontology in Finland; her enthusiasm and energy were well known, even abroad.

SGF has 115 members; 80 percent are physicians and 20 percent are chiefly psychologists and sociologists or others working in the field of gerontology, working in the care of the elderly, or generally interested in the objectives of the society. The SGF board is comprised of the president, vice-president,

*The author is indebted to Professor Eino Heikkinen, professor of gerontology, University of Tampere, and to Assistant Professor Eva Hirsjarvi, Koskela Hospital in Helsinki for valuable information regarding research programs.

secretary, treasurer, and three board members. The society is a member of the International Association of Gerontology and the Nordisk Gerontologisk Forening, a Scandinavian gerontological association.

The principal objective of the SGF is to support research in the field of gerontology, give information about research activities, coordinate research, and facilitate all efforts to improve knowledge about the problems of aging and the aged. Other objectives are to develop education in gerontology, arrange courses in gerontology, including postgraduate education, organize meetings and symposia, and establish and develop international contacts and relations in the field of gerontology. Every three years the board nominates the receiver of the Eeva Jalavisto Award for Gerontological Research.

Research Center for the Aged

The SGF's Research Center for the Aged, supervised by Professor Matti Bergstrom, professor in physiology at the Institute of Physiology, University of Helsinki, has focused its interest on studying the central nervous system and the physiological changes caused by age. It especially studies the information processing ability of the aged in relation to the level of consciousness (vigilance), using psychophysiological tests in connection with electroencephalogram measurement. The program also includes the study of the effect of environmental stimulus pressure on psychophysiological performance.

Gerontology at the University of Tampere

The academic chair of gerontology was founded at the University of Tampere, Faculty of Medicine, in 1975. The professorship is situated at the Department of Public Health Sciences, a multidisciplinary department. Research work is done in cooperation with the Department of Public Health, University of Jyvaskyla, Faculty of Physical and Health Education. Some research programs have also carried out in cooperation with Sports Research Center, University of Turku. It is currently carrying out five research programs.

The first is to measure functional aging. The normal aging of humans is not well understood, so there is a need for methods to measure functional aging (Heikkinen et al., 1974). Methods have been adapted and developed to measure skin elasticity and skin vibration threshold. Attempts have also been made to measure changes related to aging in various biopsy specimens (skin and skeletal muscle, for example). Functional aging has been measured in various populations in order to find out how aging processes appear in Finnish populations and in different regions. Variation in aging processes among men who have been in various occupations for several decades has also been studied.

The results suggest that significant differences exist in aging processes between different occupational groups (Heikkinen et al., 1975). The multivariate statistical analyses have shown that the length of education is one of the most important predictors of functional aging.

The second research program is to measure the effect of lifelong physical activity on aging. The purpose is to find out possible beneficial and deleterious effects of habitual aerobic training. The results obtained so far suggest that men in habitual physical training benefit from their interest concerning functions relevant to physical training (Suominen and Heikkinen, 1975). On the other hand the rate of aging itself seems not to be influenced by training, and no effect appeared in the parameters that are not directly involved in physical exercise.

The third program is trying to determine the physical trainability of elderly men and women and to see how such training programs should be organized. The results obtained thus far indicate that the relative trainability is good even at old age. Improvements appear in circulatory and respiratory functions, and the metabolism of skeletal muscles is enhanced (Suominen et al., 1977, in press). No untoward effects occur if training is carried out under the supervision of well-educated teachers and if appropriate medical control is done before starting the training program.

The fourth research program is trying to characterize the health status, living habits, and related social conditions among 66-year-old persons living in Jyvaskyla, a town of about seventy thousand inhabitants in central Finland. Results of the cross-sectional part of the study have been published (Heikkinen et al., 1976; Aunola et al., 1976). The cohort has now been followed for four years, and the first longitudinal investigations have been carried out to reveal living conditions and life-styles that predict longevity and/or impairment of health status and functional capability.

The last research program is investigating relations of physical activity and development and metabolism of various connective tissues. Mainly animal experiments have been carried out, but there have also been analyses of biopsy samples (skin and skeletal muscles) obtained from athletes, and their sedentary controls have been performed in addition to various physiological measurements. The results obtained thus far indicate that connective tissues respond to phyical training by metabolic and even structural alterations, and some of the effects can be interpreted to counteract age-related changes in connective tissues (Kiiskinen and Heikkinen, 1976; 1976a).

Research Programs in Helsinki

The following research programs are in progress in Koskela Hospital, the largest municipal geriatric hospital in Helsinki:

1. Epidemiological, clinical, and biochemical studies of dementia.
2. Study of the effect of pituitary peptides on senile organic brain syndrome.
3. Oxazepam, temazepam, and lorazepam as sleeping aids in psychogeriatric patients.
4. Nixotine as an antidepressant in psychogeriatric patients.
5. Follow-up study of old patients in domiciliary care in Helsinki.
6. Digoxin intoxication in hospitalized elderly patients. Correlation of age, activity (bedridden or ambulant), liver and kidney function, serum electrolytes and proteins, and medication to serum digoxin level and symptoms of intoxication.
7. Surgical mortality in patients over 70 years; effect of age, type of operation, general condition, and concomitant illnesses.
8. Postoperative deep vein thrombosis in ambulant and bedridden elderly; possible role of dehydration.
9. Effect of mental state on the operative complications and surgical mortality in the elderly.

At the Myllypuro Geriatric Hospital, the following research programs are in progress:

1. Clinical mycology in the aged.
2. Yeast fungus flora in patients in a geriatric hospital.
3. Occurrence of deep mycoses in geriatric patients in Finland.
4. Some observations of the use of lactulose in the treatment of obstipation in geriatric patients.
5. Significance of yeast fungi in aged persons.
6. The use of lactulose and the fungus flora of the microfungus flora in the aged and the use of 5-fluorocytosine in mycoses.
7. Urinary tract infections and treatment with new antibiotic especially in Pseudomonas infections.
8. Medical aspects of domiciliary care of old people.

Research Programs in Turku

At the City Hospital of Turku, the research programs cover several topics, including epidemiological research on the health of the aged in Turku (a longitudinal research program); urinary tract infection, epidemiology, follow-up, etiological factors, prognosis, and treatment, and the epidemiology of uremia in the aged; cerebrovascular diseases, extracerebral factors affecting the haemodynamics of the brain, and the effect of treatment; posopoplectic epilepsy; and epidemiology of myocardial infarction in the elderly.

Epidemiological research concerning the occurrence of diseases and different factors affecting the health of the aged, including the collection of demographic facts and estimations of the need of care, has been conducted in Turku since 1963 (Ruikka et al., 1966). The examined persons comprised four groups of women and four groups of men over 65 divided into five-year age groups. The statistical department of the National Pension Institute, where all Finnish citizens are registered, selected by computer these eight samples at random. The sizes of the groups were determined so that the number of representatives from the oldest age groups were sufficiently large. The randomly chosen persons represented about 5 percent of the total population over 65 years of age in Turku. The state of health of every examined person was evaluated on the basis of the results of the interviews, medical examinations, laboratory tests, and roentgenographic recordings. The total number selected at random was 481 persons. Of these, 405 (84 percent) arrived for the examinations.

The sample was reexamined five years later in 1968. For those who had died, the causes and time of death were registered on behalf of the authorities, and the hospital records and autopsy records were checked. The subjects still alive were called for reexamination. According to the experiences of the earlier investigation, the interest was focused on cardiovascular diseases and the analysis of the urinary findings and social circumstances. Eighty-seven percent of all subjects had died or were reexamined; 78 percent of those still alive were examined (Sourander, Ruikka, and Kasanen, 1970). The follow-up of this cohort is still in progress.

The special problem of urinary tract infection has been separately studied using the same samples (Sourander, 1966). The follow-up of the subjects continues (Sourander and Kasanen, 1972). The interest has further focused on nephrology in the aged, etiological factors in urinary tract infection, treatment, and prognosis (Sourander, 1973).

Another topic of interest in Turku is cerebrovascular disease, particularly the relations of organic brain syndromes, cerebrovascular circulation, and circulatory disorders (Sourander and Sourander, 1977). The research program includes a study of the effect of cyclandelate upon sensory parameters in patients recovering from cerebrovascular accidents (*Angiology*, in press) and a study of the correlations between electroencephalogram findings and cardiac rhythm disturbances detected by continuous electrocardiogram recording. Postapoplectic epilepsy has been studied in the aged. In progress is a research program that outlines different static and brain-scanning findings in aged patients with cerebral infarction.

A longitudinal study of renal failure in the aged in southwestern Finland was carried out in Turku, Helsinki, and Loimaa between April 1, 1973, and March 31, 1977. During the first three years all available information was collected to identify cases of uremia (patients with a serum creatinine value more than 230 umol/l) in an area that comprised the towns of Turku and Loimaa and ten rural communities where the patients were served by the Loimaa district hospital. Patients who were not hospitalized were asked to attend a nefrologic outpatient service, where they were interviewed and examined. The patients were reexamined every six months throughout the study. During the fourth year, new members entered the cohort.

Of the 191,892 area residents, 21,503 were 65 years or older; 668 cases of uremia were registered and divided in subgroups according to the diagnosis. Heart failure and hypertension was also registered. In the longitudinal approach, special attention is paid to the prognosis of uremia in the aged, the degree of uremia, renal findings, and relations to heart failure, hypertension, and diabetes mellitus. The findings in the aged are compared with the corresponding findings in the younger groups. The aim of this study is to focus on one single parameter, the serum creatinine value, and compare it with a number of clinical and social variables. The major question that this study seeks to answer is what characterizes the old uremic patients and how they differ from younger patients. It also tries to determine the prognosis during the follow-up and the recorded variables that influence the prognosis. The cohort has now been examined and followed up.

Another longitudinal research program in progress in Turku concerns the ecology of urinary bacterial flora in long-stay aged hospital patients under two regimens: a very restricted attitude to the use of antibiotics and a freer administration. The cohort comprises the patients of three hospital wards; the duration of the follow-up, which started in May 1977, is one to two years. Repeated bacteriological checks will be performed during the follow-up (Sourander, Juva, and Jarvinen).

A clinical and epidemiological study of myocardial infarction in the elderly has been performed at the City Hospital of Turku by V. Konu; it had a one-year follow-up. The study was part of a research program still in progress: the study of the characteristics of different heart diseases in the aged (Acta Med. Scand. 1977). Between March 1, 1972, and April 4, 1973, all patients from the city of Turku over 65 years with acute myocardial infarction—404 cases—were followed. Age- and sex-matched controls to 127 consecutive patients were selected by computer from the population register of Turku. In order to compare the presenting symptoms in the elderly patients with the presenting symptoms in younger patients, an additional control group was used. It was found that patients with chest pain made a better recovery from infarction than patients with painless infarction. The hospital mortality for patients with chest pain was 24 percent and for those without chest pain 65 percent; 23 percent of the patients had a painless infarction. The most common presenting symptom was acute chest pain, which was present in 65 percent. Other common symptoms were dyspnea (20 percent), loss of consciousness (9 percent), vertigo and weakness (7 percent), recurrent vomiting (7 percent), and confusional state (5 percent). Of the classical risk factors, only diabetes and a high serum cholesterol level were found to be of significance in the elderly.

Other topics that have been studied in Turku include the epidemiology, etiology, and the natural course of Parkinson's disease in the elderly (by

Professor U. Rinne and associates at the University Central Hospital); brain dopamine metabolism and the relief of Parkinsonismus (also studied by Rinne and associates); elastofibroma, a disease of the aged (studied by Professor O. Jarvi and associates of the Department of Pathology, University of Turku); and an activation program for the elderly (by Professor V. Kallio and associates, University of Turku).

A wound healing research program in progress at the Institute of Forensic Medicine, University of Turku, is making a histochemical and biochemical study of the effect of aging on enzymes in wound healing; Professor J. Raekallio is heading the work. In order to study the effect of aging on the enzymatic response to injury, an experimental study was made on young (aged 2 months) and old (2 years) rats. Histochemically the wound enzymes appeared in the same chronological order both in the young and old animals, but in the young rats, the enzyme activity was manifold in intensity. Further, old animals required approximately twice as much time to attain the maximum intensity of enzyme activity. Biochemically the enzyme activity in the wounds of the old rats was less intense that that of the young ones. The age-dependent delay in the adaptive enzyme response is an important biochemical and histochemical parameter of aging.

Muscle injury in young and old rats, histological and microangiological study, the healing of muscle injury, the inflammatory cellular reactions, the regeneration of the muscular tissue, and the formation of connective tissue and capillary vessels are being studied in young and old rats by M. Jarvinen, A. Aho, M. Lehto, and H. Toivonen at the University of Turku.

PROGRAMS

Central League on Welfare for the Aged

The Central League on Welfare for the Aged coordinates the activities of 172 member associations. It acts in close cooperation with the government and the municipal authorities. The main objective of the league is to develop the social security and welfare of the aged. Some of the member associations run homes for the aged and service centers for the aged. Research programs comprise the development of domiciliary help and preretirement education.

Geriatric Care

Geriatric medicine is not now a clinical specialty in Finland. However, in the near future it will be a subspecialty of internal medicine. The aged generally receive their health care in community health centers. In case of hospital admission, they are served by the area hospitals and central hospitals. Some hospitals have a well-developed geriatric service system: Koskela

Hospital in Helsinki, the City Hospital of Turku, the Marjatta Hospital in Tampere, and the City Hospital of Oulu. The City Hospital of Turku has developed into a modern active geriatric center in Finland under the leadership of Professor Ilmari Ruikka. Special interest has focused on the rehabilitation of the aged since the late 1950s.

Gerontological Events

Recent gerontological events in Finland include the Gerontological Symposium held in Helsinki in November 1975 when the situation of geriatric medicine was discussed and gerontological papers were read. Sir Ferguson Anderson from Glasgow gave a lecture on geriatric medicine in the modern world. In May 1977 the Nordisk Gerontologisk Forening had its third Scandinavian congress of gerontology in Turku. Another important event was Medicine 77, held in Helsinki in January 1977. Two thousand doctors participated and followed the lectures, which focused on health problems of the aged and geriatric medicine.

REFERENCES

Heikkinen, E.; Kayhty Seppanen, B.; and Pohjolainen, P. "Health situation and related social conditions among 66 year old Finnish men," *Scandinavian Journal of Social Medicine* 4, no. 2, (1976), 71-74.

Heikkinen, E.; Kiiskinen, A.; Kayhty, B.; et al. "Assessment of biological age," *Gerontologia* 20, no. 1 (1974), 33-43.

Ruikka, I. "Aims and techniques in geriatric rehabilitation," *Duodecim* 91, no. 2 (1975), 110-114.

Totterman, L. E. "Need for long term care of the inhabitants of Helsinki City," *Gerontologia* 20 (1975), 90-105.

FRANCE

J. A. HUET

and ANNE FONTAINE

The problems of the aging in France are among the most acute in Europe. In 1900, for example, those 65 or older constituted 8.2 percent of the population in France; in the rest of Europe the figures ranged from 4.7 to 6.2 percent. The aging trend began during World War I, when there were 1 million fewer births than deaths; and during World War II, more than 1 million men were killed, taken prisoner, or sent to deportation camps.

In 1961, there were 2 million people over 75; by 1975 this number had increased to 2,656,000 (592,500 over 85 years old). Now over 13.5 percent of the population is over age 65, and 18.2 over 60. These figures explain the pressure on governments when they elaborate their social budgets. Although 49 percent of the national budget is allocated to social purposes, only 10 percent is given to old people living at a poverty level; their allocation brings their annual income to a minimum of almost $3,000.

Of the 7,499,000 people 65 and over in 1975, more than 2 million received the minimum allocation. Since 1960, there has been a governmental recognition of the necessities of the aged population, and each year there is some progress.

In that year the government appointed a special commission with the mission of studying the situation of aging in France; its chairman was Pierre Laroque, and its secretary was Paul Paillat. They released an official document on a policy for the aged.

The interest of scientists in gerontology arose only around 1936, with François Bourlière (biologist) and Alfred Sauvy (demographer), Léon Binet, and Jean A. Huet. The first gerontological society, Centre d'Etudes et de Recherches Gérontologiques, was created in 1948 by Wibaux and Huet. It has been renamed the Société Française de Gérontologie, and is now the Federation of Provincial Gerontological Societies.

The only multidisciplinary research institute is the Fondation Nationale de Gérontologie.

If some hundred books have been written on gerontological subjects, the unpublished reports are more numerous. Geriatrics is not yet recognized as a specialty in medicine, but some larger universities give courses or gerontology and geriatrics. Each year some gerontological meetings or congresses, national or international, are held, attracting the French gerontologists (most of them being medical doctors).

Three publications are specifically devoted to gerontology: *La Revue de Gériatrie, Gérontologie,* and *Gérontologie et Société.*

DEMOGRAPHY

The French population by age is shown in table 9. In all likelihood, those aged 75 and over will increase during the period from 1975 to 1985, while the total over 65 will decrease (table 10). After 1985, the number over 65 will increase again.

Table 9: POPULATION BY AGE, 1975

Age	Number	Percentage of Total Population
Less than 60 years old	42,058.4	81.7
60–64	2,594.4	5.0
65–69	2,364.5	4.4
70–74	1,988.0	3.8
75–79	1,374.8	2.6
80–84	792.6	1.5
85–89	371.4	0.7
90–94	110.5	0.2
95 and over	20.1	0.03

Source: National Institute of Demographic Studies.

Table 10: POPULATION PROJECTIONS BY AGE, 1975–2000 (IN THOUSANDS)

Age	1975	1985	1995	2000
65 and over	7,498	6,866	7,989	8,436
	(13.5%)	(12.4%)	(13.7%)	(14.0%)
75 and over	2,663	3,371	3,043	3,476
	(5.1%)	(6.1%)	(5.2%)	(5.2%)

In the 1975 census, there were 4,553,000 women 65 and over, compared to 2,945,000 men of that age, and 1,990,000 women and 969,000 men 75 and over. Women comprised 61.1 percent of those aged 65 and over, and this proportion reached 68.0 percent among the 75 years old and over.

The majority of the men 65 and over were married (73.1 percent), but 51.7 percent of the women of that age were widows. The 1975 Census shows that of the 2 million old people 65 years and over who were living alone 79.8 percent

Table 11: MARITAL STATUS OF MEN AND WOMEN 65 YEARS OF AGE AND OVER, 1974

	Total	Unmarried	Married	Widowed	Divorced
Men	2,657,738	180,120	1,909,539	480,975	87,104
Women	4,256,234	425,701	1,455,444	2,237,122	137,067

were women. The number of households with a head over 75 was 1.75 million in 1975. They will be around 2 million in 1985. Twenty-five percent of the households will have a head over 65 in 1985.

Longevity differs according to sex, socio-professional categories, and location. Life expectancy is now 68.7 for men and 76.3 for women. While 35-year-old teachers or managers have 57 or 55 chances out of 100 to reach the age of 75, a worker has only 33 chances to reach that age; between these extreme categories, there is about a 7.3 year difference in life expectancy.

There is a higher percentage of old people in rural communities than in towns; old people comprise 16.3 percent of the rural population, while they comprise 10.6 percent in towns of more than 100,000 inhabitants.

In 1987, it is projected, the average life expectancy for a man will be 71.5 years and for a woman 77.2.

ROLES AND STATUS OF THE AGED

Family

In a country with a rural tradition, industrialization was a revolution. Old people with old habits, living in old houses, were suddenly displaced by the arrival of a new civilization.

Geographical mobility, due to the rural exodus and urbanization process, has condemned many old people to live isolated lives, far from their family. If cohabitation with adult children, traditionally more prevalent in rural areas than in urban ones, tends now to become less frequent, it is still an important way of living for old people in the country. Among the agricultural population 65 and over 38 percent of the men and 37 percent of the women are living with a non-married child or a young couple. This situation is not held in much favor by the children; it is found more often among people of the lowest social classes.

A recent survey found that half the children having parents 65 years old and over are living within 20 kilometers of them and only 15 percent at 500 kilometers and more. This residential proximity seems due to the children's desire to stay close to their parents. The frequency of the visits is usually weekly or monthly especially for skilled workers, the white-collar workers, and trained personnel. Among the higher-salaried staff and the unskilled workers the visits are more episodical. The visits are found to be more numerous in Paris, where retired people have a child in the vicinity more frequently than anywhere else.

The relationships between married children and parents consist of exchanges of advice, information, and services, often with financial help (half the married children received at their marriage or after substantial monetary gifts or loans).

A third of the children 3 and under with working mothers are cared for by grandmothers. Grandparents take care of their grandchildren during holidays; and if the elderly are sick, they are sometimes housed by their children. The intensity of the relationship between parents and married children is still strong.

In 1978 an experiment was conducted in the Paris hospitals of the Assistance Publique in an attempt to solve the problem of invalid old people living with their families. During the holiday period of July and August, these old people were temporarily hospitalized; the care expenses were reimbursed normally by social security.

Employment

In France, the normal retirement age is 65 for men and 60 for women who have contributed 37.5 years to social security (this since January 1, 1979). In 1975 only 10.6 percent of men and 5.0 percent of women 65 and over were still working.

There is strong pressure from the unions to lower these retirement ages, though economically it is not wise to do so. In practice, many workers are entitled to retire earlier if they are disabled or if their work is dangerous and exhausting. The retirement allocation paid by social security generally amounts to 50 percent of the normal salary. In many cases, retired workers now receive from mutual funds or complementary insurance systems 15 to 25 percent more. In France, as in most other European countries, unemployment is a very serious problem, and the young claim that old workers should retire sooner to leave their jobs vacant.

The findings of the 1968 and 1975 censuses show that activity after 65 years of age had decreased for men and increased for women. The economic sector that occupies most people after 65 is agriculture.

A special allocation is now given to those who leave the private sector between the ages of 60 and 65. They receive 70 percent of their last salary; that is to say, the equivalent of a full pension (social security and complementary pension).

Some large companies are experimenting with different preretirement systems. For example, after 60 workers can work fewer hours, month after month, with the same wages. In one automobile plant a group has been created to give some voluntary work to retired workers.

Another aspect of the French post-retirement problem is black employment, in which retirees work without declaring their income to social security and thus augment their pensions with low wages.

Community

The French policy for the aging stresses integration of elderly and younger people. It also encourages independency. The policy in favor of maintaining old people in their own homes has developed services such as home help, hospitalization and care at home, meals on wheels, senior clubs, and medical centers.

In 1971, the first Third-Age University was created in Toulouse. Since then many other cities have organized such programs with increasing success. The Sixth International Congress of the Universities of Third Age took place on June 1, 1979, in Nancy.

PROBLEMS OF THE AGED

Health

Before the age of 60 all French citizens are entitled, through the prevention services of social security, to obtain a check-up free of charge. The aged are classified as healthy, semi-invalids, invalids, or bedridden. They are all supported by social security and are generally reimbursed for 60 to 75 percent of their medical and pharmaceutical expenses. If they are afflicted by a long-term or incurable ailment, they are reimbursed completely.

In 1976, 400,000 old people aged 60 and over were in institutions. The number of institutions increased 20 percent between 1963 and 1975. In 1970, there were 352,400 beds available for old people in hospitals and institutions; the number was considered insufficient, especially for invalid people. The standard to meet was 50 hospital beds per 1,000 people above 65; of these beds 60 percent would be for invalid patients.

Since 1976, under the Seventh Plan, the gerontological organization has made a distinction between the social and medical services. There must be:

- in a district (15,000 to 50,000 inhabitants), a congregate housing (*logement-foyer*), a residence for old people in a city (*maison de retraite*), and a residence for old rurals in a village.
- in a sector (50,000 to 150,000 inhabitants), an institution, *Maison de Santé ou de Cure médicale,* for long stays of dependent people with a capacity of no more than 500 beds.

In 1975 it was decided to eliminate or modernize all the nursing homes. A survey conducted that year indicated that 47 percent of the institutions, with 29 percent of the beds, belonged to the private sector. The private retirement homes had an average of 58.3 beds. The public autonomous ones, 83.1, and the chronic sections of the public hospitals, 186.1 beds. The total was 355,565 beds for 332,893 old people in 3,728 institutions.

There was an important increase in the number of people 80 and over in institutions; the number increased by 28 percent between 1962 and 1975. On December 31, 1975, the proportion of institutionalization by sex and age was 2.5 percent for men and 3.5 percent for women over 60 in hospices and public and private retirement homes; this represented 31 percent of the total population over 60.

A 1976 survey with a nonrepresentative population sample found that 40 percent of the old people in institutions were in rooms for one or two persons; 44 percent in rooms with two, three, or four beds; and 16 percent in dormitories.

In 1975, in compliance with the new standards, 169 nursing homes were built with a total capacity of 19,856 beds. Some geriatric centers exist in major hospitals, offering medical service (20 to 100 beds) and a special service for rehabilitation (60 to 200 beds).

Several types of day hospitals exist, the most common being psychiatric. In 1975, only three were open in France; they were located in Grenoble, Ivry, and Nancy. Today about 27,500 people 65 and over are in psychiatric hospitals, and of those 19,000 are women.

Another type of day hospital is the day center. Since 1965, thirteen have opened in different towns.

There were also plans to add 8,500 beds for bedridden people between 1971 and 1975 and another 8,500 during the next five years. There would then be 89,427 beds available in 1980.

Housing

An Arab proverb says, "If you transplant an old tree, it dies." Frenchmen must have the same opinion, for it is very difficult to persuade them to leave their old and uncomfortable houses and move into modern apartments.

- 56.5 percent of the households with a head of the house 65 and over are living alone. Only 7 percent want to move.
- 54 percent of the households (2,200,000 households) own their housing; most often built before 1948 (80 percent).
- 11 percent live in social houses.
- 0.5 percent live in residences or congregate housing.
- 4.8 percent live in institutions.

Of those between 65 and 74 years old, 36.4 percent live in rural communities, while 63.6 percent live in urban communities. Of those 75 and over, 36.7 percent live in rural communities, and 63.3 percent live in urban communities. Approximately 314,000 of the elderly receive a housing allowance to help them pay their rent.

Every year France builds approximately 500,000 apartments, called social or low-cost housing. Theoretically 5 percent of these are reserved on the ground or first floor for old people, but they rarely take these units because they do not want to leave their houses. In addition, the rents in the new buildings are too high for many of them to pay, or the apartments are situated too far from where they used to live. Also, many workers have built small houses with gardens in the country where they long to retire.

Other solutions are available, but many depend on the old person's financial resources. For those with enough money, there are family or professional homes, service residences, villages for retired people. Unfortunately 3 million aged persons have little financial resources. Especially in the towns there are large sections where many single rooms located on the higher floors are occupied by old women—generally widows—who live in a sort of ghetto but do not want to move to an institution. Only one-fourth of the aged living in towns have normal comforts (with toilet, bathtub or shower, and a separated kitchen). Only 30 percent are living on the ground floor or have an elevator. And approximately 42 to 46 percent still have wood or coal heaters.

Economics

At age 60, 70.8 percent of the men and 35.4 percent of the women are still employed; while after age 65, the percentage declines to 10.6 percent of the men and 5.0 percent of the women. Between the 1968 and 1975 censuses, the percentage employed decreased for men and increased for women.

The old age pensions increased 10.7 percent in 1979. The minimum allowances will reach approximately $8 a day by the end of 1979.

The number of years a person must contribute to receive a full pension from social security is thirty-seven and a half; that is, 150 quarters. The ten best-paid years since 1948 are used to calculate the average annual base salary.

Transportation

Men 65 and over and women 60 and over are entitled to a 30 percent discount on train fares, and a 25 to 50 percent discount on some air flights.

In many towns, city buses are free of charge or 25 to 50 percent cheaper for those who receive the minimum old age allowance and do not pay taxes.

Leisure

France now has about 12,000 third-age clubs. They are organized by local authorities, private associations, religious congregations, or professional and mutual funds, and are adapted to the needs of their clients.

The general conception is that leisure can be static, dynamic, or kinetic. *Static* means that the old person cannot leave his house, so everything (radio, television, books, visits) must be delivered to him. *Dynamic* is the lot of all mobile people. They can go to the club, practice gynmastics, belong to some voluntary associations. *Kinetic* is for those who like sports, traveling, skiing, and similar activities. In summer many tours are offered, and some nonprofit associations have special programs for the aged but generally not during the summer. Financial help is given by local administrative areas to those with low incomes.

In 1954, Huet created the first municipal holidays for senior citizens. Now more than fifty cities offer similar programs for their senior citizens. And each year some institutions take their patients to the south of France for a month.

PROGRAMS FOR THE AGED

A governmental planning commission gathers the views, programs, and opinions of scientists, sociologists, medical doctors, social workers, representatives of the employers and employees, administrators, economists, and policy makers. The commission meets and works for three years and then gives recommendations to the government, which, with those of the minister of finance, are presented to the Parliament for a determination of priorities. The Seventh Plan, developed for the years 1976 to 1980, set as a priority helping the aged stay at home and giving them the means to preserve and develop their participation in the social life of the community. The program is based on the creation of three types of services: home care, third-age clubs and restaurants, and day centers.

The plan is to provide 270,000 old persons with general services near their homes, so they will not have to go to hospitals, and to enable a million more to make the best use of these services. The government wants to help the aged stay in their homes and to facilitate their social rehabilitation if they have been hospitalized. The main idea is to preserve the social life of those of the third age and help them to participate in the creation of these programs.

The decree also describes the means of organizing good information services, preretirement programs and intergeneration meetings. It insists on the adaptation of housing for impaired old people, the necessity of equipping each dwelling with a telephone and laundry facilities, and the restoration of old apartments. There are also numerous private programs, many of them with innovative plans.

RESEARCH AND TEACHING

Research

It is only since 1960 that the French government and researchers in social sciences have become aware of the problems of the aged. The first broad study of this subject was done under the leadership of Pierre Laroque. The results, published in 1962, established the bases of a national policy on aging.

It was also the starting point of the French research in social gerontology. But it is only with the preparation of the Sixth Plan, after 1968, and with its new working group, the Intergroupe Personnes Agées, that the problems concerning old people, especially their medico-social ones, have been more thoroughly studied.

For the Seventh Plan, the ministry of health and social security—administrators of agencies and pension funds—ordered research in social gerontology to help them define social policy for their organizations. These are the main sponsors of research in gerontology.

In 1976 some of the most important pension funds decided that Paul Paillat would coordinate French research in social gerontology, which represents a group of no more than thirty people.

Professor Bourlière leads the most important research group on fundamental gerontology at the Fondation Nationale de Gérontologie. At least two other groups are studying the medico-social aspects of aging and epidemiology.

Teaching

In some of the most important universities, where the most active gerontologists work, there are now two-year programs on geriatrics for medical students and specializing doctors. These universities give a diploma on gerontological competence, although this discipline is not yet recognized as a specialty. Social gerontology is regularly taught only at Paris University by Anne-Marie Guillemard, whose course is on sociology of aging, and by Jean Poitrenaud, who teaches psychogerontology.

In 1978, the Fondation Natonale de Gérontologie started a three-month introductory program on gerontology for all personnel working with the aged. Monthly seminars, organized by Michel Philibert and Robert Hugonot, take place at Grenoble. They deal mostly with the social aspects of aging.

A List of Major Research Groups

1. Association de Gérontologie du XIIIème Arrondissement de Paris, with the Groupe de Recherche Appliquée en Gérontologie (GRAEG), 49 rue Bobillot, 75013 Paris. Dr. Guillet, Dr. Balier, Xavier Gaullier, Maryvonne Gognalons-Caillard.
2. Association Gérontologique de l'Hôpital Charles-Foix, 7 Avenue de la République, 94203 Ivry. Prof. Vignalou, Prof. Betthaux, Dr. Beck.
3. Caisse Nationale d'Assurance Vieillesse des Travailleurs Salariés, Etudes et Recherches, 49 Rue Mirabeau, 75016 Paris. Claudine Donfut, Alain Rozenkier.
4. Centre d'Etudes des Mouvements Sociaux, Maison des Sciences de l'Homme, 54 Boulevard Raspail, 75006 Paris. Anne-Marie Guillemard, Rémi Lenoir.
5. Centre de Liaison, d'Etude, D'Information et de Recherche sur les Personnes Agées (CLEIRPPA), 49 rue Mirabeau, 75016 Paris. Claudette Collot.
6. Centre de Recherche pour l'Etude et l'Observation des Conditions de Vie (CREDOC), 142 rue du Chevaleret, 75634 Paris CEDEX. André et Arié Mizrahi.
7. Centre Plurisdisciplinaire de Gérontologie (CPDG), 5 Avenue de la Liberté, 38 000 Grenoble. Prof. Michel Philibert.
8. Fondation Nationale de Gérontologie: Unité de Recherches Gérontologiques, INSERM U 118; Centre de Gérontologie Claude Bernard; and Groupe CNRS. 20 rue Wilhem, 75016 Paris. Prof. François Bourlière, Dr. Yves Courtois, Dr. Pierre Aschheim, Jean Poitrenaud, Mireille Bertrand.
9. Groupe de Gérontologie Sociale, 49 rue Mirabeau, 75016 Paris. Prof. Bouzlière, Paul Paillat (scientific adviser), Fernand Clement, Christiane Delbes, Anne Fontaine. Fondation des Villes, 5 Rue de L'Abbaye, 75006 Paris. Xavier Gaullier.
10. Institut National d'Etudes Démographiques (INED), 27 rue du Commandeur, 75014 Paris. Paul Paillat, Catherine de Guibert-Lantoine, Alain Parant.
11. Institut national de la Santé et de la Recherche Médicale (INSERM), 44 Chemin de la Ronde, B.P. 34, 78110 Le Vésinet. Division de la Recherche Médico Sociale. Dr. Davidson, Dr. Hatton.
12. Laboratoire de Géographie Humaine du CNRS, 191 rue Saint-Jacques, 75005 Paris. Françoise Cribier, Marie-Luce Duffau, Alexandre Kych.
13. Laboratoire de Recherche Médico-Sociale et Centre de Gériatrie, Pavillon C, Centre Hospitalier Universitaire de Grenoble, Grenoble 38043 CEDEX. Prof. Hugonot, Mme. Israel.
14. Office Aquitain de Recherche, d'Etudes, d'Information et de Liaison sur les Problèmes des Personnes Agées (OAREIL), Maison des Sciences de l'Homme, Esplanade des Antilles, Domaine Universitaire, 33405 Talence. Dr. Colson.
15. Oganisation d'Etudes d'Aménagement de l'Aire Métropolitaine de Nancy/Metz/Thionville (OREAM— Lorraine), Rue Robert Blum, 54700 Pont-à-Mousson. Christian Henneton.
16. Université de Paris X, UER de Sciences Sociales, Laboratoire d'Anthropologie du CEDRES, 200 Avenue de la République 92000 Nanterre. Françoise Jandro-Louia, Jean Michel Louka.

Information Sources

Few books deal entirely with social gerontology or geriatrics in France, and almost no basic texts exist. The following organizations have published bibliographies on Gerontology:

1. Caisse Nationale de Retraite des Ouvriers du Bâtiment et des Travaux Publics, B.P. N 6, 06020 Nice CEDEX. Published bibliographies regularly between 1966 and 1974; in particular a bibliography of the "500 Basic Documents on Social Gerontology" by Anne Fontaine-Chevallier, Documents d'information et de Gestion, Gérontologie no. 23-24, July-October 1973.
2. Centre de Liaison, d'Etude d'Information et de Recherche sur les Problèmes des Personnes Agéeṣ (CLEIRPPA), 40 rue Mirabeau, 75016 Paris. Has published an annual bibliography since 1973.
3. Fondation Nationale de Gérontologie, 40 rue Mirabeau, 75016 Paris. Publishes thematic bibliographies in each issue of the quarterly publication "Gérontologie et Société." In 1980 prepared with two other research groups: a *Guidebook of documentation sources on Gerontology.*
4. Institut National d'Etudes Démographiques, 27 rue du Commander 75014 Paris. Published a bibliography on gerontology from 1962 to 1972 and one edited by Paul Paillat in 1973.
5. Institut de l'Environment, CERA, 1 rue Jacques Callot, 75006 Paris. Published bibliography edited by Françoise Cribier in 1973.
6. Ministère des Affaires Culturelles, Service Etudes et Recherches, BETURE-CERAU, 5 rue Bellini, 92800 Puteaux. Published "Troisième Age et Activités Culturelles" by Agnès Pitrou.

The most important periodicals are:

1. *Années-Documents CLEIRPPA,* 49 Rue Mirabeau, 75016 Paris (monthly).
2. *Documents d'Information et de Gestion, Gérontologie,* CNRO, B.P. 6, 06020 Nice CEDEX (quarterly).
3. *Gérontologie,* 64 Avenue Parmentier, 75011 Paris (quarterly).
4. *Gérontologie et Société,* Fondation Natonale de Gérontologie, 49 rue Mirabeau, 75016 Paris (quarterly).
5. *Médecine et 3ème Age,* 24-26 Rue de la Cerisaie, 75004 Paris (quarterly).
6. *Revue de Gériatrie,* 133 bis rue de l'Université, 75007 Paris (bimonthly).

SUMMARY

France is an old nation with an important aged population. It is also an aged nation, caused by high mortality during the two world wars and low birth rates lately. Thus the pecentage of aged people has increased. French demographers were successful in bringing the socioeconomic consequences of such a situation to the attention of policy makers. The government now helps the promotion of gerontology.

In 1975, more than 18 percent of the French population was over 60; that means about one man out of six and one woman out of five. This percentage will increase during the next five years. The French life expectancy at birth is now 68.7 for men and 76.3 for women.

Family problems are different in urban and rural areas. If some intergenerational conflicts exist, the relationships between parents and married children have been found to be good by three important recent surveys. The French people and their government are in favor of maintaining the aged at home or in their family as long as possible. Hospitals, nursing homes, and other institutions are considered the last solutions, and there is increasing experience with health care at home by specialized teams.

The retirement age is normally 65, but there is a very strong pressure to lower it, because of unemployment problems, and some classes of salaried people can now retire earlier. Facilities are given to those who want to retire at 60 with 70 percent of their salaries. The minimum old age allowance at the end of 1979 was around $8 a day.

The general tendency and the official policy of the Seventh Plan is to integrate the aged into the life of the community by providing all kinds of services: clubs, restaurants, day care centers, homecare, telephone. Old people rather stay in their old houses than move to modern buildings. About 5 percent of those over 65 live in institutions for the aged.

Research on the aged started in the field of social gerontology after an important survey in 1962, which established the bases of a national policy on aging. There are only a few permanent research groups in this field, however.

Two-year programs on geriatrics are available in some of the most important universities, although geriatrics is not yet recognized as a speciality. Social gerontology is taught regularly in only three universities in Paris.

For the aged, universities of third age are now open in almost every large city.

Few books deal entirely with social gerontology or geriatrics in France, although there is important unpublished material. The most important library on gerontology is located at 49 rue Mirabeau, 75016 Paris (phone number 525.92.80).

REFERENCES

Andréani, E. 1974. Indicateurs Sociaux pour la population âgée, *Documents d'information et de gestion*. Cagnes-sur-Mer: CNRO.

Attias-Donfut, C., and Gognalons-Caillard, M. 1976. *Nouvelles données d'une politique de la vieillesse*. Paris: CNAVTS, GRAEG.

Balier, C.; Ferry-Druenne, M.; and Gognalons-Caillard, M. 1976. Vieillissement individúel et vieillissement social: pour une approche dynamique de la pathologie de la sénescence. Etude de la population Centre de jour. *Cahiers de la Fondation Nationale de Gérontologie.*

Beauvoir, S. de. 1970. *La Vieillesse.* Paris: Edit. Gallimard.

Berthaux P. 1974. La mesure du vieillissement, *Gazette Médicale de France;* 20.

Binet, L. 1969. *Gérontologie et Gériatrie.* Paris: Edit. PUF.

Bourlière, F. ed. 1969. *Progrès en Gérontologie.* Paris: Edit. Flammarion.

Carette, J. 1975. *Savoir Vieillir.* Paris: Edit. du Jour.

Clément, F. 1976. *Facteurs accidentels de vieillissement.* Paris: Fondation Nationale de Gérontologie.

Collot, C., and Le Bris, H. 1975. Les aspirations au logement de retraite. *Documents d'information et de gestion.* Cagnes-Sur-Mer: CNRO.

Commission d'Etude des Problèmes de la Vieillesse. 1962. *Rapport Laroque: Politique de la vieillesse.* Paris: La Documentation française.

Cribier, F. 1978. *Une génération de Parisiens arrive à la retraite.* Paris: Laboratoire de géographie Humaine.

Gaullier, X. 1979. Politique de la Vieillesse. *Du capitalisme social à la Société post industrielle.* Paris: Fondation des Villes.

Gillette, A. 1978. *Votre commune et les personnes Agées.* Paris: Edition du Moniteur.

Guibert-Lantoine, C., and Dartiguelongue, J.P. 1974. *Flexibilité de l'âge de la retraite.* Paris: Centre International de Gérontologie Sociale.

Guillemard, A.M. 1972. *La retraite, une mort sociale.* Pairs: Edit. Mouton.

———. 1976. *La politique d'intégration de la vieillesse—génèse et usages sociaux d'un retournement doctrinal.* Paris: Centre d'Etudes des mouvements sociaux.

Henrard, J.C.; Colvez, A.; and Léonard, M.C. 1977. *Les Centres de jours—Indicateurs de Santé. Etude critique des indicateurs habituels et propositions d'indicateurs adaptés au problèmes de santé des personnes âgées.* Paris: Fondation Nationale de Gérontologie.

Huet, J.A. 1974. Grands vieillards et gérontologie sociale. *Revue Française de gérontologie.*

Hugonot, R. 1976. *La participation des personnes* âgées: *non seulement un droit mais aussi un devoir.* Brussels: 7ème Congrès du CIGS.

Jandrot-Louka, F., and Louka, J.M. 1978. *Les assistés des deux sexes en institutions d'hospice. Marginlisation des populations jeunes et âgées en éstablissements de longs séjours.* Nanterre: Université de Paris, UER Sciences Sociales.

Lenoir, R. 1977. *Transformations des rapports entre générations et apparitions du troisième âge.* Paris: Centre d'Etudes des Mouvements sociaux.

Locon, T., and Paillat P. 1971. *Conditions de vie et besoins des personnes âgées en France. II Les Agriculteurs âgés.* Paris: institut National d'Etudes Démographiqus, Edit. PUF.

Maslowski, J., and Paillat, P. 1973. *Conditions de vie et besoins des personnes âgées en France. III Les ruraux âgés non agricoles.* Paris: Edit. PUF.

Mizzahi, A. and A. 1977. *Les Personnes âgés vivant en institutions—Caractères socio-démographiques, antonomie et handicaps.* Paris. CREDOC.

Pacaud, S., and Lahalle, M. D. 1969. *Attitudes, comportements, opinions des personnes âgées dans le cadre de la famille moderne.* Paris: Edit. CNRS.

Paillat, P. 1971. *Sociologie de la vieillesse*. Paris: Edit. PUF.

————, and Wibaux, C. 1969. *Conditions de vie et besoins des personnes âgées*. I *Les citadins âgées*. Paris: Institut National d'Etudes Demographiques, Edit. PUF.

Philibent, M. 1968. *L'échelle des âge*. Paris: Edit. du Sevil.

Pitrou, A. 1979. *Vivre sans famille*. Toulose: Edit. Privat.

Poitrenaud, J. 1972. Structure des aptitudes cognitives du vieillissement. *Cahiers de la Fondation Nationale de Gérontologie*

Reboul, H. 1973. *Vieillir, projet pour vivre: essai psychologique*. Lyon: Edit. du Chalet.

Roussel, L. 1976. *La famille après le mariage des enfants. Etude des relations entre générations*. Paris: Institut National d'Etudes Démographiques, Edit. PUF.

Vignalou, J., and Beck, H. 1972. Etat actuel et perspectives de la gériatrie en France. *Revue Française du Praticien*, 22.

Zarca, B. 1974. *La retraite révélatrice du mode de vie et de la nature des relations familiales en milieu paysan*. Paris: Université René Descartes.

GERMAN DEMOCRATIC REPUBLIC
(East Germany)

U. J. SCHMIDT,

P. H. SCHULZ,

S. EITNER,

H. RICHTER,

and I. KALBE

THE POSITION OF THE ELDERLY

The position of the elderly in our society is determined by the socialist relations of production. The living conditions of the elderly are governed by the basic economic goal of socialism: a steady rise in everybody's material and cultural standard of living.

In our society, work veterans receive every possible care. Marx demanded in his "Critique of the Gotha Programme" that the elderly be given a definite place in society and be put in a position to make full use of their skills and experience to take part in public life and its development, on an equal footing with everybody else. This demand is being met in the GDR.

The basic rights of the elderly are laid down in article 3 of the constitution of the GDR: "Every citizen of the German Democratic Republic has the right to social care in case of old age and invalidity. This right is guaranteed by an increasing material, social and cultural care of elderly and disabled citizens."

The GDR's social welfare policy pursues the aim of providing social security for everybody, and in particular for the elderly. Our moral views say that everybody's duty is to assist his fellow man in the true spirit of solidarity. In consequence, the elderly have to be—and are—shown particular respect, affection, and concern. The government attempts to ensure that these people take an active part in public life. People who are growing or are old are not condemned to loneliness. Our state offers the elderly the following: the right to work until old age on request; a comprehensive system of social insurance services; full health protection; price stability, government-subsidized rents, and protection against the termination of tenancy agreements; and the socialist system of education.

The Eighth Congress of the Socialist Unity party of Germany (SED) underlined once again that the leaders of our party and government hold the elderly in high esteem. E. Honecker, first secretary of the SED Central Committee, said: "Nearly 20 percent of all GDR citizens have reached pensionable age. Many of them were first-hour activists, who successfully fulfilled the difficult task of building up a new state and a new economy after the war, and have to this day been working in production and other fields of public life. It will be important for our party in the future as well, to make use of their experience in the further construction of socialism, to improve the social conditions for all pensioners and to offer them a safe existence."

Not only the many forms of material and financial services, but also the proper behavior and attitude of all other people in our state toward the elderly and the aged help the latter to find their proper place in our society. The typical attitude toward them is rooted in the society's awareness of its obligations toward them rather than in compassion. This lofty attitude is instilled into young people in education every day. Children adopt it toward both their parents and the aged.

The fact that the leaders of the party and the government are dedicated to this policy is shown again by the latest social welfare policy program embodied in the joint resolution of the Central Committee of the Socialist Unity party of Germany, the National Executive of the Confederation of Free German Trade Unions, and the Council of Ministers of the GDR, of April 27, 1972. This resolution clearly reflects the planned nature and continuity of social services for people of advanced age. Approximately 6.5 billion marks was spent on sociopolitical policy measures through 1975 alone.

Many other countries that see people only in terms of whether they may be useful in profit making completely deny the value of old age. Since old people lose some of their previous efficiency, they are pushed to the fringe areas of society. We, however, expect these people to give us their views, make suggestions, and carry on activities, which are all based on their experience and which we cannot do without. The mode of production in some other societies makes people stop working at ever earlier ages, since there are no opportunities for employment in line with the requirements of advanced age. But our society tries to offer old people chances to pursue worthwhile and useful activities. Of course, they require special conditions, which are admittedly not only of material nature; complex care is of increasing importance.

Marx says that "the true spiritual wealth of the individual depends entirely on the wealth of his actual relations." Old people therefore suffer impoverishment, seclusion, and isolation only if they are not given useful tasks that they are able to carry out. Our public- and government-appointed management bodies in enterprises, cooperatives, and residential areas make suggestions on a continuing basis about how to make society understand the needs of old people, realize the particularities of their living conditions, and spread and generalize these insights.

Those who are old today know the bitterness of their past experience. They were first-hour activists, who offered their rich experience in order to help build up our state and our society and educate young people. We are aware of the role that grandparents play by caring for and educating our younger generation. The fact that pensioners—like working women—make up a large part of our population makes even clearer to the younger generation that the world is influenced by the stories, experience, and insights of the elderly people.

More than 600,000 pensioners work at their own request and are given every possible support and care by their enterprises and the trade unions. Scientific research results are drawn on so as to find out the best forms of and opportunities for useful work.

The support they receive from the health service is often excellent. Important guidance is provided by university staff who do research work in occupational medicine. Elderly people are happy wherever the process of aging is seen as more than a personal issue; it is also a social issue that must be settled by society as a whole.

DEMOGRAPHY

The age structure of the GDR's population is noticeably older than that of many other countries. This is shown with particular clarity by a comparison between the age groups of working age and those that have passed it. At the end of 1972, 25.4 percent of all people in the GDR were younger than 18; 50.7 percent were between 18 and 60; and 22 percent were 60 and older. A large proportion of those over 40 are women. 41.8 percent of women are over 40; the equivalent proportion of the male population is only 30.2 percent.

In 1972, 3,351,300 people—19.1 percent of the entire population—were of pensionable age. The figure for 1975 was 3,314,500—19.0 percent. There will be no significant change in this trend before 1980, when this figure will be down to 2,999,100—17.6 percent. Retirement age is 60 years for women and 65 years for men. The GDR will probably lead the world in the proportion of old-age pensioners. Even in the Federal Republic of Germany, only 18 percent of the population are older than 60. The proportion of pensioners in other major Western countries is around 15 percent. The majority of socialist countries have younger age structures as well, even though retirement age is five years earlier in many of these countries.

Another feature of the GDR's demography is that women make up a large part of the total number of pensioners: 70 percent. The reason is the outcome of the two world wars, which had a devastating effect demographically.

Since medical attendance and living conditions have improved, the average expectation of life of the elderly is increasing. This is proved by the increase—both relatively and absolutely—in the number of those over 70. Therefore there are 2.8 persons of working age to every pensioner in the GDR. The increase in life expectancy in the second half of life has not kept pace with the increase in the total life expectancy.

PROGRAMS

Social Insurance

The GDR's social insurance renders material and financial services to the extent that the national economy allows, so that the needs of working people and pensioners and their dependents, as well as for social welfare and health care, can be met in case of illness, temporary or permanent loss of the ability to work, old age, maternity, and death. Social insurance is an essential factor of social security, since it provides services that are laid down by legislation. Relevant legal provisions are decreed by competent governmental authorities. The social insurance system of the GDR is made up of the social insurance for industrial and office workers and the social insurance run by the state insurance company. The first is run by the trade unions on the basis of self-administration by those whom it insures. It provides compulsory insurance to all workers and office workers who have signed an employment contract, all students at universities, institutes of university standard and training colleges, doctors in private medical practice, all freelance artists, writers, sculptors, and those similarly employed and their dependents who are entitled to insurance services. The second is run by governmental authorities, also on the basis of self-administration by those whom it insures. It provides compulsory social insurance for all members of socialist production cooperatives and all others who have not entered into an employment relationship—such as members of lawyers' cooperatives, retail, traders, and self-employed craftsmen.

All pensioners and members of their families continue to enjoy full insurance protection without making contributions. This protection is granted by the insurance institution that insured them during their working years. They continue to be given all services free of charge and for an unlimited period of time. These include: outpatient and inpatient medical and dental treatment at public O.P.D.S., infirmaries, medical practices of the public health services, practices of self-employed doctors and dentists, hospitals, and sanitariums; nursing at home by properly qualified nursing staff provided by the public health service; spa treatment and treatment at special climatically favorable institutions; and drugs, remedies, dentures, prostheses, and other aids.

All working people who are insured pay contributions. The maximum wage or salary for which such contributions have to be paid is six hundred marks a month. The rate for workers and office workers is 20 percent of their monthly wage or salary; 10 percent is paid by the working people themselves, and the remaining 10 percent is paid by their employers. In the mining industry, employers pay 20 percent for every employee. Pensioners are exempted from the payment of insurance contributions. If they continue to work, their employers pay their part only. All services are financed from contributions and governmental subsidies. Since all improvements of social insurance services in the GDR have not been permitted to increase insurance contributions rates and the maximum wage or salary for which contributions are payable, governmental subsidies have been going up all the time. The total expenditure of the social insurance for workers and office Workers was 14.3 thousand million marks in 1972, with the government providing 5.4 billion marks of subsidies.

Pensions

Pensions form part of the comprehensive social security system in socialist GDR. The consititution guarantees every pensioner the right to public assistance in old age and in case of disability. This right is implemented through increasing material, social, and cultural services. Pensions paid by the social insurance are the principal form of material support granted to old and disabled people; they are therefore of great importance. Three facts deserve special mention in this context: First, the GDR has a very large proportion of pensioners compared to other European countries. At present there are thirty-four persons of pensionable age to every hundred persons of working age. Although the labor force will remain about the same in the next few years, the number of pensioners will rise. Second, the expansion and improvement of services has not and will not lead to a change in the maximum wage or salary for which social insurance contributions have to be paid not in insurance rates. Increased expenditure will be met exclusively by subsidies from the government. Third, one of the principles of our social policy is that every pensioner shall be guaranteed a minimum pension. This minimum pension has been steadily raised and has now reached 250 to 290 marks a month; the precise amount depends on the number of years a person has worked. In addition, the following allowance pensions are paid every month: 40 marks for children up to 18 years and 75 marks for the pensioner's spouse if she or he is not entitled to a pension.

The social insurance of the GDR grants old-age pensions, disability pensions, pensions for surviving dependents, and pensions in case of industrial accidents and occupational diseases. Pensions paid to miners, railway employees, and postal employees are governed by particularly favorable legal maxims. Additionally there are pensions for the war disabled, in addition to transitional and subsistence pensions. Resistance fighters against fascism and victims of fascism receive government-paid honorary pensions in addition to their social insurance pensions.

Working people obtain the claim to a pension through their vocational activities and the related compulsory insurance. Our society permits everybody to obtain this claim, provided he makes use of his right to work, which is laid down in the Constitution, and thus performs his duty toward society. The first condition for a claim to an old-age pension is for a person to prove that he has done a minimum of fifteen years of work for which insurance premiums were paid. The second condition is for women to be 60 and for men to be 65 years of age. Full old-age pension is paid even if the person entitled to it continues to work in his job after reaching retirement age.

Pensioners in need of nursing receive both their pension and a nursing allowance of 20 to 80 marks a month; the exact sum depends on the amount of nursing they need. Very seriously disabled persons may receive an additional special nursing allowance of 120 to 180 marks a month. Blind people receive an additional 240 marks a month.

Since the GDR was founded in 1949, there have been ten pension rises. The most important sociopolitical measures taken so far, particularly with regard to pensions, were those introduced in 1972. Under a sociopolitical program adopted at the Eighth Congress of the SED, major improvements took effect in 1972 and 1973. Thus 3.9 million people had their pensions increased on September 1, 1972. The principle was that the oldest pensioners should receive the greatest increases. The minimum pension was raised by 40 to 70 marks, with the exact amount depending on the number of years for which a person had worked. All pensions went up by an average of 47 marks in 1977. Other important sociopolitical regulations entered into force in 1973. One of them laid down that those who cannot work because of disability and therefore cannot obtain a claim to a pension have to be paid a monthly social insurance pension of 200 marks after the age of 18. If such a person also requires nursing, his pension is increased by the nursing or special nursing allowance. Since July 1, 1973, all women who have given birth to five or more children and have done no or very little vocational work receive a pension in case of diability or upon reaching the age of 60.

Another addition to the services of the social insurances was a transitional pension of 200 marks per month payable to widows and widowers for two years after the death of their spouse. The union-run social insurance for workers and office workers paid pensions to 3,123,232 persons on December 31, 1972. Social insurance in the GDR is made up to two closely related elements: compulsory social insurance and optional supplementary pension insurance. Working people who earn more than 600 marks a month—whose income exceeds the limit on which compulsory insurance contributions and services are based—can take out an optional supplementary pension insurance policy. They thus obtain the right to receive a supplementary pension for surviving dependents, increased sick pay (from the seventh week of incapacity to work), and other services. Optional supplementary pension insurance was introduced in 1971. This step was of major importance for the long-term development of the GDR social insurance.

This supplementary insurance does not imply that the limit of income that serves as a basis for contributions and services in connection with compulsory social insurance is forced by law; rather all working people who earn more than 600 marks a month may pay an additional contribution so as to obtain the right of being granted services in addition to the compulsory insurance services. This contribution amounts to 10 percent of the income between 600 and 1,200 marks a month. At the same time, enterprises are under an obligation to pay the same additional amount. The government has also undertaken to guarantee all services rendered under the supplementary insurance. Almost 80 percent of all working people entitled to do so had taken out a supplementary insurance policy by mid-1973.

COMPLEX CARE OF PEOPLE OF ADVANCED AGE

Responsibilities of Governmental Authorities and Society

Since the GDR was founded, governmental authorities, enterprises, and public organizations have been devoting a great deal of attention to the care of the elderly and their closer integration into the rest of society. This is manifest in a large number of legal norms, governmental measures, and resolutions of public organizations that aim at a steady improvement and systematic extension of the care of the elderly. The importance of the care of the elderly was underlined in particular by:

- The resolution of the Presidium of the Council of Ministers on the Improvement of the Care for Aged and Decrepit Persons of October 29, 1959.
- The resolution of the Council of Ministers on Principals and Measures Related to the Improvement of Medical, Social and Cultural Care for Citizens of Advanced Age and the Encouragement of Their More Active Particpation in the Life of Society, and on the Principal Fields of Gerontological Research of May 30, 1969.
- The skeleton agreement of Central Governmental Authorities and Public Organizations of July 24, 1969.
- The working program of the People's Solidarity Organization of April 23, 1972.
- The general instructions of the National Executive of the Confederation of Free German Trade Unions (FDGB), Concerning the Role and Tasks of Work Veterans' Commissions Affiliated to the FDGB Executive Committees, and the Tasks and Rights of Special Work Veterans' Departmental Trade Union Committees at Enterprises of April 11, 1973.

In view of the GDR's demography in general and the large percentage of persons of advanced age in particular, and the tasks that a developed socialist society has to fulfill with regard to the care of the elderly, governmental authorities and forces of society bear a greater responsibility than before for the improvement of working, living, and housing conditions. All spheres of social life are affected by this and are involved in the solution of the economic and social problems encountered in this field. The responsibilities of governmental authorities, executive organs of the national economy, and enterprises are reflected in the resolution of the Council of Ministers of May 30, 1969, which lays down a variety of tasks and specific obligations for govenmental authorities and enterprises.

The responsibilities of the social forces, especially of public organizations, clearly arise from article 3 of the GDR's constitution, which stipulates that every citizen is responsible for society as a whole and calls upon all forces of the people, which are united in the National Front of the GDR, to act in unison for the progress of developed socialist society. This obligation provided the basis for the skeleton agreement, which was concluded on July 24, 1969, between the Ministry of Health, the Ministry of Culture, the State Committee for Physical Culture and Sports, and the National Council of the National Front of the GDR, on the one hand, and the People's Solidarity Organization, the Confederation of Free German Trade Unions, the Democratic Women's League of Germany, the Red Cross of the GDR, the German Sports and Gymnastics Union, the Free German Youth Organization, and the Pioneers' Organization (the GDR's children's organization), on the other, to translate into practice the resolution of the Council of Minsters of May 30, 1969. This agreement details the specific contributions that public organizations can make in line with their special potential to the care of the elderly and their closer incorporation into society.

Similar agreements have been concluded between the councils of districts, towns, and villages, on the one hand, and public organizations and enterprises, on the other, in accordance with the resolution of the Council of Ministers and on the basis of the central skeleton agreement, so that the complex care of the elderly can become effective at the local level. These local agreements take into account the specific local conditions and contain both concrete detailed stipulations for specialized governmental agencies and obligations for public organizations, which make clear how these bodies are to improve the comprehensive care of the elderly in the region concerned. The level achieved in this care is assessed in light of the measures adopted jointly by government authorities and public organizations both locally and centrally at least once a year; and necessary conclusions are drawn for the further improvement of this care.

As stipulated in the resolution of the Council of Ministers, towns and villages have to compile complete lists of elderly persons who need attention. The lists are an essential prerequisite for the fulfillment of the many tasks that have to be performed in the care of the elderly and the improvement of their living conditions. This requires individual talks with the elderly, which are organized by local governmental authorities and attended by all forces of society, especially young people. These talks are designed to reveal the housing and living conditions, the general conditions, and the state of health of every elderly person, whether he or she receives help from dependents or social forces, whether he or she needs medical attendance, what measures are necessary to ensure the person's proper care, and what the person's desires and interests are, so that they can be taken into consideration when it comes to giving the person some work to do or getting his or her cooperation in public affairs. Persons who are alone in the world are advised on matters of contact with the people around them, especially their neighbors and co-workers. The results of such talks both help individual care and are of great importance for analytical assessments and the preparation of fundamental decisions at the regional level.

Preparation for Pensionable Age

The results obtained in the research into gerontological hygiene show that the prevention of pathological aging requires a long period of preparation during which definite aims have to be pursued. The best possible preparation is life-long education and advanced training linked with preplanning and health-promoting ways of living and working. Since the education that workers now over 55 years old received is, to a certain extent, still under the unhappy influence of educational policy of the past, the GDR tries through its health and education policies to help elderly women and men to prepare properly for retirement.

A large part of gerontological research is devoted to preparation for pensionable age. Motivation studies have been carried out at key enterprises of the national economy for a number of years. They help draft principles and outline measures with regard to the preparation for pensionable age; and these principles and measures are included in recommendations of the GDR Health Ministry in due course. Large-scale tests have been made in the mining industry, some of them at the suggestion of researchers working in gerontological hygiene. Miners, even in their 40s or 50s, were successfully retrained and then appropriately employed. Research results and practical experience also refute theories holding that there is an unavoidable decline of physical and mental abilities. These mistaken views are one of the most important obstacles to purposeful and large-scale preparation for pensionable age. Only if wrong interpretations of aging are discarded will programmed preparatory measures be successful.

The resolution of the Council of Ministers of May 30, 1969, the skeleton agreement of July 24, 1969, and the Principles and Measures Regarding the Improved Medical Attendance of Citizens of Advanced Age of February 19, 1973, are important legal foundations on which this research can successfully be carried out and practicable solutions can be found in cooperation with governmental authorities and social forces. Considerable encouragement is given by the general instructions of the National Executive of FDGB of April 11, 1973. They contain provisions on the role, structure, tasks, and rules of procedure of work veterans' commissions of the executive committees of the FDGB and industrial unions, and the veterans' departmental trade union committees of enterprises and institutions. These bodies, which represent the interests of work veterans in society, make active contributions to the drafting of preparatory measures for pensionable age.

Another prerequisite for a purposeful preparation for pensionable age is the principle of GDR social policy that says that enterprises and regional authorities have to increase their cooperation in the planning and implementation of sociopolitical measures. This cooperation is especially important to the ideological aspects of preparatory measures. We consider these aspects as the necessary basis for a democratic and scientifically founded drafting and implementation of preparatory programs. The socialist policy of complex education, training, and advanced training has led to a remarkable improvement in the qualifications of working people in the GDR. This is proved beyond doubt by a comparison bertween the results of the census in 1954 and that taken in 1971.

Better preparation for pensionable age is required if the elderly are to adapt themselves to this stage in their lives with the greatest possible ease. Preparatory measures therefore have to go hand in hand with measures related to training and advanced training, a fact that the research results obtained so far clearly prove. Finally we consider that the existence of a developed socialist society is a basic requirement for the timely planning and implementation of preparatory programs and measures for pensionable age. The basic economic fact of socialism is based not on profit making but rather on the needs of working people. Some of these needs are the preservation and promotion of the ability to work, of good health, and of efficiency until old age.

Educational policy alone is not enough if these aims are to be reached; it has to be combined with effective medical attendance, whose principles were laid down in detail by the Ministry of Health on February 19, 1973, and declared binding for everybody who works in the public health system or in the social services. Follow-up care of specific diseases using case registers is a form of long-term care for groups of persons; it begins ten years before pensionable age and lasts as long as necessary. It is given to all elderly working people who have lost part of their efficiency for organic reasons or suffer from organic or psychic disorders. Such impairment of health is revealed in the periodic mass examinations decreed by the Council of Ministers. Relevant regulations say that this kind of care has to begin well before and continue during pensionable age.

A third basic requirement is that work place and job conditions for elderly working people have to be adapted to their biological age. This requirement is met also on the basis of legal provisions issued by the Council of Ministers. At the suggestion of research workers in gerontological hygiene and on instruction of the Ministry of Health, standards have been developed that in large measure meet the demand for working conditions to satisfy the needs of the elderly. Brilliant examples have been set and splendid initiatives have been taken at a number of enterprises.

Activities for the Elderly

The incorporation of the elderly into public life is rooted in everybody's right to work and to a job, whatever his age, sex, race, or religion. This elementary right is not just a humanitarian declaration; it is laid down in a large number of laws, in particular in the GDR's socialist constitution and, in even greater detail, in socialist labor law (the Labour Code) and resolutions of the Council of Ministers and the Confederation of Free German Trade Unions.

The resolution of the Council of Ministers of May 30, 1969, says that the industrial ministers, the chairman of the GDR Council for Agricultural Production and Food Economy, other heads of competent central governmental authorities, and regional councils have to ensure the following. First, when their efficiency is decreasing, elderly people have to be given working conditions and opportunities for pursuing activities as will enable them to take part in the labor process inside or outside enterprises or carry on some other socially useful activities that harmonize with their desires so that they can be active in accordance with their skills, knowledge, and experience under the conditions of the scientific and technological revolution in their own interest and that of society. It is pointed out that rationalization credits may be granted so that protected departments and workshops can be set up. Second, changes have to be made in time at the work places of these people so that they will not have to endure difficulties and need not take on another job. Third, enterprises have to provide production facilities that will allow elderly people to do work at home or in sheltered workshops, clubs of the Association of People's Solidarity, old people's homes, and nursing homes. Fourth, people of pensionable age should not work extra hours. Whether they work shifts at enterprises, institutions, and workshops will depend on their physical fitness and personal willingness. Finally, people of pensionable age who are not able or not willing to continue working at enterprises are to be given a wide variety of opportunities for voluntary activities in their residential areas—for example, in work teams that make repairs and render other services, at clubs and meeting centers of pensioners maintained by the association, or at old people's home or nursing homes. When they retire, they must not suffer an abrupt change in their social conditions; their links with their enterprises have to be maintained.

These basic instructions for ministers of industry and for the national economy as a whole are conveniently complemented by the principles decreed by the Minister of Health on December 19, 1973, which—in accordance with the resolution of the Council of Ministers—laid down the detailed medical conditions for the employment of old-age pensioners. These conditions include:

- The participation of elderly working people (women 55 and over and men 60 and over) in the preemployment medical examinations prescribed by law and the supervision of working people;
- The follow-up care of specific diseases (including the use of case registers), which serves to supervise the psychical and physical efficiency and fitness for employment at their work places. Also under the new conditions brought about by the scientific and technological revolution, these conditions stipulate measures that may be required (such as medicinal, physical, or dietary measures, inpatient treatment, sanatorium treatment, light work, change of work place or job, or rehabilitation).
- The constant supervision of work place to ensure that working conditions are adapted to the age of those working at them, and, if necessary, the adaptation of work places to the capabilities of elderly working people.

The public health services system staff and the social services personnel, local governmental authorities, government-appointed directors of enterprises, economic authorities, and trade union bodies are thus provided with opportunities to ensure that society can fully integrate elderly working people into the life at enterprises and society.

These government measures are also complemented by the General Instructions Concerning the Role, Structure, Tasks and Rules of Procedure of Work Veterans' Commissions Affiliated to FDGB Executive Committees, Industrial Unions, and Work Veterans' Department Trade Union Committees at Enterprises and Institutions of April 11, 1973. Some of the provisions contained in these instructions follow:

- Assessments have to be made at regular intervals of how pensioners and work veterans help to fulfill the principal task set at the Eighth Congress of the SED.
- The executive committees and committees of the trade unions have to devote more attention to the further improvement of the working and living conditions of work veterans and pensioners at enterprises and, through improved cooperation with the People's Solidarity, they have to improve conditions in residential areas.
- The activities of the work veterans' commissions of executive committees have to be encouraged and accounts have to be given at regular intervals on the results that the commissions have achieved in their activities. The work veterans' commissions are instructed to contribute to the social, intellectual, and cultural care of trade union veterans and pensioners; encourage pensioners and work veterans to work at enterprises and institutions for short periods of time; encourage work veterans and pensioners to carry on unpaid honorary public activities; make proposals about the improvement of working conditions and protected work places for work veterans and pensioners; intensify contacts with pensioners who have

stopped working; and lay down such measures in enterprise collective agreements* on the basis of the labor code as will improve the social and cultural care of pensioners; and submit proposals to the enterprise trade union committee that aim at creating favorable working conditions for working people whose efficiency is declining.

Intellectual and Cultural Activities

The complete incorporation of the elderly and the aged into the life of society includes their integration into intellectual and cultural activities of society. The term *socialist culture* refers to the intellectual, moral, aesthetic, and emotional levels of development of each person; it thus incorporates one's entire knowledge, skills, talents, behavioral patterns, attitudes, convictions, social habits, and pleasures.

This rather wide concept of culture entails complex cultural tasks for developed socialist society. Even old people can use the vehicle of art to gain new intellectual and emotional understanding of certain processes and developments. The experience that art provides can be of great help to them in everyday life when they try to maintain and deepen their relations with other people. Thus culture has a great bearing on the human relations and the moral and ethical behavior patterns of elderly people and also those of younger age groups, which is reflected in the way younger people behave toward older people. The reason is that art refines everybody's ethics, encourages humanitarian behavior, and allows the individuals and society to lead full lives. If relations among people in society are to reach their optimum, especially for the benefit of the elderly, the enjoyment of art by both elderly and young people has to be given a great deal of attention.

Art also satisfies the human need for joy at everything that is beautiful and noble in life. Yet this is not always possible; it depends rather on the content and forms of art. Art can also engender hatred, which has an unfavorable effect on relations among people. Everything is done in the GDR to prevent old people from being discredited. The resolution of the Council of Ministers, May 30, 1969, and the skeleton agreement quite clearly seek to incorporate elderly people fully into intellectual and cultural life. This is increasingly becoming the most important job for the Association of People's Solidarity, which was deliberately freed from tasks that prevented it in the past from making full use of the potential of socialist society and its own potential. The needs of many elderly people for pursuing cultural activities and attending cultural events have risen considerably. The elderly participate in hobby groups, working groups, and hobby circles, and they display a great readiness

---

*An enterprise collective agreement is concluded once a year between the management and the trade union branch of an enterprise and contains measures related to the fulfillment of plans and social conditions for the employees of the enterprises.

to become familiar with treasures of culture. In 1972, 10,233 local branches, 302 clubs, and 254 meeting centers of the Association of People's Solidarity held 105,599 political and cultural events. They were attended by 7,480,000 persons of advanced age.

A wide variety of cultural activities, joint attendance at art events, penetrating discussions, and social gatherings have given rise to new intellectual and cultural participation by large numbers of elderly people. The Association of People's Solidarity and its committees have realized that the development of an interesting intellectual and cultural life in its local branches, clubs, and meeting centers has become a primary objective. Experience has shown that changes in the cultural life of a people cannot be effected overnight. Therefore, the mobilization of elderly people in connection with this kind of care is a long-term job and a continuous process of great importance.

The principal goal of the process is that attention be given not only to the passive enjoyment of art but also to active artistic creation, which is in line with the wide concept of culture defined above. This refers not only to culture at the work place but also in the homes of elderly people. This effort forms part of the complex socialist rationalization scheme that determines the organization of working and living conditions in terms of gerontological hygiene. The GDR's cultural policy is guided by the principle that only what becomes part of our everyday life and habits really counts in terms of culture.

The wide range of intellectual and cultural activities under socialism includes the acquisition of a wide general knowledge, a variety of social gatherings, and a life marked by cheerfulness, joy of living, recreation, relaxation, and sports. Thus the intellectual and cultural life of a person takes place in production work, public activities, and the organization of his environment and the relations among men. Socialist cultural needs comprise those for meaningful creative activities in material production, the participation in running and planning the development of society, and the establishment of genuine fraternal relations among people at work places and during spare time; a wide general education and best job qualifications, and the utilization in everyday work and life of the knowledge gained in general education and advanced training; clean and beautiful residential areas, flats, enterprises, and work places; and sports and recreation of various types, including social events, dances, conversations, and relaxation.

At enterprises, intellectual and cultural activities are initiated and pursued by production collectives in the main and by all working collectives, party branches, institutions of training and advanced training, art circles, and clubs. Regionally they are carried on by families, communities of tenants occupying the same block of flats, public organizations, restaurants, sports grounds, clubs, artistic institutions, museums, and memorial places. The integration of the elderly into these activities is one of the principal tasks of government-appointed managers and forces of society, with the Association of People's Solidarity playing a prominent part.

The principles governing the comprehensive care for people of advanced age were given the form of theses by the People's Solidarity. They include the following suggestions on methodical procedures:

1. Discussions should be launched at clubs and meeting centers so that lively exchanges of views can be held with leading public figures, including party and government officials, deputies to Parliament and regional assemblies, and cultural workers. The subjects of these discussions should include current political affairs and important matters of the conduct of life.
2. The plans of enterprises that deal with working and living conditions and with intellectual and cultural activities should produce an effect on the enterprises themselves, on areas under the direct supervision of local governmental authorities, and on residential areas.
3. Cultural events arranged by other segments of society should include more elderly people. Village clubs, agricultural production cooperatives, and associations of villages should help to reach these aims in the countryside.
4. An increasing number of clubs are open on Saturdays and Sundays in more and more counties and districts. On these days, hot food should be served for lunch.
5. Creative cultural activities should be intensified at clubs and meeting centers of the People's Solidarity. These activities should take the form of singing, music, do-it-yourself work, collecting, gardening, chess and so forth. Heavy emphasis is laid on the foundation of hobby groups for gymnastics for the elderly; for this purpose, contacts should be established with the section for sports for the elderly of the German Sports and Gymnastics Union.
6. Social gatherings and entertainment should be of high quality. First-class cultural workers, musicians, and other artists should be secured for important occasions.
7. Television should adapt its programs to the needs of the elderly.

These principles also include specific forms of cultural activities, such as outings and excursions, tributes paid to elderly persons, the membership of such persons in club committees and discussions with young people at schools, Pioneer Clubs, youth clubs, apprentice workshops, and young people's homes. Their cooperation in club commissions, local branches, and meeting centers of the People's Solidarity proves to be another important way of mobilizing the elderly to take a more active part in intellectual and cultural activities. All these efforts and programs are not allowed to develop spontaneously in the GDR; they are planned, discussed, and adopted by vote in a democratic manner. They are also checked upon by progress reports. Since elderly citizens take an active part in their planning and management, they help find solutions adapted to their needs and thus contribute to the humanitarian aims of national culture.

Medical Care

The medical care of people of advanced age, especially those who are alone, is systematically extended. This is one of the permanent top priorities of basic outpatient care. Its principal objective is preventing and combating chronic diseases. Elderly people receive medical care, like everybody else, under the socialist health protection system.

Medical care for the elderly includes:

- Adequate information and documentation for every doctor about the elderly persons living in his or her area.
- The gradual integration of these persons into a system of follow-up care for the aged (which is independent of the medical supervision of working pensioners provided by doctors at their enterprises).
- The organization of care for elderly persons in the residential area concerned who require nursing. The potential represented by public organizations and neighborly help is drawn on for the purpose.
- The organization of care at home before elderly persons leave hospital. This care is agreed on with the doctor who is in charge of following-up outpatient treatment.
- Expert advice for the elderly on how to improve their health and raise their efficiency. This advice is given under health education schemes and serves to help them to prepare for old age.
- The organization of specific geriatric care by consulting physicians at district and county level. It includes coordination of care potential and promulgation of special knowledge and research results in the field of geriatrics among doctors, nurses, social workers, and other personnel looking after the elderly.

Some of these stipulations refer to the first directive, issued on March 16, 1970, to implement the resolution of the Council of Ministers. It is headlined the Improvement of Medical, Social and Cultural Care for Citizens of Advanced Age and the Encouragement of Their Increased Participation in Public Life. Although this directive deals mainly with social and cultural aspects, the Decree on Principles Regarding the Improvement of the Medical Care of Citizens of Advanced age of February 19, 1973, is primarily concerned with medical aspects. GDR scientists who are concerned with these affairs say that there is no similar legislation in other countries.

The medical care of persons of advanced age is the job of all doctors who administer outpatient and inpatient treatment. Doctors are assisted by nurses, predominantly district nurses, and by social workers. The heads of institutions of the public health system and the social services show understanding and care of the elderly and, in consequence, ensure excellent outpatient treatment. Particularly noteworthy are the efforts made to spare old people irritatingly long periods of waiting and troublesome long walks or travels to doctors. Any inpatient treatment necessary is given in close coordination with the institutions of the inpatient health system.

Doctors who administer outpatient treatment know about the people of advanced age who live in the areas they serve. This information is obtained in a joint effort of the doctor, the district nurse, and the social worker of the area concerned. Wide-ranging assistance is also provided by the voluntary staff of the People's Solidarity and the Nursing and Social Service of the Red Cross. Doctors also have recourse to reports prepared by the councils of urban districts, towns, and villages that contain information about the care in the particular region. The doctor who administers treatment to an elderly person is in charge of this person's whole medical care and has to initiate nursing, if required.

Outpatient nursing is done by district nurses, who are in close touch with the elderly. They take medical measures, nurse the sick, and attend to the personal problems of elderly persons. Their work gives the aged a sense of comfort and security. The staff of the Association of People's Solidarity and the Nursing and Welfare Service of the Red Cross are important forces of society that help fulfill these humanitarian tasks. The elderly know that if they fall ill, their cases will be diagnosed properly and speedily, and they will receive constant medical supervision and treatment, often in their homes. How frequently they are visited depends on their state of health.

Doctors treat elderly persons in their own homes when necessary. Patients of advanced age who are capable of walking can see doctors during consultation hours, which are held at offices of district nurses, doctors' practices, old people's homes, and nursing homes. Sometimes doctors go to clubs of the People's Solidarity to give advice. These services make it easier for patients to consult a doctor and to shorten any walks or travels to him. Experienced doctors who are no longer in active service often provide assistance in this respect.

When an elderly person is admitted to a hospital, the hospital gets in touch with the doctor who provides the outpatient treatment. Such contacts are particularly important when a patient is about to leave the hospital so that subsequent care (medical treatment and nursing) can be arranged. An integral part of the medical and social care for the elderly is rehabilitation.

Medical and social care also covers advice for the elderly on how to promote good health and efficiency and recommendations on intellectual and physical activities they should pursue to maintain their personal and public activities as long as possible. District centers for health education fulfill these special tasks of health education. Cases deserving special mention are those in which working people of 55 to 66 years are given follow-up care for specific diseases by the enterprise health service. In this way, care of persons of advanced age is begun that is continued in their residential areas or enterprises after they have stopped working. As long as elderly working people are in full-time or part-time employment, their work places and jobs are continuously adjusted to the needs of their age. The factors that are taken into consideration include fitness, abilities, and interests. The district medical officer of health is responsible for all measures that serve to coordinate the activities of outpatient and inpatient institutions of the public health system.

The further improvement of the medical care of elderly people required that a suitable specialist, who primarily administers outpatient treatment and has a thorough knowledge of matters related to geriatrics and gerontological hygiene, assist and advise the district medical officer of health. One of the tasks of this doctor is to spread research results and domestic and foreign experience in the field of geriatrics among doctors, nurses, and social workers in the district he is in charge of. District medical officers of health have ensured that in a large number of cases doctors are employed full time at old people's homes, and especially at nursing homes, to look after their occupants. Today this is particularly true of large homes; in other cases, one doctor looks after the occupants of several homes.

The advanced training required for all personnel concerned with the medical and social care of elderly people has to be ensured by the district medical officer of health as well. It is usually provided by competent institutions of health care and consulting physicians. Their work ensures that the opinion that pathology is caused by old age is gradually being eroded.

The GDR Academy of Advanced Training for Doctors runs a course every year that provides instruction and advanced training to doctors who work in geriatrics and give advice in districts and counties. This system encourages an early application of new knowledge, regular advanced training, and exchanges of experience at lower levels. The basic medical training provided at universities and medical academies in the GDR and the basic training given to medium-level medical personnel provide a systematically increased amount of knowledge in gerontology and gerontological hygiene. In the standards for the training of specialists, more and more attention is paid to the tasks involved in giving elderly people medical attention and arming these specialists with the relevant knowledge.

The advanced training given to doctors, nurses, and social workers serves to spread knowledge in geriatrics and gerontological hygiene in line with the latest findings of medical science and practical experience. There has been a remarkable improvement in the medical care of these persons over the last few years.

Social Care

Home help organized by local councils, the People's Solidarity, the National Front, and other forces of society in residential areas serves to make life more comfortable for elderly people who are in need of attendance and nursing and to relieve them of household duties and any other work involved in looking after themselves if they are not capable of doing so. This care is geared to the individual requirements of elderly people and is provided by means of a wide variety of measures. Its primary objective is to give sick people help if they need it rather than to leave them to their own devices and to prevent loneliness by encouraging their contacts with the people around them.

The growing sense of responsibility for one another among people in the GDR is a precondition for elderly people's being offered care by their neighbors, in particular by tenants in the same block of flats, volunteers of the People's Solidarity, the Democratic Women's League, and the Red Cross. Most blocks contain an occupant who is supported by the residential area commission of the National Front and attends to the needs, interests, and problems of elderly people.

Help and services are organized for the elderly by governmental authorities and public organizations to an ever increasing extent in every residential area. These include: practical and financial help when flats in old buildings are being renovated; repairs; laundry service at reduced rates or free of charge and the organization of a laundry collecting and delivery service; help by neighbors; housekeeping and flat cleaning by the People's Solidarity; help in everyday activities organized by the socialist children's and young people's organizations, among others; the provision of technical aids for running the household, additional sanitary and hygienic installations, aids for dressing and undressing, and so forth; the provision of hot meals brought to the flats of persons who are without a family and require nursing; the distribution of meals at reduced prices at factory canteens, restaurants, clubs, the People's Solidarity, institutions of the public health system, and the social services; and the use of bathing and shower equipment and pedicure at regular intervals.

The People's Solidarity, which has a membership of more than 1.6 million and employs a voluntary staff of about 119,000, does a tremendous job of helping elderly people at home; it continually upgrades its help. About 21,000 elderly persons who require nursing are at present assisted by 14,700 housekeepers of the organization. In 1968 these figures were 11,200 and 8,500, respectively. The government provided more than 20 million marks for this purpose in 1972.

Old people's and nursing homes are important in social care. They demonstrate the GDR's concern about the well-being of its citizens and their constitutional right to security and care in old age in practical terms. Old people's and nursing homes provide full board and lodging, social care, cultural care, nursing, and medical attention to people who need this kind of help. The homes offer all the conveniences of flats. They are the permanent (and usually last) residence of their occupants. These factors determine the way the occupants live together, encourage the preservation of their mental faculties, and inspire their cultural activities. These homes also serve as centers at which old people in surrounding areas receive care.

Since the GDR was founded, new government-sponsored homes have been built and suitable buildings have been converted so that the total number of places at these homes has risen from 38,000 to 79,500. In addition, there are about 17,300 places at denominational homes. Thus 3 percent of all people of pensionable age were accommodated in such homes in 1972; within the next few years, this figure will rise to 5 percent. The proportion of places for the aged at nursing homes has gone up from 32 percent (24,000 places) in 1955 to over 57 percent (55,600 places) in 1972. This increase has taken place mainly in the last few years in response to the rising demand. The government provided a total of roughly 210 million marks of subsidies in 1972 to support government-sponsored homes and to render services to denominational homes. The monthly expenditure for every occupant is 230 marks at old people's homes and 330 marks at nursing homes. The occupants themselves pay only a small amount toward the expenses—up to 90 marks at govenment-sponsored old-people's homes and up to 105 marks at government-sponsored nursing homes. Occupants who need public relief receive a monthly allowance of 60 marks from the government. Admission into a home is based solely on a person's need for help and nursing; financial conditions are never considered.

Since the GDR has a large proportion of people over 70 years, governmental authorities face the important task of increasing the number of places, especially at nursing homes, within the next few years. In the wake of World War II, the GDR found itself in a situation in which it had to provide nursing for a large number of people in a very short period of time, but it did not have suitable buildings. Therefore a large number of old people's and nursing homes had to be set up in rather old buildings, such as large blocks of flats, former castles, and manor houses. Many of these buildings have been thoroughly renovated to include modern conveniences and to permit first-class care. For this purpose the Ministry of Health issued minimum requirements on June 24, 1970, which have to be met in the renovation of old homes. Newly built homes have to comply with the General Instructions for the Planning, Designing and Equipment of Old People's Homes with Nursing Wards of July 12, 1973.

Housing

Housing conditions are a very important factor of complex care. Elderly people try to keep up their independence in, and responsibility for, running their households, managing their lives, and organizing their relations within their traditional surroundings as long as they can. Therefore they have to be given flats that meet their needs and make life easy for them. This principle underlies the resolution of the Council of Ministers of May 30, 1969, which places local governmental authorities under an obligation to provide elderly people with suitable housing space. Statistics show that about 30 percent of all flats in the GDR are occupied by pensioners who run independent households. Yet these pensioners represent only 13 percent of the population. Many of them live on upper floors, although physical disability and old age make it very difficult for them to climb stairs.

In areas of towns where there are virtually nothing but old buildings, the proportion of old-age pensioners has been increasing steadily, since generally only fairly young working people have moved into new residential areas. The resultant gradual concentraton of elderly people in certain residential areas and their subsequent separation from the younger population would be a trend that did not meet the interests of the elderly and was incompatible with their position in socialist society. Therefore this trend has to be vigorously resisted. Elderly people who have stopped working do not wish to be isolated from the rest of the population; they prefer to keep in touch with the working population, to live near their children or other relatives, and to take part in community affairs. They have proved that they can be useful to society; for example, they can render help to working people by looking after their children and doing cleaning work and repairs in flats. Therefore for the last few years, local governmental authorities have been providing more and more suitable housing space for elderly people in new residential areas.

The number of residential homes and apartments for elderly people continues to increase. Their planning and designing is regulated by recommendations issued by the Ministry of Health on May 13, 1971. These homes and buildings offer all the necessary advantages for the elderly, especially since they permit occupants who are without a family to be in constant touch with the people around them and, if necessary, to get help from neighbors. Old people who require care or nursing all the time receive assistance from the People's Solidarity in the form of home help or from a public meal distribution center.

In addition to subsidized rents for flats in new buildings, they benefit from other government subsidies, which allow them to move into flats that meet the requirements of old age.

GERONTOLOGICAL RESEARCH

A central gerontological research project launched by the Ministry of Health in 1969 has been continuing the long-standing traditions of German gerontological researchers under new conditions and in line with their ideas on clinical and experimental gerontology. Work on this project is done by 250 scientists and other staff of various specializations from institutions of higher education and the public health system. Some of the project's top priorities are more effective forms of social, medical, and gerohygienic care of old people; the combating and prevention of diseases frequent in old age; the investigation of reasons for, consequences of, and influences on functional disturbances in old age; contributions to research into the causes of aging processes; the maintenance of efficiency and the ability to work in advanced age; and the preparation for pensionable age.

The project helps prepare training programs that guarantee a systematic advanced training of doctors and an adequate training of students in practical gerontology. Special lectures are read by those working in internal medicine and other fields of medicine, and compulsory advanced training is given in gerontology and geriatrics in the clinical training of specialists.

The project forms part of an international research effort. International cooperation is carried on mainly with the Research Institute for Gerontology of the Academy of Medical Sciences of the Soviet Union in Kiev and with many other national institutes in the world. Agreement was reached in the Coordinating Committee of Socialist Countries in the Field of Gerontology on comprehensive cooperation with other socialist countries. The Gesellschaft für Gerontologie der DDR ("Society of Gerontology of the GDR"), which is affiliated with the Gesellschaft für Klinische Medizin der DDR ("Society for Clinical Medicine of the GDR"), makes tremendous efforts to spread new knowledge and to encourage exchanges of information among doctors working in gerontology, and to plan and give training in this field. The society holds a national conference every two years, which is also attended by scientists from abroad, and it sends members to other conferences in this field. A large number of papers were read by GDR delegates at the World Gerontological Conference in Kiev in 1972. In a joint effort with gerontological societies of all other socialist countries, it publishes the *Zeitschrift für Alternaforschung* ("Journal of Gerontological Research"), which discusses theoretical aspects and practical clinical aspects of gerontological research and describes the position of aging and old people in the GDR and other countries.

Since gerontological research is so important, the gradual establishment of a center for gerontology is planned in the GDR. This center will be a national place of reference for everybody engaged in this work.

Under the research project, a lot of work of great practical importance has been accomplished to help improve the care of old people. As an example, the program for the prevention and control of cerebrovascular disease helps make use of the latest scientific findings. The research results from this project have helped to draft new hygienic requirements and norms—for example, flats for old people—and to boost the efficiency of such people in their activities for the benefit of society. These results also show that old age does not necessarily lead to a decline in efficiency and the ability to learn; instead the integration of old people into the life of society is a social and medical necessity. The results prove the correctness of the thesis that work is indispensable for people. Useful work adapted to the change in efficiency in old age, the encouragement it gives to the devlopment of each person's personality, and the proof it furnishes of each person's social value are of decisive importance in the delay of the process of biological aging.

The fact that approximately 600,000 people of pensionable age make use of their right to work proves that this opinion has by and large established itself in practice. The changes taking place in the GDR, a modern industrial state, as a result of scientific and technological progress do not restrict our view that work is important for the elderly. The socialist relations of production objectively offer every opportunity to elderly people to make use of their constitutional rights.

REFERENCES

Demmler, H. "Soziale aspekte der Gestaltung der Arbertsbegingungen für Altere Werktatige," *Zeitschrift für Alternaforschung* 31, no. 2 (1976), 107-141.

Eitner, A. "Zu Einigen Aufgaben, Zielen und Programminhalten der Geropsychohygiene bei der Vorbereitung auf das Alter," *Zeitschrift für Alternaforschung* 33, no. 2 (1978), 127-140.

Eitner, S., and Richter, G. Rehabilitation und Gerontologie," *Zeitschrift für Alternaforschung* 33, no. 3 (1978), 213-226.

Schmidt, U. J., and Bruescke, G. "A preventive programme for people on advanced age in the GDR," *Giornale di Gerontologia* 23, no. 11 (1975), 973-977.

GREECE

JOHN ZARRAS

The population of Greece is estimated at 9,268,000 currently. Of this number, some 1,173,000 persons are 65 years of age or more, including approximately 196,000 persons who are more than 80 years old.

Greece has not yet determined the nature and extent of the needs of its aged population or the number of old persons who are incapable of coping, either on their own initiative or even with the help of their families, with their personal problems. Moreover no attempt has been made to define and evaluate such problems or to weigh their importance. Yet day by day, the government, and indeed society as a whole, particularly in the larger urban agglomerations, are made aware of the constant growth in the number of aged persons who stand in imperative need of some form of assistance—financial, social, or psychological. In many cases such assistance is either not forthcoming or is deficient in quantity or quality.

Greece is thus beginning to be aware that it has done very little toward meeting these needs. The country is face to face with a new and quite distinct problem of many facets to which it has not hitherto given serious attention. It is beginning to understand that it can no longer confine itself to the protection of a restricted number of aged persons who undeservedly find themselves in distressed circumstances. It is called upon to take a serious interest in and systematically care for a large segment of the population—to attend to their welfare and happiness and make sure that they have an active and respected place in the community.

DEMOGRAPHY

The Greek population is steadily aging. The aging index (percentage of those 65 and over), which today stands at about 12.3 percent, is estimated to reach 16 percent by the year 2000. The expectation of life at birth, at present calculated at about 70 years for men and 73 years for women, is expected to reach 72 and 76 years, respectively, by 1985. According to certain forecasts, in the year 2000, the total population will be 10.5 million. Of these, 1,675,000 will be 65 and over, and 336,000 will be 80 and over.

The needs of so substantial a segment of the population—in relation to Greece's resources—will inevitably be extensive and diverse; they will, moreover, swell progressively in volume. It is thus evident that the aging of the Greek population and the ensuing consequences, economic and social, are now beginning to be of growing importance to the country.

The aging of the population in Greece is similar to that prevailing in other European counties. It is due to a decreasing birthrate. In addition, the high rate of emigration is accelerating the trend in Greece (table 12).

Table 12: PERCENTAGE DISTRIBUTION OF POPULATION, BY AGE AND YEAR

Age	1961	1971		1980	
			a	b	c
0–14	25.9	24.9	24.2	22.7	23.0
15–64	65.7	64.0	65.9	63.9	64.4
65 and over	8.4	11.1	9.9	13.4	12.6

Source: G. Siampos, *Demographic Evolution of Modern Greece, 1821-1980.* Athens, 1973, p. 185.

Note: Column a assumes no migration in the period 1961–1971.
Column b projection takes into account emigration from 1966–1980.
Column c assumes no migration in the period 1966–1980.

During the twenty-year period 1951–1971, the number of aged persons nearly doubled, rising from 500,000 to almost a million. The proportion of aged persons rose from 7 percent to 11 percent in the same period (table 13). It is estimated that if no emigration movement had taken place, the proportion might have been lower. The main cause of aging remains the low birthrate of the postwar period coupled with low mortality.

Table 13: POPULATION 65 YEARS AND OVER

	Absolute Numbers			Percentage of Total
Year	*Males*	*Females*	*Total*	
1951	227,020	287,079	514,099	7.0%
1961	295,774	390,880	686,654	8.4
1971	418,656	538,460	957,116	11.1
1980	553,000	686,000	1,239,000	13.4

Source: G. Siampos, *Demographic Evolution of Modern Greece, 1821-1980.* Athens, 1973, p. 185.

The large number of surviving aged people is the result of the low mortality, as reflected in the high expectation of life. Expectation of life at birth is 70.1 years for males and 73.8 years for females; these levels are similar to those of other European countries (table 14). At age 65, the expectation of life during the twenty-year period 1950–1970 increased from 12.7 to 14.3 for males and from 14.6 to 16.3 for females. A newborn infant gained more than seven years during this period, while an old person of 65 gained fewer than two years.

Table 14: LIFE EXPECTANCY BY SEX

	At Birth		At Age 65	
Year	Males	Females	Males	Females
1950	62.84	66.30	12.72	14.63
1960	67.00	70.38	14.00	15.58
1970	70.09	73.79	14.25	16.30

Source: G. Siampos, Demographic Evolution of Modern Greece, 1821-1980. Athens, 1973, p. 185; Office National de Statistique de Grèce, "Mouvement Naturel de la Population de la Grèce." Athens, 1974, p. 202.

That there are more surviving females age 65 and over results from a higher mortality and more emigration among males. The ratio of the aged stood at 778 males to 1,000 females in 1971. In 1961 and 1951, the respective ratios were 757 men to 1,000 women and 791 men to 1,000 women.

The number of divorced persons and single persons among the elderly is small. The majority of males are married; a small proportion is widowed. Among females, the majority are widowed. (See table 15.) These differences are due to the fact that average age at marriage was much lower for females than for males and to the higher male mortality.

Table 15: MARITAL STATUS OF THOSE 65 AND OVER

Marital	Percentage Distribution			Absolute Numbers, 1971	
Status	1951	1961	1971	Males	Females
Total	100.0	100.0	100.0	418,656	538,460
Single	3.5	4.0	5.0	20,520	27,268
Married	50.9	51.7	56.9	334,048	210,152
Widowed	45.4	43.8	37.3	60,980	296,292
Divorced	0.2	0.5	0.8	3,108	4,748

Source: G. Siampos, Demographic Evolution of Modern Greece, 1821-1980. Athens, 1973, p. 185; National Statistical Service of Greece, Statistical Yearbook of Greece, Athens, 1977, p. 423.

DEVELOPMENT OF GERONTOLOGY

Numerous experts have sought to trace the origins of gerontology and geriatrics to classical times, citing texts that refer to the old age of Homer, Solon, Hippocrates, and, from a later period, Galen. The ancients, of course, were not familiar with the phenomenon of aging insofar as its grave social and economic consequences were concerned, a phenomenon that has led to the recent rapid development and advancement of gerontology as a special branch of knowledge.

In 1953 the Society for the Protection of Old Age was founded in Athens. Although its aims included the study of the problems of old age, the society in fact confined its activity to the provision of medical care to a limited number of indigent old persons.

Only in recent years has public opinion in Greece become aware of the problems of old age and of the need to take systematic action to cope with them. During 1968, the Ministry of Coordination set up the Commission on Demographic Policy, which in turn appointed a special working group. That November, the group's report described the increase in the proportion of aged persons in Greece as being "not only the gravest—in its adverse consequences —among the problems affecting the contemporary demographic evolution of the country, but the one of which least is known generally." In 1973 Greece introduced the first legislative instrument—legislative decree 162—relating to measures for the protection of persons of advanced age. This decree, however, merely enunciated general principles of policy in this particular sector. Nevertheless a fairly general interest in the problems of old age had begun to manifest itself, in various ways, much earlier. The reason is simple: at no time had the state withdrawn its traditional interest in a largely institutional protection of needy old people, even as—by the same token—charitable initiative strove unceasingly to provide a variety of services for them.

In Greece—by contrast with other countries—senior citizens have not yet set up organizations designed to study and deal with their particular problems. The sole form of organization among aged persons in Greece is to be found in the pensioners' unions, whose main purpose is to defend the social insurance rights of their members. These unions constitute what is known as "pensioners syndicalism."

The movement toward collective organization and collective action in the sector of gerontology has assumed importance only since 1976. It is supported principally by members of the learned and liberal professions—doctors, biologists, demographers, psychologists, sociologists, and social administrators— who direct their attention to the various facets of the problem of old age.

As a result of this movement, two learned societies have recently been founded: the Greek Geriatric Society (1976) and the Hellenic Association of Gerontology (1977). It is expected that the two societies will provide the requisite impetus to the development of gerontology in Greece.

STATUS AND ROLES

Emigration and Urbanization

The urban population of Greece shows a tendency toward a continuous increase in relation to total population: it rose from 38 percent in 1951, to 44 percent in 1961, and to 53 percent in 1971. A dearth of land holdings, chronic underemployment, a marked feeling of financial insecurity, and a low standard of living are the main reasons why large numbers of Greek farm workers have abandoned the land to seek a better life either abroad or in urban areas in Greece, principally the Athens district and the Salonica conurbation. Thus the greater Athens area is today estimated to represent 32 percent of the population of Greece and 56 percent of the country's total urban population. Furthermore, in the period since 1952 there has been a tremendous increase in emigration, both overseas and to western Europe, a trend (particularly from 1952 to 1973) that has been the most extensive in the modern history of Greece. The large majority of the emigrants come from agricultural regions and belong to the economically active population.

The intensified flight from the land has altered the old social structure of the Greek village and created new conditions for the rural family and its aged members. No less serious in their impact on family life and on aged persons have been the changes in living conditions that have inevitably occurred in urban centers that have absorbed the migratory flow.

Family Structure

A few decades ago, the patriarchal family constituted the characteristic model of Greek social organization. Today the extended family is no longer the rule. The tendency toward the nuclear family started to manifest itself many years ago, initially in the cities and later in rural areas. Nevertheless the patriarchal family continues to be of some importance—albeit to a reduced degree—in rural areas, particularly as a center of productivity, and there are still cases in which children, even after marriage, remain in the parental home.

In urban areas, there are progressively more cases in which both the parents and the married children find it necessary or preferable not to live under the same roof. A sample study made in 1966 indicated that the nuclear family is the family type most often encountered in Greece (66 percent of the sample in the Athens district). Cases in which parents or other relations of one spouse share the home represent no more than 18 percent.

Family Cohesion

Quite apart from the question of whether aged parents live with their married children, the ties between them and their children remain strong, in town and in country alike.

A sizable proportion of the young people who leave their villages try not to cut themselves off completely from parents and relatives. Whenever opportunity offers, they visit them and continue to care for them.

Frequently once the children are satisfactorily settled in an urban center, they take steps for their parents to join them in the new home. At the same time, cases do arise in which old people, fearing the turmoil of city life, prefer to remain in their village. Cases of widowed women living with their children and grandchildren are far commoner than widowed men living in those circumstances. In Greece, the grandmother plays a useful role in the rearing of the children and in maintaining tradition, and this is true in both the rural and the urban areas.

Although cases in which children in the large towns show indifference to or even abandon their parents are constantly growing in number, it is nonetheless generally regarded as incumbent upon the children to concern themselves with their parents' problems and to help them in every possible way.

In keeping with Greek tradition and custom, the care of parents in their old age continues to be a sacred duty for the children; it is deemed a token of honor. Conversely, the total neglect of an aged parent and his admission to an old people's home—particularly if the home is among those maintained for indigent persons and which often fall far short of acceptable standards—entail a grave social reproach for the children.

Thus if the problem of the protection and care of aged persons in Greece has not yet assumed the magnitude and gravity that are implicit in so heavy an incidence of aging, this fact is mainly attributable to the Greek family and to the care it devotes to its older members.

Role, Status, and Living Conditions

In rural areas cases of families in which the parent maintains the traditional role of head of the family are not uncommon. At the same time the mechanization of agriculture and new methods of cultivation, to which the young are more adaptable, have inevitably diminished the role played by their elders.

Since 1961, the adoption of a general measure providing for the award of pensions to farm workers over 65 years of age has served to lend support to the faltering status of the elderly. This pension, though small, has raised the morale of a whole group of persons who previously had to look to their families for even their petty expenses. The measure has also enhanced the position of the elderly not only within the family but within the community as a whole.

The life of the aged in rural areas is a tranquil and simple one. They continue, to the extent of their ability, to undertake light work, and their recreational demands are small. Their recreation resides in the family circle, radio and television, and sitting on the front porch—a pastime they can enjoy almost the whole year because of the mild climate.

Elderly men find pleasure in frequenting the village coffeehouse, playing cards or backgammon, taking part in discussions, and offering their views, their experiences, and their reminiscences. In the villages, even the old men who have no relatives feel less lonely than they would in the cities; their long, honest life has earned them respect, the atmosphere of the coffeehouse is congenial, and they enjoy the daily companionship of their fellow villagers.

Living conditions for the elderly in the large urban centers, Athens in particular, cannot be considered satisfactory. The reasons are many: crowded conditions in apartment houses, the polluted air, the noise, the incessant traffic in the streets, the lack of parks or sheltered areas for the elderly, the long distances between points of the city, the shortage of house servants, and similar problems. In such an environment, the adjustments confronting the elderly upon retirement are difficult, especially those whose pension is small by comparison with past earnings. Those who have children and relatives who still show an interest in their well-being escape the feeling of total isolation to some extent. But those who are alone and who feel unwanted become dejected.

Unlike their counterparts in the villages, old men in the large cities constantly see their role and their authority dwindling. They do not understand the changing patterns of family and social life in the city. They move unnoticed amid crowds of strangers. They do not, of course, encounter any feelings of hostility or even unkindness, but the marks of respect formerly shown by the young toward the old in public places are gradually disappearing.

Elderly people who migrate to the large cities, either in search of employment or to join their children, have to face difficult problems. Leaving the open spaces and the clean air of the countryside, they find themselves abruptly compelled to spend their days in dark, crowded, squalid dwellings since the income of their children—usually manual workers—is low. They are doomed to idleness either through lack of special skills or because of age. They are forced to change their everyday habits radically, together with the tempo of their lives, losing thereby the feeling of personal freedom. Within an alien social milieu, they are incapable of forming new ties to take the place of the friends, the church, and the coffeehouse of their native village.

All these factors have an adverse influence on their health, tending to nurture dejection and hasten the onset of the physical exhaustion of old age. It is not rare to come across cases in which old people decide to part from their children in the city and return to their village.

PROGRAMS

Pensions and Social Insurance

Reference has been made to the interest—by and large, the warm interest—that the Greek family normally continues to evince toward its older members. In addition, one other factor has hitherto served to retard the more acute manifestations of the problem of old age: an intricate system of social insurance of extremely broad scope.

The social insurance structure, based on a large number of sectorial schemes, follows these general lines:

1. All wage earners in urban areas not covered by a sectoral insurance agency are insured by the Social Insurance Institute against disability, old age, sickness, and death.

2. Certain categories of salaried persons in urban areas are insured against the fore-going risks by independent sectoral agencies.
3. All wage earners in urban areas are insured against unemployment and in respect of dependency benefits by the Labor Force Employment Organization.
4. A special insurance applies to civil servants and the armed forces in respect to pensions and medical care.
5. Persons engaged in the professions (with few exceptions) come under separate insurance funds.
6. In addition to the benefits offered by their main insurance system, a large proportion of the urban population are entitled to supplementary benefits offered by various auxiliary insurance funds and provident funds.
7. Farmers and farm workers are insured by the Agricultural Insurance Organization against disability, old age, and sickness, as well as against crop damage due to natural causes (such as hail and frost).

Thus almost all aged Greek persons, particularly those over 65 years of age (and many even below that age, depending on the insurance agency to which they belong), either receive a monthly pension or rely indirectly on such a pension for their maintenance (for example, through a spouse entitled to a pension).

Nevertheless the prevailing system of old-age pension grants is full of discrepancies and inequalities that should be studied and removed. Extensive differences are found in the legislation and statutes governing the various insurance agencies regarding pensionable age, the general conditions applying to pension entitlement, the method of calculation, and the question of the accumulation of pensions and salaries. Auxiliary insurance covers only part of the population and in a far from uniform manner.

For many categories of pensioners, the amount of the pension at the lowest levels remains unacceptably small, particularly if compared with cases of large or multiple pensions that are in payment. Pensioners who were at low points in the wage scale and who reached pensionable age before completing sufficient years of contributory service receive an inadequate amount. Until recently and with only a few exceptions—for example, the civil service, the public sector, banks—Greek legislation did not make provision for the automatic adjustment of pensions to wage rises. Generally there was a long delay before any such adjustment was authorized. On January 1, 1979, Law 815/1978 came into force. It provides for an automatic reajustment of pensions every time there is a rise in the minimum wage rate.

There has long been a need to reorganize the social insurance system and establish certain general principles and norms. The task has proved to be far from simple. Similarly a solution has been awaited for many years to the question of granting pension entitlement to all aged persons without exception who, for a variety of reasons, have been excluded from the protective frame-work of social insurance.

Meanwhile indigent persons not covered by the insurance system find themselves in a dire situation. Their case is aggravated by the fact that Greece has not organized a public assistance system providing for regular cash allowances to the needy; relevant legislation, however, prescribes that "social protection" may be available to those in need on an individualized basis to cover "specific needs."

Age of Retirement

The pensionable age depends on the insurance organization covering each category of workers. In many such organizations the pensionable age is 65 for men and 60 for women. For the agricultural population the age is 65, irrespective of sex. Where certain professions and certain insurance organizations are concerned, the pensionable age is variously 62, 60 or 55. In the case of a number of insurance organizations, the benefit is not linked to age or to compulsory retirement from work. The person insured is entitled to a reduced pension upon completion of a given period of service or a given number of contributions. Recently, all persons covered by the Social Insurance Institute were given the right to retire voluntarily with full pension at the age of 58 provided they had completed thirty-five years of pensionable service.

For civil servants, compulsory retirement is set at the age of 65 in the case of senior officials and 62 for officials at lower grades. Since 1965 retirement on full pension has been obligatory upon completion of thirty-five years of service irrespective of age. In Greece there is a widespread demand, on the part of both the elderly and the young, for a lowering of the age of retirement, though on differing grounds. The spirit informing the maxim "Make room for the young" has prompted the dismissal from the country's labor force of persons still fit for work—to the detriment not only of the national economy but of the welfare and psychological health of aged persons anxious to continue working.

Closely related to the question of the pensionable age is that of the employment of pensioners: should this be forbidden or discouraged or, on the contrary, facilitated? And if the latter, under what specific conditions? The present position is that most insurance organizations insist on retirement from the profession as a condition of pension entitlement. This, however, depends as a rule on the choice of the person concerned.

Legislation applying to certain insurance organizations looks with disfavor on the employment of pensioners. Thus it provides for deferment of the pension if the earnings from the salaried employent exceed a given figure.

Questions relating to pensionable age, compulsory retirement on pension after thirty-five years of service, productive employment of ablebodied pensioners, early retirement with reduced pension sometimes on the basis of several incompleted pensionable years, and accumulation of pension and wages have been treated in Greece in an improvised and at times contradictory manner. Nevertheless the problems at issue are of exceptional importance; they have an impact on the financial bases of social insurance in Greece. As a matter of social and financial policy, it is imperative that efforts be made to tackle the problems without delay and in a new spirit.

The employment bureaus have not taken steps to organize a special system for helping persons of advanced age or a fortiori pensioners to find work suited to their capacities, nor are there any facilities to which aged persons can turn for professional reorientation or technical retraining. There is also a lack of special centers for assisting aged persons in the process of readjustment or in finding full-time or part-time employment; efforts in this direction are of limited scope and are mainly confined to the sector of institutional care.

Medical Care

The regulatory provisions in the sector of medical care are analogous to those applying to pension entitlement. Almost all Greek citizens are covered, either fully or partially, against sickness under various systems and agencies: the working urban population (compulsorily insured), the agricultural population, the dependent members of the families of the foregoing groups (indirectly insured), the pensioners, and the indigent. Thus aged persons are entitled by law—either as insured persons, if still working, or as pensioners, or as indigents—to medical, pharmaceutical, and hospital care. This health care, as provided by the insurance organizations or the state, is not uniform in kind, quality, or volume of services. For a substantial proportion of old-age pensioners, whose medical needs tend to increase with the passage of time, the health services placed at their disposal constitute an essential element for the maintenance of their standard of living.

The organization and procedures for providing medical and related care to indigent persons present a number of serious weaknesses. In fact, the difficulties that aged indigent persons encounter in order to receive the hospital care to which they are legally entitled usually prove insurmountable. The problems connected with the reorganization of sickness insurance and the establishment of a general program of national health are currently engaging the close attention of the Greek government and the nation's medical circles.

Greece lacks special health services reserved for aged persons; adequate facilities for the treatment of old people suffering from psychological disturbances; geriatric hospitals, clinics, and units for elderly persons in the large hospitals; hospital facilities for the treatment of outpatients; and ancillary services (such as convalescent homes and disability and physiotherapy centers). The lack of special services for the elderly sick is generally considered the reason for the long average duration of hospitalization in Greece as compared with other European countries.

Geriatrics is not taught systematically in Greek medical schools, nor is it among the specialized branches recognized in Greece. The number of Greeks who have qualified as geriatricians in foreign countries is very small.

Nutrition

For a number of reasons, including the raising of the standard of living, the nutrition of the Greeks has improved both in quality and in quantity during the last few years. In 1963, the proportion of animal proteins in the Greek diet was already double that of the prewar period. This improvement covered all age groups including the aged.

There is no information available concerning the nutritional problems of elderly Greeks, and no steps have been taken with regard to their problems. With the exception of isolated efforts in the voluntary sphere or within the ambit of institutional care, nutritional and dietary problems relating to the aged have failed to attract serious attention in official or private circles. Yet many old persons face acute difficulties in obtaining adequate nutrition. Among these persons are those who are in straitened circumstances, those who are living alone, those who are unable to do their own shopping or cooking, and those who are mentally disturbed. The problem merits the attention of all concerned, including voluntary circles, and calls for policy decisions on the part of the state.

Housing

So far the state has not addressed itself to the specific problems of the housing needs of the ever-growing number of old people, single or couples.

There does not appear to be any acute housing problem for old persons in rural areas. Most farmers and farm workers own their homes, and a fairly strong element of family cohesion still persists. In those areas, however, there remains the broader problem of the modernization of a substantial proportion of old houses that lack essential facilities.

The situation is different in the large urban centers, particularly in Athens and Salonica, where there is a pressing demand for housing for old persons, both those living alone and couples. Furthermore exceptional difficulties confront aged people in the large cities who occupy rented accommodation and whose income and pension are small.

A veritable impasse awaits those who live in dilapidated dwellings of the kind that are constantly being torn down in the large urban centers to make room for modern apartment buildings. When that happens, they find themselves in a truly tragic situation, because there may be no place for them to go.

Thus the housing question and the concomitant question of social services for the steadily growing population of old persons are beginning to assume disquieting proportions in the larger cities.

Social Welfare

Although there has been a marked improvement in the matter of old-age pensions and sickness insurance, Greece has lagged behind other countries in providing social services for the aged. Until a few years ago, the general view was that the only services of which Greece stood in need in the sector of the protection of old age comprised the building of further old-age homes. Accordingly state and voluntary action for the protection of old age until recently had not gone much beyond institutional care for indigent old persons.

In consequence, there is scarcely any trace in Greece of the manifold social welfare services that function in other countries—for example, clubs and meeting places of various kinds, educational and recreational programs, artistic and cultural projects, counseling and referral services, housekeeping services, friendly visiting and entertainment centers, distribution of food in the home, transport facilities, mobile libraries, legal assistance and advice, services for the protection of old people from exploitation, and sundry other services designed to help the elderly adjust to the far-reaching changes in mode of life associated with old age, to dispel feelings of isolation and dejection, and, as far as possible, to make their lives more interesting and agreeable.

There is a need to study without delay the possibility of introducng at least some of these services, principally in Athens and Salonica, for all of the elderly. The danger exists that if the state remains supine in the matter for much longer, Greece may find itself abruptly confronted by an accumulation of difficulties and with a sizable segment of the population overwhelmed by acute social and psychological problems.

At the same time, a tribute must be paid to the determined efforts—albeit of limited scope—that the voluntary sector has long since started to make in order to organize social welfare services, mainly for impoverished old persons, both in Athens and in the provinces. Some of the benevolent societies associated with these efforts are carrying out an invaluable pioneering task for the country in the sphere of the protection of old age; they are receiving financial support from the state.

Since 1968 the archdiocese of Athens has initiated special programs for the protection of aged persons whose financial means are slender or who are totally impoverished. Special mention may be made of the Spitia Galinis Tou Christou homes ("Homes of the Tranquility of Christ"). These are parochial day homes for old persons accommodating twenty-five to thirty persons. The aged of the neighborhood who have no family milieu may gather for a midday meal, and occasionally for an evening meal as well, receive medical care, enjoy recreation, and receive any needed assistance. In addition, some parishes have what are known as Groups of Elderly Persons Living Independently; the members have an opportunity to meet twice or thrice a week for either a meal or a recreational program. For a number of years the Foundation for Social Work has run a community-based program for needy aged in two metropolitan areas. The services given include medical care, cash assistance for medication and living expenses, case work and group work, and recreation activities.

In 1977 the nursing department of the Greek Red Cross initiated a small program of home care for the aged organized on a neighborhood basis. This program, using the services of public health nurses, registered nurses, and volunteers, is mainly concerned with certain vital problems of the aged in the neighborhood, including problems of health, nutrition, and home help.

Institutional Care

For old persons requiring institutional treatment and whose financial means are partially or wholly inadequate, there are ninety-three old people's homes with some forty-five hundred beds. The ones with the largest number of beds are in Athens, Piraeus, and Salonica; the remainder are scattered in the capitals of territorial departments and other towns. The largest of the Greek institutions of this kind is the Old People's/Poor People's Home of the Charitable Society of Athens, which can accommodate about eight hundred. It has a long tradition of service.

Of these ninety-three institutions, which include the Homes for Elderly Refugees, seven are public-law entities financed by the state; the remainder are run privately by local authorities, the church, voluntary agencies, and other groups.

Mention should also be made of five more old age homes with 260 beds for the aged and 330 for the chronically ill. Three of these homes are public entities financed by the state. The government has entered into special agreements with eight of the private old people's homes under which it may lodge a certain number of old people in the homes against payment of an agreed sum per person. Moreover the government defrays part of the cost of forty-five more private old people's homes through regular subsidies. Thirty-three homes have private resources or special sources of income; these function without state subsidy.

It is now generally felt that, with a number of exceptions (including some sincere efforts at modernization), the services offered by many old people's homes are far from being satisfactory in quality or in quantity. Steps should be taken immediately to improve the conditions under which the homes function.

Because of the insufficiency of available facilities in public and nonprofit institutions, private enterprise has undertaken to meet the need for housing and care of old people in the middle and upper income brackets. Some years ago commercial boarding houses or rest homes for the aged were unknown in Greece. They have grown in number in the past ten years, especially in the Athens area and to a more limited extent in Salonica.

Chronic Invalids

A particularly acute problem concerns the question of caring for old persons who are bedridden or semi-invalid and for whom there is no hope of recovery. This problem represents a grievous burden for the Greek family and the social services.

There is a lack of centers equipped to offer home care—medical treatment and social services—as well as of nurses specialized in the care of old people. It is difficult to find household help. And the number of institutions, public and private, for the care of chronic sufferers is insignificant in relation to growing demands. For all of Greece, there are eleven such institutions, with 1,278 beds available plus the 330 mixed homes mentioned above. Estimates indicate that there are perhaps ten times this number of persons who should be admitted to institutions for incurable invalids. As has been stated, very little has been done regarding the care of invalid or semi-invalid aged in their own home. In 1968, the archdiocese of Athens took the initiative and set up three mobile medical units for the home treatment of the chronically indigent aged, together with two hostels for invalid persons, where the more difficult cases are treated.

The prospects in this area are far from encouraging, however. According to some forecasts, by the year 2000 about 100,000 old persons will be bedridden and require suitable medical and social care.

Reference has already been made to the growing number of commercial homes for the aged in the middle and higher income brackets. Many of these homes provide care for invalids, semi-invalids, and bedridden persons. They serve an urgent need, but sometimes the standards of care are low.

Legislation Relating to Old Age

Legislative decree 162 of 1973 is the first piece of legislation in Greece specifically related to the protection of persons of advanced age and which encompasses in its aims the financial, social, and psychological needs of the aged population as a whole. It represents the first official recognition of the imperative obligation, which devolves on Greece also, to attend to the organization of a network of services in favor of elderly persons analogous to those functioning in various advanced countries. The decree in question is a pilot or framework instrument that lays down the basic principles and basic directions of national policy in respect of the protection of old age, both institutional and extra-institutional. Clearly, however, the mere announcement of general principles cannot be deemed sufficient. What is of paramount importance is the application of the principles and the prompt elaboration of specific programs to give them substance.

Special mention may also be made of legislative decree 1118 of 1972 concerning establishments for the care of persons of advanced age and chronic invalids. Under this decree all such establishments came under state control and supervision, the terms and conditions of their lawful functioning being subsequently stipulated thereunder. These conditions include licensing, suitability of premises, standards of services, qualifications of personnel, and size of staff.

A second piece of legislation on this subject, law 877/1979, recently come into force. It prescribes the obligation of commercial establishments for the aged: those offering boarding house services, those designed for chronic invalids, and those concerned with both categories of elderly persons.

Administration

The development and application of an appropriate policy in the field of the protection of old age requires an adequately staffed and able administration. In Greece the Ministry of Social Services is responsible for questions concerning health, social insurance, housing, and social welfare. Between the various services of the ministry, however, there is a lack of a coordinated approach to matters of common interest. The ministry has never taken up the study and elaboration of comprehensive and cohesive measures designed to serve the elderly, at least insofar as the spheres of its own competence are concerned.

Toward the end of 1976 a small administrative unit in the General Directorate of Social Welfare that had been dealing with questions concerning aged persons was raised to divisional status as the Division for the Protection of Old Age. It is hoped that this new unit will undertake the task of ascertaining the needs and expectations of aging Greeks and of promoting appropriate programs for their welfare.

It would certainly be salutary to make arrangements to study the possible establishment of a special, semi-independent agency, with enlarged administrative terms of reference and adequate staffing, to undertake the task of developing a comprehensive and well-coordinated old-age policy. Meanwhile there is need to strengthen the relevant services of the Ministry of Social Services by engaging outside experts (of every branch); their cooperation is indispensable if this intricate problem is to be tackled in a global and interdisciplinary manner.

Training of Personnel

The personnel problem of the institutions and the various welfare services concerned with the aged is especially acute. In several cases the personnel needed in this field, both professional and auxiliary, is insufficient in number and inadequately trained for the functions to be performed. The only organized facilities for training in these functions are the existing schools of social work, which train multi-purpose social workers and place students for field work practice, both in case work and in group work, in facilities for the aged. None of these schools is oriented toward the specific social, psychological, or medical problems of the old, however.

Elements of gerontology and geriatrics are taught in the schools for clinical and visiting nurses, but these schools do not train specialists in geriatric nursing.

Schools of home economics provide general courses on nutritional needs at various ages, but they do not have any indigenous teaching material related to the particular needs of the elderly population of Greece. Nor do they train specialized dietitians.

In view of future prospects for the welfare of the aged in Greece, close attention should be given to organizing programs for the training of the personnel needed in both the professional and the voluntary sector and at all levels.

STUDY AND RESEARCH

The various facets of the problem of old age have not yet been the subject of specialized, systematic study and research in Greece. With the exception of isolated inquiries undertaken from time to time by specialists, none of the recorded studies of a social or psychological nature is directed to problems relating to old age and its protection.

Certainly occasional limited studies on the special problems of old persons have been carried out in recent years by a number of bodies, among them the archdiocese of Athens, the Iake School of Social Work, the League of Greek Volunteers, the Foundation for Social Work, and the Gerontological Center of Dourghouti.

The body that is most competent to conduct sociological studies—the National Center for Social Research—has included the problems of old age in its syllabus since 1970; it has not, however, issued any publications so far.

Recently, the Social Services Section of the Center for Planning and Economic Research studied the needs of the elderly and the measures that should be adopted to cover such needs. It did so within the framework of the drafting of the Program for Economic and Social Development, 1976-1989. The program proposes that in the field of social welfare priority should be given to services for the aged and for children, and that particular emphasis should be given to care at home rather than institutional care. In continuation of this work, the center is now starting a more comprehensive study of the problems of the aged in Greece.

The Center of Studies of Age-Related Changes in Man has been functioning in Athens since 1962; it was founded by a small research team and is presently supported by the Ministry of Social Services. A number of original studies prepared by the center concern age-related functional changes of the human system.

In preparing this chapter, I have relied mainly on the material I gathered for a survey on the aged in Greece in 1971 on behalf of the United Nations. I consulted the publications of the National Statistical Service of Greece, various official reports, and certain bibliographical sources related to the subject of aged people. I have also collected data regarding the status and needs of aged persons through interviews with officials associated with social services and programs, with experts and research workers, and with community leaders in certain rural areas, among others. The 1971 survey, completed and brought up to date, was published in Greek in 1974 by the Council for Training in Social Work as *The Problem of Old Age in Greece*. For this chapter, I have taken account of up-to-date statistical data and of all relevant developments since 1974.

SUMMARY

The demographic evolution of Greece during the past twenty-five years has been marked by a low level of annual population growth; a steady fall in the birthrate; an expanding urbanization, coupled with a progressive diminution of the rural population; a swelling population in Athens and Salonica; increased emigration; and an accelerated rate of aging of the population. The last factor, combined with the social changes induced by industrialization, urbanization, and emigration, have resulted in a general interest in the problems peculiar to old people. Until recently, these problems were not particularly acute in Greece, nor did national policy reserve any significant place for them. The reason was not so much that persons of advanced age were relatively fewer in number but that tradition and custom laid upon the family the burden of maintaining and protecting them. Although the family still comes into play, there is a steady increase in the number of old persons who are separated from the family unit and in the number of those among them who have to face the problems of old age alone and unaided.

For some years, the financial and health problems of old people have been substantially alleviated through the comprehensive award of old-age pensions and the extension of sickness insurance. Nevertheless there remain immense and urgent problems to be solved with a view to the improvement of health services—for all ages but particularly for impoverished elderly persons—and the radical reorganization of the social insurance system, with special reference to old-age pensions. The question of providing a minimum income for all Greeks over 65 years of age is of particular importance.

Although there have been improvements in respect to old-age pensions and sickness insurance, those achieved in many sectors of the social services have been few in number and limited in scope. State action is still restricted to financial support for certain voluntary private activities and programs and to the continuance of established institutional protection for indigent old people, mostly on the basis of somewhat outdated methods.

There is an urgent need to organize services of every kind for the aged, who, on the one hand, exchange a life of full activity for one of unrelieved leisure, and on the other hand, have to cope with social, psychological, and other problems of many different kinds. Decisive steps must be taken for the proper housing of the various categories of aged persons, particularly in Athens and Salonica, where the problem may soon become especially acute.

The rapid pace at which the aged population has increased and continues to increase, coupled with the weakening of the traditional ties within the Greek family, has annulled the margin of time during which further inaction is acceptable. Accumulating problems are clearly gathering into a whirlwind, and if Greece remains unprepared, it seems likely that it will face immense difficulties and unforeseeable consequences for its economic and social life. Hence there is an imperative need to study promptly the problem of old age in all its aspects—demographic, public health, economic, social, civic, administrative—and to ensure that its solution is embodied in a comprehensive, lucid, and coordinated national program, based on conditions in Greece and corresponding to Greece's needs and capacities.

REFERENCES

In Greek

Angelis, I. *The Problem of Old Persons*. Bulletin of I.K.A. KST No. 6, Athens, 1976.
Archdiocese of Athens. *Activities and Targets of the "Special Care for the Aged."* Athens, 1971.
————. *What Is the Special Care for the Aged?* Athens, 1972.
Center of Planning and Economic Research. *Perspective Development Plan of Greece 1972-1987*. Report by the Committee for the National Development Model. Part A. "General Development Orientations." Athens, 1972.
————. *Perspective Development Plan of Greece 1972-1987*. Report by the Committee for the National Development Model. Part B. "Orientations for Development of Sectors and Regions." Athens, 1972.

————. *Programme of Long-term Perspectives 1970-1985.* Final report of Committee of the Ways of Living. "Development in the Ways of Living." Athens, 1972.

————. *Programme of Long-term Perspectives 1973-1987.* Final report of the Committee on Health. "Health." Athens, 1972.

————. *Perspective Development Plan of Greece 1973-1987.* Final report of the Committee on Social Welfare. "Social Welfare." Athens, 1972.

————. *Development Program 1976-1980.* Report of the Working Group on Health. Athens, October 1976.

————. *Development Program 1976-1980.* Report of the Working Group on Social Security. Athens, December 1976.

————. *Development Program 1976-1980.* Report of the Working Group on Social Welfare. Athens, October 1976.

Charitable Society of Athens. *The Old People's Home, A Century of Action.* Athens, 1964.

Dontas, A. "Social Problems of Elderly Patients," *Maderia Medica Greece,* 6, no. 6. Athens, 1978.

Gedeon, Sophia. *Pro senectute.* Athens, 1966.

Marcoyannis, Chr. "Care for the aged". In *Positions and Ideas.* Athens, 1969.

Marcoyannis, G. *Welfare of the Aged in Greece.* In Bulletin of I.K.A. IST No. 9, Athens, 1966

Mastroyannis, I. *Social Welfare History of Modern Greece.* Athens, 1962.

————. *Social Welfare.* Athens, 1969.

Ministry of Coordination. "Reports on Population Policy" (mimeographed). Athens, June and November 1968.

Ministry of Coordination, Center of Planning and Economic Research. "Population in Greece: Review and Developments." Report of Population Committee. Athens, May 1978.

————. "Economic and Social Development Program 1978-1982: Preliminary Guidelines." Athens, 1979.

Ministry of Social Services. *Social Budgets of the Years 1969-1978.* Athens, 1979.

National Research Institute. *Social Protection in Greece.* Athens, 1970.

National Statistical Service of Greece. *Statistical Year-book,* Athens, 1977.

Pantras, L. *Social Policy. Planing.* Athens, 1970.

Pylarinou, P. *The Consequences of the Progressive Increase of the Aged Population.* Athens, 1959.

Roussou, Ch. *The Problems of the Third Age.* Bulletin of I.K.A. 29 Nos. 1-2. Athens, 1979.

Siampos, G. *Demographic Developments in Greece 1950-1980.* Athens, 1969.

————. *Demographic Evolution in Modern Greece 1821-1985.* Athens, 1973.

————. "Demography." Athens, 1979.

Tsakonas, A. *Old age, the Mind, and Longevity.* Athens, 1934.

Tsoukas, A.; Veleheris, N.; and Gousgounis, F. *Gerontology and Geriatrics.* Athens, 1960.

Valaoras, Vas. *Human Hygiene.* Athens, 1962.

————. *Demographic Problem of Greece.* Athens, 1973.

————. *Economic Development and the Human Factor.* Athens, 1976.

Vassiliou, V. *A Preliminary Exploraton of Variables Related to Family Transaction in Greece*. Athens, 1966.

Vayas, Chr. *Abstracts of the Dourghouti Social Study*, Foundation for Social Work-Volunteers Association (FSW-VA). Athens, 1977.

Yatra-Iliopoulou, T. *The Life after 50*. Athens, 1968.

Zarras, I. *The Problem of Old Age in Greece*. Athens, 1974.

Zavitsanos, Th. *Old Age and Old Age Mortality in Greece*. Athens, 1963.

In English

Campbell, J.K. *Honour, Family and Patronage*. Oxford, 1964.

Doxiadis, C.A. *City for Human Development*. ACE Publication No. 12. Athens, 1972.

Friedl, Ernestine. *Vassilika—A Village in Modern Greece*. New York, 1962.

Moustaka, Calliope. *The Internal Migrant. A Comparative Study in Urbanization*. Social Sciences Centre. Athens, 1964.

Psomopoulos, P. *Human Disability and Human Settlements*. ACE Publication No. 90. Athens, 1972.

———. *Disabled People in Disabling Settlements*. ACE Publication No. 120. Athens, 1973.

Safilios-Rothschild, C., and Gerogiopoulos, J.A. "A Comparative Study of Parental and Filial Role Definitions." *Journal of Marriage and the Family*. August 1970.

United Nations. *Report of the Urbanization Survey Mission in the Mediterranean Region—November to December 1959. Annex: Urbanization in Greece and the Athens-Piraeus Conurbation*. New York ST/SOA/SER T/I.

Wood-Ritsatakis, Anne. *An Analysis of the Health and Welfare Services in Greece*. Center of Planning and Economic Research. Athens, 1970.

In French

Office National de Statistique en Greèce. *Mouvement Naturel de la Population de la Greèce*, Athens, 1974

HUNGARY

EDIT BEREGI

DEVELOPMENT OF GERONTOLOGY

Life-expectancy at birth is increasing all over the world, and the proportion of older age groups within the entire population has risen. Gerontology, the science concerned with the aging of the organism, dates back to ancient Greece and Rome. The considerable increase of average life expectancy has raised numerous medical and sociological problems and enhanced the spread of scientific gerontology.

Gerontological research in Hungary is based on an old tradition. The first Hungarian work on geriatrics dates back to 1692. Its author, Koleseri, established that aging may be influenced by hygienic regulations. Since then, several more pertinent works have been published by Hungarian scientists. Koranyi's work (1937) represents a landmark. He established that the decrease of adaptation should be considered as the first sign of senescence, a conclusion valid up to the present. Koranyi found that symptoms of senile decay have to be searched for at the initial stage, not when severe changes have already developed. Koranyi also initiated the First Hungarian Congress on Gerontology in 1937, held in Budapest. Pioneer work in Hungarian gerontological research has been performed by Haranghy, who reported on the difference in water purification ability of young and old mollusks (1938).

Organized gerontological research began in 1954 by the foundation of the Gerontological Committee of the Hungarian Academy of Sciences, under Haranghy's presidency. Gerontological research in the country was coordinated and sponsored by the committee, which also organized scientific sessions and courses.

Some important events of Hungarian gerontological research may be summarized as follows:

1956: Hungary joined the International Association of Gerontology and participated in its conferences.

1958: The Gerontological Section of the Hungarian Biological Association was formed and organized meetings and congresses.

1967: The Hungarian Gerontological Association was formed to deal with the biology of aging, medical relations, and social problems. At the same time the Gerontological Committee of the Hungarian Academy of Sciences stopped its activity.

1965: The Research Department of Gerontology sponsored by the Ministry of Health, was founded, an important advance in gerontological research.

1970: The Center of Social Institution was formed with the aim of methodological counseling of old people's homes.

1978: The Research Department of Gerontology became Gerontology Center of the Semmelweis Medical School, Budapest.

1957: Laszlo Haranghy was awarded the CIBA Foundation Prize for his work, "The Senile Changes in the Spleen and Bone Marrow."

1969: Edit Beregi with her paper, "Comparative Morphological Studies of the Allergic Reactions of Young and Old Animals," shared the Karger Prize with Alex Comfort (United Kingdom).

DEMOGRAPHY

In Hungary, as in most other countries, the number of persons aged 60 years and over has been increasing. At present the number of persons aged 60 years and over exceeds that of 1960; the proportion amounts to 18.2 percent of the entire population, as compared to 13.8 percent in 1960, 11 percent in 1950, and 10 percent in 1940. In addition, because of the lower birthrate, the number of children has decreased. Currently 20 percent of the population is under 15 years of age; from 1940 through 1960, the comparable proportion was over 25 percent (Klinger, 1974).

The present demographic conditions in Hungary are characterized primarily by a low birthrate, which has occurred within a short period and has shown substantial fluctuation. The birthrate of about 14.5 to 15 per thousand is somewhat under the European average and is about half of the rate observed fifty years ago. Accordingly the number and proportion of aged increase while that of children decreases. The remarkable unevenness of the age pyramid (Huszar, 1974), is an unavoidable feature of the process.

The demographic situation of Hungary is determined primarily by the number of births. Between 1870 and 1880, the birthrate in the territory of today's Hungary was still high—over 40 per thousand. A slow decrease began during the 1890s, and the decline accelerated in the years preceding World War I. In the last year of peace preceding World War I, the ratio of live births per 1,000 inhabitants was already 10 per thousand below that in the 1890s. This downward trend started in Hungary, as in other central and eastern European countries, substantially later than in most of the western European countries. The slow and late decrease in fertility was a consequence of the late and moderate industrial development in Hungary (Huszar, 1974). The decline of the birthrate accelerated during the interwar period. With a birthrate of about 20 per thousand before World War II, Hungary occupied an intermediate position among the European countries. Birth statistics of the last thirty years have the following characterics (Huszar, 1974):

1. Between 1947 and 1950, the birthrate increased to about 21 per thousand.
2. In consequence of population policy measures—economic, social, health, and legal—the birthrate increased in 1954 to its peak of 23 per thousand.
3. From 1955 until 1962, the birthrate decreased, falling steeply to 12.9 per thousand in 1962, the lowest rate in Hungarian history.
4. In 1966 and 1967, the birthrate increased to 15 per thousand. This rise was the consequence of the stimulating effect of govenmental measures—the introduction of child welfare allowances, an increase of family allowances, an acceleration of house construction, and a modification of the distribution of flats, among others. The increased proportion of women of childbearing age contributed additionally to the increase in birthrate.
5. Since 1970 the birthrate has remained around 14.7 per thousand.

Table 16 shows the percentage distribution of the population according to age and sex from 1920. Compared to the 9 percent of the population 60 years old and over in 1920, there were 18.2 percent by 1976. The proportion has thus doubled.

Table 16: DISTRIBUTION OF POPULATION BY SEX AND AGE (IN PERCENT)

Year	Under 15	15–39	40–59	60 and Over	Total
1920	30.6	41.3	19.1	9.0	100.0
1930	27.5	42.6	20.1	9.8	100.0
1941	26.0	40.6	22.7	10.7	100.0
1949	24.9	38.8	24.7	11.6	100.0
1960	25.4	36.8	24.0	13.8	100.0
1970	21.1	37.0	24.8	17.1	100.0
1975	20.2	37.2	24.2	18.4	100.0
1976	20.5	37.0	24.3	18.2	100.0
Men	21.7	38.5	23.9	15.9	100.0
Women	19.3	35.6	24.7	20.4	100.0
Number of women per 1,000 men	944	981	1,097	1,365	1,062

Source: Hungarian Statistical Pocket Book (Budapest: Statistical Publisher, 1976), p. 36.

A review of the proportion of pensioners is presented in table 17. Compared to the 6.4 percent of pensioners in 1960, the proportion rose to 17.0 percent by 1976.

The sex composition of active and inactive workers has been analyzed (Klinger, 1974). It has been found that the number of men capable of earning their living diminished 4 percent between 1960 and 1970. During the same period, the proportion of inactive men of working age showed a near threefold increase, from 5 percent to 12 percent of the population. The economic

Table 17: PENSIONERS AS A PERCENTAGE OF TOTAL POPULATION

Year	Percentage
1960	6.4
1970	13.4
1974	16.1
1975	16.6
1976	17.0

Source: *Hungarian Statistical Pocket Book* (Budapest: Statistical Publisher, 1976), p. 156.

structure of the female population showed a more positive change. The last decade was characterized by the regular increase of actively working women and the decrease of dependent women. Between 1960 and 1970, the number of actively working women increased 360,000 and reached 40 percent of the female population in 1970; the figure was 33 percent in 1960. In 1970, somewhat less than half of the female population was dependent; 3 percent were on child-welfare allowance, and 11 percent were pensioners and other inactive women of working age. During the last forty years, the number of actively working men increased almost 20,000 although their proportion decreased, while the number of actively working women more than doubled. Almost a million women worked in 1930—about 20 percent of the female population—and the number was over two million in 1970 (Klinger, 1974).

Table 18: AVERAGE LIFE EXPECTANCY AT BIRTH

Year (average)	Men (in years)	Women (in years)
1920–1921	41.0	43.1
1930–1931	48.7	51.8
1941	54.9	58.2
1948–1949	58.8	63.2
1955	65.0	68.9
1959–1960	65.2	69.6
1968	66.6	71.9
1970	66.3	72.1
1972	66.9	72.6
1974	66.5	72.4

Source: *Hungarian Statistical Pocket Book* (Budapest: Statistical Publisher, 1978), p. 46.

Calculations on the development of the average life expectancy at birth performed by the Central Statistical Office are presented in table 18. The evidence shows that, from 1920 on, average life expectancy at birth has always been longer for females than for males, and the sex difference has increased in recent years. The average life expectancy increased in both sexes until 1960. Since that time there has been a stagnation, particularly in male life expectancy. Table 19 shows mortality ratios according to age, and table 20

Table 19: MORTALITY ACCORDING TO AGE

Age	Mortality Rate[a] 1959–1960	1969–1970	1975	1975 Percentage Distribution of Deaths
In the first year of life	50.1	35.8	32.6	4.8
1–2 years	2.9	1.4	1.0	0.2
3–6 years	0.7	0.5	0.4	0.2
7–14 years	0.5	0.4	0.4	0.3
15–39 years	1.4	1.3	1.3	3.9
40–49 years	4.0	4.0	4.6	5.0
50–59 years	9.9	9.9	9.5	8.3
60–69 years	25.6	25.5	25.3	21.5
70 years and over	92.2	90.1	89.6	55.8
Total	10.3	11.5	12.4	100.0

Source: Hungarian Statistical Pocket Book (Budapest: Statistical Publisher 1976), p. 45.

a. Rate of death per 1,000 of the same age group (in the first year of life per 1,000 live births).

Table 20: MORTALITY ACCORDING TO MAIN CAUSES OF DEATH AND AGE GROUPS, 1975 (PER 10,000)

Cause of Death	First Year of Life	1–6	7–14	15–39	40–59	60 and Over
Tuberculosis		0.1		2.4	22.8	74.7
Syphilis				5.5	27.8	66.7
Malignant tumors	0.1	0.2	0.2	3.1	19.8	76.6
Heart disease and hypertension		0.1	0.0	1.5	11.5	86.9
Cerebrovascular disease		0.0	0.1	0.9	7.5	91.5
Influenza	1.7	0.5	0.5	3.2	6.3	87.8
Pneumonia	32.0	3.4	0.7	3.7	7.8	52.4
Peptic ulcer	0.1			3.2	18.5	78.2
Ileus and hernia	3.8	0.1		2.4	11.8	81.9
Cirrhosis of liver			0.1	5.5	33.2	61.2
Nephritis and nephrosclerosis	0.5	0.2	0.3	6.4	15.9	76.7
Malformations	87.8	9.1	1.3	1.8		
Birth injury, complicated delivery, and other anoxic and hypoxic states	100.0					
Other causes of perinatal mortality	100.0					
Accidents	1.1	2.3	2.3	20.4	19.6	54.3

Source: Hungarian Statistical Pocket Book (Budapest: Statistical Publisher, 1976), p. 49.

displays the main causes of death according to age groups. Cerebrovascular diseases were the leading causes of death in the population aged 60 years and over in 1975 (91.5 per thousand), followed by influenza (87.8 per thousand), and heart disease and hypertension (86.9 per thousand).

In conclusion, life expectancy at birth, as well as the proportion of persons aged 60 years and over within the population, has increased in Hungary while the ratio of children has decreased. Therefore birthrate has to be controlled by population policy measures for the time being, as well as in future decades.

ROLES AND STATUS OF THE AGED

Reaching retiring age and being pensioned often brings changes with which the elderly find it difficult to cope. Those doing heavy physical labor usually have to retire from such labor. The situation is entirely different for individuals whose job does not demand hard physical work, who have an intellectual occupation, or who need the psychological stimulation connected with their work because it helps them to retain their mental faculties. The lack of such stimulation after retirement often brings rapid senescence to such people; doing adequate work keeps them in good condition both mentally and physically.

In certain industries where there is a shortage of manpower, a so-called delayed retirement bonus has been introduced; thus individuals of retirement age may continue in their job, and for every additional year they work, their pension increases. The age of retirement does not mean the loss of work capacity. Accordingly individuals who have reached the age of retirement are entitled to postpone retirement and to keep their jobs. Retirement age is generally 55 for women and 60 for men.

Taking into consideration the fact that the retirement age group increases and the working age group decreases, employment after retirement is of national economic interest. In addition, the experience and professional skill of the elderly would be sorely missed in some cases.

The employment of the aged takes two fundamental forms: employment in addition to the pension and uninterrupted employment without making use of the pension. The number of employed pensioners amounts to about five hundred thousand. A characteristic feature of the employment in addition to pension is that of taking up a job other than the original one.

The Central Bureau of Statistics has performed a survey to find out from those involved whether they approve of the retirement age being 55 and 60 and to discover the reason why they continued to work after having reached retirement age. The bureau also examined who the people were who continued to work. The majority of those questioned thought it important to do active work in old age, but only a few favored raising the retirement age. These answers show that the elderly think it important to be ensured the chance of retiring under existing conditions, as well as the possibility of work to those who so wish. When asked what they missed most after retirement, those who had done physical work missed the income, regular occupation, and the companionship of their co-workers. Intellectuals missed the work itself, the pleasure of performance, and the social recognition accorded for their achievement; earnings played a secondary role.

In old age mental alertness is promoted by continuous activity. Moreover close contact with members of the family and society is also important. The family is still of decisive significance in the lives of most elderly people because it implies social relationships, intensifies activity, and stands for security of livelihood. Not only are the members of the family who share the home important; so are sons and daughters living in separate homes and other relatives with whom a permanent connection is maintained.

Table 21: PERCENTAGE DISTRIBUTION OF PENSIONERS BY LIVING ARRANGEMENTS

Living Arrangement	Percentage of Total
Alone	21.9
With spouse only	33.9
With spouse and children	7.9
With spouse and child and the latter's children	5.5
With child	7.5
With child and the latter's family	11.8
With grandchild	1.0
With relatives	6.0
With nonrelatives	2.0
In a social home	1.0
Unknown	1.5

Source: "The Situation of Pensioner." In *Book of the Central Statistical Office* (Budapest: Statistical Publisher, 1963), p. 2.

As table 21 shows, 21.9 percent of pensioners live alone, 33.9 percent live with their spouses only, and most of the rest live with children and their families. The problems of aged individuals who have to be provided and cared for have to be solved within the family; this is the most suitable way from the individual's point of view. An aged person who does not live with his family is best off remaining in his own environment and being given care on this basis.

The situation of the older generation has also been considerably influenced by the deep changes that have taken place during the past decades in the structure and role of the family. The large families have disappeared, and instead of the family system with one wage earner, two or more wage earners have appeared. This process is connected with the increase of urbanization and industrialization. The other important factor is women's increased employment, which means that the aged who live in the family lack care during the day and live in solitude despite the fact that the family returns home in the evening; even then the others are occupied with housework, learning, and other individual business.

Families can, some with difficulty, take care of the aged at home, but additional difficulties arise because of the small size of modern flats. This must not mean a reduction of the family responsibility in supporting and caring for the aged person, but it does mean that the family may need help. These are the factors that increasingly call for state and social collaboration in the care for the aged.

PROGRAMS

The care of aged individuals presents a serious problem all over the world. In Hungary this task has been assumed increasingly by the state, though the family also plays an important role.

The care of aged individuals is directed by the Social-Political Committee of the Ministry of Health. The work of the ministry is promoted by the Center of Social Institutions, which is the methodological department of the Ministry of Health. A social gerontological and a welfare department are active in this institution; they help the country-wide work of the ministry by devising appropriate conceptions and furnishing information.

We summarize as follows the forms of social care systems in the country.

Day Centers

Day centers or clubs for aged people offer one form of district care. In the morning, elderly individuals in need of help go to the day center where they are provided for, under strict health control. The physically still active but solitary pensioners or married couples generally go to those day centers, which have libraries, newspapers, radio, television, parlor games, organized occupations, and meals. At present, there are 593 day centers with room for 16,029 elderly persons. For every 10,000 inhabitants 60 years or older, 88.7 places are available.

Many active elderly individuals have joined with pleasure in devoting their energies to various forms of care. For instance, in many cases pensioners have initiated and, with the support of the community, participated in setting up day centers. They also take part in organizing the day-to-day programs. The most active individual is elected to take on responsibility for keeping order in the club and to smooth over differences or settle disputes. Members of the club organize the home's cultural programs, which may be quite varied, by arranging lectures on medical and educational subjects; playing folk and classical music; hearing reports on experiences during travels; showing short documentary films; arranging meetings with young people; going on excursions; establishing connections with other clubs; and arranging competitions between clubs.

In the organization and maintenance of day centers for the aged, the Hungarian Red Cross is the most active group. It finds premises, gathers financial contributions, and organizes cultural and hygienic care and activities for the aged.

Social Care at Home

Another form of district care is social care at home, which is given to aged people who are ill but wish to remain in their own homes. Besides professional nurses, social care activists also take part in home care; some receive a fee for their work.

Table 22: PERCENTAGE DISTRIBUTION OF SOCIAL WORKERS AND INDIVIDUALS UNDER CARE

Type of Care	Social Workers (N=6,427)	Individuals (N=19,539)
Professional care by local authorities	9.6	40.3
Social care, salaried	40.5	22.3
Social care, not salaried	44.4	18.2
Care connected to other activity	0.5	3.3
Other	5.0	15.9

Source: P. Bajaczi and T. Daniel, eds., *Information Year Book* (Budapest: Statistical Publisher, 1975).

Table 22 demonstrates on a country-wide scale the distribution and ratio of those who do care work and those who are attended to in various care forms. Care may be provided by a professional branch of the county or municipal council, or in connection with some other work, by social care for a fee, and by social care without payment. Social care at home is given to 19,539 individuals, and the work is done by 6,427 social workers.

Active, healthy elderly individuals share in the work of care at home. They visit those who need such support, help with the housework, go with the person under care to the doctor, if necessary, see that the patient takes medicines as prescribed, and helps with meal preparation.

The Red Cross also helps here. They find those in need of care, submit proposals to the councils concerning the respective needs, and find persons willing to carry out the work of care.

The work of the Red Cross youth groups of primary and secondary schools is most effective. They do shopping, read books and newspapers to the aged, and talk about their school life and plans, so that a sort of family connection gradually develops.

Residential Homes

When the aged give up their homes, they can go to a central institute—residential homes—where adequate housing, food, and medical care are provided, thus freeing the aged person from essential burdens. If a person is healthy and physically active, it is necessary to find an occupation for him or her. This may be realized in two ways; those under institutional care are drawn partly into helping with the housework and partly into the work of committees managing the home. Since 1971, at the recommendation of the Ministry of Health, three committees are active in most residential homes with the co-operation of aged individuals. The Food Committee deals with the menu of the social home and fixes it in agreement with the requirements of the community. The Cultural Committee helps residents spend their leisure time usefully by arranging such activities as common programs, excursions, and visits to theaters. The Safeguarding Committee takes up problems of the residents, endeavors to solve them, and tries to resolve differences that may arise.

In Hungary 28,247 individuals are taken care of at four types of homes: general care is arranged for 39.2 percent; care of bedridden patients for 36.7 percent; psychiatric care for 23.1 percent; and tuberculosis care for 1 percent.

As to organization, day centers for aged people, social care at home networks, and residential homes are superintended by county and municipal councils, and the care network is directed by centers at county towns.

Homes for the Elderly

The fourth form of social care, homes for the elderly, represents a completely different category. These houses are for elderly married couples or individuals who have no relatives, do not need financial aid, and wish to remain independent. The residents are given independent but smaller apartments than their original homes. The upkeep of this apartment costs less than did their former flat, and it provides more comfort. Elderly individuals may keep house or avail themselves of such facilities as dining rooms. Housekeeping and medical care are provided. There are also a common club room where residents meet and workrooms where the aged are paid for work that does not require much effort.

Care in old age is a many-sided task that has to be shared by the family, society, and the state. Every form of care can function satisfactorily only if directly involved aged people are drawn into the work. This promotes the useful occupation of elderly active individuals who, being familiar with their own problems, can contribute valuable assistance in improving the care.

Other Programs

Active pensioners are provided other advantages. To be able to spend their leisure time usefully, they can purchase tickets at reduced prices to museums and cinemas; purchase monthly tickets for trams and buses and half-fare railway tickets; receive rent contributions; and take advantage of low-priced accommodations for holidays. They can spend their time in the Garden of Retired Persons and be members of the Picture Club for pensioners. To lessen daily expenditures, they receive cheaper meals at restaurants, legal advice free of charge, which has been organized in every part of the country by the National Council of Lawyers, and free consultation at the Gerontological Research Group at the Medical University.

One of the daily papers has a pensioners' column where elderly individuals are informed on subjects of special interest to them and are apprised of openings, excursions, and similar events. Elderly people learn about activities through personal communication, information transmitted officially, and the mass media. "Life to the Years" is a monthly television program. The radio program "How Are You?" is an entertaining program for pensioners. As far as the press is concerned, the Hungarian Red Cross writes monthly about gerontology. Articles dealing with the problems of aged people are frequently published on a variety of themes in a weekly column. In addition, nationwide daily and weekly papers, as well as radio and television, handle the problem of elderly people through medical and legal advice, letters to the editor, and similar avenues.

According to statistical data, daily papers are read by 49 percent of retired men and 39 percent of retired women. The proportion of those who listen to the radio is 90 percent for both men and women (Palos, 1976).

Organized programs at the pensioner clubs, such as educational lectures, films, health education, and club competitions, help the elderly spend their time profitably. Social organizations cooperating with local councils organize Old People's Day or Old People's Week each year. On these occasions, the aged receive presents, they are celebrated, and those who cannot leave their homes are visited. In schools the children are told about the life of the aged and discuss their problems.

RESEARCH

In Hungary, organized research started in 1954 with the establishment of the Gerontological Committee of the Hungarian Academy of Sciences. The activity of the committee included organization of scientific meetings, coordination of gerontological research, and development of postgraduate courses. In 1960 a gerontological team examined persons aged 100 and over.

The Gerontological Committee of the Hungarian Academy of Sciences emphasized repeatedly the importance of establishing the Research Institute of Gerontology. The plan was accepted and sponsored by the Ministry of Health.

The Gerontology Center of the Semmelweis Medical University, Budapest, is now the center of gerontological research. Longitudinal studies of healthy aged have continued since 1965 at its fifteen-bed department. Problems of resorption are studied at the biological laboratory; the hormonal regulation of

calcitonin and age-related changes of serum lipids at the biochemical laboratory; immunological reactions and age related changes of T and B lymphocytes
at the histochemical laboratory; age dependence of humoral and cellular
immunity at the immunological laboratory; age-related changes of retinal
accommodation at the electrophysiological laboratory; and age changes in the
function of the nervous system in the psychiatric laboratory.

In addition, basic research is carried out at several University Research
Institutes, as well as geriatric research at several clinical departments and
hospitals and in residential homes.

The main lines of gerontological research in Hungary include age-dependent
changes of cells and cell organelles, of immune function and the immune
system, prolongation of life expectancy, biological changes in different
organs, resorption and adequate nutrition, arteriosclerosis research, respiratory and cardiovascular changes, neural changes, drug therapy in old age,
alterations of bones and joints, osteoporosis research, retirement preparation,
employment of the aged, and old-age care.

Many young scientists are showing interest in gerontology. Up to now six
scientists have obtained the degree of C.M.Sc. with their dissertations on
gerontological subjects, and one scientist has obtained the degree of D.M.Sc.

The Hungarian Gerontological Association organizes about five scientific
meetings yearly. Conferences with international participation were organized
in 1962 and 1976. Numerous scientists from foreign countries participated. In
1972 a satellite symposium was organized in Budapest that preceded the
Congress of the International Association of Gerontology in Kiev.

As far as possible, Hungarian gerontologists participate at international
meetings. Hungarian delegates have been elected to the executive committee
of the International Association of Gerontology, as honorary secretary at the
European Clinical Section of the International Association of Grontology; and
as members of the Board of Directors of the International Center of Social
Gerontology in Paris. Hungarian gerontologists are also members of the
editorial board of foreign gerontological journals.

Much gerontological research is in progress, and the variety of research
topics points to the manifold interests of biologists, physicians, and sociologists in gerontological research. Research, primarily basic research, is considered most important since its results might be helpful in the prolongation of
active life. An additional aim is to improve old age and to prolong activity.

REFERENCES

Beregi, E. 1970. Comparative morphological studies of the allergic reactions of young
    and old animals. *Gerontologia* 16: 141-150.
————. 1976. The care system of aged individuals in Hungary and their participation in
    care work. In: Centre international de gérontologie sociale. *7ème Congress
    International de Bruxelles*. Compte-Rendu des Exposes. pp. 160-167.

Haranghy, L. 1938. Experimentelle beitrage zur kenntnis der wasserreiningungs und wasserklarungswirkung der seemuscheln. *Publicationi della Stazione Zoologica di Napoli* 17: 58-91.

———, ed. 1965. *Gerontological studies on Hungarian centenarians.* Budapest: Publishing House of Academy.

Haranghy, L.; Racz, P.; Harsfalvy, E.; and Kiraly, F. 1958. Altersveränderung an Milz und Knochenmark. *Medizinische und Soziologische Altersproblem.* 2: 45-63.

Huszar, I. 1974. Up-to-date questions in our population policy. In *Population policy and problems of the world population*, pp. 337-353. Budapest: Kossuth Publisher.

Klinger, A. 1974. Population policy in Hungary. In *Population policy and problems of the world population* pp. 249-334. Budapest: Kossuth Publisher.

Koranyi, S. 1937. Aging. *Orvoskepzes* 27:356–368.

Koleseri, S. 1692. *Tractus brevis de mediis quibus vitae sanitatis conserverentur et prolongaretur.* Budapest: National Press.

Palos, M. 1976. The role of information in the care of the aged. In *Congress abstracts of the Congress of the Hungarian Gerontological Association with International Participation*, p. 51. Budapest.

Volgyi, L. 1975. The organization for the social provision of disabled old people in Hungary. *Actuelle Gerontologie* 5:637–645.

IRELAND

JOHN F. FLEETWOOD

In common with the rest of the Western world, Ireland is faced with an ever-growing number of elderly and retired people requiring supportive medical and social services so that they may have reasonable comfort. But the problem is not exclusively of the twentieth century. The pre-Christian Brehon laws contained several sections relating to the care of the aged and infirm (Joyce, 1906). These included provision for old people who were unable to support themselves. They might retire and give up status and land either to their own children or to a third party. The duty of supporting old people fell primarily on their children, who could be punished if they failed to do so. In the absence of childen, the tribe as a group was responsible.

Christianity was introduced to Ireland in 432 A.D., and many of the religious orders untertook as charitable work the care of poor disadvantaged persons, who inevitably included many of the aged. This tradition continues to the present day, though administrative and funding details have changed.

The Poor Law Act of 1838 was intended to "provide relief for the destitute poor of Ireland by affording them temporary residence and support in work-houses." Under section 57 of this act, children were held liable for the support of their parents, and monies expended for relief of the latter could be recovered from the former. This act was often administered in an arbitrary and inhumane fashion. It came into effect at the time of the terrible famines of the 1840s, a combination of circumstances which left a bitter race memory that has not yet entirely disappeared. I remember once advising an elderly man to go into what is now the county home. He declined the suggestion with an oath and snarled, "Is it the poor house you mean? I hope you die there yourself!"

In 1922 Ireland was partitioned. The six northeastern counties remain legally part of Great Britain; any further legislative references in this section are to the southern (Republic of Ireland) part of the country only.

The over-65 population of Ireland has steadily increased from about 3 percent in 1841 to over 11 percent at present. The increased proportion of elderly people has been due to several factors. The main ones are these:

1. Heavy emigration following the famines of the mid-nineteenth century and again in the first half of the twentieth century, through the 1950s. This emigration predominantly involved the young, active, and potentially fertile.

2. Birth control was, up to recent years, not a major factor in Ireland, but the average age of marriage was often so late as to result in no offspring. While the average age of marriage is now much lower, family limitation is commonly practiced so that any major changes in age proportion are unlikely to be noted in the future.
3. Particularly in rural Ireland, delayed delegation of parental authority in the running of a farm or business often resulted in a child's emigrating to a land of greater opportunity. This situation has been recognized even internationally for many years; Lipset (1950), quoting Arensberg, stated: "One important approach which may give us some insight on the position of the old in American society is a cross cultural comparison. In rural Ireland, for example, the peculiar social structure may keep a middle-aged Irishman of 40 or more in the status position of an adolescent in our society. Only when an individual takes over the family farm and marries is he an adult sociologically, and this does not usually occur until the father dies or retires. As a result, people who are chronologically and socially old in our society are in the flower of adulthood among the rural Irish. There age is something to be looked forward to, as it brings with it a higher status and a full adult role."

A factor peculiar to Ireland is the large number of old people living in rural areas as shown by the following percentages for rural persons over 65 living in the four provinces: Leinster, 58 percent urban and 42 percent rural; Munster, 33 percent urban and 67 percent rural; Connaught, 12 percent urban and 88 percent rural; and Ulster (Republic area), 9 percent urban and 91 percent rural. Leinster includes the capital city of Dublin with a population of almost 900,000 (about 23 percent of the country), as well as several other relatively large towns with a total population of about 158,000.

The Poor Law Act remained the main adminstrative instrument of relief for several years after partition. Minor changes were made, but it was not until after World War II that major improvements in both the letter and spirit of administration showed the way to more humane treatment of the underprivileged generally and specifically the aged, particularly in the field of residential care.

An act of 1924 established the Department of Local Government and Public Health as the central authority. Old-age pensions were administered partly by the revenue commissioners.

In 1925 a commission was appointed to inquire into the laws and administration relating to the relief of the sick and destitute poor. When the commission reported in 1927, an important recommendation was that the original intention to reserve the county homes for the aged and infirm poor as well as for chronic invalids should be revived and that standards should be raised. The many demands on the new government's treasury and the outbreak of war in 1939 meant that very little was done until the late 1940s.

An interdepartmental committee set up in 1949 recommended that county homes should be suitably reconstructed and reserved for the aged and chronic sick. The findings and recommendatons were similar to those of the 1925 commission.

A report issued in 1951 indicated that the government had accepted the recommendations of the 1949 interdepartmental committee. It stated that, while in general it was not intended that there should be a multiplicity of homes and hospitals for the accommodation of the aged and chronic sick in any area, sympathetic consideration would be given to proposals for a limited number of subsidiary institutions, provided by adaptation of existing local authority buildings or country houses, in a few of the very large counties where hardship would result from removing old people too great a distance from their friends. To assist in the reconstruction of county homes, the government undertook to make state grants available for the purpose of carrying out approved works. The grant was at the rate of 50 percent of approved loan charges.

Following this, several of the old county homes were greatly improved and modernized. Although there was a parallel improvement in the personal care given to the patients, most of the homes had inadequate numbers of nurses and paramedical staff so that the amount of active treatment was, and often still is, limited.

PROGRAMS

Health

Local health authorities maintain a number of district, county, regional, and psychiatric hospitals. All of them have elderly patients who require active treatment or for whom there is no alternative accommodation. A number of elderly persons are maintained on a long-term basis in voluntary and private general hospitals, small nursing homes, and similar establishments. According to the 1968 report of an interdepartmental committee, the total numbers involved were 20,217; about 5,400 were in general hospitals, homes, and other institutions. Probably there has been an overall increase since then. The figures given represent some 7 beds per 1,000 total population or 62 beds per 1,000 of the over-65 population. The distribution of these beds throughout the country was uneven, and the committee recommended a uniform ratio of 40 geriatric beds per 1,000 of the over-65 population as a practical target and suggested that even this number could be reduced with better domiciliary social services. About 20 to 25 percent of the beds should be reserved for active diagnosis and treatment.

The committee also recommended that 20 places per 1,000 of the over-65 population should be made available for welfare as distinct from sick admissions. It was recognized that this number might have to be increased because people outside the lower income group would make increasing demands for nonmedical admission.

The official policy has been well summarized in a recent letter from the Department of Health to the author (Mulvihill, 1977);

The general picture will be familiar to you. It is that community services (domiciliary medical and nursing care, home help, meals-on-wheels, laundry facilities, assistance with minor home decorations and repairs, day centres, outings, occasional holidays and so on) are provided by local health boards throughout the country—or by voluntary agencies subsidised by the health boards, under the general direction of the Minister of Health. The central idea is that it is better for people, in terms of personal dignity and happiness, to be retained in the community, while this is possible, rather than to be placed in hospitals or other institutions.

In addition, local housing authorities operate a scheme of grants for the repair, reconstruction or adaptation (e.g. the provision of a ramp for a wheel-chair) of the homes of elderly people, and they also provide demountable dwellings and mobile caravan-type homes for those whose own homes are dangerously unfit.

Perhaps the most important contribution made by local housing authorities (and by voluntary agencies subsidised from public funds) to the care of the elderly is the provision throughout the country of sheltered housing schemes—usually a small group of houses featured by amenities such as handrails, non-skid surfaces, special bath and toilet facilities and an alarm system to alert the resident warden in case of any mishap by day or night. It is usual for the local health board to provide a community centre adjacent to a sheltered housing scheme to act as a meeting place for the residents and for other old people in the vicinity and also as a convenient clinic for the provision of paramedical services such as chiropody and physiotherapy.

In addition, local health boards provide Welfare Homes for the aged. The Homes are intended for persons who although not ill nevertheless require a measure of general supervision in an institutional setting. They are provided on the basis of a standard plan designed to provide 40 places for residents. To-date 25 such Homes have been built and occupied throughout the country.

Voluntary effort (a very significant part of the Irish community care programme) is organised under the general guidance of the National Social Service Councils—each a fusion of voluntary groups, including Old Folks Associations, acting in concert with one another and with the statutory authorities.

In general it is proposed to continue to develop community care of the elderly on the foregoing lines subject to budgetary considerations and to the outcome of periodic reviews of the various aspects of the programme. (You will appreciate, of course, that the health programme does not embrace Social Welfare benefits, such as old age pensions, free travel, free TV licenses, cheap fuel schemes and so forth).

Two pilot schemes now at the experimental stage may be of interest to you. In one, a number of elderly persons have been boarded out with private families. The placements were made on the advice of social workers and public health nurses, great care being taken with "matching" of the persons and families concerned. Weekly payments are made by the health boards in respect of maintenance, while the clients retain appropriate sums for personal spending. The second scheme involved the placement of a number of elderly persons on a bed and breakfast basis in a guesthouse. The old people are conveyed each morning to a Day Centre where they have mid-day and evening meals and recreation before being brought home.

It is likely that these schemes will be developed when economic circumstances permit.

It is unfortunately fashionable to decry the efforts of statutory bodies, but it is only fair to state that every effort is made to implement the humane aspirations of the letter quoted though the desired results have not always been achieved.

It is impossible in geriatrics to separate social from medical care, but inevitably various welfare agencies, both statutory and voluntary, will pay more attention to one or other facets of the overall problem. In general, in Ireland statutory agencies concentrate on the essentials, while voluntary bodies provide the amenities that make the difference between existing and living a full life. There is an increasing amount of cooperation as outlined in the letter quoted above so that there are fewer gaps and less duplication of valuable services.

Financial

Under the social welfare acts, practically all employees aged 16 years and over must be covered by social insurance, regardless of the level of their earnings. The cost of weekly contributions is shared on a roughly two to one basis by the employer and employee. Eligibility for contributory pensions depends on a certain number of contributions having been paid within a specified period prior to the sixty-sixth birthday. The contributions are income linked.

The central government, through the Department of Social Welfare, is responsible for old age and retirement pensions, which, though not munificent, are a great improvement over the recent past when many old people were on the borderline of malnutrition unless their pensions were supplemented by voluntary welfare bodies. O'Cinneide (1972) estimated that 24 percent of the total population of Ireland fell below the poverty line and that 32.98 percent of these were over 65 years of age. There are now three principle statutory types of pension: retirement pension, contributory-old age pension, and noncontributory old-age pension.

A retirement pension is payable to a person insured under the social welfare acts, from the age of 65 on, provided he does not then engage in employment that is insurable under the same acts. He may, however, continue to be self-employed up to the age of 66, when he becomes eligible for an old age pension and may, if he wishes, resume work. In principle, if there is a discrepancy at 65 between the amounts to which a pensioner is entitled under the two forms of pension, he will receive the higher amount. The maximum rates of pension per week in April 1979 were £18.60 for pensioners under 80 years and £20 for pensioners 80 years and over. Additional amounts are payable as follows for dependents: £11.90 for adults under 65 years and £14.05 for adults over 65 years. A retired pensioner living alone receives an extra £1.30 per week. On the death of a retired pensioner, the surviving widow is entitled to a widow's pension.

A contributory old age pension is payable to an insured person from the age of 65 years onward provided he has an adequate number of insurance contributions paid. The pension is payable throughout the pensioner's life and is not affected if he remains in employment or has other means, including nonstatutory pensions. The maximum personal rates of pension are the same as for a retired pensioner.

A person who is not eligible for a retirement or contributory pension may qualify for a noncontributory old age pension, which is a social assistance benefit. The amount payable depends on several factors, including the individual's income. Broadly a single person can have £6.00 per week and qualify for a full pension of £15.80 per week. If his income is over £15.00 per week, he does not qualify unless he has dependent children. If his income lies between the extremes, he will receive a pension reduced pro rata. All assessable amounts are doubled for a married man and subject to an increase for other dependents, and an additional £1.20 per week is payable after the eightieth birthday.

Elderly people who are paying income tax are entitled to certain small concessions even if they are in one of the upper-income groups. They are also entitled to certain valuable benefits from public facilities.

1. Free travel on the state transport system is available to all persons aged 66 years or over residing permanently within the state. Pensioners automatically receive a travel authorization; nonpensioners must apply. This facility extends to the pensioner's spouse when accompanying him or her.
2. Old-age and certain other pensioners receive a free ration of electricity and a free television license.
3. A small (£8.80) allowance is payable to an incapacitated pensioner over 67 years of age who is receiving full-time care and attention from a relative if certain conditions are satisfied. Pensioners living alone may be entitled to an extra £1.30 per week.
4. Persons of any age in the lower income group may apply for what is known colloquially as a "medical card." This entitles them and their dependents to free general practitioner treatment from the doctor of their choice, free medicine, and free hospital treatment and investigation.
5. Special cost-of-living-index–linked state savings bonds with a guaranteed minimum return may be purchased by persons aged 65 and over as a hedge against inflation.
6. Centenarians receive an ex gratia payment of £50 on their birthday with a message of congratulations from the president.

Geriatric Nurses and Physicians

Increasing numbers of public health or community nurses are being recruited. As might be expected, there is a preponderance of old people under their routine care. This fact is recognized in their training program, which emphasizes the care of elderly patients in their own homes. The Nursing Board is, in fact, ahead of the medical and general nursing schools in its recognition of the importance of geriatrics in total patient care.

Physicians interested in geriatrics have complained for many years that medical students, student nurses, and paramedical workers do not receive adequate exposure to geriatric problems and their solutions. Some teachers still correlate "old" with "hopeless" and believe a geriatric ward is a dumping ground that provides minimal care to hopeless cases at the hands of therapeutic nihilists.

In the last few years the eight regional health boards have been empowered to appoint physicians with specific geriatric responsibility. So far only a limited number of appointments have been made, notably in the eastern, southern, and western regions and on a temporary basis in the midland region. (In Northern Ireland, nine geriatric consultants deal with a smaller and more compact population with essentially the same age distribution as the Republic.)

The stated objectives in appointing these geriatric physicians are:

- To assess rehabilitate, and resettle elderly patients in the community by making the best use of existing resources currently caring for the elderly, by providing outpatient clinics, by providing a domiciliary consultant service for general practitioners, and by providing extended care beds for nursing dependent patients who have been assessed.
- To assist in the promotion and operation of community and special care programs by attending committees concerned with the development of welfare homes, day centers, district nursing services, and so on.
- To promote the specialty of geriatrics by teaching medical students, nurses, paramedical personnel, welfare workers, and the general public.

RESEARCH

County Homes

A number of regional medicosocial studies have been undertaken in an effort to identify different local needs. One of the most extensive of these (MacDevitt, Brett, and O'Connor, 1975) was published by the Medico-Social Research Board.

The over-65 populations of three county homes in predominantly small-town and rural areas were selected for investigation in April 1972. A one-in-four random sample of 140 individuals between 65 and 98 years was studied. The study included a questionnaire filled in by the nurses and, where the patient's mental and physical state permitted, a personal interview. In 43 cases relatives were also interviewed.

The authors admit that extrapolation from their small sample to the community as a whole may not be accurate, but they believe that the picture presented fairly accurately reflects the situation throughout the country; probably the findings are not grossly different from those obtained from similar surveys in other Western countries.

Only 4.3 percent of the sample were married with living spouses. One third-of the married and widowed had no children. Of the widowed in the general community, 92.68 percent lived with either a son or daughter compared with 50 percent of the widowed later admitted to the homes. The mobility of children and other relatives is an important factor in isolation and consequent admission to institutions in old age.

There are marked differences in the self-care capacities of people in the homes and outside. The authors discuss whether this resulted from individual variations in the aging process, lack of care prior to admission, or postadmission deterioration.

Over 41 percent of the home sample had been living alone before admission as compared with less than 25 percent in the outside community. It appeared that adverse changes in household composition sometimes precipitated admission.

Primarily social admissions made up 60 percent of the total and primarily medical admissions the balance, though there was an overlap. The average length of stay was 4.65 years. The authors stress that rehabilitation without the support of community services is futile.

Most of the persons admitted were in the lower socioeconomic categories. Almost three-quarters had no income other than the old-age pension, and a quarter of those admitted said that they had had financial problems.

Many of the sample had very poor housing conditions, and none were living in specially built accommodation for the aged. None of those in the homes had a telephone, a factor that must have seriously increased their sense of isolation and desire for admission.

One of the authors of the original work (Brett, 1975) carried out a further detailed study on institutionalization and aging in which he analyzed the sociological theory of institutionalization and its application to a geriatric home situation. He undertook six weeks of observation in the three homes that provided the original material. He then spent a further two months in a fourth home, during which a more intensive analysis took place and some detailed case studies were made with the object of tracing the progress of newly admitted patients through various stages until the old person adopted the role of the institutionalized patient.

The fourth home was superior to the others in facilities and staffing. There were also more stringent admission regulations, which meant that it did not tend to become a dumping ground for unwanted old people, an image often associated with the county home. As a result, the general atmosphere among both patients and staff was considerably better than in the other units studied.

In the course of his work in the fourth home, Brett came across a poem written by a pupil of the workhouse primary school whose father was, in fact, master of the institution. It explains, better perhaps than more sophisticated treatises, the still common aversion to using the county homes:

They carved the name above the gate, 1849
When they built the Workhouse on the hill
Of limestone tall and fine.

A plague wind blew across the land
Fever was in the air
Fields were black that once were green
And death was everywhere.

People came to drink the soup
Ladled from greasy bowls:
They died in whitewashed wards that
Held a thousand Irish souls.

And still the Workhouse looks to
Heaven—the hills high-windowed dome
The same for all its name is changed
Today to the County Home.

Athlone Survey

Athlone is a town of ten thousand in the center of Ireland; it lacks heavy industry and has a large rural hinterland. In 1973 the local community services council carried out a survey on the needs of old (over-65) people in the town. Its findings are probably comparable to those that could be obtained elsewhere.

The fieldwork was conducted by a team of professional interviewers working on a voluntary basis with the assistance of local volunteers. The sample used was a stratified random sample with uniform sample fraction. The following are the most significant results of this survey:

1. Three-quarters of the sample suffered from at least one serious medical complaint and a further one-fifth had two such complaints.
2. Rheumatism and heart conditions were the most frequently mentioned illnesses. Over one-tenth of the sample had impaired and another one-fifth slightly impaired hearing. While only 2 percent admitted total blindness, another 40 percent wore glasses all the time. Three percent were bedridden and another 12 percent slightly restricted in their physical movement.
3. A quarter were cared for during illness by their spouse and almost a third by some other household member. Two-fifths of the sample visited the doctor regularly.
4. A quarter lived alone, a fifth with a spouse, a tenth with spouse, children or children-in-law, or grandchildren.

5. Almost half of the respondents' households had no bathroom and the same proportion had no running hot water. Nearly 40 percent of the households experienced
difficulty in getting repairs done. Forty percent thought improvements needed to be
done; plumbing was the most frequently mentioned.

6. The vast majority of the sample had some kind of recreational activity at home,
television and/or radio being the most popular for one-third and reading for
one-quarter of them. A quarter of the sample went out walking daily, but most went
out very infrequently.

7. Eighty-seven percent never attended the local old folks' club. About half were
interested in a new center for old people.

8. A quarter of the respondents expressed interest in receiving voluntary visitors. The
majority of those living alone spent every evening of the week alone. Twenty-five
percent of the total and 40 percent of those living alone said that they sometimes felt
lonely.

9. A third felt that laundry, shopping, and cooking services would be of benefit to all
old people. Less than one-fifteenth said they would benefit personally from
shopping and cooking services, although 30 percent thought that they themselves
might use a laundry service. When the interviewees ranked three services from a
list of nine in terms of their importance for all old people, meals-on-wheels,
laundry, and chiropody were ranked highest. Nearly 60 percent were in favour of
voluntary activity on behalf of old people.

10. Half of the sample were using the travel and electricity services, two-fifths availed
themselves of free television licenses, and one in twenty-five of free fuel. Very few
of the nonusers of these services were in that category because of ignorance about
the services or their entitlements.

11. One-sixth of the sample approved of residential care for old people and one-quarter
conditionally approved. One hundred and thirty respondents gave their opinions
about central government policy. Over half of them considered financial and
economic matters the most important, and one-quarter of them made various
suggestions about aspects of housing.

Dublin Survey

The National Prices Commission published in 1977 the results of a survey of
139 people over the age of 51 years living in a low-income area of central
Dublin. The authors were a multidisciplinary team with experience in social
medicine, behavior, economics, and nutrition. They showed that 73 percent of
the sample had diets that were nutritionally inadequate in at least one respect.
A third of the over-65 group were not eating enough to satisfy their daily
energy requirements. Protein intake was inadequate in some 12 percent, and
almost half the subjects had an insufficient iron supply. Over a half were
deficient in vitamin C, and 18 percent were not taking enough calcium.

The authors argue that their findings point to nutritional deficiency existing
in up to twenty thousand elderly people in Ireland, though I feel that the
findings may not be applicable to rural areas.

An ironic finding was that nutritionally adequate diets were sometimes cheaper than inadequate ones. In some cases, the food purchased and its cost were materially affected by the nearness of shops, the presence of cooperative friends or relatives, and the type and quality of food available locally. With frequent price fluctuations, it is difficult for anyone to calculate the best buys in terms of both nutritional value and price.

It has been said that a community's degree of true civilization can be measured by the care it gives to the handicapped, the underprivileged, and the old. At a recent meeting in Dublin a speaker startled the audience by bluntly declaring that old-age pensioners had never had it so good and that fringe benefits brought their standard of living to a very respectable level. There is a certain truth in this claim. From the material point of view, for example, the elderly person is better off than ever before, but unfortunately the relatively generous benefits provided by the state have resulted in a slow erosion of family responsibility. Other factors, including working wives, smaller houses, lack of domestic help, inflation, and emigration of family members who would otherwise be available, all play a significant part in the increased demand for social geriatric services.

Survey of Relatives

MacDevitt et al. (1975) studied the opinions of relatives about the elderly patients either admitted to homes or remaining in the community. The relatives of those elderly who remained in the community saw the age of the elderly as less of a burden to the relatives than did the relatives of those who had been admitted. The differences were most obvious in the perceived effect on mental and physical health of the relatives, and there was a lesser impact on the financial situation and social life. The smallest effect was on household routine and on children, a point with which many general practitioners might not agree.

A majority in both groups said they were unaffected financially by the presence of the old person in the house. Only 4 percent were receiving the old-age allowance. In fact very few were eligible for this payment. I believe that answers to the question about financial stress should be treated with caution, for the natural pride of many people, particularly in rural Ireland, could encourage them to be overoptimistic in their reply to this part of the questionnaire.

In a survey of two hundred admissions to a long-stay unit, Fleetwood (1974) noted that about 25 percent could have stayed at home had better domiciliary services been available. In these cases, the relatives would have willingly cooperated. The point is also brought out in MacDevitt's study.

Despite many pressures, family coherence is still more stable in Ireland than in many other Western communities, and neglect is often due to thoughtlessness rather than callousness. The status of the aged is generally good, and there is overall recognition of their special needs. Because they are not a united voting force, however, their impact as a political pressure group is less than it might be.

A measure of the community's awareness of the importance of social service to the aged can be seen from a perusal of the 1976 People of the Year awards. Of the twelve awards, two were for work with the aged and two were for work with a large geriatric content.

Most towns have some form of geriatric welfare committee to provide recreation and social amenities for senior citizens. In addition to these groups, many charitable organizations have undertaken work with the elderly over a long period. These include church groups and the Irish Red Cross Society, which has, through its Geriatrics Committee, actively encouraged its units to provide welfare and recreational services throughout the country for many years.

In all communities, some people are too proud or too apathetic to use the services provided. Case finding is by far the most difficult problem in geriatric work, a feature by no means confined to Ireland. It is here that the general medical practitioner has a very important role to play, for the old person will trust his doctor, who may be able to induce him to recognize that acceptance of statutory services does not bear what is still regarded as the taint of a work-house handout.

Despite the appointment of regional geriatricians, most of the day-to-day clinical care of the aged falls on the general practitioner. His success in keeping people out of hospital is in direct proportion to the availability of ancillary services, but he must also be aware of technical advances in geriatric medicine. There is an increasing number of courses, symposia, lectures, and discussions relating to geriatrics available every year in Ireland.

Irish Gerontological Society

The Irish Gerontological Society was founded in 1950 to provide a discussion ground for physicians and others interested in gerontological and geriatric problems. One or two meetings are held anually, though many papers that could properly be presented are in fact read to other groups with a wider audience. Papers presented over the years have included "Carbohydrate Tolerance in Elderly Subjects," "Urinary Obstruction in the Aged," "Maternal Age and Foetal Defects," "Nutrition and Aging," and "Hypothermia in Old Age," as well as several dealing with the social problems of an aging population.

The society is represented on the Council of the International Association of Gerontology, and a number of physicians interested in geriatrics are members of the British Geriatrics Society.

There have been few major gerontological research studies carried out in Ireland. Work now underway includes a study by John Lavan of confusion in five hundred geriatric admissions, research by R.E. Moore on the responses of aged men to cold stress, and a study by Geraghty, Sheridan, and Healy of a test technique to determine the presence of brain failure, modified for use with a rural Irish population. The test consists of asking questions, which if incorrectly answered may indicate a degree of brain failure requiring specific measures in management.

At Our Lady's Manor, a private geriatric home in the suburbs of Dublin, a study of different levels of skeletal deformities and their consequences has been initiated by A. Meade. The investigations are to include radiological screening, biochemical assay of bone physiology, and bone biopsy. It is hoped that the project will provide information about some of the factors rendering senile bones liable to fracture.

At the Psycho-Endocrine Unit of the Department of Psychiatry of University College at St. James Hospital, Dublin, there is a twelve-bed clinical unit with complete facilities for undertaking metabolic and sleep laboratory studies with remote electroencephalogram and remote blood sampling equipment. The program is designed to evaluate the available techniques for monitoring sleep pattern, endocrine profile, and mental performance indexes in normal subjects under varying conditions (A. Darragh). It is proposed to extend this program to study changes in these indexes in different age groups.

The predominant interests of the center lie in the field of hypothalamic pituitary function and the influence of physiological, pharmacological, and pathological processes on the functioning of this integrated psychoneuroendocrine complex.

In recent years increasing emphasis has been placed on preparation for retirement and old age. The civil service, large corporations, and businesses generally now organize preretirement courses and seminars for their employees. Unfortunately these are not provided early enough in the individual's career. Employers might disagree, but it is not excessive to say that from the earliest days of work, an employee should be helped to cultivate a retiring mind so that he would look toward his arbitrary retiring date as marking a move to something rather than from something.

Significantly, at least one of the community welfare groups for the elderly now operates an employment bureau for retired persons who wish to take up a part-time occupation either voluntarily or for a salary. The number of applicants for jobs far exceeds the posts available.

REFERENCES

Athlone Community Services Council. 1973. *A survey of the aged*. Athlone.
Brett, T. D. 1975. Master's Thesis. Social Science Research Centre, University College, Galway.

Corridan, John P. 1965. Demographic aspects of the geriatric problem. *Gerontologia Clinica* 1976. 7:370.

Department of Social Welfare. 1976. *A national income related pension scheme.* Dublin.

———. 1977. Summary of social insurance and assistance services. Dublin.

Fleetwood, J. F. 1974. Communication to the Seventh European Congress of Clinical Gerontology.

Hensey, B. 1959. *The health services of Ireland.* Dublin: Institute of Public Administration.

Joyce, P. W. 1906. *A smaller social history of ancient Ireland.* London: Longmans Green.

Kaim Caudle, P. S. 1972. Senior citizens in Irish history. *Administration* 17.

Kelly, P. 1972. From workhouse to hospital: The role of the Irish workhouse in medical relief to 1921. Master's thesis, University College, Galway.

Lipset, S. M. 1950. *Proceedings of the Pacific Coast Committee on Old Age Research.* Stanford, Calif.

MacDevitt D.; Brett, T. D.; and O'Connor, M. E. 1975. *Admission to county homes.* Medico Social Research Board.

Mulvihill, M. 1977. Personal communication.

National Prices Commission. 1977. *Report on nutrition.* Dublin.

O'Cinneide, S. 1972. The extent of poverty in Ireland. *Social Studies* (August): 381–400.

O'Neill, T. P. 1958. The Irish workhouse during the great famine. *Christus Rex* 12.

Poor Law Act 1838. 1, 2 Victoriae 1 Chap. 56.

Rynne, Catherine. 1973. *Enjoying retirement.* Torc Books.

Summary of Social Insurance and Assistance Services. 1977. Dublin: Department of Social Welfare.

ISRAEL

SHIMON BERGMAN

Israel defies an easy standard classification as a traditional, developing, or modern Western society. By virtue of the region in which it lies and in the composition of its population, it no doubt contains elements of all three. Its successful blend of these elements has earned it the fame of a paradise for sociologists and anthropologists and of the ideal living laboratory for social experiments.

Israel is one of the few examples of a modern society that did not evolve from an existing institutional structure. Rather it is the result of a conscious process of building a society from institutional elements that were partly planned, partly brought by immigrants from their cultures of origin, and partly came as an answer to immediate needs or emergencies. From this point of view, the major components of Israel's being were immigration, planning, improvisation, fusion of backgrounds and cultures, and responses to pressures accompanying the process of forming a new Jewish society in the years before Israel was established in May 1948 (Eisenstadt et al., 1970).

IMMIGRATION AND AGING

Immigration is the central phenomenon of Israel's existence. Without it, Israel could never have come into existence, nor can it sustain itself without its continuation. In it lies the nation's historical raison d'être as the haven for those in need and as the spiritual, cultural, and historical center it can offer to Jews in other countries.

Immigration to Israel has to be considered primarily in noneconomic terms because for the early settlers, it really meant lowering the standard of living and a trend to deurbanization. The motivation for immigration was ideological. It was a highly selective group, unigenerational or two-generational at most. There was no host society to absorb them, no cultural milieu in which to assimilate. The emerging values emphasized human and social equality, idealization of work, orientation to group rather than family, stress on the future (hence an idealization of youth, of pioneering spirit and activity), and vision of an ideal society, with health and social protection of the worker, and insurance for his old age, in the very distant future (Eisenstadt et al., 1970). The share of the aged in that process was minimal. Those aged who were in the country were a reminder of the past rather than a factor in the present or a significant forecast for the future. Their share in the slowly growing Jewish population did not exceed 3 percent, with a part of these aged belonging to the generation of old religious Jews centered mostly in the holy towns (Bergman, 1969). It was on these values that a host society was built for the absorption of future immigration waves.

The emergence of Israel was a turning point; for many, it was an act of messianic fulfillment. Immigration, conceptualized as the supreme national value, was institutionalized as one of the first basic laws of the country. Its practical effect was a nonselective immigration by right, permitting all types, among them the sick, handicapped, and aged, soon to become clients of the fledgling health and welfare services of the new state. Over 1.6 million people, more than twice the original population in 1948, have since come from over seventy countries: 47 percent from Africa and Asia and 52 percent from Europe and other Western areas. The implications of the figures and of continents of origin are obvious considering the differences in values, demography, standard of living, education, and skills.

Research generally shows that the aged are reluctant movers unless activation is strongly religious or emotional or whole communities move. The rather high presence of the elderly in this mass movement after 1948 is unique. Some 8 percent of all immigrants were at least 60 years of age on arrival (about 130,000 persons, 60 percent of them from Europe). Some 85,000 persons were 65 or over (5 percent of the total immigration since 1948) at the time of their arrival in the country. Those between 45 and 64 years old at immigration have constituted 18 percent of the total immigration movement since 1948.

The unique features of that enormous immigration were its dominant national-emotional motivation, the sanctioned right to immigrate, the principle of nonselectivity, the rapidity of its implementation, and the inclusion of categories normally excluded from migration movements to pioneering countries —the sick, the handicapped, and the aging.

About 45 percent of all immigrants and 34 percent of all immigrants aged 65 and over arrived in the country between 1948 and 1951, years of economic austerity, postwar shortages, and the earliest stages of the organization of the new state. Close to 700,000 immigrants—among them 30,000 aged 65 and over—had a tremendous impact on the limited absorptive capacity of the small host society (650,000 people) in these three years.

Sixty percent of the aged immigrant group were of European and Western origin and 40 percent were from Asia and Africa, compared to 52 percent and 47 percent, respectively, in the overall immigration into Israel. Sociologists of immigration in Israel point out the following characteristics of the immigration from Asia and Africa: relatively extended families and intensive kinship relations; traditionalism, with strong emphasis on the authority of the elders;

collective responsibility of the family; limited occupational differentiation; relatively rigid occupational structure; and specific social differentiation. These characteristics were confronted by those of the host society based on orientation toward the young, the small nuclear families, the future, high social mobility, and developed occupational differentiation (Eisenstadt et al., 1970).

For immigrants from Asia and Africa, the process of adaptation to the host reality led to a transformation of the internal structure of the family and the social participation of its members. These transformations were particularly sharply perceived by the elderly, whose status was undergoing serious change. The confrontation with the negative impact of the new material, organizational, and informal social environments was often very traumatic, particularly the "dis-aging" effect of bureaucracy, which conferred no status on the aged, and the "asymetric relationship" between young bureaucrats and elderly clients (Bar Yosef, 1967). The resulting inability of the elderly to cope with the demands of the new environment often brought them frustration, which they expressed in aggressive behavior toward social institutions (Bergman and Amir, 1973).

The aged immigrants from Europe faced no fewer difficulties even though they were closer to the main cultural and social features of the host society dominated by European values, norms, and structural characteristics. Their recent past was burdened by the horrible experience of war and Nazi persecution. Many arrived alone, having no spouses, children, siblings, or other kin to turn to. (Of the structurally most isolated group of aged in Israel—those who have no relatives—more than 80 percent were of European origin.) They too showed the symptoms of stress inherent in immigration and in the interaction with the material, organizational, and informal environments. Studies on mental hospitalization in Israel in those years showed that at least 15 percent of the immigrant hospitalized aged showed adjustment disorders; this figure held equally for European and non-European aged immigrants (Miller, 1970).

The establishment of Israel and the ensuing mass immigration created two rather distinct groups of aged: those born in the country (about 4 percent of those 65 and over) or settled in Israel in the years before 1948 and whom we may define as old settlers or local aged; and those post-1948 aged immigrants whom we could define as imported aged. Socioculturally they fall into two additional groups: Western and Oriental. This gives us four subgroups—Western local; Western imported; Oriental local, and Oriental imported—for analysis.

The local aged consist almost exclusively (96 percent) of the early pioneers who immigrated in their youth (between 18 and 30) and have now reached old age. Theirs is the first generation of pensioners whose retirement process is similar to the one of the industrialized countries based on contributory or budgetary pensions secured under labor agreements. This group constitutes only about one-third of all aged in the country; 85 percent of them are of European origin. Their roots in the community are of longer duration; their living conditions are of higher standards; their education is better; their community integration fuller; and their self-image and their expectations of society more positive, clearer, and more demanding than the imported aged.

Immigration up to 1948 was highly selective toward young persons without families. As a result, the majority arrived at old age at the same time. Most of them matured away from filial responsibility, and most of them did not impart to their children the experience or example of the presence, interaction, and/or care of the older person in or close to the family. Research indicates that some of the symptoms of undesirable intergenerational behavior may be associated with the lack of socialization opportunities to interaction with and care of older people within the family context. In a way, what happens on the microlevel of the family could be observed on the macrolevel of a society deprived of previous experience with aged persons as an integral part of the host society. This phenomenon is particularly evident in the smaller-sized communities of the collective settlements (kibbutzim) (Musham, 1975).

Today's elderly were the founding generation of the state; they created and entrenched the value system and the norms of Israel as the absorbing society, which include the importance of work, a high regard for achievement, an idealization of pioneering work, and a youth orientation to the future. For them, retirement is unwelcome and perceived as a disruptive factor in their social functioning. Parting with leadership roles and with active involvement in affairs of the society they helped to found is very difficult; the transition from active membership in the old-settlers group to a marginal role of a pensioner is often traumatic.

Many of the foundations for the social security and welfare of that group were laid before 1948 or soon after the establishment of the state. Patterns were developed for some financial basis of retirement (today's pension funds), for their medical care, and for other social provisions. They also enjoyed better conditions and a higher standard of living than did their post-1948 counterparts.

The imported aged consisted of the post-1948 elderly immigrants. The pattern of aging of the Oriental elderly reflects different social, cultural, and economic characteristics. Caught in the process of the acculturation of the younger generation, the aged Oriental found himself exposed to the tribulations of a double process of adjustment: that of an older person in a traditional family that undergoes rapid changes in a predominantly Western society and that of an older immigrant in a new community. The Oriental family has always played a more important role in the life of the elderly. More aged of Oriental than European origin live with their children, and this applies also to the married aged. Many aged live with their sons; Oriental widows tend to remain with the family rather than live in separate households.

The impact of the new social environment was negative. Change in the status of women, acculturation of grandchildren, and the conservatism of the aged often clash, leading to various consequences, including reactive behavior on the part of the aged and requests for placement in old-age homes.

THE GROWTH OF GERONTOLOGY

The background developments following the establishment of the state and the explosion of aging as a result of the immigration of elderly explains Israel's growing interest in aging. Pragmatic needs to create services, provide care, organize and train manpower, and obtain basic data even for short-term planning brought about the emergence of a small nucleus of doctors, social workers, and nurses who began to explore and develop the operational basis for services and foundations for gerontological development.

In 1954, Israeli delegates attended the International Association of Gerontology Congress in London. In 1956 the first National Conference on Aging was held, and the Gerontological Society was founded. In the same year the first Gerontological quarterly L'et Zikna ("Old Age") made its appearance and continued until 1961 (in 1973 it was renewed as Gerontologia, the quarterly of the Israel Gerontological Society). In 1959 a second conference took place with the participation of mayors, members of parliament, and heads of social services. Since 1957, regular participation in IAG congresses put Israel on the international gerontological map, including involvement in the activities of the European Social Research Comittee and the European Clinical Section. In 1966 two public committees (government and trade unions) were charged to prepare blueprints for national policies in the area of services to aged and in retirement. The published reports became important documents of social policy on the aging. The establishement of the National Association for the Planning and Development of Services to the Aged gave additional large-scale impetus to practical activities in the area of aging. In 1970 and 1971, gerontology began to be taught at some of the universities, including Tel Aviv and Haifa. In 1975 the Tenth International Congress of Gerontology convened in Jerusalem, and in 1974 and 1975, the Brookdale Institute of Gerontology was established in Jerusalem. Two volumes of the Annotated Bibliography on Aging in Israel were published by the Gerontological Sociey in 1966 and 1976, and the number of gerontological publications (articles, research reports, special issues of professional magazines, and so forth) showed constant increase. In 1975 a government-appointed committee (headed by a supreme court judge) studied again the issues of aging (such as employment and retirement) and published its recommendations. A health service insurance bill and a bill of national pensions are still under consideration and will soon be submitted to Parliament.

DEMOGRAPHIC TRENDS

As a classic immigration country, Israel shows a steady increase in population. Since 1919, slightly over 2 million Jews have entered the country. Since the establishment of Israel in 1948, the Jewish population has increased over fourfold (430 percent). The number of aged has increased almost eightfold; at the end of 1977, it stood at 9.1 percent of the Jewish population as compared to 3.8 percent in 1948.

The non-Jewish population (15 percent of the total inhabitants of Israel)—Muslems, Christians, and Druzes—is considerably younger; those 65 and older constitute only 3.3 percent of that group. Due to a very high rate of fertility and improved social and health conditions, the percentage of those 65 and over has gone down in the last several years. While the non-Jewish population more than trebled in the last thirty years, the number of aged only doubled.

The analysis of sources of population increase among Jews for the period 1948–1977 shows that natural increase accounted for 35 percent and immigration for 43 percent with the basic population in 1948 providing 22 percent (in round figures).

The Jewish population of the country has become increasingly native. Fifty-three percent of the present population is Israeli born; 10 percent is Asian born; 11 percent is African born; and 20 percent is European and Western born.

The mean age in the population has gone up in the last decade from 28.7 to 30.3, whereas the median age has gone down during the same period from 26.7 to 25.6.

Our aged population (65 plus) is relatively young, with 42 percent between 65 and 69, 28 percent between 70 and 74, 17 percent between 75 and 79, and 12 percent 80 and over.

Jews are a larger proportion of the aged than are non-Jews as can be seen from the following comparison: Jews are 85 percent of the total population and 93.7 percent of those 65 and over; non-Jews are 15 percent of the total population and 6.3 percent of those 65 and over.

The Jewish aged population is mostly foreign born. Locally born elderly are only about 4 percent of the aged; 15 percent come from Asia, 9 percent from Africa, and 72 percent from Europe and West. The group aged 45–64, those to become aged within two decades, has a similar composition, with an increase in the percentage of locally born. The locally born are about 9 percent, Asia born 18 percent, Africa born 16 percent, and Europe born 56 percent. The implications for patterns of retirement, service requirements, and for other aspects of planning are obvious.

The population aged 0–29 is well balanced between sexes with no change in the ratio over the last twenty-five years. A shift in the direction of decrease of ratio of males per females occurs in the remaining age groups with the exception of those 65 and over, which shows an increase from 861 males (in 1950) to 986 males (in 1974) per 1,000 females. The increase in the dependency ratio of Jews can be seen from the following data: the ratio of those under 14 years to those 65 and over in 1950 was 0.45 and in 1975 was 0.48; the ratio of those 65 and over to those 15 to 64 in 1950 was 0.06 and in 1975 was 0.13; and the ratio of those under 15 plus those 65 and over to those 15 to 64 in 1950 was 0.51 and in 1975 was 0.61.

Israel is rather high on the list of countries with low mortality; it has insignificant infant mortality and high life expectancy at birth (table 23). The highest gain at birth, as in other countries, is evident from figures for the last quarter of a century (table 24).

As for marital status, Israel's population shows trends similar to those in other developed countries. As age goes up, the percentage of married males goes down but stops at almost 60 percent at the age of 30 as compared to 11 percent for married females at the age of 80. At the age of 80 there are twice as many widows as there are at the age of 65 (86 percent and 42 percent respectively) but almost five times as many widowers (39 percent and 8 percent respectively) (table 25).

The forecast of population for Israel is complicated by the factor of the unknown extent of immigration in the years to come. Using two estimates (25,000 immigrants per year and 50,000 per year) the forecast for 1993 shows that Jewish aged, 65 and over, will go up from the present 9.1 percent to 9.7 percent or 9.9 percent, respectively, and there will be a further decrease in the population of elderly in the non-Jewish sector from 3.3 percent to 2.7 percent, respectively. The reason for the contrasting trends has already been mentioned. In the overall population, those aged 65 and over by 1990–1993 should bring Israel very close to the category of aging societies.

This review of the demographic trends can be summarized: up to 1948 immigration of individuals mostly without adult families; after 1948, population transfers of families or whole communities with considerable aging presence (the former mostly of European origin and the latter mostly of non-European background characterized by lack of previous exposure to modern social structure). As a result, serious cultural, social, and economic differences with many tensions have arisen in the patterns of intercontinental and intergenerational relations (young members of new immigrant waves in relation to old members of their own waves and in relation to old members of old immigration waves—the host society). Another important confrontation is that between cohorts of previous immigrant groups—the current leadership of the country who are reaching old age and are under pressure to retire—versus their sons and daughters and the sons and daughters of more recent immigrants. In the non-Jewish sector, although the elderly are still a small minority, the growing trend of Westernization is gradually resulting in changes in inter-

Table 23: MORTALITY AND LIFE EXPECTANCY

Year	Mortality per 1,000	Infant Mortality per 1,000	Life Expectancy Male	Female
1933–1935	9.3	78.0	59.5	61.8
1951	6.4 (8.8)[a]	39.2 (48.8)	67.2	70.1
1961	5.7 (7.3)	24.3 (48.0)	70.7	73.5
1975	7.5 (5.4)	19.2 (37.0)	70.5 (69.4)	73.6 (72.6)
1977	6.9	17.8	71.9 (68.5)	75.4 (71.3)

Source: Composite table derived from tables iii/1 and iii/34, *Statistical Abstract of Israel,* 1975, and tables iii/34 and iii/35, *Statistical Abstract of Israel,* 1978. Jerusalem.

a. Figures in parentheses are for non-Jewish inhabitants.

Table 24: LIFE EXPECTANCY AT SELECTED AGES

Age	1950 Males	Females	1974 Males	Females	1977 Males	Females
At birth	66.5	69.5	70.5	73.7	71.9	75.4
At 55	20.4	22.2	21.1	22.3	21.5	23.4
At 65	15.4	14.6	13.8	14.5	14.1	15.5
At 75	8.3	9.0	8.3	8.4	8.6	9.1

Source: U. O. Schmelz, ed. *Society in Israel: Selected Statistics.* Jerusalem: Central Bureau of Statistics, 1976.

Table 25: MARITAL STATUS

Age	Sex	Married	Widowed	Other
65–69	Males	87.9%	8.1%	4.0%
	Females	52.6	42.3	5.1
70–74	Males	82.0	14.5	3.5
	Females	36.7	58.7	4.6
75–79	Males	74.6	22.2	3.2
	Females	24.3	72.0	3.7
80 and over	Males	58.0	38.8	3.2
	Females	11.2	85.8	3.0

Source: Derived from Table 22/B, *Statistical Abstract of Israel,* 1975, Jerusalem, p. 48.

generational relations and in the strong status of the older person in the traditional extended family (Rizeq, 1978).

Musham has summarized these problems: "Israel is faced with a host of problems arising in an aging population. Israel obviously shares with all other countries a low or decreasing fertility in the trend of aging. But as a country of immigration and one containing substantial national minorities, these problems assume some unique peculiarities. Some of them alleviate the burden or delay its impact. Others, on the other hand, preclude easy solutions to the problems of aging of the population."

ROLES AND STATUS OF THE AGED

Israel's two distinct groups of elderly—local and imported—are molded by different attitudes and environments. They now coexist spatially as a result of immigration, but they demonstrate a variety of sentiments, attitudes, and life-styles.

Immigration involves desocialization, disorganization of a person's role system, loss of social identity. Adjustment to the new environment requires understanding the new role system and building a new role and a new identity. Two concomitant processes take place: desocialization intertwined with attempts to salvage the previous sociopersonal system, and the rebuilding activity, with ensuing conflicts between the two, leading to situations of tension (Bar-Yosef, 1967). The new material, organizational, and informal social environment play an important part in this process of retention and/or rebuilding of one's role in the new society.

The process of salvaging and of adapting was especially characteristic of the elderly of the traditional societies with the pattern of extended families. They have retained, in general, strong family orientation and traditional life-style. There is not much change, nor is there much striving for it. Yet research shows that many, particularly the widowed living with their children, feel lonely and dissatisfied. There the break in life-style is possibly the strongest because their central role as mother, wife, and senior housekeeper is lacking or is seriously curtailed by the invading social change. Their participation in decision making and child rearing is reduced; the young daughters-in-law acculturate quickly and resist interference. Social agencies have found that there is an increase of requests from such three-generational families for relocation of the elderly into old-age homes. It is these role-reduced Oriental women who rate their health poorest and feel lonely more often than their Western counterparts. Their link with the family is still strong; more aged of that group share households and are part of family life with their children; up to 75 percent of unmarried Oriental aged—as compared with 50 percent of European aged—in urban areas live with their children. Of those married, some 50 percent share households with their children compared with 17 percent of their European counterparts. In rural areas shared households are even more frequent. Yet this fact cannot hide the highly reduced role of the older person, who often sees himself as the guardian of the old ways and mores and runs into conflict with the younger generation. There is increasing evidence of the threat to gerontocracy in Arab villages and the weakening of the extended family ties. This is even more evident in urban areas.

The old settlers aged evidence the process of role reduction in a way similar to that in other Western societies. Salvaging previous roles of active mastery in work and decision making the family, community, political life, and other areas is a major challenge. The increasing involvement of society in the provision of welfare and the generally better economic situation of that group makes these aged less dependent on the younger generation and more aggressive or demanding in regard to their position and their role. In this sector that organization of the aged has appeared. These people provide the active leadership in the political organization of aged over such issues as pensions, representation in professional unions, and retirement conditions.

A considerable percentage of Israeli aged men continue their work role beyond the age of 65—some because of economic need, some because of inherent value and importance ascribed to the role of a working person in a society in which work was elevated to the status of religion, and some because they still fill an active role as parents (late postwar remarriages among survivors of the holocaust and the need to provide help to their late-born sons and daughters). In 1977, 17 percent of all persons 65 and over were still in the active civilian labor force (29 percent of males 65 and over). This represents a decrease in comparison with a decade earlier. But this is a drastic transition at 65 from the work role to retiree role (the percentage of working males in the age group 55–64 is 85 percent as compared to 29 percent in the males 65 and over).

Oriental aged tend to retire earlier and generally see themselves as less able to continue working than the old settlers. The Oriental aged perceive discontinuation of work in terms of loss of income rather than as loss of status. The old settlers, in contrast, give up their work life reluctantly. Therefore their capacity for role reorganization become a key issue in the formation of a life-style in later years. Their expectations of retirement are rather negative despite a growing awareness of the need for retirement planning and preparation. Theirs is the first generation of elderly to depart from work in an institutionalized manner. Imbued with reverence for work, with no retirement patterns and leisure roles to fall back upon, they see themselves facing a serious role reduction in society. Ongoing trade-union affiliation, volunteer involvement in the community, and some beginnings of self-organization are some of the expressions of the search for revised role identity.

Education has been found to be highly correlated with many aspects of the aging issues, including employment, role transition, and role reorganization. Here too is a contrast between the two aged groups (Western and Oriental). In the total Jewish population in 1977, 7 percent were defined as illiterates, women showing a rate twice as high as that of men (9 percent versus 4 percent). As age rises, so does the percentage of illiterates because of immigration from less-developed societies. In the age group 55–64, there were 13 percent illiterates, and in the group 65 and over, 19 percent illiterates. However, whereas among the aged of European background there were only 3 percent illiterates, the Asia-Africa regions showed 22 percent illiterates. Aged of Oriental origin with lower education are more frequently those who describe their health in negative terms, are less involved in activities, assume no active roles, favor separate services to aged people, have a lower self-image, and see older people as dependent, vulnerable, and more in need of preferential treatment and protection by society when compared with other groups in society (Bergman, 1977).

Involvement and roles in the local and national arena are changing for the elderly. The founding generation of society—old settlers now 65 and over—is recognized for its historical role and contribution, but leadership is passing to younger hands, painfully and at an accelerating pace. This process is particularly interesting in the cohesive small communities of the collective rural settlements (kibbutzim) where generational proximity makes confrontation more acute. In Parliament, the rest of the governement, the bureaucracy, the political parties, and economic institutions, among others, the replacement process is progressing at a quicker pace, though the elderly presence is still felt. In the traditional Arab sector, the emancipation of the younger generation from the political, economic, and social gerontocracy is even more pronounced. Many of the imported elderly of non-European origin have found their previous status of power center, parent, authority, and patriarch completely upset. In a restatement of Burgess's "roleless role," one could speak here of the "beheaded heads of families" in a society that is remote from their way of life and therefore can offer no meaningful roles of involvement on the macrolevel of social activity.

PROBLEMS OF THE AGED AND SOLUTIONS SOUGHT

Immigration also causes a sharp dividing line between the two major aggregates of aging in areas of income, health, housing, institutional care, leisure, and service-providing activities.

Income

The aged in Israel, an economically vulnerable group, form one of the three major poor groups in society. A considerable incidence of poverty and economic dependence on income maintenance programs is characteristic, with all the ensuing consequences for health, perception, service utilization, and social involvement by the elderly. Contributory occupational pensions and social security (national insurance old-age allowances) are the two fundamental components of maintenance for the aged. The majority of the aged are not eligible for occupational pensions and have not accumulated sufficient years of pension rights (because of their high age on arrival and their short period of employment). They are therefore in poor economic circumstances; for many social security is the only or major source of income.

Excluding occupational pensions, the income (earnings, interest, dividends, and rent) of an older person (in 1971) did not exceed 15 percent of the average earnings of a prime age employee. The incidence of poverty is the highest for the aged who live alone, most of them women. About one-third of the cases handled by local welfare offices are over 65 years of age. Western aged have higher incomes than Oriental aged; men are better off than women; and old settlers are better off than newcomers. Only 25 to 30 percent of the aged are believed to enjoy a comfortable economic situation.

The level of income is related to education, length of stay in the country, degree of physical mobility, and the type of household. Inability to manage economically was found to be one of the major reasons for seeking institutional placements. On the other hand, some surveys show that improved financial conditions were a factor (29 percent) in the decision for self-discharge from old-age homes and return to community living (Bergman, 1973).

Three out of four aged receive old-age insurance pensions (statutory and nonstatutory). Close to half of them also receive noncontributory supplementary benefits (social betterment allowances), which are given only to those for whom the national insurance pension constitutes the only or the major source of income. The pension rate for single aged is defined as 16 percent of the average wage for a single person and 24 percent for a couple. The minimum income guarantee (the national insurance pension plus the supplementary benefit) is defined as 25 percent of the average wage for a single person and 37.5 percent for a couple. Linkage to average wage in an economy of rising inflation provides a partial protection against loss of purchasing power. However, it will take a long time before more aged will achieve a firmer basis of income consisting of the occupational and national insurance statutory old-age pension. The rate of increase of these recipients is slow. If it continues at its present rate of 1 percent increase yearly, only in the next generation will half of all social security beneficiaries have accumulated the right to receive their occupational pensions.

Some surveys indicate that 55 percent of the aged have an income level comparable to the lowest decile in the income distribution for the general population, and 80 percent have an income level comparable to the three lowest deciles. The latest changes in the minimum income level have brought it up to the poverty level (in 1969 it was only 80 percent of the poverty level), a condition that will eliminate the remaining traces of groups of older people with incomes below the poverty line (Shamai and Rotter, 1975). Under consideration by the administration and Parliament is a draft for a statutory nation comprehensive pension program, which will offset the deficiencies of present programs and ensure a further improvement in the economic situation of the retirees.

Housing

In a country of immigration, housing is of unusual importance. Ownership of housing is valued and encouraged, and the percentage of house owners among the aged is higher among old settlers than among newcomers. Because housing is primarily a problem of allocation by authorities, the choice of housing by older people is extremely limited unless they are financially independent. Often nonvoluntary separation or distance from other members of the family results from housing allocation practice. In larger cities there are pockets of poor housing in older neighborhoods where the aged continue to live; often they are the last ones to leave. Some neighborhoods in the inner city show high concentrations of aged—up to 20 to 25 percent—most of them old settlers. These areas are characterized by deteriorating safety and social withdrawl.

The overwhelming majority of all aged live in separate households. Many of those who share households live in crowded conditions. Close to 89 percent of those 65 and over live in households of one to two persons compared to 53 percent in the age group 55–64 and to 36 percent in the general population. In comparison with the 89 percent of Jewish aged, only 64 percent of elderly non-Jews in Israel live in one- or two-person households.

In shared households, the ability of ambulation of the aged to walk is of utmost importance to mutual relationships, family climate, and probability of continued presence of the aged in the family. Over half of the aged live in the community in regular housing. Voluntary relocation is rare at high age except for reasons of health or crisis. The proportions of aged living in shared households are highest among the widowed (some 40 percent), females (about 25 percent), and aged Orientals (about 20 percent). Of those who share households, many would prefer to live separately if they could afford it. The preference for independent living should have serious bearing on policy and future planning of housing for the elderly (Weil et al., 1970).

Problems arise in regard to the aged unmarried immigrant for whom no housing is readily available close to large cities. Temporary congregate arrangements are provided, but this practice causes hardship and absorption difficulties. No specially planned housing for aged in sufficient variety and number is available to absorb those in need of a protective environment, and no statutory provisions have been formulated to ensure sufficient housing for the aged within the extensive programs of public housing.

Institutional Care

Only about 4 to 5 percent of the aged live in institutional settings of various types and sponsorships (for example, well aged, infirm, and nursing wards). Preference for institutional living is rather low, and admission policies favor illness and mobility limitations as primary criteria for admission. Two decades ago, ambulatory aged (well aged) constituted close to 85 percent of the residents of institutions. Today only 30 to 40 percent of the beds are occupied by them, the rest serving frail ambulatory and nursing-care elderly. The average age of the residents is high: those aged 80 and over constitute close to half of the aged institutional population, whereas they are only 12 percent of the total aged population in the country.

Nine out of ten residents are widowed, divorced, or were never married. Those of European origin are overrepresented, and those of Oriental origin are underrepresented, though their share in institutional placement is constantly on the increase (Doron, 1976).

Opinions are divided as to the real demand for institutional placement. Surveys of the aged in communities indicate low preference. Demand as registered by institutions may have its sources in pressure by families, by care givers in the professional community, or by a formal registration of the older person, many of whom never really intend to enter and never do.

Considerable modernization and professionalization of institutional care have taken place. New models are being tested (such as trilevel homes, regional care centers, and old-age homes as centers of gerontological services in the community). There is a growing awareness of the need to do away with the dichotomy of institutional versus noninstitutional services and to replace it by the concept of a broad continuum of community-based services aimed at providing the services needed by an individual at any level of functional capacity with a flexible movement from type to type of service in either direction (from more to less protective services and vice versa). This philosophy would result in greater individualization of service and selectivity of admissions to various kinds of services based on careful professional assessments of health, social conditions, and functional capacity of the older person (Eshel, 1974).

Health

Surveys of national or local samples show that the overwhelming majority of the aged are ambulant (85 percent); some 13 percent are homebound, and 2 percent are bedridden. The latter two categories are strongly correlated with age, economic status, education, and ethnic origin (European and Asian-African). To what extent being bedridden is culture bound should be investigated because nonmobility seems to have some cultural sanction in old age in some groups.

Positive self-evaluation of health is not very high, even among the ambulatory aged. We do not have sufficient data on the possible effect of migration, past experiences (such as war and concentration camps), or cultural factors on the self-evaluation of health. Studies show that the younger aged, males, the working, and those with better education, of European origin, and of long residence in Israel have a more positive health image of themselves than others do of themselves. Women rate themselves lower than men, and non-Europeans see themselves as less independent in many of the functions of daily living and environmental mastery (Bergman and Bar Zuri, 1977; Weil et al., 1970).

Those 65 and over account for 17 percent of all hospitalizations (about twice the percentage in the general population). Their hospital stay is double the average duration. The order of magnitude of groups of pathology (rates per

100,000 population in each age group) is ischemic heart disease (14 percent), malignant neoplasm (10 percent), cerebrovascular disease (6 percent), infectious and parasitic diseases (3 percent), pneumonia (2 percent), and external causes (6 percent). The order of causes of death (on a one in a hundred thousand cases rate) is ischemic heart disease, 220; malignancies, 139; and cerebrovascular diseases, 104.

Utilization of medical services varies with education, sex, degree of ambulation, length of residence, and ethnic background. The percentage of aged interested in separate health services for the elderly (such as special clinics) is about 30 percent of those 60 and over (Bergman, 1977). Hospitalization of the aged for assessment and treatment is not always easy. Discharge is often premature in relation to the possibility of ensuring continuation of care and provision of environmental adjustment in the community.

Long-term treatment, convalescence, and rehabilitation facilities are not yet sufficient. Home care and day hospital care are showing some increase. Regional health offices and their nursing services are becoming more involved in chronic care and rehabilitation of the elderly. Conversion of maternal health clinics into family care centers should benefit the elderly. The family continues to be the almost exclusive provider of personal care in times of crisis (up to 95 percent), and provision of incentives for supportive care should be a major health policy improvement. Supportive services (such as meals on wheels, housekeeping, and luncheon clubs) are developing at an accelerated pace, primarily under local authority auspices.

Health education and preventive measures lag behind curative facilities. Psychogeriatric problems in an immigrant society are numerous, and facilities for care are not catching up with demands, either on an ambulatory or an institutional basis. In addition, the availability of services does not ensure their full utilization by the aged. Aggressive outreach and health education programs, where practical, enhance effective service utilization.

Practically all aged (some 94 percent) have health service coverage for ambulatory and hospital care through voluntary, local authority, or Ministry of Health sponsorship. A bill to provide health services insurance is under consideration by Parliament to provide almost full coverage of all health services, including chronic hospitalization. In general, considerable improvement in curative and in public health measures has taken place. However, insufficient attention has been paid to preventive measures in regard to preretirement groups in the country.

Leisure

Patterns of living and leisure are an important aspect of the aged. The Oriental aged are family oriented. Despite changes, they find most of their outlets in that framework. Synagogues, informal gathering places, formal clubs for older people, and similar groups are also serving a useful role.

Western aged are peer and community oriented. Their involvement in extra-familial activities is more intensive, though limited. Despite their preference for separate living arrangements, they maintain a web of interfamily contacts. Social contacts of the elderly are enabled by networks of clubs (serving 7 to 10 percent of the aged population), neighborhood organizations, political groups, self-organizations, and religious activities, among others. Leisure education is limited; leisure is not yet sufficiently sanctioned as a legitimate life-style in old age. There is considerable preference for integrated all-ages leisure services, especially among the European aged.

Voluntary agencies, local authorities, government services, trade unions, immigrant associations, adult education groups, and self-help groups of elderly are increasingly involved in creating more opportunities for recreational, cultural, and communal activities by and for the elderly. Preretirement preparation is gaining popularity as a possible additional avenue for providing meaningful associations, roles, and reengagement opportunities.

Service-providing Agencies

Three major institutions are involved in the provision of programs to meet the needs of the elderly: government (national, and local), trade unions, and voluntary organizations.

A number of ministries (Labor and Welfare, Health, and National Insurance Institute) are directly responsible for some of the most important programs, either directly administered or supported and implemented through local authorities. Through its Services to Aged Department, the Ministry of Labor and Welfare provides planning, assistance in organization, and financing of services to the elderly, such as admission to institutional care, clubs, day centers, meals on wheels, and housekeeping. These are implemented by the local authorities responsible under the law for the establishment and provision of welfare services to the population. The Labor and Welfare Ministry is also responsible for the implementation of the provisions of the law of supervision of institutions (1965) through establishment of standards and supervision of operation of the various facilities.

The Ministry of Health is responsible, through its Department of Aging, Chronic Diseases and Rehabilitation for provision of institutional placement of nursing cases and nursing care to the chronic ill and aged at home and in family health care centers. The Ministry of Labor and Welfare is involved in operating a special agency for employment of the elderly and support for retraining the elderly. Government labor exchanges register aged job seekers and assist them in job placement, but few aged actually seek this service or are effectively helped by it. The National Insurance Institute is the major income maintenance agency.

Other ministries are not yet sufficiently involved in or aware of the need of activities in this area. There is no central coordinating, planning, or directing unit in government bureaucracy in charge of activities for the aged although recommendations in this direction have repeatedly been made. A recently established national authority on retirement and pensioners has not yet been legislated by Parliament and has so far concentrated primarily on practical activities connected with preretirement preparation.

The government is also partner with a voluntary relief agency, the National Association for the Planning and Development of Services for the Aged in Israel (Eshel, 1974) engaged in developing new models of regional homes for aged, service delivery systems to the aged in communities, and manpower development in servicing older people.

The Trade Unions Federation of Israel (Histadrut) is an important factor in indirect and direct services to the aged. Its sick fund is the major health agency in the country. Seven principal pension funds belong to the Histadrut; so do old-age homes and congregate housing facilities, as well as a network of clubs for aged members of the trade unions.

Voluntary agencies with a variety of sponsorships (national, local, and immigrants' associations, for example) have been actively involved in setting up institutions and clubs for their aged members and developing sundry services over the years. Mutual help groups of aged have also begun to be active in the field.

There is no overall coordinating agency, although a number of attempts have been made to set up such a structure. The Israel Gerontological Society, at various points, has served as the meeting ground, and its Committee for Professional Services has made many valuable contributions to patterns of coordination between agencies and organizations.

LEGISLATION ON AGING

There is no special or specific legislation on the aged. However, a number of laws have a special bearing on the overall welfare of the aged: the law of National Insurance for old-age pensions; the Licensing and Supervision Law of Institutions, which regulates the level of institutional care; the Law of Employment, which prohibits employment discrimination because of age; the Law of Alimonies, which provides for filial responsibility; the Inheritance Law; the Law of Protection of the Dependent; the Tenant Protection Law; and others.

TEACHING

The growing concern with problems of aging and the constant development of services have brought about demands for a professionalization of care of older people through manpower development and training. The Gerontological Society has played a prominent pioneering role in this field. Seminars, courses, institutes, and study conferences have paved the way. Assistance and guidance have been extended to professional groups and schools to develop curricula and syllabi for various professions.

Aging, theory, research, and practice are taught at several universities. Numerous extension courses in aging are provided in community colleges, professional organizations, kibbutzim, and large service organizations.

A number of teaching aids have been developed and published by the Gerontological Society (the quarterly *Gerontologia* and the two-volume *Aging in Israel*, with annotated bibliographies) and by the Tel Aviv University *(Case Book on Aging, Community Work with Aged*, and an annotated bibliography, *Social Work with Older People*). Over 2,500 articles and research reports by Israeli researchers and writers have been published in the last twenty years in Hebrew and in foreign-language journals abroad.

RESEARCH

Background

Although the special character of the country and of the problems of older people in Israel have almost from the beginning aroused the professional interest of researchers from Israel and other countries, systematic and well-founded research in gerontology has been relatively slow in coming. The explosion of aging as an urgent social problem demanded immediate symptomatic care before etiology, prevention, and other aspects of the problem could be tackled. Practice preceded theory, experimentation came before empirical evidence, and use of imported models and knowledge was dominant before local efforts began to draw from and analyze the enormous wealth of cultural, social, and health knowledge that the immigrants brought with them.

Historically there are three periods in the research development in gerontology in Israel, each roughly covering a decade. In the first period (1949–1958), primary attention was given to production of statistical data by the Central Bureau of Statistics, General Federation of Labor, Jewish Agency (on immigration, absorption, and settlement), Malben-JDC (absorption and rehabilitation of the elderly, handicapped, and chronic ill), Kupat Holim (hospitalization and utilization of health services), and various organizations of immigrants. These constituted the major resource for reports, reviews, and analysis of problems and services to the elderly.

There was also a growing awareness of the need to formulate research questions and delineate explanation areas. A few descriptive studies analyzed institutional aged populations, reviewed problems of chronic diseases, or surveyed activities of agencies serving the elderly. However, the real development of gerontological research in that period was hampered by a number of factors: the urgency to concentrate on practical issues, lack of funds, research preference for other areas, and scarcity of researchers interested and/or trained in gerontology.

In the second period (1958–1969), two major research areas began to emerge: the special characteristics of the Israeli society and what might be called the issues in regional pathology and morbidity patterns in culturally heterogeneous groups of immigrants and old settlers. The establishment of the National Institute of Insurance and the introduction of the old-age pensions (1957) opened up new areas of exploration about the aged. At this time also Israel became involved in cross-national studies that produced the first major profile of its aged population (Weil et al., 1970), and the first major contribution to international gerontological exploration of aging in a planned society. During that period the first studies of the biology of aging were undertaken (aging of red blood cells), and the results were published by Danon et al.

The third period (1970 to the present) is characterized by high research awareness, sensitivity, interest, and activity in all four major areas of gerontological research: biology, medicine, social-behavioral sciences, and applied social research in welfare and care of the elderly. Research seems to go in two principal directions: areas and subjects specifically related to Israel (social and medical) and areas of universal and/or cross-national interest. This development is reflected in the growing number of publications by Israeli researchers at home and in foreign periodicals; the holding of research symposia by the Gerontological Society and various academic bodies; the establishment of prizes for young researchers; and the increasing number of graduates—such as biologists, psychologists, nurses, and social workers—who select aging as the topic of their research. The establishment of the Brookdale Institute of Gerontology in 1974 was an important contribution to the promotion of research in aging in Israel (over thirty discussion papers published by the institute are valuable additions to the growing research literature in this country). The extensive bibliography *Aging in Israel* (Bergman, 1967, 1976) and especially the excellent *Guide to Israeli Research in Social Gerontology* (Kretzmer, 1976) provide guidance for those interested in a closer exploration of the subject by areas of topics and chronology of development. A similar guide to biological and medical-clinical research is in preparation.

Major Research Areas

Biology

A major area in which pioneering research work was done in the early 1960s was that of biophysical aspects of red blood cell aging. From 1961 through 1963, Danon studied and described changes in the structure of the membrane of old versus young cells (in human cells) and the reduction of negative charges on membranes of old erythrocytes. He also explored how the macrophage distinguishes between the young and old cells in order to eliminate the old cell. In recent research the macrophage in the old animal has been studied from the point of view of the cell in charge of removing old cells as deteriorated self-cells and from other deteriorated self-cells (such as those that become malignant). Another aspect now under study is that of the substance produced by the macrophage and which promotes proliferation of fibroblasts, formulation of collagen, and more rapid wound healing.

D. Gershon, using nematodes as a model, studied structural or enzymatic alterations as possibly responsible for functional deterioration leading to death. Studies showed possibility of extending the life span of nematodes by protecting them at certain stages of their life against the oxydative denaturation.

The aging of bacterial cultures was studied by Sempolinski. Structural alterations of membranes of mice plasma and, more recently, changes in membranes of fibroblasts aging in vitro have been researched by Rasin at Hebrew University.

Cellular aspects of decline in the immune capacity of the aging animal are another area of exploration. Globerson found that old animals have potentially active cells in the immune system. Their potential is not fully expressed, though experiments show that it can be improved. Gershon found no decline of capacity in cell division in old animals after specific stimulation. There is a decline in the general immune direction and in the number of cells that react. However, cells that react do so normally. Trinin at Weitzmann Institute has studied the decline of the thymus and the THF (timing, humoral factor). Recent studies proved that spleen cells of old animals react to the THF by improving the cellular immune capacity. Yagil, also at Weitzmann Institute, researched the induction of enzyme activity in aging animals and the role played by errors in the protein-synthesis mechanisms in aging animals.

A growing number of experienced and younger scientists at the Weitzmann Institute at Rehovot, at the Technion in Haifa, at the Hebrew University in Jerusalem, at the Bar Ilan University in Ramat Gan, at the University of Tel Aviv, and at other centers of high learning show great interest in research in the biology of aging. The biological research section of the Gerontological Society has also shown increased activity. At the 1976 Conference on Aging, some twenty research papers were presented in three sessions in the biology of aging: cellular models in aging research, deficiencies in the immune system, and deficiencies in the subcellular level in aging cells. A national symposium on teaching aging in biology was held in 1978 under the auspices of the Gerontological Society and various university institutions.*

Clinical Medicine and Public Health

Israel's ethnically heterogeneous population and the observed differences in patterns of morbidity and health behavior between the two major constituent groups have influenced the major direction of the clinical gerontological research of the first and particularly second decade of gerontological exploration in Israel.

*The author appreciates the assistance of Prof. D. Danon in the preparation of this section.

Atherosclerosis was extensively studied, with a special accent on nutritional aspects as a contributing factor to the disease. Comparative studies were conducted on the sectors of the Jewish population of the country—the old settlers and the Yemenite immigrants (1940–1950). The major assumption was that the differences in life-style, environmental factors, and dietary regimes accounted for the lower level of cholesterol and for the lower incidence of arteriosclerosis found among recent Yemenite immigrants. Studies conducted on Yemenites after a prolonged stay in Israel showed a narrowing of the differences between the two groups, probably as a result of changes in the dietary patterns of the Yemenites: a case of dietary acculturation. Comparative studies were also conducted on various ethnic groups in the country, including bedouins, on various aspects of diabetes. Strokes were researched from the clinical, psychological, social, and rehabilitational aspects (Adler, 1969; Geltner, 1972).

Cardiovascular diseases received considerable attention on intergroup differences in Israel and on cross-national level. Librach compared the prevalence of ischemic heart diseases among elderly Yemenites and Europeans in an institutional setting. Kallner and Groen studied differences in coronary and cerebral atherosclerosis among Western and Eastern immigrants in Israel, as well as mortality patterns from coronary heart diseases among Eastern immigrants. Brunner and his associates studied the physical fitness of trained elderly and the physiologic and anthropometric parameters related to coronary risk factors in Yemenite Jews who had lived different lengths of time in Israel. He also conducted an epidemiological study in kibbutzim on physical activity and the incidence of myocardial infarction, angina pectoris, and death due to ischemic heart disease in Israelis of European and Yemenite origin.

Librach and associates conducted a number of studies on myocardial infarction—immediate and long-term prognosis, initial manifestations, and assessment of incidence and risk factors—among diverse groups of the institutionalized aged.

A longitudinal study was conducted on cardiovascular diseases and hypertension among ten thousand civil servants in Israel (Medalie, Neufeld, Kahn, et al. 1968, 1973, 1975). Antonovsky studied the social and cultural factors in coronary heart disease, an aspect of the Israel-American sibling study.

War and holocaust experiences in Europe, upsetting effects of relocation, difficulties in adjustment to new environments and norms, and the disengaging effect of the Israeli social structure, among others, were areas of considerable interest to Israeli researchers. Innovative elements of functional diagnosis in mental disorders among the aged were introduced in treatment (Tramer, 1961; Pliskin, 1958; Margulec, 1960, 1962); suicides among the aged of various cultural backgrounds were analyzed (Gampel, Shichor, Bergman); and deviant behavior and criminality were researched for their association with immigration (Bergman and Amir, 1973, 1975).

Pioneering research was developed in gerodontics. Langer and associates (1961) studied factors influencing satisfaction with complete dentures in geriatric patients, diverse cultural reactions to dental rehabilitation among the aged from different cultural backgrounds, tooth survival in multicultural groups, and physiologic and psychologic considerations in oral rehabilitation.

In the area of public health, a number of important studies have been conducted. Kaufman (1974) studied nutritional aspects in institutional settings. Gugenheim and associates examined food consumption and nutritional patterns of the aged living on public assistance; they found no malnutrition. Accidents among the aged in old-age homes (Margulec, 1970), utilization of health services by residents of institutions (Librach, 1965) and those living in the community (Weil, 1970; Cohen, 1976; Bergman, 1977), extent of disability in Jewish and Arab rural areas (Margulec, 1976), and the prevalence and causes of blindness among the aged (Abramson, 1971) are some topics examined by researchers in the last decade. However, a number of important aspects of health needs and patterns of health behavior in urban and rural areas are yet to be studied.*

Social, Behavioral, and Applied Research

Old age in Jewish thought, culture, and lore had not frequently been the topic of research. Over a half-century ago E. Simon (1924) contrasted the Jewish concept of reverence for old age and its spiritual value with the Hellenistic veneration of youth and physical beauty. Recently M. Kurtz (1977) studied the meaning of the concept of the aged person as reflected in scriptures and in commentaries of the eleventh and twelfth centuries and identified interpretations of old age as a phase in life with a number of subdivisions highly reminiscent of the recent concepts by Neugarten on young-aged and old-aged persons.

Demography and Immigration

Musham (1965, 1966, 1975), Schmelz (1971), and others have dealt with various trends and aspects of the demographic structure of Israel, such as dynamics of aging, differential mortality, and modes of longevity. Antonovsky (1967) and Cohen (1971) analyzed social class, life expectancy, and overall mortality, as well as selected causes of death, in different immigrant groups. Harpaz (1975) analyzed demographic changes in the aged population of a big city. Berman (1974), Atar (1970), and others described rural populations of Israel, including collective settlements in which the rate of aging progresses rather rapidly.

Although immigration is the crucial issue in Israel, not many researchers have centered on the aged immigrant. Shuval and associates (1975) studied the

*The author wishes to acknowledge the assistance of Prof. I Margulec in the preparation of this section.

adjustment of immigrants from the Soviet Union and found that some areas, such as identification with host country, are positively related with age. Technicek (1976) studied the absorption problems of older immigrants (from Eastern Europe as compared with those from the West); and Antonovsky (1970) studied the factors in the adjustment of American immigrants to Israeli society (up to the age of 65). The differences in attitudes to welfare services, self-image, and preferences for separate services between aged new immigrants and old settlers were identified by Bergman and Bar-Zur (1977). Lack of sufficient knowledge and orientation of elderly immigrants in regard to services especially created for them were shown to result in their inability to utilize them fully or surmount the bureaucratic difficulties they face (Eran, 1975).

The living conditions, family relationships, patterns of work, retirement, and leisure of the elderly were studied primarily in urban settings on national and local samples. The study by Weil, Nathan, and Avner (1970) was rightly termed "the broadest sociological profile to date on the elderly" in Israel; it provided the first reliable data and portrait of elderly Israelis in urban areas in which over 90 percent of all Jewish aged reside. A number of local surveys, including a full survey of an agricultural area, were highly useful for the identification of needs and for planning community and service interventions. Patterns of leisure among the elderly have been the subject of several studies (Katz, 1975; Harpaz, 1974; Weil, 1977; Lowenstein, 1977), two of which (Bergman, 1965; Appel, 1977) centered on clubs for older people.

Work and Retirement

Considerable attention has been devoted in the past few years to problems of work and the emerging issues of retirement and the need to prepare for it. The centrality of work in the life of adult males was studied by Manheim (1972, 1976) who concluded that "in no occupational category was the oldest age group found to be less work centered than any other age group." The same problem was studied by Levitan (1976) in regard to elderly workers in the communal settlements. A group of researchers at the Brookdale Institute are involved in studies on various aspects of occupational and industrial mobility. Retirement attitudes and patterns have been given growing attention. During the last decade, since the first study on the topic was published (Jacobson, 1967–1968), a number of researchers have devoted their attention to the problem: Manheim, Kraemer, Bronfield and Honig, Peri, Bergman-Bar Zuri, Levitan, Atar (kibbutzim), Nir-el (executives), Eran, and Gutman. The propensity to retire, planning for postretirement roles, readiness to use preretirement counseling, and inclination to return to work are some of the major problems explored along the analyses of the differences among various groups of subjects (white and blue collar, new immigrants and old settlers, European and non-European, male and female, level of education, and so forth.

The economics of aging has also been receiving considerable attention. Researchers at Brookdale Institute and at the National Insurance Institute have analyzed the problems of income maintenance, protection of pensions against inflation, the role of savings and wealth in determining economic status over the life cycle, and similar areas.

In the area of psychological research, less has been attempted. As in other countries, the years betwen 40 and 60 have not been given sufficient research in human development. The major works in this area are those of Shanan (1968, 1972, 1974, 1975), which center on the concept of active coping as meaningful for the understanding of the interaction of culture, personality, and the process of disengagement. Data were gathered on samples of those between 40 and 60 and analyzed in terms of possible relationships between structure and function in the process of growing old. Stress is laid upon the possible importance of information on aging in the middle years for the shaping of retirement and placement policy, as well as the potential mental hygiene value of such information for parent and adult education. A number of younger researchers have investigated age and sex differences in the perception of the life cycle from maturity to old age, factors explanatory to differences in intelligence between adult women and men, and time perception in aging.

Attitudes to aging in Israel are a new research area. Bergman has studied attitudes of political parties to problems of the elderly (1966) and attitudes of nurses to working with older people in clinical settings (1970, 1974). More studies in this area are now being completed.

The dramatic rise in the number of elderly as a result of immigration and of aging among the old-settler population has brought about a rapid increase in the number, types, and scope of services. This process raises a number of basic questions not yet fully examined in applied gerontological research here: integrated versus separate services (S. Pelz, 1976; Bergman-Bar-Zuri, 1977), institutional versus noninstitutional (Weil, 1973, 1975; Bergman, 1973; Silberstein, 1970; N. Baruch, 1976), the knowledge of and ability and readiness to utilize services (Eran, 1975; Markus, 1976), centralized versus decentralized ranges of planning, and typology of sponsorship and preparation of manpower for professionalization of care and services. Some of these questions await research investment in the near future.

CONCLUSIONS

There are three major trends in the gerontological development in Israel: the rapid—imposed and natural—aging of the population; the increased awareness among the population, planners, and decision makers of the importance of the problem and therefore a greater readiness to allocate more public and non-government resources for services to the aged; and a growing involvement of academics in the field of aging through practice, teaching, and research.

While aged population forecasts until the end of the century have been worked out, their translation into long-term planning in terms of priorities in allocation of resources, location of services, types of services to be created, and manpower needed is not developed extensively. There is growing need for greater investment in analysis and evaluation of services and activities already in operation, better data on the aged population of today and of the aging group, and of greater involvement of scientists and researchers in exploring the etiology of some of the phenomena in aging in Israel to contribute to greater welfare and better social policy for the elderly.

SOURCES OF GERONTOLOGICAL INFORMATION

- The Israel Gerontological Society (1956), P.O.B. 11243 Tel Aviv. Publishes a quarterly information bulletin, *Yedi'on*, and *Gerontologia*, an interdisciplinary quarterly (four issues in Hebrew, one issue annually in English).
- Brookdale Institute of Gerontology and Adult Human Development, P.O. Box 13087, Givas Ram, Jerusalem, founded by the American Joint Distribution Committee. Publishes a series of discussion papers on diverse gerontological topics based on research planned, conducted, or completed by the institute research staff. Papers are published in English and/or Hebrew.
- Association for the Planning and Development of Services for the Aged in Israel, 10 Shlom Zion Hamalka, Jerusalem, Israel. Publishes annual reports on its activities (in English and Hebrew).
- University courses or concentration areas in aging are available at School of Social Work, University of Tel Aviv, Tel Aviv; School of Social Work, University of Haifa, Haifa; Department of Nursing, School of Continuing Medical Education, University of Tel Aviv; Sackler School of Medicine, University of Tel Aviv; Department of Psychology, Hebrew University, Jerusalem; Department of Social Medicine, Hadassa Medical School; and Hebrew University, Jerusalem.

For sources of material in the research section of the report and for detailed references on other bibliographical information, the reader is referred to the following bibliographical sources in English:

Bergman, S. *Aged in Israel*, a selected bibliography, Israel Gerontological Society, Tel-Aviv. Vol. 1, 1966, Vol. 2, 1976.

Bergman, S. *Aging in Israel*, Gerontology (Israel), 1975, 4:76-80.

Brookdale Institute of Gerontology. *Publication Abstracts*, Jerusalem, 1978-1979.

Kretzmer, M. Guide to Israeli research in *Social Gerontology*, Brookdale Institute of Gerontology, Jerusalem, 1976. Discussion Paper No. 21-76, p. 62.

REFERENCES

Bar-Yosef, R. 1967. Social absorption of immigrants in Israel. In H. Davis, ed., *Migration, mental health and community services*. Geneva: American Joint Distribution Committee.

Bergman, S. 1969. The rights of the aged. In *Human rights and social welfare*. New York: Columbia University Press.

———. 1973. Facilitating living conditions for aged in the community. *Geriatrics* 1.

———. 1978. Aged in Israel. *Society and Welfare*, Special English Issue. Jerusalem: Ministry of Labor.

Bergman, S., and Amir, 1973. Crime and delinquency among aged in Israel. *Geriatrics* 1.

Bergman, S., and Bar-Zuri, R. 1977. *Attitudes of aged in welfare services*. Tel Aviv: Histadrut Research Department.

Doron, A., 1976. *Community of the aged*. Jerusalem: Ministry of Welfare.

Eisenstadt, S., Bar-Yosef, and Adler, H., eds. 1970. *Integration and development in Israel*. Jerusalem: Israel Universities Press.

Eshel, 1974. *Guidelines for services needed for the aged, 1975–1980*. Jerusalem: Association for Services to Aged in Israel.

Histadrut. 1967. *Retirement age in Israel*. Report of the Committee of Specialists. Tel Aviv: General Federation of Labor.

Jewish Agency. *Activities of the Social Service Department for the years 1974, 1975*.

Kanev, I. 1968. *Social and demographic development and the shape of poverty in Israel*. Tel Aviv: Kupat Holim Research Institute.

Miller, L. 1970. The mental health of immigrants. In A. Yarus, ed. *The child and family in Israel*. New York: Gordon and Breach.

Musham, H. 1975. On dynamics of aging of the population in Israel. *Gerontology* 4:

Rizeq, S. *Aging in Nazareth: Life situation and service needs*. Haifa.

Schmelz, U., ed. 1976. *Statistical abstract of Israel, 1975*. Jerusalem: Central Bureau of Statistics.

Shamai, N., and Rotter, R. 1975. *The economic circumstances of aged in Israel*. Jerusalem: National Institute of Insurance.

Weil, E.; Natan, T.; and Avner, U. 1970. *Investigation of family life, living conditions and needs of the non-institutionalized urban Jewish population aged 65 in Israel*. Jerusalem: Ministry of Welfare.

Weil, H. 1973. *Homes for the aged in Israel, 1971*. Jerusalem: Ministry of Welfare.

The statistical data in this chapter (unless otherwise indicated) were drawn from two major sources:

Statistical Abstracts of Israel, The. 1975, 1978. Jerusalem: Central Bureau of Statistics (published annually).

Schmelz U., ed., 1976. *Society in Israel* (selected statistics). Jerusalem: Central Bureau of Statistics, pp. 172 ff.

ITALY

AURELIA FLOREA

In the last few years, old age in Italy has been recognized as a national social problem. It is being discussed not only at the level of sociological analyses but among the public at large. The difficulties of the third age, the old person as a social problem, the isolation and role of old people—these and similar expressions make their appearance well beyond technical circles and are entering everyday language.

The mass media have played a role in this popularization, even if their approach is guided in general by the need to make news and/or shake public opinion about some aspect of it. Nevertheless the subject needs a deeper discussion and a more thoughtful approach, particularly at the level of training and participation. There may be more interest in the problems of old people today than in the past, but it is still true that the rejection of old age and of old people is one of the contradictions of our society that we all experience. Science and technology enable us to live longer; the last period of life, retirement, can last more than a quarter of a century; but it can be a quarter of a century given to the "useless age" or to the "rejected age," as it is sometimes called.

Adults delude themselves that old age can be put off until an indeterminate moment; and for young people, this moment does not exist at all on their horizon. Old age is considered an event even less probable than death; people declare they will die first or that they would rather die. And in any case, everyone thinks that he is going to cope with this event better than other people, forgetting that old age is not just an individual problem and that the various solutions depend also on the system of the society to which one belongs.

The heroes of society, the young and the strong, are flattered by the manipulation of propaganda to which they are subject in their role as instruments of production and consumption. To be young has become one of the dominant values; it is enough to think of the use made by publicity of the word *young*: a young fashion, a young drink, a young face. Thus while everybody is emotionally certain that old age does not concern them, they are at the same time victims designated for social isolation as soon as the magic moment of exploitation of their energy and their youth is over. Those who survive will inevitably be victims of a negative old age, the result of the cultural-economic conditioning inherent in that society to which they themselves have contributed. The negative content of the condition of old age derives directly from the relationship of individuals and society: the absence of a role, the isolation from significant social life, the marginality in family relationships, and the lack of commitment, partly induced, partly forced on old people. Even the material aspects, such as economic and health needs, are an inevitable consequence of the relationship between individual and society, of mutual distrust and exploitation, once the problem is considered in a global way.

DEMOGRAPHY

The number of Italians 65 and over reached 6,101,820 at the date of the last census in 1971, one million persons more than in the previous census in 1961 (table 26). The percentage of the population 65 and over had reached 11.36 percent in 1971; the percentage of the population between 60 and 65 is only 5.2 percent. The importance of these figures, particularly in their relation to the other age groups, can be assessed from tables 27–29 which show the development of the ratio of old people to the total population from a century ago. In particular, they show the progressive increase during the last century of the older age groups in the total population. The percentage of people older than 60 was almost three times as high in 1971 as it was in 1861 (from 6.4 percent to 16.7 percent), and the same hold true for the age group 65 and over, which has increased from 4.0 percent to 11.3 percent. The highest increase—3 percentage points—is found in the 60–65 group. The successive groups follow in decreasing order: 65–69, +2.3 percent; 70–74, +2.1 percent; 75–79, +1.5 percent; 80–84, +1 percent; 85–90, +0.3 percent.

Table 26: POPULATION BY AGE GROUP

Age Group	1961	1971
15 and under	12,404,900	13,227,663
15–59	31,169,816	31,983,496
60–65	2,227,437	2,823,468
65 and over	4,827,416	6,101,820
Total	50,623,569	54,136,447

Source: "Sommario di Statistche storiche d'Italia 1861-1975." Rome: Instituto Centrale di Statistica, 1976.

Other phenomena have contributed to the progressive aging of the Italian population. There is a progressive decrease in the percentage of the 0–15 group in respect to the total population. This percentage dropped from 34.2 percent in 1961 to 24.4 percent in 1971 (table 26). This decrease appears also, though in lesser degree, in the age group 15–35, which was 33.0 percent in 1861 and is now 28.3 percent. The aging of the population appears quite clearly also from the direct relation between the older and younger groups in the population. In

Table 27: POPULATION PERCENTAGES BY AGE GROUP

Age groups	1861	1871	1881	1891	1901	1911	1921	1931	1941	1951	1961	1971
0–14	34.2	32.4	32.2	34.0	34.4	34.0	31.3	30.0	28.6	26.2	24.7	24.4
15–35	33.0	33.7	32.6	31.9	30.5	31.1	32.8	33.6	33.1	31.4	30.7	28.3
36–59	26.4	26.2	26.3	25.2	25.5	24.6	25.4	25.6	27.3	30.1	30.7	30.6
60–64	2.4	3.0	3.8	3.5	3.5	3.7	3.7	3.5	3.5	4.0	4.4	5.4
65–69	2.0	2.2	2.1	2.4	2.6	2.8	2.8	3.0	3.0	3.2	3.5	4.3
70–74	1.0	1.3	1.7	1.8	1.8	2.0	2.1	2.2	2.1	2.4	2.8	3.1
75–79	0.7	0.8	0.8	0.7	1.1	1.1	1.2	1.3	1.4	1.6	1.9	2.2
80–84	0.2	0.3	0.4	0.5	0.5	0.5	0.5	0.6	1.0	0.7	0.9	1.2
85–89	0.1	0.1	0.1		0.1	0.2	0.2	0.2		0.3	0.3	0.4
90 and over										0.1	0.1	0.1
Total 60 and over	6.4	7.7	7.2	8.9	9.6	10.3	10.5	10.8	11.0	12.3	13.9	16.7
Total 65 and over	4.0	4.7	5.1	5.4	6.1	6.6	6.8	7.3	7.5	8.3	9.5	11.3

Source: "Sommario di Statistiche storiche d'Italia 1861-1975." Rome: Instituto Centrale di Statistica. 1976.

Table 28: MALE POPULATION PERCENTAGES BY AGE GROUP

Age groups	1861	1871	1881	1891	1901	1911	1921	1931	1941	1951	1961	1971
0–14	34.6	32.7	32.7	34.7	35.1	35.2	32.3	31.1	29.6	27.6	25.8	25.5
15–35	32.2	33.1	32.1	32.1	30.2	30.1	32.1	33.8	33.9	31.8	31.6	29.2
36–59	26.5	26.2	26.3	24.3	25.2	24.5	25.2	24.5	26.1	29.4	30.3	30.6
60–64	2.5	3.1	3.8	3.3	3.5	3.7	3.7	3.4	3.4	3.6	4.1	5.1
65–69	2.0	2.2	2.1	2.4	2.6	2.8	2.8	3.0	2.8	3.0	3.0	3.9
70–74	1.1	1.4	1.7	1.9	1.8	2.0	2.1	2.1	2.0	2.2	2.4	2.7
75–79	0.7	0.8	0.8	0.8	1.1	1.1	1.2	1.3	1.3	1.5	1.6	1.6
80–84	0.3	0.4	0.4	0.5	0.4	0.5	0.5	0.6	0.9	0.7	0.8	0.9
85–89	0.1	0.1	0.1		0.1	0.1	0.1	0.2		0.2	0.3	0.4
90 and over											0.1	0.1
Total 60 and over	6.7	8.0	8.9	8.9	9.5	10.2	10.4	10.6	10.4	11.2	12.3	14.7
Total 65 and over	4.2	4.9	5.1	5.6	6.0	6.5	6.7	7.2	7.0	7.6	6.2	9.6

Source: "Sommario di Statistiche storiche d'Italia 1861-1975." Rome: Instituto Centrale di Statistica, 1976.

Table 29: FEMALE POPULATION PERCENTAGES BY AGE GROUP

Age group	1861	1871	1881	1891	1901	1911	1921	1931	1941	1951	1961	1971
0–14	33.8	32.1	31.6	33.1	33.6	32.8	30.4	28.8	27.6	25.1	23.7	23.3
15–35	33.7	34.3	33.0	31.8	30.9	32.0	33.6	33.4	32.4	31.0	29.8	27.7
36–59	26.1	26.2	26.6	26.2	25.8	25.0	25.5	26.9	28.4	30.8	31.1	31.0
60–64	2.3	2.9	3.9	3.6	3.6	3.7	3.7	3.5	3.7	4.3	4.7	5.5
65–69	2.1	2.1	2.0	2.4	2.6	2.7	2.8	3.0	3.1	3.5	3.9	4.5
70–74	1.0	1.2	1.7	1.8	1.9	2.0	2.1	2.2	2.2	2.5	3.1	3.6
75–79	0.7	0.8	0.7	0.7	1.0	1.1	1.1	1.4	1.5	1.6	2.1	2.4
80–84	0.2	0.3	0.4	0.4	0.5	0.5	0.6	0.6	0.1	0.8	1.1	1.4
85–89	0.1	0.1	0.1		0.1	0.2	0.2	0.2		0.3	0.4	0.5
90–94										0.1	0.1	0.1
95 and over												
Total 60 and over	6.4	7.4	8.8	8.9	9.7	9.2	10.5	10.9	11.6	13.1	15.4	18.0
Total 65 and over	4.1	4.5	4.9	5.3	6.1	6.5	6.8	7.4	7.9	8.8	10.7	12.5

Source: "Sommario di Statistiche storiche d'Italia 1861-1975." Rome: Instituto Centrale di Statistica, 1976.

238

1911 there were 29.1 old men for every 100 boys; in 1971 there were 57.9 (table 30). In the case of women, the figures were 31.7 in 1911 and 78.9 in 1971. The other main collateral phenomena that have accompanied and favored the increasing percentage of the old population in respect to the total population can be seen in table 31, where the data concerning the birthrate and the average life expectancy are presented. The birthrate fell by almost half between 1911 and 1971, and life expectancy grew steadily. In 1911 the average life expectancy for men was 46.6 years and for women 47.3 years; in 1971 the average length had grown respectively to 70 years for men and 75 for women.

Table 30: RATIO BETWEEN THOSE OVER 60 YEARS OF AGE AND THOSE UNDER 15 YEARS (OVER 60 FOR EACH 100 UNDER 15)

Census	Male	Female	Total
1911	29.1	31.1	30.1
1931	34.0	38.3	36.1
1951	40.9	52.3	46.5
1961	48.1	65.9	56.8
1971	57.9	78.9	68.1

Source: Sommario di Statistiche storiche d'Italia 1861-1975." Rome: Instituto Centrale di Statistica, 1976.

Table 31: BIRTHRATE AND AVERAGE LIFE EXPECTANCY AT BIRTH

Year	Birthrate	Average Life	
		Male	*Female*
1911	31.4	46.6	47.3
1931	24.5	53.8	56.0
1951	18.4	63.7	67.4
1961	18.3	67.2	72.7
1971	16.8	70.0	75.0

Source: Sommario di Statistiche storiche d'Italia 1861-1975." Rome: Instituto Centrale di Statistica, 1976.

STATUS AND ROLE OF OLD PEOPLE

Work and Retirement

If it is true that work is the central aspect of the individual's existence insofar as it is the main instrument of self-realization and social participation, as well as the main means of survival, it is easy to understand that its sudden, compulsory, and definitive end, even when it does not cause economic hardship, can constitute the basis of the so-called retirement crisis. The forms this crisis can take, and their intensity, do in fact vary with the type of work. However, it is a general fact that old age begins legally with retirement, and this fact alone, in a society like ours where people are valued in proportion to their productivity, means that one is expelled from the world of the people who are valued. It means being rejected in a private isolation, which does not entail a link with the social world.

In Italy different situations exist as far as retirement age is concerned because of a large number of laws concerning special categories of workers. For some public agencies, retirement is at 60; in other, especially in the civil service, retirement is at 65; while some special groups (university professors and high judges) do not retire until 70. Women are usually retired five years earlier than men, but in some occupations (such as civil service) they retire at the same age as men. In industry, for some years, there has been a tendency to encourage early retirement because of the economic crisis and the restructuring of various industries. In fact, these operations have taken into account only productivity problems; from the point of view of the individual, once he is out of productive life, he is also out of all processes leading to change, out of the bargaining procedures for economic and social success; therefore he is excluded also from the possible benefits that may derive from it.

Often early retirement is caused by ill health, which in turn is a consequence of the environmental factors, the fast pace, and the organization of work previously done. For this reason, the debate in Italy over early retirement or flexible retirement age (earlier than usual, delayed, or keeping full job responsibilities) has focused first on the issue of a different work quality—of work conditions that would be less damaging and more moderately paced. In fact flexible retirement has not been looked at favorably by industrial sociologists or by the trade unions. The latter maintain that old workers need their rest, and that in an economy based on profit, it is not acceptable to create a reserve of labor, probably cheap labor, according to the wishes of the employers. It is true that work today is exhausting because of the environmental conditions and because of its rhythms. The reasonable solutions, therefore, is to change these conditions. More recently, the two positions have appeared to be less sharply contrasted, and at least in theory it is accepted that there could be an occupation policy oriented to the full employment of all people who wish to work with a different distribution of tasks and different work conditions. It seems inevitable in this case to give up the productivity logic, according to which work activity lasts a given time, and to start anew from a conception of work that includes considerations of the goals of the activity itself and the satisfaction of human needs.

Family Relationships

Since the two pillars of organized life are work and family life, once the old person has been excluded from the world of work, there remains only the private space of the family world. But the present organization of family life, itself conditioned by the rhythms and models imposed by the capitalistic organization of society, is such that the relationships of the old person with the family are unequal; the old person is necessarily the loser. This problem certainly concerns our country, particularly in the more industrialized centers and in large towns. The average adult, torn by a series of roles, jobs, and tasks in an intensive and neurotic rhythm, may find himself faced by an old person whose life horizon is limited to the family ghetto and demands affection and communication from him. Inevitably the younger adult is incapable of satisfying the demands except partially and with little attention. This unequal relationship is a source of frustration and tension on both sides. To this we must add the practical difficulties—sometimes the impossibility—of giving the needed care when the old person is ill or not self-sufficient.

The isolation of old people within their family sometimes constitutes a source of frustration even greater than if the old person lived alone. The situation of old women is even worse unless they can contribute to family life with their help in the home. They are even less admitted to participation in the life and interests of their children and relations. They are considered even more estranged and on the margin of the society.

The problems of all old people cannot necessarily be linked to their family situation. Many have no family or children. The ratio between the increase in life expectancy and the decrease in the birthrate shows that the group of old people living alone is bound to increase. Many old people live with their spouse alone; many others are widowed or were never married. According to ISTAT data, 40 percent of old people live alone or with their spouse only. Of these 55 percent are unmarried or widowed. The squalor and grimness of the life of the old people living alone in a large town is appalling. Research by the St. Vincent of Paul Association of Turin showed that half of the old people studied lived throughout the year in complete solitude, with no opportunity of human relationshps. Their loneliness and isolation derives also from the fear of anonymous violence in the town. At the stage of community study, it was discovered that old people, and in particular old women in a working-class area of Rome, never went out in the evening nor received visitors. In fact, they would not even open the door to the social worker, whose voice they knew.

The situation is better in rural areas where the old people still have a different sort of relationship with their families and are better adjusted to the community. Even in these areas, however, there is a crisis of the traditional role, linked to the disappearance and the transformation of the old-style patriarchal family. Even in Italy there is a widespread conviction that the solution to the problem of old people's family relationships cannot be found within the family; it can be only the result of a deep transformation of society as a whole.

Social Relationships

In Italy, as much as in other countries, old age is characterized by an objective condition of social, economic, and family marginality, by a role crisis, and by an identity crisis. Once they are outside the productive process, old people feel—at least in the present generation—that their horizon has become very limited. In particular they lack the social recognition that was an important part of the satisfaction connected closely with the role of a productive person.

Several studies have shown that as a result of this state of affairs, old people in Italy suffer from anomie reactions, expressed in particular by renunciation. Renunciation becomes a form of adaptation, which consists of practically abandoning both the cultural goals and the institutionalized means to reach them. These resigned old people, according to these studies, are apathetic as far as the present is concerned; they are nostalgic for the past and tend to avoid entering into social relationships with other people. Because of the loss of their main role, they also experience a sense of isolation. Renunciation is the answer to a situation of acute anomie, following a breakdown of the normative system, of the family system, and of the system of social relationships already established. This condition is particularly serious because, to the individuals concerned, it appears that it must continue indefinitely.

Social organization makes it difficult for old people to find their place again in the community and minimizes their opportunities of relationships with others. If social relationships are closely linked to the roles individuals have, once the roles are lost, the loss of social relationships follows closely. In Italy, very little has been done so far to face and solve this problem. It is only recently, since social services have been conceived as instruments of socialization, that some new hypotheses are beginning to emerge, as well as the possibility of exploring other solutions, which may avoid the paternalistic (or oppressive) character of past experiences (such as residential homes for old people).

PROBLEMS

The needs of the elderly in Italy are many and complex. They range from problems of a practical and financial nature, to problems of housing, health, isolation and loneliness, and lack of services.

Economic Problems

The first aspect of this serious problem for old people is the income level. The existing data are incomplete, but they illustrate part of the problem. There is a progressive decrease of the average individual income beginning from age 50. At age 65 and over, the income level is less than half the average individual income for the age group 31–40. There are close links between income, educational attainment, area of residence, and size of the town of residence. In the northern and central regions, incomes are higher at every age level, though the differences become smallest in the older age groups and in correspondence with the lower levels of education. This one difficulty indicates how general the needs of old people can be; they are made more serious by an extremely complicated and inadequate system of pensions. In fact, retirement coincides with a definite lowering of the standard of life.

According to the Italian pension system, there are different types of pension—old age, disablement, survivors, cumulative pensions—to which one can be entitled at different ages. Law 153 (1969) established a social noncontributory pension for all persons over 65 whose income is below a given level fixed by law. The number of people benefiting from this pension in 1973 was 850,000, of whom 87.9 percent were women. The minimum of the noncontributory pension at present is 53,600 lira monthly; the minimum level of contributory pension (for the salaried and self-employed) is 66,950 monthly. This is barely enough for subsistence. The significant fact is that about 75 percent to 80 percent of the Italian pensioners receive only the minimum pension.

Housing Conditions

Another important aspect for the global assessment of the life situation of the elderly population and its needs concerns housing conditions, both for all old people and for those living alone or with other old people. Given the low level of average income of old people and the situation of the housing market in Italy, old people usually are in no position to compete. They therefore find themselves among the citizens who have to accept the poorest sort of housing.

The last census data, for example, show that dwellings occupied by a family with a nonprofessional head of the family (most old people are in this category) lack such services such as a separate bathroom and central heating. This group also has the highest incidence of inadequate dwellings, which lack electricity or inside plumbing.

Health Problems

The low income level of old people leads necessarily to poor health conditions (already shaky because of old age itself), due partly to inadequate diet, partly to bad housing conditions, and partly to the psychological depression linked with financial insecurity. The elderly frequently request admission to hospitals, requests that derive not only from their low income but also from loneliness and the lack of social services and different health services as alternatives to hospitalization. Persons over 60 constitute 17 percent of the total hospital population and 50 percent of the patients in departments of internal medicine. In 1970 it was calculated that stays in the hospital of old people for reasons of a social, economic, or family nature amount to 6.4 million days in general hospitals and 9.2 million days in psychiatric hospitals.

At the same time, a progressive transformation of pathology is occurring: degenerative illnesses and accidental injuries are replacing infectious diseases. The transformation of an agricultural society into an industrial one has produced a new series of illnesses linked to work conditions and environment, as well as new habits linked to urbanization. In addition, the extension of life expectancy has caused a new and greater morbidity. Health services, however, have not changed with the change in pathology. Degenerative illnesses, for example, could be treated in clinics and outpatient departments or at home, which would cost much less than hospitalization, but new structures are needed. It is estimated that 10 percent of hospital patients with acute illness and 90 percent with chronic illnesses would benefit from rehabilitation treatment in order to become again at least partially self-sufficient. Because of a lack of such services, 40 percent of the elderly suffer chronic disability; had there been timely rehabilitation intervention, the percentage with chronic disability could be as low as 5 percent. Rehospitalization rates for cases discharged into situations of poverty, poor housing, lack of family, or poor family relations can grow to 95 percent. The same is true of situations where the family is unable to give help, and there are no supportive services in the health and social field. Until there is a reform of the health and social services, a vast number of old citizens will face poverty, illness, or chronic disability.

Loneliness and Institutionalization

The usual alternative to loneliness (or to tensions in family life) today is admission to a rest home or to a traditional institution; they also constitute a guarantee against financial need, and the certainty of having some care available in case of need. The traditional institutions were custodial and authoritarian. Today many rest homes have become a welfare service asked for by the old people themselves; they meet some needs that would go unsatisfied in a situation of living alone or even of living with the family. In a situation of general crisis and multiple frustrations, with a lack of supportive social services, old people often do not feel that the rest home is a consequence of their being rejected by their family. They may feel that in fact it is a substitute for the family, an institution that has proved incapable of performing the functions ascribed to it. Nevertheless many old people prefer staying in the family or on their own. This choice often means ignoring or minimizing the frustration of living within a structure unable to give much care or affection and ignoring and minimizing the insecurity and isolation of the city where community and social relationships have dwindled and then disappeared. In effect no single solution can be adequate if the more general problems responsible for the uneasy conditions of old age are not solved first.

PROGRAMS

The problem of care for the aged has been increasingly recognized in Italy in the last few years. This may be for two reasons: on the one hand the problem has become more serious because of the increase in the numbers of old people and the backwardness of the social services; on the other hand, Italian society has become much more aware of social problems in general and especially of those concerning the isolation of particular groups of people. As a result, new trends have appeared, both in the practice of existing social services and in the attempt to create new services, which would be quite different from the traditional ones; their main objective would be avoiding the institutionalization of old people. The new trends have begun to appear, particularly in some sectors concerning housing, domiciliary services, financial assistance, day hospitals, and day centers.

Housing

Public interventions in housing by the regional governments have taken two forms: providing residential facilities of a more traditional type (homes, service flats, and group flats) and providing ordinary housing reserved for old people (flats reserved in subsidized housing projects, contributions and grants for the improvement of dwellings, grants toward the rent, and offers of flats owned by local authorities at prices related to the income of the aged). One of the most popular facilities is the service flat building. They are very small flats meant for individuals or couples. They have centralized services of the type found in hotels but no specific geriatric social or health services; instead they have links with services operating in the same district. They are located in residential areas of towns and often have a multiple use; for example, handicapped young people may live in them. The group flat is a form of communal dwelling but indistinguishable from ordinary lodgings. It has room for eight to ten people and is usually a large flat in an ordinary building; it has no special health or welfare services.

Domiciliary Services

In connection with housing and with services aimed at the general population in a situation of need, several regional governments have considered or are already establishing domiciliary services. There seem to be three types of such intervention: home help to facilitate the personal and home life of old people (for example, personal cleaning, house cleaning, and shopping); home nursing given by health visitors, physiotherapists, or other rehabilitation personnel under the guidance of the general practitioner in charge of the case; and social work care both in the sense of casework treatment for special cases and general promotional work, organization, and coordination of the various service.

Financial Assistance

In some cases financial assistance is considered a particular form of domiciliary care, in others as a separate service or as a grant for housing needs. Generally it takes the form of personal or family benefit, which can supplement other types of pension when the benefit would not be replaceable by some form of care (residential or home based).

Day Centers

Day centers may include health services or be limited to social and cultural activities, or sometimes social work. In general, they offer, at the district or the borough level, supportive services (canteens, baths, and showers, for example), use of leisure time and cultural enrichment, and other services that may help an old person to lead an autonomous life. Day centers give priority to the needs of the aged but are open to all citizens. They are connected to other structures (such as health, social services, and cultural services) and other centers of collective and associative life (other neighborhood centers, trade union and political parties branches, public parks with facilities for sport or for old people, and so forth).

Day Hospitals

Since the responsibility for hospital planning has been given to regional governments, day hospitals have become part of the Italian health and social services. They are a key element of the new program of hospital care because they can be the link between outpatient services and hospital care proper. Day hospitals have not been thought of specifically for the aged, but when they function also as rehabilitation centers, it seems quite likely that the aged will be the main users. For patients who need only a few hours of treatment or care every day, day hospitals provide a great advantage by avoiding the psychological shock of hospitalization. The experience of day hospitals in Italy is still very limited, and they should be considered as at an experimental stage.

Not many reliable data are available at present on the implementation of these services, but there is no doubt that a step forward has been made in the way of conceiving of social services. There are many gaps and partial interventions, but Italy still lacks a national law dealing with the reform of the social services. A bill that has been pending in Parliament for years has been delayed again, this time in order to coordinate some of its provisions with the national health service bill.

In the meantime regional governments have had the unquestionable merit of stimulating the national government and of offering the first examples of open services, from which it will be possible to draw some conclusions based on experience. In particular, two characteristics seem to be essential for any type of service: democratic participation, both of users and of social organizations, in the management of the services and the participation of the users in service delivery. Another important aspect is the need to adjust the architectural features of services to the needs of aged people so as to keep barriers to free movement to a minimum. Regional legislation has considered this point in the planning of the new centers. No doubt there is still a long way to go before we have a satisfactory social services system capable of satisfying citizens' needs, but at least some basic principles have been established.

LEGISLATION

The lack of a national law makes it very difficult in Italy to define the general orientation of welfare policy. However, a turning point was reached in 1970 when regional governments started their legislative activity. The different strategies chosen by different regions have followed the lines of some of the more advanced projects of reform, and they all show the intent of offering a range of services to the aged. These are characterized by the objective of avoiding admission to institutions or hospitals by offering domiciliary services and by being organized at the level of maximum decentralization. However, not all of the principles on these issues have been equally accepted and assimilated among the regions, thus pointing to the need to avoid isolation, to develop a coordinated and comprehensive intervention, and to give priority to prevention over restoration. Some of the old formulas appear just to have been brushed up; others are new only in terminology; sometimes enunciations that are correct theoretically fall down in implementation.

Eight regions have made laws on the aged, and some others are preparing new legislation. With the exception of Emilia Romagna—where every intervention seems directed to citizens in general rather than special categories and where the social policy is oriented to comprehensive interventions at the geographical level—the other regions still seem to be very attached to models that are becoming obsolescent.

One issue has concerned admission to institutions and homes for the aged. Admission has been considered by almost all the legislations, but it is in general thought of—in the words of the Regione Umbra—as the last solution "when it has become impossible to provide in other ways for their welfare" and "admission in a home does not necessarily exclude other financial or welfare benefits." A wealth of detailed regulations exists concerning admission to a home, but the provision for other services are much less precise.

The common denominator to all the regional laws concerning the welfare of the aged is represented (with the exception of the Molise region and the first two laws of Trentino-Alto Adige) by domiciliary services. They are considered a synonym of deinstitutionalization and are represented as the basic alternative service. But in order to keep the old person in his own social context as an active member of the community and to avoid the danger of keeping him in his own house with no other contacts than his spouse or the personnel of the services, domiciliary services cannot be enough. They are essential if the aged are to be placed in a situation where they can be part of the community, but they are only one aspect of the situation. For example, very often inadequate housing conditions are responsible for admission into a home, besides being a cause of ill health. Housing is a primary need, and together with domiciliary services they are often not considered; housing services often are not implemented or adequately financed.

The regions of Liguria, Lombardy, and Umbria provide grants toward rent; Liguria also encourages "in the framework of the programs for subsidized housing, the building of dwellings for the aged, located in ordinary buildings, and structured in such a way as to meet the special needs of the aged." Lombardy, waiting for the implementation of law 865 on subsidized housing, encourages the allocation of free dwellings owned by local authorities (municipalities or provinces), by associations of local authorities, and by municipal assistance agencies and also provides for grants for the restoration or the purchase of dwellings. It is clearly preferable to have public intervention in the housing system so as to favor the construction of suitable dwellings for the aged rather than grants toward rents for dwellings found in the free market; often these are both expensive and not suitable for the aged tenants.

Only in Umbria and Piedmont are domiciliary services established by a law that concerns the aged, the disabled, and children in order to encourage their being kept in their ordinary family and life environment. Not all the regional laws coordinate domiciliary services with the health services, and particularly with home nursing. The coordination of health and social services at district level is paramount for preventive action and timely intervention in situations of need; in the special case of the aged, it may mean avoiding admission to a home. The connection with the basic health services concerns not only the domiciliary services but also the housing service and other services that are basic to an integrated policy.

So that the aged have a choice of residence according to their needs and wishes, intermediate residential services are of equal importance. Halfway between ordinary dwelling and institutions, they include service flats building (small flats with centralized services but not welfare service) and the group flat (small communal groups, with home help and home nursing). The first of these has been planned by Trentino Alto-Adige and by Lombardy (where the service flats are considered together with health resorts). The regional law of Umbria provides for small communal groups, including the aged, the disabled, and the minors. Here is another example of nonsectorialization of services coming from the same region; these atypical community homes would allow different age groups to live together.

Another important service in connection with integration beween different age groups is the one of recreational centers. But often they appear to be exclusively for old people (Friuli, Venezia Giulia, Trentino Alto Adige, Lombardy, Piedmont), thus establishing a single category of users and their segregation. In other sectors there are indications of the need to do away with the isolation of the aged to help them to remain in their natural social and community context. Suggestions include providing the aged with free transport passes and free installation of telephones. These certainly are positive interventions as long as they are part of an integrated policy. But in reality, none of these laws can be considered fully integrated; they ought to take into consideration every aspect of community structures.

As far as the aged are concerned, there has been a break with the previous system, even if it is at different levels for different regions. We must hope that regional legislators will come back to these issues to deal with the neglected aspects and improve the existing ones and that the regions that have not yet produced any legislation for the aged will do so shortly, benefiting from the experiences of the others.

RESEARCH

Gerontological studies in Italy have followed basically the same lines of those taking place abroad, with some cultural specifications. Some components of the problems of old age may have been magnified more than others—for example, the concern for family life. Essentially the interest in the problems of old age, both of the social scientists and the workers in the field, has been focused on the definition of needs and indications for interventions in the social and welfare field.

We can divide the literature into two large periods: before and after the beginning of the debate on the reform of the social services. The first studies were concerned mostly with spreading information on the needs of old people in fairly general and superficial terms. They were writings to denounce a situation, sometimes in rhetorical and repetitive terms, but useful nonetheless in a totally uninformed environment where even the workers in this field seemed unaware of the social problems they met every day.

The second group of writings deal with the need for reforming the structures and for developing new approaches to welfare action. The need for a global, planned social policy is repeatedly stated, so that social, health, and social security problems of old age can be dealt with. There is a search for the instruments of an effective social planning; social isolation of old people is denounced, as well as the dangers of institutionalization. The problems of readjusting to a different life in society for old people are identified. Open services and more adequate pensions are fought for. It was during this period (between 1966 and 1970) when the role of the regional governments became part of the debate. Any form of service for the aged was seen as necessarily integrated, and the position of old people in society was recognized as no different from that of any other citizen: paternalistic attitudes must be avoided, and no distinction should be made between citizens on the basis of belonging or not belonging to the world of production. A network of open services was demanded.

The largest number of studies in the beginning dealt with problems of old people in institutions; the efforts led to improvement in the institutions. During the last five years, the most common study has been a survey describing for a given geographical area (district or borough) the characteristics of the local aged population; most of these have been sponsored by the local authorities as a basis for future alternative services.

Many papers have been written on the subject of social security. The tendency to deal with pensions in a global way by doing away with categories appears fairly late and only very timidly. There is a great deal of uncertainty on the issue of old people who continue to work, even part time, after retirement, much perplexity on the effective utilization of old workers, and a search for substitute activities that allow a good social adjustment. An issue that has created much interest is the one of holidays for old people, where social rehabilitation could occur through the organization of a service for leisure time, limited to a period, and unfortunately often unsupported by other services.

Various symposia and conferences on the problems of old people have been effective in popularizing the subject. Among the most important are the ones organized by ONPI (opera Nazionale Pensionati d'Italia, the national agency for pensioners), by the Institute for Social Medicine, and by the Society for Gerontology and Geriatrics. There are quite a number of specialized periodicals, including *Longevita, Giornale di Gerontologia,* and *Medicina Geriatrica.* Also quite important has been the production on the part of Attivita Assistenziali Italiane e Internazionali, a semigovernmental agency, of books and teaching material, which in the last few years was collected in two series, "Sussidi tecnici" and "Indagini e documentazioni sociali." AAI also has operational activities in the field.

The contribution of sociological and psychological research has not been extensive. Psychological research has centered its interest on the issues of adaptation or maladjustment in old people (Trentin et al.; Burgalessi, 1975) on mental activity (Cesa-Bianchi), on the maintenance of self-conception (Crespi), on the problem of roles and psychology of aging (Maderna). For the sociologists, the initial orientation established by Pagani with his writings and research has had a great influence. His interpretations of the crisis of old age rest on the change from a rural to an industrial urban society, with the attending demographic transformation and the changes in the institution of the family. His research (and that of his collaborators) on poverty published in the periodical *Longevita* before 1960 has been a major contribution. In the early

1960s, some studies on the position of old people in the family that were made in different areas of the country showed also a difference in socioeconomic development (Corsini, 1962), on leisure time use among retired workers in large towns (Florea, 1964), on the problems of life in an institution (Mariotti, 1969), on health conditions and attitudes to health problems (Florea, 1964), on the condition of old age and role loss (Burgalassi et al., 1975), and on old people in a changing society (Guidicini et al., in press).

After 1970 there was a definite increase in book production in all fields: journalistic reports on institutions, hospitals, and rest homes (Franco, 1974); medical diaries (Musmeci, 1974); urban studies (Venturicci, 1971); social policy studies (Foschi, 1975); textbooks on old age (Vischer, 1971; Brize and Vallier, 1972); the series of INCRA (II sistema anziano); and a book containing all the current information on work, social security, and social relationships of old people (Columbo et al., 1975).

The crisis of old age has been dealt with both as a whole and in the context of the most relevant components, such as work, retirement, family life, and leisure time, although the number of research agencies is very small, and the research tradition still very young. Many of the data may not be comparable, and some may be useless for sociological or psychological analysis. Examples are the way in which the Central Institute for Statistics groups occupations so that research on suicide and attempted suicide of old people becomes impossible; the difficulties in reconstructing not only the global income of old people but even the average income from pensions; the lack of census data on housing stratified by age group; and the lack of data on cohabitation in the same household elaborated by age groups. There is a lack of research on the conditions of life of old people (taking into account the extreme heterogeneity of this so-called age group), on isolation and loneliness, on social participation, on aging in women and its problems, on sexuality, on economic poverty, on antisocial behavior in old age, on the problem of death, and on the idea of time and social behavior. These are all issues to which research could contribute greatly and provide some indications for interventions.

A critical assessment of the research should take into consideration not only the topics covered but methodology. In comparison with research studies made abroad, where often the biological components have been given more attention than the social constraints on old age, studies in Italy have always given major attention to role loss, noncommitment, and isolation in ghetto-like situations, which are mentioned but not always underlined in studies abroad. However, gerontological studies in Italy are still quite a long way from the social reality of the country; their analysis of social, cultural, and economic dynamics of Italian society, of its gaps and contradictions, which determine the inconsistency and the pathology of social phenomena, is not pushed far enough. It is not sufficient to state that the crisis of old age derives from the changes in society and that our society is changing; nor is it enough to denounce injustices, often in a moralistic or paternalistic tone, even when the denunciation does not become an exercise in political rhetoric or demogogy. This transformation is in fact uneven, with an imbalance between real society and legal society; individuals are obliged to live in a constant conflictual situation where their own needs and the needs for interpersonal relationships are often frustrated by their day-to-day experience of confusion and repetitive monotony. The contradictions and deep conflicts created by the uncontrolled change endanger both individuals and institutions. The crisis also affects young people searching for values, women torn by conflicting models, fighting themselves and others, adult males against whom they all protest, threatened in their insecure balance. Who are the problem carriers? Is it legitimate to assume that the change in function and social position of the aged is merely a symptom of the social system's change? These are problems still unsolved in Italian gerontological research.

REFERENCES

Brize, P. R., and Vallier, G. 1972. *La terza età*. Florence: Sansoni.

Burgalassi, S. 1975. *L'eta inutile*. Pisa: Pacini, p. 184.

Columbo, V. 1975. *Gli anziani*. Milan: Giuffrè, 1975, p. 747

Corsini Florea Martinelli. 1962. *L'anziano in famiglia*. Rome: ISTISS.

Florea, A. 1975. *Bibliografia della Gerontologia Italiana*. Rome: A.A.I., p. 265.

———. 1964. Condizioni di salute del soggetto anziona e suo atteggiamento verso il problema sanitario. *Giornale di Gerontologia* 10.

———. 1964. *Risultati di un'indagine sul tempo libero di un gruppo di operai pensionati*. Atti del IV Convegno ONPI. Rome: Il Pensiero Scientifico, pp. 112-130.

———. 1977. *Anziani e società industriale*. Naples: Liguori Editore, p. 160.

Foschi, F. 1975. *Gli anziani nella comunità*. Rome: Cinque Lune, p. 209.

Franco, A. 1974. *Il vecchio in Italia o merce o rifiuto*. Rome: COINES, p. 117.

Guidicini, P.; Giovannini, G.; Palmieri, G.; and Stagni, E. 1977. *Condizione urbana e cultura della terza età*. Milan: Franco Angeli, p. 178.

Malfatti, M., and Tortora, E. 1974. *Gli anni negati*. Milan: Mursia, p. 269.

Mariotti, M. 1969. *Il ghetto per i vecchi*. Florence: Scwaryz.

———. 1971. *Note sulla condizione dell'anziano: il ruolo dell'edilizia e della pianificazione*. Genoa: Istituto di Architettura e Tecnica Urbanistica della Facoltà di Ingegneria dell'Università di Genova.

Musmeci, L. 1974. *L'ultima età*. Milan: Feltrinelli, p. 121.

Pagani, A. 1964. *Sociologica della vecchiaia*. Milan: ANEA

Venturicci, P. 1971. *L'età anziana: assistenza e architettura*, Pisa: Pacin.

Vischer, A. L. 1971. *ABC della terza età. Aggiungere anni alla vita*. Milan: Ferro.

JAPAN

DAISAKU MAEDA

The Japanese economy has made great progress during this century. Between 1900 and 1970, the Japanese manufacturing industry expanded 150 times; during the same period, that of the United States expanded 14 times, Italy 17 times, Germany 9 times, and France 6 times (Oouchi et al., 1971). The development has been especially conspicuous since 1955. Between 1955 and 1970, Japan's industrial production expanded 6.7 times.

Industrialization inevitably brings about urbanization. Thus the speed of our urbanization has also been very fast in these twenty-five years. These two factors—very fast industrialization and urbanization—caused a drastic social change in the life of the Japanese people. This change, sometimes referred to as the Westernization of life, deeply affected both the social and economic life of the people of all classes in both rural and urban communities. Thus Japan's old people of today have lived under two completely different sets of national goals and ideologies. They also went through very rapid changes in standards of living with the shift from an agricultural country to an industrialized country.

An American anthropologist once wrote, "Aging in Japan, as elsewhere, is a matter for deep human ambivalence" (Plath, 1972). In fact, because of the very fast and drastic social changes, there coexist two contradictory factors in the many aspects related to aging in Japan. For example, while respect for the aged is still regarded as one of the essential virtues of Japanese society (Palmore, 1975), the social services for the aged, which are indispensable for their well-being, are much less developed compared with those of the countries of the Western world. Thus it is very difficult to give a clear picture of aging in Japanese society.

Japanese people used to define old age as persons 60 years and over, as did most of the other societies under the influence of Chinese culture. The sixty-first year after birth, called *kanreki* ("return of the calendar"), used to have a special meaning; it was often regarded as the beginning of second childhood. People 60 years of age and over were thus permitted to be dependent on others, mainly their grown-up sons. In reality, however, most Japanese old people continued to work, either for money or for the sake of the satisfaction in continuing to have a meaningful role in life.

But today the concept of old age is changing greatly. According to recent nationwide research, three out of four middle-aged persons between 30 and 45 think that old people are those aged 65 and over (Office of the Prime Minister, 1975a). Moreover, about 40 percent of the interviewees answered that old people were those aged 70 and over.

Like most gerontologists in Western countries, Japanese gerontologists tend to use age 65 as a dividing line between middle age and old age. The main reason is that the population aged 65 and over seems to be appropriate for considering social programs. But in many actual programs, persons aged 60 and over are generally treated as old people. In fact, the pensionable age of the largest public pension program, *Koseinenkin-hoken* (Welfare Pension Insurance Program) is 60 for men and 55 for women, five years younger than the average pensionable age of Western countries.

DEMOGRAPHY

Currently the total population of Japan is about 111.9 million (1975 national census). The number of old people aged 65 and over is 8.9 million, 7.9 percent of the total population. Though this percentage is the highest among the countries of Asia, it is lower than the industrialized countries of Europe and North America.

The age structure of Japan's population was quite stabilized from the beginning of the twentieth century to the mid-century (table 32). The very high birthrate (promoted by the national policy) offset the gradual increase of the aged population resulting from the advancement of medicine and public health and the general improvement of the standard of living. Since 1950, the birthrate has decreased very sharply; now Japan belongs to the second-lowest-birthrate group in the world. This low birthrate, combined with the extension of the life expectancy of old people (table 33), which increased their number, especially that of very old people (table 34), brought about a very sharp increase in the proportion of the population aged. This tendency is expected to continue until the beginning of the next century when the proportion of the aged in Japan will become one of the highest in the world.

Another important demographic factor concerning the aging population is its geographic distribution. Mainly due to the enormous migration of the younger population from the rural areas to the industrialized areas, the proportion of population aged is much larger in rural areas than in the metropolitan areas. For example, in 1975, the proportions of old people aged 65 and over in Tokyo and Osaka, the two largest metropolitan areas of Japan, were 6.2 percent and 5.9 percent, respectively. On the other hand, there were several rural prefectures whose proportions of old people aged 65 and over already exceeded 11 percent. This discrepancy is predicted to continue to exist or even be enlarged in the future (Society for the Study of Population Problems, 1972).

Table 32: THE AGED POPULATION

Year	Total Population (in thousands)	65 Years and Over (in thousands)
1920	55,391	2,917 (5.3%)
1935	68,662	3,189 (4.6%)
1950	83,200	4,109 (4.9%)
1955	89,276	4,747 (5.3%)
1960	93,419	5,350 (5.7%)
1965	98,275	6,181 (6.3%)
1970	104,665	7,393 (7.1%)
1975	111,934	8,858 (7.9%)
1980	118,012	10,327 (8.8%)
1995	131,427	16,276 (12.4%)
2005	138,397	20,757 (15.0%)
2015	141,760	25,091 (17.7%)
2025	142,963	24,853 (17.4%)

Source: For 1920–1975, *Reports of National Censuses.* Tokyo: Office of the Prime Minister, 1920–1975; for 1980-2025, *Estimation of Japan's Future Population.* Tokyo: National Institue of Population Problems, 1975.

Table 33: LIFE EXPECTANCY AT AGE 65

	Male	Female
1965	11.86	14.59
1974	13.38	16.18

Source: Table of Life Expectancy, 1965 and 1974. Toyko: Ministry of Health and Welfare, 1966, 1975.

Table 34: INCREASE OF THE ELDERLY POPULATION BY AGE (IN THOUSANDS)

Age	1950	1970
60–69	4,075	6,718(+65%)
70–79	1,967	3,381(+72%)
80 and over	371	949(+156%)

Source: Estimation of Japan's Future Population. Toyko: National Institute of Population Problems, 1975.

It is feared that this difference may make the development of the services for the rural aged very difficult because many more people will be scattered in extended areas where the population of younger people who can work in the services for the aged will be limited.

WORK AND RETIREMENT

One of the major problems related to aging in Japanese society is the very early fixed mandatory retirement age practiced in most large firms. Two-thirds of enterprises having more than thirty employees have a fixed mandatory retirement age (table 35). Fixed mandatory retirement age itself is a problematic practice in light of the welfare of the aged. The problem is much more serious in Japan because of the low mandatory retirement age (table 36). In over 70 percent of enterprises having such a system, the age is between 55 and 59. According to the same government survey, it is clear that among those whose fixed retirement age is 60 and over, more than nine-tenths set the age at 60 years old (Ministry of Labor, 1973).

Table 35: PROPORTION OF ENTERPRISES PRACTICING FIXED MANDATORY RETIREMENT AGE

Size of Enterprise (number of employees)	Enterprises Having Fixed Mandatory Retirement Age System (in percent)
Total	66.6%
5,000 and over	100.0
1,000–4,999	99.0
300–999	94.3
100–299	90.4
30–99	55.0

Source: Survey on the Employment and Administration of Enterprises. Tokyo: Ministry of Labor, 1973.

Table 36: AGE OF FIXED MANDATORY RETIREMENT (IN PERCENT)

Size of Enterprise (number of employees)	54 and Under	55	56–59	60 and Over
Total	0.3	52.0	12.3	35.4
5,000		38.0	51.0	11.0
1,000–4,999		42.7	37.4	19.9
300–999		49.5	27.7	22.8
100–299	0.2	53.6	16.7	29.5
30–99	0.3	52.3	6.4	41.0

Source: Public Opinion Survey about the Problems of Old Age. Toyko: Office of the Prime Minister, 1973.

In 1974, one year after this survey was done, 69 percent of the total labor force was employed by someone else. Among these, roughly 70 percent were working in enterprises having more than thirty employees and thus with a fixed mandatory retirement age. It can safely be said that more than half of the total labor force of Japan is under a very early fixed retirement age.

Because Japan's public pension has not matured yet and the pensionable age is 60 for men and 55 for women (except for government employees), the majority of persons must try to find another job when they first retire. With but a few exceptions (very high government officials and executives of reputable firms), jobs after their first retirement provide a much smaller income, have a much lower social status, and are often unstable and/or irregular. Thus in spite of the early fixed mandatory retirement age, 81 percent of old people aged between 60 and 64 are working (table 37). The labor force participation of old people over 65 is also much higher compared to other industrialized nations.

Table 37: INTERNATIONAL COMPARISON OF THE MALE LABOR FORCE

Country	60–64	65 and Over	Pensionable Age
France (1968)	65.7	19.3%	60
Italy (1971)	40.6	13.4	60
Canada (1961)	75.8	28.5	65
The Netherlands (1971)	74.8	13.1	65
Sweden (1970)	75.7	15.2	65
Great Britain (1971)	80.7	15.8	65
United States (1970)	73.0	24.8	65
West Germany (1973)	67.1	15.1	
Japan (1973)	81.0	46.7	55

Source: *Survey on the Planning for Later Life*. Toyko: Office of the Prime Minister, 1975.

Note: Includes participation of men only.

The major cause of the higher labor force participation of Japanese old people seems to be a lack or shortage of income, but most of these people are willing to work in their later life. According to recent research more than 40 percent of old people aged between 60 and 69 want to continue the job that they have been engaged in from younger days as long as they can. It should be noted that the percentage of middle-aged persons who think thus is about the same as that of older persons (Office of the Prime Minister, 1974a). This suggests that the labor force participation of older persons will not decrease over the next twenty years if other conditions are held constant.

LIVING ARRANGEMENTS

One of the most conspicuous differences between the life of old people of Western countries and that of Japan can be seen in their living arrangements. Table 38 shows that although four out of five old people live with their children in Japan (Ministry of Health and Welfare, 1973a) less than one-third, or even one-fourth, of them live with their children in Western countries (Shanas et al., 1968).

The difference is especially startling when we compare the number of persons living with married children. In Western countries, about half of those living separately from their children do live geographically near their children (Shanas et al., 1968; Cowgill, 1972). If we take this type of living arrangement into consideration, the difference becomes significantly smaller, though there

Table 38: COMPARISON OF LIVING ARRANGEMENTS IN WESTERN SOCIETIES AND JAPAN

	Denmark (1965)	United States (1965)	Great Britain (1965)	Japan (1969)	Japan (1973)
Old people living with a child	18%	25%	33%	79.2%	74.2%
Married child	4	8	12	61.0	
Unmarried child	14	17	21	18.2	
Old people living with other relatives	3	7	8	0.5	
Old couples living alone	45	43	33	13.1	
Old individuals living alone	28	22	22	5.2	
Other	6	3	4	2.0	

Sources: E. Shanas et al., Old People in Three Industrial Societies. New York, Atherton Press, 1968; Survey on the Opinion about Life after Retirement. Toyko: Office of the Prime Minister, 1969; and Survey on the Actual Living Conditions of the Elderly. Toyko: Ministry of Health and Welfare, 1973.

Note: The statistics for Japan are for those 60 and over; for the other countries, they are for those 65 and over.

still remains a considerable gap. A hypothesis can be made that Japanese old people live with their children because of the housing shortage. It is certainly true that in large metropolitan areas there is still a serious shortage of houses. However, a more careful examination discloses the fact that the proportion of old people living separately is significantly larger in those metropolitan areas than in smaller cities and rural areas (Ministry of Health and Welfare, 1973a). In other words, older people tend to live with their children even in the localities where there are fewer housing problems.

A number of other factors seem to be significant in influencing the living arrangements of our older people, but none is a definite answer to the difference. In other words, the very high proportion of old people living with their children in Japan seems to be due to the unique attitude of Japanese people, both young and old, toward the living arrangements of older persons.

This attitude of Japanese people is clearly shown by a recent nationwide survey (Office of the Prime Minister, 1974a). Seventy percent of those aged 60 to 69 think that "it is natural to live together" or "it is better to live together, if possible." The percentage of middle-aged persons who answered thus is only slightly smaller than older persons. According to similar research of younger generations, 46 percent of the persons aged 30 to 34 answered that one of the children, even if married, should live with the parents if possible. In addition, 21 percent of them answered that married children may live separately from the parents if the two generations can visit each other very often (Office of the Prime Minister, 1974b).

This research shows that younger generations still hold a sense of strong filial duty to satisfy the parental expectation to live together or very close to each other and to take care of them. Thus if other conditions hold constant, even twenty years from now, the proportion of older persons living with their children will not change very significantly.

THE ECONOMIC LIFE OF OLD PEOPLE

It is difficult to give a clear-cut picture of the economic life of Japanese old people because the overwhelming majority live with their adult children and are more or less dependent on them economically. In most cases, it is impossible to separate the household of old people from that of their children. The money the child earns is shared with his retired parents.

First, let us look into the economic life of households whose heads are aged 65 and over (in the case of women, aged 60 and over) and all the other members are younger than 20. According to research done by the Ministry of Health and Welfare (1973b), 80 percent of these households belong to the lowest quartile group in the distribution of income.

The very small income or the lack of income of old people comes mainly from the fact that our public pension programs are not yet matured and that the number of old people receiving a substantial pension is very limited. The proportion of people aged 60 and over and receiving the benefit of the public contributory old age pension is only 22 percent (Office of the Prime Minister, 1974a). Therefore the number of old people who can live an economically independent life is very small in comparison with Western industrialized countries. Recent research on this issue (Office of the Prime Minister, 1973) disclosed that only 31 percent of the old people aged 60 and over thought that they could live an economically independent life. Among them, 59 percent have a sizable earned income, 35 percent have adequate pensions, and 27 percent have income from their property.

Another important source of income of the Japanese elderly is financial assistance from their children. A recent nationwide survey (Office of the Prime Minister, 1974b) showed that 45 percent of old people who have living children (both living with and separately from them) are receiving financial assistance from them. Even in the case of the elderly living separately from their children, 27 percent are receiving some financial assistance. Among the persons receiving financial assistance from their children, 59 percent receive a substantial amount, 19 percent receive some part of their living expenses, and the remaining 21 percent receive just pocket money. In short, most of the Japanese old people cannot live on their own income. In this sense they are poor, but, because most of them receive financial support from their children, their actual life is not miserable.

Many old people who have no children to rely on are dependent on public assistance. In 1973, 3.7 percent of old people aged 65 and over who are members of families received public assistance; the percentage of public assistance recipients in the total Japanese population was only 1.2 percent. The economic distress of these people can be seen more clearly by looking at the public assistance statistics of aged households. In 1974, 15 percent of aged households throughout Japan were receiving public assistance. Incidentally, the proportion of aged households in all the families receiving public assistance has been gradually increasing from 22 percent in 1965 to 35 percent in 1974. Now in Japan, the second most important cause of poverty, next to illness and/or disability, is old age (Health and Welfare Statistics Association, 1976).

ROLE AND STATUS*

According to recent nationwide research on hours spent daily on various activities, old people aged 70 and over average about 9.5 hours a day in bed. They work for about 2.5 hours, and they spend about 3 hours doing household chores and personal care. They usually spend about an hour and 40 minutes in eating three meals. To meet friends, neighbors, and relatives, they usually spend 50 minutes a day. The rest of the time is spent engaging in leisure activities, among which watching television and listening to the radio are for the longest periods of time—about 4.5 hours. Other types of leisure activities take about half an hour. For reading they usually spend slightly less than half an hour.

I have no comparable data at hand about the daily life of the elderly in Western societies, but my personal observations and reading lead me to these conclusions. Japanese old people spend more time working, more time watching television and listening to the radio, and less time on active leisure activities like visiting and hobbies. Generally, Japanese old people are less active or more socially withdrawn than those in Western countries. In fact, the Japanese people tend to expect the elderly to be quiet and meditative rather than bustling and active.

That Japanese old people are socially less active than younger people does not necessarily mean that they have no meaningful roles. On the contrary. Most usually live with their children and grandchildren, even in urban areas, and thus have some roles in their homes. According to recent research of urban old people aged 65 and over (Tokyo Metropolitan Institute of Gerontology, 1974), 33 percent of them (both sexes) take the full responsibility of housekeeping; 12 percent have more than four roles; and 35 percent have one to three roles. The percentage of those who have no role is only 20 percent.

Many old people help in their children's work. This is especially true when the family is self-employed—farmers, retail dealers, and small restauranteurs,

---

*This section deals with people over 70 years old because many persons, especially men, are still working in their 60s.

for example. Most of the old women help in taking care of their grandchildren, sometimes finding satisfaction. When the grandchildren are big enough and do not need their care anymore, watching them grow up becomes an important source of life satisfaction.

Most of the old people are satisfied with their present life. This means that to have many duties to accomplish even after retirement does not mar the happiness of Japanese old people. Indeed they are carrying out their duties in the family life quite willingly.

Japanese old people seem to spend a limited length of time on leisure activities, which include a number of folk arts and hobbies suitable for them. Generally, these activities are easy to begin, and as people develop their skill, they bring them satisfaction and a sense of achievement. Some of these activities are *haiku*, a very short poem of seventeen syllables; *waka*, a short lyric poem of thirty-one syllables; *shodo*, calligraphy; *ikebana*, flower arrangement; *sado*, tea ceremony; *shigin*, recitation of poems and many other Japanese styles of classic singing; *bonsai*, growing of live miniature trees in small pots; Japanese classical dancing; Japanese folk dancing; *shogi*, Japanese chess; *go*, Chinese chess; and various traditional and modern handicrafts. Many of these can also be enjoyed by oneself, perhaps one of the reasons why Japanese old people are less socially active.

In spite of the availability of various arts and hobbies suitable for older people, the actual number of persons enjoying them is rather limited. According to the nationwide research of 1969 (Office of the Prime Minister, 1969), less than half (48 percent) of Japanese old people have some kind of hobbies.

LIFE ATTITUDE IN MIDDLE AND OLD AGE

Over 80 percent of Japanese people aged 60 and over feel that their life and circumstances are more or less satisfactory (Office of the Prime Minister, 1974a). No marked differences are seen by the age brackets, though the proportion of those who are fully satisfied increases with age.

According to a research project done in 1960 on the happiness and worries of American adults (Riley et al., 1968), 27 percent of people aged 55 and over were classified as feeling "very happy" and 55 percent as feeling "pretty happy." That is, 82 percent were judged as feeling more or less happy. "There is a striking similarity between the feelings of American older persons and of Japanese. It is very interesting to note that in a society where most of the old people do not have any substantial income, must continue to work, are dependent on their children, over 80 percent are satisfied with life and circumstances.

The Japanese situation and the happy feeling of older people may seem to be contradictory. A number of interpretations can be made. First, it may be due to the psychological need of mature persons to accept themselves and their life situations and be happy with them. This interpretation can explain the similar percentage of happy and satisfied persons of the two completely different societies. The second possible interpretation is that the unique living arrangements of Japanese old people offsets the lack or shortage of income in old age. Because of the life-style of living together with their children, Japanese old people rarely feel isolated or deserted and more often feel that their life is meaningful.

Most Japanese old people are also feeling happy with their past life (Office of the Prime Minister, 1974a). Over 60 percent of Japanese people aged 60 and over feel that their past life was "very fruitful" or "pretty fruitful." And 60 percent or more of middle-aged persons aged between 40 and 59 predict that their future life would be "bright" or "rather bright" (Office of the Prime Minister, 1974a). Thus it might be said that most of the middle-aged persons in Japan are well-adjusted psychologically to old age. But in the light of social policy, attention should be placed on the fact that over 10 percent of them are afraid that their future life will be dismal, and about 25 percent are uncertain about the prospect of old age.

PROGRAMS FOR THE AGED

The most frequently expressed demand by persons aged 50 and over for the improvement of specific public measures was the increase of the amount of pension (Office of the Prime Minister, 1973). Over 60 percent of them expressed this demand. The second most frequently expressed demand was the lowering of the age limit of the free medical care program, which at present is 70 years old (38 percent). Other expressed demands were for job-finding services, an increase of facilities for leisure activities, an increase of home helpers, an increase of good homes for old people, and an increase of beds in geriatric hospitals.

Since the end of World War II, especially after the enactment of the law for the welfare of the elderly in 1963, the Japanese national government has been making considerable efforts to meet these demands. The progress has been certainly remarkable. Nevertheless programs for old people still have to be improved and/or expanded.

Income Maintenance Programs

Like other industrial countries, Japan's income maintenance programs for the aged consist of public pensions and public assistance. The coverage of public pensions is excellent for the younger generations, including both the employed and self-employed. But because of its late start—especially in the case of the program for the self-employed, which was started in 1961—the public pension programs have not fully matured yet. Although several measures were taken for their faster maturation, the proportion of people aged 60 and over receiving the benefit of the contributory old-age pension is still only 22 percent. Even taking into account those older persons who are receiving the noncontributory old-age pension and the special war pensions, the total percentage is still only 61 percent (Office of the Prime Minister, 1974a). The amount of the noncontributory old-age pension in August 1968 was only 16,000 yen (U.S. $69) a month.

Thus public assistance is still playing an important role in the income maintenance programs for the aged in Japan. In 1976 3.2 percent of old people aged 60 to 69 and 4.9 percent of those aged 70 and over were receiving public assistance, while the rate of public assistance recipients in general was only 1.2 percent (Health and Welfare Statistics Association, 1976).

Health Services

Health check service. All those aged 65 and over, including those who are bedridden, can receive a free health check once a year. If a problem is discovered, further close examination will be given also free of charge.

Free medical care service. Old people aged 70 and over who cannot afford to pay their share of public medical insurance (generally 30 percent of the medical care cost) can get necessary medical care free of charge. Over 80 percent of those aged 70 and over are eligible for this program.

Community rehabilitation training service. This is an experimental and demonstration project. In 1977 there were 147 such centers throughout Japan.

Health education services for the elderly. This is a new program that started in 1975. In 1977, 1,325 local governments (40.7 percent of all local governments) were receiving the national subsidy for this service.

Services for Life Satisfaction

Job-finding service. In addition to the general exployment service centers, which usually serve those under 65, there are about 125 job-finding service centers throughout Japan.

Old people's clubs. These are the community-based organizations of the elderly themselves. In 1976, there were about 108,000 such clubs throughout Japan, and 48 percent of those aged 60 and over participated. In 1977, 100,000 such clubs were receiving the national government's subsidy.

Community welfare centers for the elderly. In 1976 there were about 655 community welfare centers for the elderly throughout Japan.

Neighborhood welfare centers for the elderly. In 1975 there were about 1,400 such centers throughout Japan.

Vacation hostels for the elderly. These are reasonably priced hostels for the elderly in vacation spots or at hot springs. In 1976 there were 65 such centers throughout Japan.

Care Services for the Elderly in the Community

Home-help services. In 1977, there were about 12,600 (full-time equivalent) home helpers throughout Japan, 75 percent of them full-time workers. This service is given free of charge, but the income limit is rather strict.

Provision of special equipment. Special beds and mattresses, bathtubs, gas hot-water heaters, air-cushions (for the prevention and treatment of bedsores), and other aids are provided (or lent free of charge) to bedridden old people or other severely handicapped old people with limited income.

Temporary personal care services. This service is given to an old person or an old couple living alone (with limited income) when they need temporary personal care due to illness and the like. The elderly themselves purchase the services with stamps previously given free of charge by the local government. The service is given by the neighbors appointed by the local government.

Telephone installation and telephone reassurance services. These rather new programs are expanding rapidly. By the end of 1977, 27,500 telephones were installed throughout Japan. Telephone reassurance services are implemented mainly in the communities of the metropolitan areas, but the number of such communities is still very limited. These services provide someone to call elders regularly to see if they are alright.

Meal services. Fewer than a hundred communities have this service, still in the experimentation and demonstration stages.

Loan funds. Those who want to add a new room or improve an existing room for the aged parents can borrow money from the local government at a very low interest rate or none at all.

Institutional Care

In 1976 about 128,700 older persons—1.4 percent—were in some kind of institution for the aged. This rate is very low compared to industrial countries in the Western world. This seems to be mainly due to the characteristic pattern of living arrangements of Japanese old people. The small number in institutions does not necessarily mean that there are enough of these homes, however. Especially in the large metropolitan areas there is a shortage of nursing homes for bedridden or severely handicapped old people. In 1976 there were 911 homes for the aged (for those who are ambulatory), 25 homes for the blind aged, 627 nursing homes, and 132 homes for the aged with moderate fee (for those who are ambulatory).

Other Major Public Measures

Housing for the elderly is not well developed in Japan. There are only a very limited number of specially equipped housing for the elderly.

The adult education program for the elderly is administered by the Ministry of Education. Almost all local governments are providing this service.

The aged person as well as the person who is taking care of aged parents or relatives has his taxable income reduced. If the aged parents or relatives are bedridden or severely handicapped, the amount of reduction will be greater. The tax reduction for those who are taking care of aged parents or relatives is designed to preserve Japan's traditional family support and care of aged persons.

RESEARCH IN GERONTOLOGY

Historical Review

In Japan research on aging is a relatively new field. Organized scientific research on aging was started in the 1920s in the field of medicine at the Tokyo University School of Medicine and the Yokufukai Institution, a large multi-functional voluntary institution for the aged. Until recently they were the two major centers for medical research on aging in Japan.

In 1953, after the long sterile period of World War II and the ensuing economic distress, the National Society for the Study of Geriatrics was organized. This is the forerunner of the present Japan Geriatrics Society (Nihon Ronen Igakukai). Modern psychological research on aging was also started at the Yokufukai Institution in the 1930s, but the number of psychologists devoted to this area was quite small until recently.

The organized effort for the development of the social science of aging and related problems was also started very late—the beginning of the 1950s. In 1954 the Japan Society for the Study of Longevity (Nihon Jumyo-Gaku Kenkyukai) was established, enlisting the participation of most of the leading researchers in the social and behavioral sciences interested in gerontological study at that time.

In the meantime, the activities of the International Association of Gerontology, which was organized in 1950, gave rise to the awareness of the necessity of interdisciplinary efforts in the study of aging. In 1956 the Japan Geriatrics Society and the Japan Society for the Study of Longevity co-sponsored the first nationwide interdisciplinary congress of gerontology. Four years later in 1960, under the initiative of these two organizations, the Japan Gerontology Society (Nihon Ronen Gakukai) was organized as a federation of the two independent societies—the Japan Geriatrics Society and the Japan Social Gerontology Society (Nihon Ronen Shakai-Kagakukai). The first National Congress of the Japan Gerontology Society was held in 1959, a year before the formal establishment of the federal society. Since then the joint national congress has been held every two years, and in a year between the joint congresses, each of the two societies has a national congress of its own.

In 1972, twelve years after the Japan Gerontology Society was organized, the Tokyo Metropolitan Institute of Gerontology was established by the Tokyo metropolitan government. This is a multidisciplinary research institute dedicated solely to the study of aging and the related problems. Many outstanding gerontologists of various fields cooperated in the establishment of this research institute, and some of them joined its research staff.

The establishment of the Tokyo Metropolitan Institute of Gerontology gave a great impetus to the gerontological researchers in the related fields, especially physiology, pathology, biology, and other fundamental studies, because the institute placed a strong emphasis on such fundamental studies. Previously these studies had been engaged in only sporadically by a limited number of researchers, who had few chances to discuss the issues among them; cooperative efforts were seldom made. In 1974, a group of biologists, physiologists, biochemists, pathologists, and some physicians started a multidisciplinary exploratory study on the mechanism of aging with a special grant from the Ministry of Education, Science, and Culture. Parallel with the activity of this group, an effort was made to organize a national association devoted to this end; early in 1977 the Japan Society for Biomedical Gerontology (Nihon Kiso Roka Kenkyukai) was organized. In 1975, the Japan Science Council (Nihon Gakujutsu Kaigi) set up the National Committee for Aging Research (Roka Kenkyu Renraku Iinkai), which is now playing an important role in the promotion of gerontological research in Japan.

Recent Trends

It is almost impossible to describe the recent trends of the gerontological research in Japan within a limited space. I have chosen to do so by classifying the papers presented to the national congresses of the Geriatrics Society and Social Gerontology Society held in 1976 according to the major topics in the fields.

Medicine

At the 1976 National Congress, 286 papers were presented. They are classified by the major topics as follows:

Cerebral infarction	27
Neurology	8
Hypertension	24
Arteriosclerosis	17
Cardiology	53
(electrocardiography, arhythmia, and block, 11; ischemic heart disease, 26; others, 16)	
Respiratory organ	16
Digestive organ and surgery	21
Urinary organ	4

Hematology	11
Internal secretion	13
Metabolism	44
(carbohydrate metabolism, 13; lipid metabolism, 21; others, 10)	
Immunology	6
Motor organ	4
Physical strength	6
Geriatric psychiatry	9
Aging in general	10
Health examination	8
Medical care system	2
Causes of death	3

Psychology

At the 1976 National Congress of Social Gerontology, twenty psychological and psychiatric papers were presented. They are classified by the major topics were as follows:

Personality	2
(empathy, 1; Rorschach test, 1)	
Perception	2
Memory	3
Association	1
Adaptation	1
Morale	1
Psychotherapy	1
Mental retardation	1
Psychological functioning in general	4
Other	4

Sociology and Social Welfare

At the 1976 National Congress of Social Gerontology, thirty-two papers related to sociology and social welfare were presented. They are classified by the major topics as follows:

Demography	1
Family structure	1
Life history	4
Living alone	1
Leisure activity	2
Food and nutrition	2
Needs for social welfare service	2
Medical care	4
(community medical care, 3; other, 1)	
Nursing	5
(visiting nursing, 1; other, 4)	
Institutional care	3

Assistance to a dying person	4
Suicide	5
Others	2

Fundamental Studies

The major topics of the biomedical study group are damage and repair of DNA in aging, the alteration of enzyme in aging, cell aging in vitro, cell aging in vivo, aging of supportive structure, aging in intercellular communication, aging and biological surveillance, and models for aging of the individuals.

Major Organizations and Agencies

Japan Gerontological Society (Nihon Ronen Gakukai)

This is a federation of two societies. Its function is to sponsor a biennial joint National Congress of Gerontology. The permanent office is located in the office of the Japan Geriatrics Society.

Japan Geriatrics Society (Nihon Ronen Igakukai)

Membership: 3,300
Congress: Annual (including a joint congress)
Address: c/o Geriatrics Section, the School of Medicine, Tokyo
               University; 3-chome, Hongo, Bunkyo-ku, Tokyo.

Japan Social Gerontology Society (Nihon Ronen Shakai-Kagakukai:

Membership: 420
Congress: Annual (including a joint congress)
Address: c/o Sociology Department, Tokyo Metropolitan Institute of
               Gerontology; 35-2, Sakae-cho, Itabashi-ku, Tokyo.

Japan Society for Biomedical Gerontology (Nihon Kiso Roka Kenkyukai)

Membership: 300
Congress: Annual
Address: c/o Department of Biology, Tokyo Metropolitan Institute of
               Gerontology; Sakae-cho, Itabashi-ku, Tokyo.

Tokyo Metropolitan Institute of Gerontology

This is the only independent institute in Japan that deals directly with research on aging. It is established and fully supported by the Tokyo metropolitan government. It has eleven research departments: biology, pathology, clinical pathology, biochemistry, pharmacology, physiology, behavioral science, sociology, epidemiology, rehabilitation research, and integrated research. In addition it has the following independent sections: nutrition and nursing. It employs about seventy full-time research specialists, more than eighty part-time research specialists, about a hundred full-time research assistants, and a number of clerical and maintenance personnel. The address is 35-2, Sakae-cho, Itabashi-ku, Tokyo.

Medical Schools

Some of the medical schools are noted for their outstanding contributions to research on aging. Among them are the medical schools of Tokyo University, Kyoto University, Osaka University, Kanazawa University, and Nihon Medical College (Nihon Ika Daigaku).

Geriatric Hospitals

Some of the geriatric hospitals are also functioning as research institutes. Among them, the Tokyo Metropolitan Geriatric Hospital, which is working very closely with the Tokyo Metropolitan Institute of Gerontology, and the Yokufukai Geriatric Hospital, which is part of a multifunctional gerontological institution run by a voluntary organization, are outstanding. The addresses of the Tokyo Metropolitan Geriatric Hospital is 35-2, Sakae-cho, Itabashi-ku, Tokyo. That of the Yokufukai Geriatric Hospital is 1-12, Takaido-nishi, Suginami-ku, Tokyo.

Periodicals

Journal of the Japan Geriatrics Society, quarterly (in Japanese).
Journal of Social Gerontology, semiannual (in Japanese and English).
Geriatric Medicine, monthly (in Japanese), Life Science Publishing, Co., Tokyo.
Bulletin of the Geriatric Research of the Yokufukai Geriatric Hospital, annually (in Japanese).
Annual Report of the Welfare of Senior Citizens (in Japanese), Japan Welfare Fund for the Elderly (Nihon Rojin Fukushi Zaidan), Tokyo.

SUMMARY

The improvement of the living standard and the advancement of modern medicine, with the decreased birthrate, in Japan as in the countries of the Western world, have resulted in a growing proportion of old people, especially very old people.

Mainly due to the rapid increase of the older population, Japan's tradition of very early mandatory retirement age has not been changed yet. Neither has the traditionally high percentage of labor force participation of older persons changed yet.

In Japan as many as 75 percent of old people still live with their children. This percentage probably will not decrease much in the near future.

Because of the immaturity of the public pension programs, most of the Japanese old people are not economically independent, but most of them are satisfied with their present life and circumstances. As Plath (1972) has pointed out, the later life of Japanese old people naturally entails suffering. Japan's social measures to alleviate them are not well developed, though vigorous effort has been made by the governments at all levels, as well as by a variety of voluntary organizations.

In Japan research on aging was started in 1920 in the field of medicine. Organized efforts for the advancement of gerontological research in other fields, however, began only recently, though the development has been fast and encouraging.

REFERENCES

Cowgill, D., and Holmes, L. eds. 1972. *Aging and Modernization*. New York: Appleton-Century-Crofts.

Health and Welfare Statistics Association. 1976. *Trends of the welfare of the people*. Tokyo: Health and Welfare Statistics Association.

Ministry of Health and Welfare. 1973a. *Survey on the actual living conditions of the elderly*. Tokyo: Ministry of Health and Welfare.

————. 1973b. *Survey on the actual conditions of the life of people*. Tokyo: Ministry of Health and Welfare.

Ministry of Labor. 1973. *Survey on the employment and administration of enterprises.*. Tokyo: Ministry of Labor.

Office of the Prime Minister. 1969. *Survey on the opinion about the life after retirement*. Tokyo: Office of the Prime Minister.

————. 1973. *Public opinion survey about the problems of old age*. Tokyo: Office of the Prime Minister.

————. 1974a. *Survey on the life and opinion in later years*. Tokyo: Office of the Prime Minister.

————. 1974b. *Survey on the family support and care of aged parents*. Tokyo: Office of the Prime Minister.

————. 1975a. *Survey on the planning for later life*. Tokyo: Office of the Prime Minister.

————. 1975b. *Statistical information on the problems of the aged*. Tokyo: Office of the Prime Minister.

Oouchi H.; Arisawa H.; Wakimura G.; Minobe R.; and Naito M. 1971. *Illustrated Japanese economy*. 5th ed. Tokyo: Iwanami Publishing Co.

Palmore, E. 1975. *Honorable elders*. Durham: Duke University Press.

Plath, D. 1972. Japan: The after years. In D. Cowgill and L. Holmes, eds., *Aging and modernization*. New York: Appleton-Century-Crofts.

Riley, M. W., et al. 1968. *Aging and Society*. New York: Russell Sage Foundation.

Shanas, E., et al. 1968. *Old people in three industrial societies*. New York: Atherton Press.

Society for the Study of Population Problems. 1972. *Prediction of population distribution among regions*. Tokyo: Society for the Study of Population Problems.

Tokyo Metropolitan Institute of Gerontology, Sociology Department. 1974. *Research on the object and functions of the community welfare centers for the aged (II)—A comparative study of users and non-users*. Tokyo.

MEXICO

MANUEL PAYNO

DEVELOPMENT OF GERONTOLOGY

The Mexican Geriatric Society was founded on December 22, 1950, and the Mexican Academy of Gerontology in February 1951. Because erroneous conceptions about gerontology were widespread in Mexico, even among the medical profession, the society decided in 1951 to institute fifty conferences by specialists on the problems of people over 60. During the following years we arranged a successful one-year course with eighty-five two-hour conferences. More than 130 physicians, medical students, and professional people from other fields attended each. We have succeeded in giving the medical profession and the public in general a correct idea of gerontology and its importance. Today the problems of the aged are widely discussed.

From 1951 to 1976, Castro Villagrana, Rodriguez Rodriguez, Meneses, Hoyos, Pino Quintal, Bravo Garcia, Barrera Rosales, Hernandez Ramfrez, Carrillo Azcarate, Velilla Zavazola, Sanchez Malariaga, and I have published over 480 articles in professional magazines and newspapers. We have addressed many national and international conferences, directed primarily to medical professionals, social workers, nurses, and the public interested in gerontology in Mexico. The National Assembly of Surgeons of Mexico asked for the collaboration of the Mexican Geriatrics Society in the preparation of a division of their 1952 convention dedicated to geriatrics. Since then, all medical conventions have dedicated part of their time to the problems of aging.

Local societies of geriatrics have been established in different states of Mexico as sections of the Mexican Geriatric Society: one in Torreon, state of Coahuila; another in Monterrey, state of Nuevo Leon; recently one in the state of Mexico; and there is the Pasteur Institute in Puebla, recently founded by a private donation. The Centro de Retiro de Torreon has been established by a group of physicians.

The first Pan-American Congress of Gerontology was held in Mexico, in September 1956 under the sponsorship of the secretary of health of Mexico. Subsequent to the congress the following developments in the field of social gerontology have taken place:

1. Some labor contracts contain better provisions for retiring laborers.
2. The national railways have set aside $350 million (pesos) for experimental farms for retired workers.
3. In September 1958, retired railway workers received half of the total raise given to active workers.
4. Retired civil servants and other organizations are working for increased pensions as the cost of living rises.
5. Social security of Mexico has accepted one of the points of the first Pan-American Congress of Gerontology that pensions should be movable with the costs of living.

We believe that the aged, and all other Mexicans, have a right to be able to use all that is necessary and sufficient to satisfy their needs and to be able to live in a modern society that respects their dignity and permits them to use all the advances—social, moral, and scientific—that the modern civilization has created to benefit man. This progressive conception is the basic idea of our revolution, which has obliged the government to take steps to be able to make the necessary studies and propose solutions to the uncertain situation of millions of Mexicans 40 years or older. In our country, the elderly are important because of their technical knowledge.

Gerontology is a science that has most rapidly advanced. It has implications for the social and political future of Mexico and Latin America. We believe that an advanced social organization is one whose government cares for social welfare, which is the basic ideal of Mexico. It is necessary to prepare Mexicans for aging by preclinical or preventive treatment, which should start early in life. It is also necessary to prepare the aged psychologically for the changes they will face in their rapidly changing environment. It is also necessary to prepare the family for the changes they will observe in the elderly.

The aged need some activity appropriate to their biosocial condition; in many cases it will help to resolve their financial situation so that they will not be an economic burden to their family or the authorities. Each case should be studied and treated in accordance with the individual needs and the capabilities of the government.

Nobody should leave work prematurely because we need all possible help to teach and prepare the younger generations. Inactivity or leaving work prematurely accelerates the process of aging if there is not adequate psychological preparation for retirement; it should start at least ten years before retirement.

Mexico has thousands of men and women who fought in our revolution to make possible the social and political progress that we today enjoy. The younger generation has the obligation to repay them by permitting them to grow old in a dignified way, by respecting their independence, and by helping them achieve freedom from financial worries.

DEMOGRAPHY

Although only 15.9 percent of all Mexicans are over 60 (table 39), Mexico has one of the fastest growing populations of the continent. Its population has increased from 26 million in 1950, to 56 million in 1970, to 63 million in 1978, to 69 million in 1979, and the population is calculated to be 152 million in the year 2000. This has obliged the authorities to take steps to be prepared and look for solutions in health problems and occupational activities.

Table 39: POPULATION BY AGES, 1979 (in thousands)

Ages	Total	Percent	Men	Percent	Women	Percent
All ages	69,381	100	34,621	49.9	34,759	50.1
40–44	2,635	3.9	1,315	1.9	1,320	2.0
45–49	2,188	3.3	1,085	1.6	1,102	1.9
50–54	1,745	2.8	857	1.2	888	1.6
55–59	1,318	2.6	640	1.2	678	1.4
40–59	7,886	11.0	3,897	5.2	3,989	5.8
60–64	1,000	1.5	481	0.6	519	0.9
65–69	808	1.2	386	0.5	422	0.7
70–74	629	1.0	298	0.4	331	0.6
75 and over	775	1.2	355	0.5	420	0.7
Totals 40 and over	11,098	15.9%	5,417	7.2%	5,681	8.7%

Sources: Agenda Estadística, 1978; Proyecciones de la Población Mexicana 1970 a 2000; Emcuesta continua sobre ocupación, 1978; Secretaria de Programación y presupuesto, Dirección General de Estadística e Información, 1979.

We cannot expect a normal aging if we have not had adequate medical attention during our childhood and adolescence. Medical science is responsible for longevity because we have better health and a better environment as a consequence of the dispositions given by the authorities, such as better housing and nutrition.

Mexico now has 1,688,732 women 60 years and over and 879,815 men who are economically inactive, making a total of 2,548,550 inactive. Of these, 3,222 are receiving economic help from private foundations in homes for the aged, and 2,335 are in official institutions. There are a large number of private institutions that help the aged in different parts of the country.

RETIREMENT INCOME

About half of the 2,548,550 inactive elderly receive pensions or retirement funds. The great majority of the aged represent a heavy burden on their families and the federal government. The situation of the retired aged represents a great burden on the nation, especially since our country needs to use the technically prepared to teach the younger generation.

Some pensions are 100 percent of the last salary; some take into consideration an average of the last three to five years' salaries; and some are 75 percent of the last salary, which in most cases is insufficient to cover the needs of living. During the last devaluation of the peso, the government ordered a 2.3 percent increase in salaries and pensions, which is not enough to cover the high cost of living. The Mexican Academy of Gerontology believes that pensions should move with the cost of living. Today all new contracts with unions take into consideration retired workers, who receive an amount agreed to by the organization and the owners. To help the aged when they retire, we have proposed that every worker should have an insurance policy so that when he retires, he will receive a good bonus.

PROJECTS

Geriatrics Course

In view of the success experienced with the previous courses in geriatrics for physicians and students, the society plans to establish a two-year course in geriatrics. One of the reasons for arranging it at a high professional level is to curtail the work of those who lately have made false promises of rejuvenating people, even back to the age of 30. We have received many requests from officials and physicians in Latin America for participation in such a course, but one of the major problems is financing the project. The course will include studies in the physiology of the aged, pathology, laboratory analysis, cardio-pathology, internal medicine, cancerology, radiotherapy, isotherapy, surgical procedures, psychiatry rehabilitation, hospital practice, and social geriatric medicine. We have a large amount of clinical material available for the course and will use the state hospital, rest homes, chronic hospitals with more than six hundred beds, and the private asylums, which house about twenty-five hundred aged residents. All these patients need medical attention and rehabilitation from a geriatric point of view.

The course should cover a minimum of two years. Four months a year will consist of theoretical work in the form of conferences, round table discussions, and laboratory work. Six months will be spent on clinical investigation, with treatments, rehabilitation, and an evaluation of results. Weekly meetings will discuss the cases under treatment. In addition, there will be special conferences on the other clinical aspects and on active programs. After the two years' work, six months will be allowed for preparation for the final examination for a degree in geriatrics.

National Institute of Gerontology

We have completed a plan for the organization of the National Institute of Gerontology, which was approved by the First Pan-American Congress of Gerontology, with the recommendation that every country of our continent should have an institute to coordinate work done on the problems of aging.

The Mexican Academy of Gerontology and the Mexican Society of Geriatrics have well-founded hopes that the current president of Mexico, José Lopez Portillo, who has studied all of our social problems, will take a decisive stand in favor of resolving old-age problems.

During my service as medical adviser in gerontology for the secretary of health, we prepared a plan to establish gerontological units of fifty beds, complete with yards, plants, individual rooms, day rooms, and a place for meditating. We proposed to construct one unit in each state, but up to now, the work has not been possible because of our financial difficulties. These units are to be self-administered by retired professionals, principally physicians and nurses, under the supervision of the S.S.A. In this way some occupations for the elderly retired would be provided.

We are trying to unify the clinical studies and the medical examinations of the aged so that they can be analyzed by computer.

We believe that solutions to gerontological problems can be found by organizing an institute, a department, or an independent commission, which is within the power of the president to establish. The organization would include administration, inspection and control, technical committees, professional advisers, and the following divisions:

Medicine and Investigation

Medical services by doctors, nurses, social workers, and other professionals.
Homes for mental patients.
Units for toxicological patients.
Centers for psychophysical rehabilitation.
Centers for geriatric rest.
Mobile units.
Coordination of medical, biological, and social investigation.
Short-term geriatric hospitals.
Hospitals for chronic and incurable diseases.
Consulting offices for officials and establishments.
Private and cultural centers.

Social Aids

Organization of activity units.
Geriatric homes.
New jobs or productive activities for aged.
Voluntary auxiliary committees.

Medical-legal assistance.
Advisers on grants, pensions, and other aids.
Distribution of medicines, food, and other aids to people in need.
Preparation projects and organization of complementary industries using retired personnel.
Centers for production and occupational therapy.
Geriatric colonies.

Planning, Information, and Statistics

Office of Educational Preparation.
Orientation for the families.
Education for adults and preparation for retirement.
Reorientation in new socioeconomic activities.
Courses for doctors, nurses, social workers, and auxiliary workers.
Conferences at different cultural levels.
National and international grants.
Office of Planning and Financial Aid.
Coordination of occupational units, advisers to labor organizations, and employers on problems of aging.
Office Of Information and Statistics (national and international).
Library.

Recently the Asociación Pro-dignificación del Anciano, formed by Dr. Emma Godoy and others, has been active in television and in preparing programs and publications.

In March 1979, Dr. Jose A. Zapata V. presented a project, "Asistencia Medico-Social Gerontologico," to the ISSSTE (social security for government employees). It is a complete study for the attention of federal employees.

The Academia Mexicana de Gerontologia presented to the authorities a project for the use of hydroponics as an activity helpful for the aged. There are centers for this activity in different parts of the country, reporting to the National University of Mexico, government Agrarian Offices, and other organizations.

Dr. Manuel Payno, as a professor and delegate of the Faculty of Medicine of the National University of Mexico, presented a paper, "The University and the Third Stage of Life," to the second congress of the association of academic personnel of the university. This paper, which was accepted and approved, suggests that the retired and elderly return to the university in a program that will help reunite the younger and older generations in round table discussions, seminars, courses, etc., and will enable the elderly to give their opinions on the problems of today's world.

Dr. Payno has also been asked to put the final details on a two-year course at the National University of Mexico for the master degree in gerontology for medical professionals, social workers, nurses, and auxiliary personnel.

REFERENCES

Del Pozo, Efren C. The Mexican Institute for Social Security, *American Journal of Public Health*, 55 (December 1965): 1957-1963.

Payno, Manuel. *El problema gerontológico de México*, 1974.

————. El 12% de la poblaciíon tiene disposiciones genéticas a sufrir desordenes generales como consecuencias de la edad. Gaseta Facultad de Medicina Núm. 39. November 30, 1975.

————. Los factores ambientales tienen importancia en el procedimiento de envejecimiento. Gaseta Facultad de Medicina Núm. 32. October 30, 1976.

————. Trabaja para personas mayores hidroponia. Gaseta de la Facultad de Medicina Núm. 7. March 15, 1977.

————. Adecuada atención médica requieren las personas senicientes. Gaseta de la Facultad de Medicina Núm. 51. May 1976.

————. 6000 millones de habitantes en el mundo para el año 2000. Gaseta de la Facultad de Medicina Núm. 74. May 15, 1977.

———— El 50% de los médicos padecen enfermedades cardiovasulares. Gaseta de la Facultad de Medicina Núm. 76. July 30, 1977.

————. La mayor longevidad se encuentra en los hombres de ciencias. Gaseta U.N.A.M., 11. November 29, 1976, p. 5.

————. Anemias en geriatría. Gaseta de la Facultad de Medicina Núm. 90. June 15, 1978.

————. Desaprovechamiento de la mano de obra de los ancianos. Gaseta U.N.A.M., 34. May 1978, p. 14.

————La incomprensión hacia los ancianos les producen serias trastornos psicologicos. Gaseta Facultad de Medicina. 94. August 1978.

————. El envejecimiento, alteraciones del sistema nervioso. Atención Médica. September 1978, pp. 2-6.

————. La Universidad y la Tercera Etapa de la Vida. Segundo Congreso de las Asociaciones Autónomas del personal Académico. U.N.A.M., November 1978.

————. Agenda estadistica. Gaseta U.N.A.M., 1978.

————. Proyecciones de la población mexicana de 1970 a 2000. Encuesta continua sobre ocupación. Sría. de Programación y Presupuesto, 1978.

————.Dirección General de Estadística e información, 1979.

THE NETHERLANDS

R. J. van ZONNEVELD

About 11 percent of the population of the Netherlands—like that of the industrialized nations of Europe, North America, Australia, and New Zealand —is aged 65 years or more. Like these other countries, the Netherlands can be further characterized by rapid urbanization, increased bureaucracy, specialization, automation, and often miniaturization of working activities. These aspects of population, technological development, changes in ethics and in concepts of the role of the aged (so-called generation gap), the greater value attached to youth, and the ever-growing absolute and relative number of aging and old people have led, like elsewhere under the same conditions, to the so-called problem of the aged. Whether there actually exists such a problem or whether the problem has originated and lives on in the minds of certain people who are overconcerned with the lot of old people remains to be seen.

Several features of its population are unique to the Netherlands. The first is that it has the youngest population of all Northern, Central, and Western Europe (except Ireland). For example, the percentage of persons 65 and over in is the Netherlands is 11.2 (1979); already in 1972 this percentage was 13.6 in Belgium, 13.5 in the Federal Republic of Germany, and 13.2 in Great Britain. The most important reason for this phenomenon is clear: the birthrate has been relatively high in the Netherlands and has steeply fallen only in the last decade (in 1977 it was 12.5 per 1,000 inhabitants; between 1955 and 1964 it was 21.1).

Another special feature is that for the past four or five centuries, certain groups of the elderly have been taken care of. From about the fifteenth century, many Dutch communities have had *hofjes* ("small courts") built by employers, for certain of their former employees or servants, or by churches or other charitable religious organizations. Such hofjes consisted of one or more rows of small dwellings, often grouped around a courtyard, where old people could live free or for a very low rent. Often they were also provided with free food, fuel, clothes, and other necessities, although special medical care was probably not given. In the sixteenth and particularly the seventeenth century in a great many cities in the Netherlands—including Amsterdam, Haarlem, Leiden, Delft, The Hague, and Groningen—quite a number of hofjes were centrally located so that the old people who lived in them were not shut off from their community. The advantage of living in a hofje was that some surveillance of their physical and mental health could be maintained. This system of sheltered housing, which still exists, could be found in other countries too— among them Flanders and Germany.

A third special feature is that for a long time private organizations—in the beginning mostly under the auspices of the church (first the Roman Catholic church and later also the Protestant church)—gave attention to the lot of particularly poor and sick old people. In addition they often worked as semigovernmental institutions in providing accommodation. Although private initiative is amply valued, profit making from social services, such as health care, is not.

Local public authorities also provided for care of the aged, but generally to a lesser degree. Only in the last few decades have both central and local governments undertaken a great many activities to help the elderly. Private organizations still play a very important role.

A fourth feature is the existence of a great number of nursing homes that provide, as one of their main functions, long-term care, mostly geared to the needs of sick and/or disabled elderly. (Fifteen percent, however, is younger than 65.) Long-term and chronic cases are treated and cared for mainly in these somewhat small hospital-like (100–300 beds) institutions, and not in general hospitals. A very important part of the work in nursing homes is reactivation of the elderly through physical, recreational, and occupational therapy (Braadbaart and Spruyt, 1977).

The fifth unusual feature is the General Exceptional Medical Expenses Compensations Act, which since 1968 has provided for virtually all residents of the Netherlands for the expenses associated with long-term illness.

A sixth feature is that almost 10 percent of the aged (65+) in Holland live in care-rendering old-age (residential) homes and nearly 3 percent in various sorts of nursing homes. This percentage of institutionalized old people is the highest in the world; it is about, or more than, twice the percentage in Great Britain, the Federal Republic of Germany, Belgium, and France.

But there is also considerable extramural care for the aged. This is the seventh special feature. Extramural health care has existed for several decades on a large scale, and since the 1950s a great variety of social provisions for many old people has come into existence. These services are often provided by private organizations, but primarily with substantial financial support by the central or (in most instances) local government. Local public authorities themselves also provide more and more services.

DEVELOPMENT OF GERONTOLOGY

Growth of Research

Before and during World War II, very little scientific research was undertaken in the field of gerontology. After the war, J. G. Sleeswijk, a professor in physiology who edited the first Dutch handbook, *Old Age from the Medical Point of View* (1948, 1949), with some others took the initiative to found the Netherlands Society for Gerontology in 1947. For several years this society's membership increased only from about forty to about eighty. But in 1950 the Netherlands Society was among the relatively few national societies that founded at Liège (Belgium) the International Association of Gerontology. After 1955 the membership of the society increased steadily to about four hundred in 1967 and then remained on that level or somewhat higher.

The society gradually founded three sections: medical, social sciences, and biological. The last remains small and participates mainly in the national congresses of the Federation of Biological and Medical Societies. The clinical section, with the largest membership, meets once or twice a year. The social sciences section has become gradually more important, partly because of the foundation of the Gerontological Center at Nijmegen, which undertakes mostly studies in the field of social gerontology. During the early 1970s, the society organized annual national congresses, and later—mostly sponsored by the Social Sciences Section—the Gerontological Days, two-day meetings organized around a central theme.

In 1970 the society started the publication of the quarterly *Nederlands Tijdschrift voor Gerontologie* ("Netherlands Journal of Gerontology"). It produces about 260 pages per year, with articles from various disciplines on research, policy, practical care, documentation about congresses, abstracts of newly published books, and so forth. The chief editor is Dr. J. M. A. Munnichs.

Very little research that could be called gerontological in nature was done until the beginning of the 1950s. Then the Organization for Health Research TNO (*TNO* stands for applied scientific research that is partly organized in a semigovernmental research organization) established a Committee on Gerontological Research, with a full-time coordinator. This committee has stimulated and financially supported several scientific investigations, mostly of a biomedical nature. The first thesis in the field of gerontology, *Health Problems of the Aged*, concerning a sociomedical survey on the health care needs of three thousand people, by R. J. van Zonneveld, and financially supported by TNO, appeared in 1954. Following that survey the committee decided to sponsor a nationwide interview and examination survey on health and a number of sociopsychological variables as a basis for policy for future research. The survey was performed by 374 general practitioners, who examined 3,149 old people all over the country on the basis of eight random samples according to sex and five-year age groups. The results were published in English (van Zonneveld, 1961). This survey was then extended into a longitudinal study, in which the subjects were reexamined by the same doctors, using the same methods and questionnaires, after five, eight, eleven, fourteen, sixteen, and seventeen years. The report on the first eleven years of follow-up was published in 1976 (Beek and van Zonneveld). The same survey was undertaken in the total population of old people in one general practice (Fuldauer, 1966) and, on a longitudinal basis (four examinations in eleven years), was performed among 480 male inmates of a large residential home (Beek and von Zonneveld, 1969, 1972). Gradually more medical doctors, including general practitioners, nursing home directors, psychiatrists, and internists, became interested in gerontology and geriatrics, and thus a series of larger investigations have been laid down in theses (among others, Burger, 1971; Cahn, 1964; Fennis, 1973; Leering, 1968; Merkus, 1974; Oostvogel, 1968; Tonino, 1969; Welten, 1968) or in books and articles in medical and gerontological journals. These investigations were partially financed by TNO and partially by other organizations and/or by the universities.

The TNO committee also supported as early as 1951 biological research in old animals at the Netherlands Cancer Institute. The first thesis in this field was "Ovaria van oude muizen" ("Senile Mouse Ovaries") by P. J. Thung (1958). Gradually this experimental gerontological research expanded, and in 1971 TNO decided to establish the independent Institute for Experimental Gerontology TNO at Rijswijk, closely connected with the Radiobiological Institute TNO and the Primate Center TNO. Director of the institute is Dr. C. F. Hollander, special professor (under the auspices of the Netherlands Society of Gerontology) in medical gerontology at the State University of Utrecht. This institute, with about twenty-five academic staff members, is widely known. Hollander succeeded in the special chair Dr. J. Th. R. Schreuder, an internist, who is considered the pioneer of clinical geriatrics in the Netherlands. Although much clinical geriatrics is being performed, particularly in nursing homes, still very little biogerontological and geriatric research is done in the medical schools. Geriatrics is, in spite of several attempts, not yet recognized as a medical specialty. As yet there is still only one special chair in medical gerontology. Thus medical (clinical) gerontological research is still very underdeveloped.

Research in the field of social gerontology has fared somewhat better. Although barely started fifteen to twenty years ago, a great number of studies of a psychological, sociological, sociomedical, evaluative, economic, and operational nature have been undertaken. Various larger studies have been undertaken or stimulated by the Gerontological Center at Nijmegen, a cooperative of a number of university departments and nonuniversity institutes. The director is Dr. J. M. A. Munnichs, a psychologist and lecturer in psychogerontology at the Catholic University of Nijmegen. Dr. Munnichs's thesis, "Ouderdom en eindigheid" (1964), which later appeared in English as "Old Age and Finitude, dealt with attitudes to finitude during old age. This was the first major research project in psychogerontology. At Nijmegen Catholic University an interdisciplinary social gerontology group is also being developed.

Another important thesis appeared in the same year. It was a study on "Intelligence and age, in adults and old people" (Verhage, 1964). It was performed on 1,621 subjects between 12 and 77 years of age, a representative sample of the Netherlands. One of the results was the development of the "Groningen Intelligence Test."

Two registers of social gerontological research have been published, one on the years 1945–1964 and one on the years 1965–1973. The first contained 149 reports on research and 36 on policy; the second 404 research reports and 94 policy reports. Although there has been an increase in the quantity of this type of research, the quality has not improved much.

During the last fifteen years or so, more than a hundred very small, often rather unscientific surveys have been undertaken on a local or regional level to measure the needs for various services and to learn more about attitudes (toward certain services, for example) and opinions of the aged, about their health, about nutritional habits, and other aspects of their life. Several of these studies have been carried out as scriptions (a smaller study than an academic thesis) of students of universities or "academies" for social work. (Social work is not a university discipline in the Netherlands.)

Apart from the Institute of Experimental Gerontology TNO (for biological research) and the Gerontological Center and the Guter Faculty Group at Nijmegen (primarily for sociogerontological research), there are only a few scattered nuclei of gerontological research; some are in the Department of Social Gerontology of the GITP (Communal Institute of Applied Psychology) at Nijmegen, the Department of Physiology of the Free University at Amsterdam, and the Department of Psychology at the State University of Utrecht and of Groningen. In 1977 the Amsterdam Institute for Gerontology was founded, but it has not undertaken any major research so far. Some clinical gerontology research is undertaken in a few hospital departments and in a few nursing homes.

In 1967 the state secretary for public health requested the Health Council to advise on the necessity of expanding gerontological research. A special committee, set up by the council for this purpose, advised in 1971 that much more research should be undertaken in all the major fields of gerontology. The report of this committee was finally published in 1973, but in the first years afterward the government did not do much with these recommendations or with the Council for Medical Scientific Research's statement in 1973 that far too little research was undertaken in the field of medical gerontology . Only recently has some more action by the government been undertaken; for example, some financial support has been given for the Netherlands Institute of Gerontology. At present it has only a staff of a director (an economist), temporarily a sociologist, and a secretary, and its main goal is fund raising and taking stock of and coordinating ongoing research. In 1978 the government established the Planning Group for Gerontological Research. This group, consisting on a tri-partite basis of government representatives, researchers, and "users of research," is to present in 1979 a national program for gerontological research, to be partially financed by the government. Furthermore because a majority in the Second Chamber (House of Representatives), when discussing the revised memorandum on policy for the aged (1975), requested more research, some more activity may be expected.

Education and Training

In the university departments, education in gerontology is still very scarce, although there are some promising developments. The medical faculty of the State University of Leiden has had a committee on geriatrics for several years, which has succeeded in including in the normal curriculum a one-week block of medical gerontology for third-year medical students and a one-week block of clinical geriatrics for fourth-year medical students. In addition, a special coordinator-gerontologist is to be appointed. At several other universities gerontology, although mostly also on a rather small scale, is included in the medical or psychological curriculum. A second special chair at the University of Amsterdam will probably be established soon, as well as a special chair on nursing home care at Nijmegen. The medical faculty at Maastricht is considering a chair in gerontology.

Practical problems in caring for the aged are dealt with more in the education and training of nurses (particularly district or public health nurses), social workers, and specifically of the *ziekenverzorgster* (a nursing aide with almost 2½ years of training), most of whom work in nursing homes. Also several ten thousand "Helpers for the aged," who work in residential homes and in the community, and home helpers have received special training in dealing with old people. Thus in the lower ranks of treatment and care givers, the situation regarding education and training in care of the aged is much more favorable than among university-trained professionals.

DEMOGRAPHY

Table 40 gives the population, in percentages, in 1975 and estimations for the future, by sex and age groups. The predictions are based on the assumption that the fertility pattern will be 10 percent below the replacement level. At the end of 1976, 636,000 men and 879,000 women (11.0 percent of the population) were 65 years and older. Seventy-four percent of the men but only 45 percent of the women were married. The percentage of old women who are married will further decrease in the years ahead.

In the year 2000, the Netherlands will have 1.95 million old people (12.8–13.7 percent), an increase of about 26 percent in twenty-five years. The very old (those 80 and over) will number 390,000 (increasing from 1.9 percent to 2.5 percent in the total population) in 2000. This means that they will form nearly 20 percent of all old people. The following conclusions can be drawn

Table 40: PRESENT AND FUTURE POPULATION (IN THOUSANDS AND IN PERCENT)

Age Group	Men				Women			
	1975	1985	2000	2020	1975	1985	2000	2020
0–19	2372	2259	2169	1988	2266	2158	2068	1895
20-34	1651	1757	1679	1590	1548	1689	1617	1528
35-64	2113	2497	3036	3135	2152	2455	2960	3134
65-69	230	231	276	387	282	287	323	455
70-74	174	186	206	325	230	263	288	427
75-79	115	127	145	181	165	206	244	269
80 and over	103	118	126	154	143	215	263	296
total	6758	7175	7637	7760	6796	7274	7963	8003
65 and over	622	662	754	1047	837	972	1117	1447
Age Group	**Men**				**Women**			
	1975	1985	2000	2020	1975	1985	2000	2020
0–19	35.1	31.5	28.4	25.6	33.3	29.7	26.6	23.6
20–34	24.4	24.4	22.0	20.5	22.8	23.2	20.8	19.1
35–64	31.3	34.8	39.8	40.4	31.7	33.8	38.1	39.2
65–69	3.4	4.6	3.6	5.0	4.1	3.9	4.2	5.7
70–74	2.6	2.6	2.7	4.2	3.4	3.6	3.7	5.3
75–79	1.7	1.8	1.9	2.3	2.4	2.8	3.1	3.4
80 and over	1.5	1.6	1.7	2.0	2.2	3.0	3.4	3.7
65 and over	9.2	9.2	9.9	13.5	12.2	13.4	14.4	18.1

Source: Central Bureau of Statistics. 1973. *The Future Development of the Dutch Population after 1972.* Voorburg.

from table 40 and from other statistical data (Report 13 of the State Committee on Population):

1. The aged will continue to increase absolutely and relatively in numbers (in 1900 there were only 308,000 old people, or 6.0 percent; in 1930, 484,000 and 6.2 percent; and so on).

2. Within the group of the aged, the very old (80 and over) are increasing relatively more than the old (65–80).

3. Women live longer than men.

4. There are more old women than old men.

5. There are more married old men than married old women.

6. The percentage of married old men will continue to increase and that of married old women to decrease.

7. More old men remarry than old women do;

8. Half of the old men are married to younger women; for old women this percentage is 10.

9. Among the very old there are very many unmarried old women (including widowed).

10. The mortality of married people is lower than that of unmarried people, a difference that decreases with increasing age.

One more demographic fact may be given here: the ratio between the so-called nonproductive group (0–19 and 65 and older) and the productive group (20–64) was 0.82 in 1975; it will be approximately 0.77 in 1985, 0.66 in 2000, and 0.67 in 2020. The nonproductive group was 45 percent of the total population in 1975; it will decrease to about 40 percent and then again increase to 42.5 percent.

The number of the aged is now about a third of the number of young people (0–19); in 2000 it will be three-sevenths. One can only guess about the impact of this development on manpower for the care of the aged.

Life expectancy data are given in table 41. From this table a few conclusions can be drawn. First, the life expectancy of men was, as in many other countries under similar conditions, decreasing because of the increase in mortality through accidents), cardiovascular diseases, and cancer, but it is now increasing slightly (through some decrease of fatal heart infarctions and accidents). Second, the life expectancy of women at various ages is still increasing slightly. And third, as a whole, the increase of life expectancy is almost negligible at the moment; it will only increase substantially if cardiovascular diseases and cancer are greatly reduced as causes of death.

Table 41: LIFE EXPECTANCY

Year	At Birth	At 1 Year	At 50 Years	At 65 Years	At 80 Years
Men					
1951–1955	70.9	71.7	25.8	14.1	5.8
1956–1960	71.4	71.8	25.7	14.1	5.9
1961–1965	71.1	71.4	25.3	14.0	6.0
1966–1970	71.0	71.1	24.9	13.7	6.2
1975	71.2	71.1	24.9	13.6	6.2
1976	71.5	71.4	24.9	13.5	6.2
Women					
1951–1955	73.5	74.0	27.4	14.9	6.1
1956–1960	74.8	75.0	28.1	15.4	6.2
1961–1965	75.9	75.9	28.8	16.0	6.6
1966–1970	76.4	76.3	29.2	16.4	6.8
1975	77.2	77.0	29.8	16.9	7.1
1976	78.0	77.7	30.4	17.4	7.4

Source: *Statistical Pocketbook 1978* (The Hague: Central Bureau of Statistics, 1978), p. 37.

The death rate in the Netherlands was 7.9 in 1977. Table 42 indicates the major causes of death among the aged. The largest killers are the same as in other countries. First are cardiovascular diseases (43 percent of all deaths, of which 54 percent occur in men and 84 percent occur after age 65). Second are malignant neoplasms (cancer) (25 percent of all deaths, of which 58 percent occur in men and 71 percent occur after the age of 65). Third are accidents, violence, and poisoning, and fourth are diseases of the respiratory tract.

Source: Pocket Yearbook 1978 (The Hague: Netherlands Central Bureau of Statistics, 1978), p. 47.

Table 42: MORTALITY BY CAUSE AND AGE

Cause of Death[a]	45–64 Years	65–74 Years	75 and Over	Total	Total of Male Population	Total Mortality per 100,000 Population
Total 1965	20,077	24,313	43,018	98,026	54,484	797.3
Total 1976	21,258	28,916	55,621	114,454	63,963	830.9
Infectious and parasitic diseases	139	137	269	736	401	5.4
Neoplasms	8,214	8,731	10,105	28,561	16,507	210.9
Endocrine, nutritional, and metabolic diseases	298	419	842	1,707	603	12.6
Diseases of blood and blood-forming organs	34	43	134	241	118	1.8
Mental disorders	95	111	444	786	367	5.8
Diseases of the nervous system and sense organs	328	363	449	1,481	819	10.9
Diseases of the circulatory system	7,813	13,015	27,654	49,430	26,565	364.9
Diseases of the respiratory system	799	1,555	4,050	6,693	4,287	49.4
Diseases of the digestive system	710	894	1,705	3,540	1,751	26.1
Diseases of the genitourinary system	222	451	1,425	2,179	1,259	16.1
				26		0.2
Diseases of the skin and subcutaneous tissue	9	9	85	109	32	0.8
Diseases of the musculoskeletal system and connective tissue	92	156	244	531	166	3.9
Congenital malformations	61	25	24	875	452	6.5
				1,059	605	7.8
Symptoms and ill-defined conditions	818	851	2,070	4,280	2,503	31.6
Accidents, poisonings, and violence	1,201	825	2,189	7,016	4,170	51.8

a. International Statist. Classification of Diseases, Injuries and Death Causes, 1965.

286

Today in the Netherlands 25 of every 100 who die do so between the ages of 65 and 75, and 49 do so after the age of 75.

Some trends can be discerned in these mortality patterns. Cardiovascular diseases are increasing in men between 30 and 55 years and after 65 years, and decreasing between 50 and 60 years (slightly); in women they are increasing between 20 and 45 years (a slight decrease between 40 and 45), and decreasing under 20 and above 45 years. Malignant neoplasms among men are increasing in the age group 5–20 years and over 50 years; among women, they are decreasing under 30 years, remaining steady between 30 and 70 years, and increasing after 70 years. Accidents are increasing among men and women in all age groups except men around 50 years.

A great number of old people (probably about 12,000 per year) die of cerebrovascular disease. Because death often occurs only after a prolonged time, a great many of these patients have to be treated and cared for in nursing homes.

Calculations made by the Central Bureau of Statistics indicate that it is expected that in 1980 about 22,300 men 65 and over and 18,200 women 65 and over will die of cardiovascular diseases and that 13,500 old men and 9,000 old women will die of cancer annually.

Since there is no existing single or continuous national health survey in the Netherlands, comparatively little is known about diseases and disability among the aged. A system of about fifty surveillance points (manned by general practitioners) is improving this situation somewhat gradually. A few surveys shed some light on this issue. First, the survey by van Zonneveld (1961) gives an idea about prevalent groups of diseases. Tables 43–46 give data respectively, on the frequency, by sex and five-year age groups, on the kind of principal affliction for which old people received their last medical treatment, for which a physician was regularly consulted, for which a specialist was consulted after the age of 65, and for which hospitalization occurred after the age of 65.

Cardiovascular and renal diseases were the principal affliction for which old people received their last treatment (19 to 33 percent), with a significantly higher percentage for women than men in all age groups with the exception of the group 80 to 84 years old. The group of ''other diseases'' followed (18–28 percent) with almost identical percentages for both sexes. The group of diseases of the respiratory system (excluding neoplasms and tuberculosis) was very important (12–24 percent), with the men leading significantly in all age groups but one.

Almost half of the men and women who saw a doctor regularly did so for cardiovascular and renal diseases. On this point there was no important difference between the sexes. Among the remaining groups of diseases for which a doctor was consulted regularly, there was none with remarkable frequency. Rheumatic afflictions took second place among women, and respiratory afflictions were second among men and third for women (table 44).

Table 43: KIND OF PRINCIPAL AFFLICTION FOR WHICH LAST MEDICAL TREATMENT WAS RECEIVED (IN PERCENT)

Age	Cardio-vascular and Renal Diseases	Malignant Neoplasms	Cerebral and Mental Diseases (Suicide), Apoplexy	Gastro-intestinal Diseases	Diseases of the Respiratory System	Tuber-culosis	Infectious Diseases	Prostate Complaints	Rheuma-tism	Diabetes	Other Diseases	Total Percent	Total Number
Men													
65–69	20.7	1.2	1.5	10.7	21.6	0.9	3.7	2.1	7.0	2.4	28.2	100	328
70–74	21.7	1.3	3.4	10.4	21.1	1.3	2.9	3.4	7.0	2.1	25.4	100	383
75–79	25.4	1.6	3.4	10.9	21.7		4.1	4.7	8.0	1.3	18.9	100	387
80–84	29.4	1.8	1.1	5.1	24.2	0.4	4.0	5.8	4.0	4.7	19.5	100	277
85 and over	19.1	4.6	3.1	8.4	19.8		3.8	8.4	3.8	0.8	28.2	100	131
Total	23.9	1.7	2.5	9.4	21.8	0.6	3.7	4.3	6.4	2.3	23.4	100	1,506
Women													
65–69	26.5	3.9	3.9	11.4	12.3	0.3	1.8		11.4	3.0	25.5	100	333
70–74	31.7	3.4	3.7	7.9	13.1	0.8	2.1		10.5	3.7	23.1	100	382
75–79	33.4	2.4	3.2	11.2	12.3		2.1		8.6	4.0	22.8	100	374
80–84	28.6	2.3	5.6	10.5	12.8	0.8	2.3		10.2	2.6	24.3	100	266
85 and over	29.4	3.3	5.3	7.3	24.0		4.0		4.7	4.0	18.0	100	150
Total	30.0	3.1	4.1	9.9	13.8	0.4	2.3		9.6	3.5	23.3	100	1,505

Source: Zonneveld, R. J. van. 1961. The health of the aged: An investigation into the health and a number of social and psychological factors concerning 3149 aged persons in the Netherlands, carried out by 374 general practitioners under the direction of the Organisation for Health Research TNO,* Assen: Royal van Gorcum, p. 68.

Table 44: GROUPS OF PRINCIPAL DISEASES FOR WHICH A PHYSICIAN WAS REGULARLY CONSULTED (IN PERCENT)

Ages	No Regular Consultations	Cardiovascular and Renal Diseases	Malignant Neoplasms	Cerebral and Mental (Suicide), Apoplexy	Gastrointestinal Diseases	Diseases of the Respiratory System	Infectious Diseases	Prostate Complaints	Rheumatism	Diabetes (only)	Other Diseases	Total Percent	Total Number
Men													
65–69	64.6	15.1	0.9	2.0	4.3	3.4		0.9	2.3	1.4	5.1	100	351
70–74	68.5	14.3	0.5	2.0	2.5	4.4	0.5	1.2	1.7	1.0	3.4	100	406
75–79	62.0	18.0	0.5	3.2	1.9	5.4	0.5	1.7	1.2	3.9	3.9	100	411
80–84	57.9	20.3	0.7	0.7	1.7	4.7	0.3	3.1	1.4	4.1	4.1	100	295
85 and over	59.2	13.1	2.9	0.7	2.2	7.3		2.9	2.2	7.3	7.3	100	137
Total	63.2	16.4	0.8	2.1	2.6	4.8	0.3	1.8	1.8	4.4	4.4	100	1,600
Women													
65–69	50.9	19.8	3.2	2.9	5.7	1.1	0.3		6.6	3.2	6.3	100	348
70–74	42.4	27.4	2.0	2.3	2.0	2.0	3.8		6.4	3.1	10.3	100	391
75–79	42.4	27.0	1.3	1.0	4.7	4.5			5.2	3.7	10.2	100	382
80–84	43.1	23.6	1.8	4.4	3.0	3.7	0.4		6.3	4.1	9.6	100	271
85 and over	47.3	23.7	2.6	6.6	2.0	5.3			4.6	2.6	5.3	100	152
Total	45.0	24.5	2.1	2.9	3.7	3.5	0.2		6.0	3.4	8.7	100	1,544

Source: Zonneveld, R. J. van. 1961. The health of the aged: An investigation into the health and a number of social and psychological factors concerning 3149 aged persons in the Netherlands, carried out by 374 general practitioners under the direction of the Organisation for Health Research TNO.* Assen: Royal van Gorcum, p. 69.

More women than men consulted a specialist after the age of 65, although the difference is less marked than might have been expected. The specialist was most often consulted for disorders in the category of cardiovascular and renal diseases, though the group of "other diseases" was much more important here than in the preceding case. This latter group, however, usually includes the consulting of an opthalmologist for eyeglasses. Men consulted a specialist for a prostate disorder in 4, 8, 13, 18 and 27 percent in the successive age groups (table 45).

Sixteen to 45 percent of the men and 21 to 40 percent of the women in the sample were admitted to a hospital one or more times. Age was an important factor. Those who had only recently reached 65 had much less chance of hospitalization than those who had long since passed this age. Not only may the younger aged have had less illness requiring hospitalization but they may also have had more possibility of being nursed elsewhere than in a hospital (table 46).

The data in these tables came from a nationwide survey. Some local surveys (Fuldauer, 1966; Tonino, 1969) or examinations done on old people admitted (or on waiting lists for admission) into hospitals (Welten, 1968) and nursing homes (Oostvogel, 1968; Merkus, 1974; Leering, 1968) give additional insight.

Van Zonneveld and Fennis in 1962 undertook large surveys on the health and chronic conditions in random samples of people over 40 years of age in a city (Leiden) and in a province (Friesland). Fennis (1973) worked out the data for the *aged* persons. According to the surveys, one patient in eight 65 years and over had suffered from a cardiovascular disease; one in five from a digestive disease; one in fourteen had become chronically ill due to an accident; and one in seventy a malignant tumor. The hospital statistics for 1968 give these ratios as 1:8, 1:7, 1:15, and 1:7, respectively, showing reasonably good agreement, with the exception of tumors.

In Leiden and ten rural municipalities of Friesland at least 15 percent of the aged indicated that they were suffering from one or more disorders with a disease duration of at least four weeks. Among old men in the city of Leiden, the prevalence of all chronic diseases (more than four weeks) in the age groups 65–69, 70–74, 75–79, and 80 and over was 15, 12, 14, and 16 percent; in the province of Friesland 13, 12, 13, and 13 percent. For women, prevalences in Leiden were 10, 15, 16, and 20 percent and in Friesland 14, 18, 20, and 21 percent.

The main causes of chronic diseases in men and women in Leiden and Friesland were (in order): diseases of the respiratory system, circulatory system, digestive system, and nervous system. Together they form 54 percent of all chronic diseases in Leiden and 56 percent in Friesland. In total 8 percent of the male aged and 10 percent of the female aged population of Leiden were suffering disabling diseases.

Table 45: GROUPS OF PRINCIPAL DISEASES FOR WHICH A SPECIALIST WAS CONSULTED (IN PERCENT)

Ages	No Consult-ations	Cardio-vascular and Renal Diseases	Malignant Neoplasms	Cerebral and Mental (Suicide), Apoplexy	Gastro-intestinal Diseases	Diseases of the Respiratory System	Infectious Disease	Prostate Complaints	Rheuma-tism	Diabetes	Other Diseases	Total Percent	Total Number
Men													
65–69	62.7	8.3	1.1	1.7	4.8	2.8	0.6	1.7	2.6	0.6	13.1	100	351
70–74	47.6	10.8	1.7	2.7	8.6	2.7	0.5	4.2	3.4	1.5	16.3	100	406
75–79	42.7	8.3	2.4	2.4	7.1	4.9	0.2	7.6	3.2	1.2	20.0	100	409
80–84	44.0	7.1	2.0	1.0	7.8	3.7	0.7	10.2	2.7	3.1	17.7	100	294
85 and over	44.2	2.2	4.3	0.7	5.1	2.2		15.2	2.2	1.4	22.5	100	138
Total	48.8	8.2	2.1	1.9	6.9	3.4	0.4	6.6	2.9	1.5	17.3	100	1,598
Women													
65–69	54.2	7.5	3.5	2.0	6.9	1.4	0.3		4.9	2.6	16.7	100	347
70–74	39.8	11.5	3.6	2.0	7.7	2.3	0.8		5.9	3.6	22.8	100	391
75–79	37.4	11.6	3.2	0.5	13.2	2.4	0.8		2.4	3.2	25.3	100	380
80–84	46.6	7.4	3.7	0.4	5.9	2.2			3.7	2.6	27.5	100	269
85 and over	50.0	4.6	2.0	2.6	7.9	1.3				2.0	29.6	100	152
Total	44.7	9.2	3.3	1.4	8.6	2.0	0.5		3.8	2.9	23.6	100	1,539

Source: Zonneveld, R. J. van. 1961. The health of the aged: An investigation into the health and a number of social and psychological factors concerning 3 149 aged persons in the Netherlands, carried out by 374 general practitioners under the direction of the Organisation for Health Research TNO.* Assen: Royal van Gorcum, p. 71.

Table 46: GROUPS OF PRINCIPAL DISEASES FOR WHICH HOSPITALIZATION OCCURRED (IN PERCENT)

Age	No Hospital-izations	Cardio-vascular and Renal Diseases	Malignant Neoplasms	Cerebral and Mental (Suicide), Apoplexy	Gastro-intestinal Diseases	Diseases of the Respiratory System	Infectious Diseases	Prostate Complaints	Rheuma-tism	Diabetes	Other Diseases	Total Percent	Total Number
Men													
65–69	83.9	3.7	0.9	0.9	2.0	1.1	0.3	1.4	0.6	0.9	4.3	100	351
70–74	70.8	5.2	1.5	1.2	5.4	2.5	0.7	3.4	0.7	0.5	8.1	100	407
75–79	63.0	4.1	2.0	1.0	6.1	2.4	0.2	7.1	0.7	0.7	12.7	100	410
80–84	55.5	3.7	1.0	0.7	7.5	1.4	0.7	12.2	0.3	1.4	15.6	100	295
85 and over	58.0	1.4	2.2	0.7	8.0	2.2		13.8	0.7	1.4	11.6	100	138
Total	68.0	4.0	1.4	0.9	5.4	1.9	0.4	6.4	0.6	0.9	10.1	100	1,601
Women													
65–69	79.5	3.2	2.0	0.9	4.3	0.6	0.3		1.1	0.6	7.5	100	348
70–74	66.6	4.8	3.6	1.5	4.8	2.6	0.5		1.3	1.8	12.5	100	392
75–79	59.9	6.6	3.2	0.5	11.1	1.8	0.8		0.8	1.8	13.5	100	380
80–84	64.0	4.1	3.0	0.7	7.0	1.5			0.4	1.9	17.4	100	380
85 and over	63.1	2.6	2.0	2.0	6.6	2.0	1.3			0.7	19.7	100	152
Total	67.2	4.5	2.9	1.0	6.8	1.7	0.5		0.8	1.4	13.2	100	1,542

Source: Zonneveld. R. J. van. 1961. The health of the aged: An investigation into the health and a number of social and psychological factors concerning 3149 aged persons in the Netherlands. carried out by 374 general practitioners under the direction of the Organisation for Health Research TNO.* Assen: Royal van Gorcum, p. 72.

To an old person, how he feels is especially important. In the nationwide survey (van Zonneveld 1961) the large majority of the subjects examined (78 percent of the men and 64 percent of the women) thought that they were in good health. With increasing age, the percentage of those who subjectively rated themselves as healthy dropped only slightly. In almost every age group, significantly more women than men complained about their state of health. It is possible that the generation to which these oldest individuals belong did not find it proper to complain or to admit that there was anything wrong with their health, which might imply helplessness. The percentage of the aged who found their own health poor was very small—2 percent for men and 4 percent for women. That of women rose somewhat in the successive age groups. These percentages are only a little lower than in a survey on the health status and needs of three thousand old people performed in Groningen in the 1950s (van Zonneveld, 1954).

These data are not to be considered entirely accurate, but they give an impression on the amount of disease and disability among the aged in the Netherlands. It seems probable that these numbers will not differ greatly from those in adjacent countries. They demonstrate once again that chronic disease and disability are relatively prevalent among old people, and the more so with increasing age. More old women than old men have chronic diseases and disability. The practical implications of these demographic and morbidity data are clear: aged women need more medical provisions than aged men do, and the need for these provisions increases progressively with age in women more than in men.

ROLES AND STATUS OF THE AGED

In the media and in many reports and speeches, it is stressed time and again that the aged form an integral part of the Dutch population, that they should not be segregated or discriminated against, and that they should be supported in any conceivable way to remain independent (or to regain independency). In practice, though, in spite of this lip-service, old people often do not have much voice in general matters or in matters concerning themselves.

In general it appears that attitudes toward the elderly in the Netherlands, as in other countries under similar circumstances, are theoretically rather positive but often rather negative in practice. Few tasks are entrusted to the aged, with a consequence that they can claim few rights on income and prestige. Since the provisions often needed cannot be paid for by the aged in low-income groups (and that is the great majority), they have to become dependent on their social environment, which leads to stereotyping.

In general it is doubted that many old people have a secure place in the family. A practical reason is that much new housing offers too little space for an old father and/or mother to provide both themselves and their children and grandchildren sufficient privacy. The general tendency is for young parents to want to live alone with their children, and—partly perhaps as a reaction—the oldest generation finds privacy a great asset. In fact, in Holland only 5 to 10 percent of all people over 65 still are living together with children and/or grandchildren. Nevertheless there is much contact between the generations— the so-called extended family relations can very often be found—though the tendency to listen to the advice of aged relatives is certainly much less prevalent than half a century ago.

In the community in general, the roles and status of the aged are usually not important. On many boards, after a certain age (65 or 70), the old person has to step out. This was even so in some political parties rather recently. The old are considered to be unable to keep in step with developments in modern society. Only recently (1976) the Central Committee Homes for the Aged has published a report in which it advises that the residents of such homes should have the right (ensured by law) to organize a committee of residents, which should have some sort of authority. The board and the committee of residents should consult each other and the residents should have a right to participate on the board itself. In many old-age homes, this situation already exists, but in far more it does not, or only in a small degree. In recent years in a few old-age homes, the residents have insisted on more rights and participation in matters of policy regarding their home through "occupation" of the building.

On the other hand, quite a few important positions are kept by people over 65. There is also a growing tendency to provide old people with more informa- tion, with more financial means, and with other facilities to enable them to participate more fully. The general policy of the government is to encourage and enable old people to go on living independently as long as medically and socially possible in their own environment and participating fully in social life.

With regard to employment, aging and old aged persons contribute very little. The age of retirement is still fixed for men and women at 65, with a few exceptions for lower or higher ages. In reality, however, hundred of thousands quit their job earlier than 65 through the channel of the Disablement Insurance Act. In spite of this, investigations have shown that many aging and old people have problems in retiring or being retired, among them the loss of status and prestige and the loss of social contacts. Preretirement courses are partly geared to help the aging to cope with such problems.

The tendency is to lower the retirement age. Many, especially labor unions, advocate it as a way to lower unemployment among younger people in spite of the claim that everybody should be entitled to choose his own retirement age, even if it is higher than 65. The changing attitude toward the value of gainful work will perhaps ease the position of the retired in that prestige and role will not be so linked with being gainfully employed.

A few words should be added with regard to the role and status of aging members of minority groups. Although there are various minority groups from several parts of the world living in Holland, a distinction should be made between those who came to the Netherlands with the expectation to live there until death and those who came (and come) to work temporarily and then return to their homeland. These latter migrants offer no great problems with regard to aging and old age, at least at the present, because most leave Holland before old age. Among those who expect to stay (such as most people from the South Moluccas, Surinam, and the Dutch Antilles) extra problems may arise when growing old. In general, little is known about this issue because little research has been done in this field. However, problems in this regard may be less because many of these people still live in the traditional way as in their original countries. That may signify that the minority old have a somewhat more respected role and status than old Dutchmen. But for some who have lived twenty-five to thirty years in Holland, serious problems now arise since their children, born and raised in Holland, no longer listen to their parents, who then lose even more contact because they have few encounters with aging Dutch people.

PROBLEMS OF THE AGED

Health Care

In 1970–1971, one in seven patients discharged from general (acute) hospitals was 65 and over; in 1969 one in four patients in general hospitals was 65 or over; in 1972 almost one in three patients in mental hospitals was 65 or over. It is estimated that the general practitioner spends 30 to 40 percent of his time on the aged; for district nurses this percentage may sometimes be between 50 and 60. Both the processes of aging and the increasing rate of long-term and chronic diseases as the years go by in old age have brought with them many problems of how to cope with long-term disease. Examples of such problems follow:

1. General hospitals are not suited for and are too expensive for treatment and care of long-term patients, of whom the aged form by far the greater part.
2. Mental hospitals often can do relatively little for old people.
3. Medical doctors, nurses, and physiotherapists are insufficiently educated and trained for long-term treatment and for care of the aged.
4. The costs for treating and caring for the elderly sick are soaring.
5. The reservoir of manpower for caring for the aged sick and invalid is decreasing because of the falling birthrate.
6. Although Holland has a high rate of social welfare, the attitudes of many people toward long-term disease and disability, particularly among the aged, form a constraint to proper care.
7. There is still far too little knowledge of the process of aging and the etiology and natural history of many long-term diseases, so we do not know how to prevent these ailments and how to treat them adequately.

Nutrition

Surveys have demonstrated that nutrition and the nutritional state of old people in Holland is no great problem. Of course, there are a number of related problems among the aged in this respect—the state of their teeth or dentures and their apathy may result in not cooking and consuming adequate food, for example, and may lead to such problems as anemia and osteoporosis.

Housing

Accommodation of the elderly has become a major problem as the aged have increased so quickly in number over the past forty years. The attitudes of the young toward keeping their parents with them has changed, and the income of the aged has often remained too low to allow for better housing. Also the migration of young people to the suburbs or small towns away from the old city or from the loosely populated rural areas, the increased traffic, the decline in goods delivered at home, and the insufficient and inadequate facilities in the older houses make housing of the elderly a major problem.

Transportation

Although public transport is relatively well developed in the Netherlands, it is a problem for quite a few old people because of high costs, difficulty of access to buses and railway carriages, density of traffic, and the fact that only a few old people have a car and can drive. In certain areas public transport is diminishing its services also.

Inactivity

Physical, mental, and social inactivity may cause such problems as the promotion of disease, disability, immobility, fewer contacts, fewer interests, loneliness, isolation, demotivation, and disengagement. It is difficult to say how many old people and in what degree and for which aspects inactivity is a major problem.

PROGRAMS FOR THE AGED

Institutions

Between about 1945 and 1965, many people believed that putting old people in institutions was a good solution. This attitude is changing, yet many institutions have been built.

General (acute) hospitals have not changed much, at least with a view toward the rapidly increasing number of long-term and/or aged patients. Whether general hospitals should have a special geriatric department is still a controversial issue. Although many new hospitals have been built since World War II and several had plans for such departments, only four or five general hospitals have geriatric wards where certain old sick people are examined and treated, but only for a relatively short time.

Because of the unsuitability of acute general hospitals for long-term care and their disinterest in this respect, and the circumstance that so many old people could not be treated and cared for either by their own family or in residential homes, the nursing home system was developed. A few nursing homes existed before the war (called rest houses then), mostly on a profit-making basis and offering very little else than nursing. The modern nursing home increased rapidly after the introduction in 1968 of the Exceptional Medical Expenses Compensation Act (AWBZ). This law provides the financing of treatment in a recognized nursing home from the very first day if this is considered necessary.

After 1955 a few specially designed nursing homes for mentally disordered old people came into existence. At the moment the prevailing idea is that a combined nursing home may offer the best solution, provided that the units for the physically and for the mentally impaired patients are separated. At the end of 1978 more than 300 recognized nursing homes with over 43,700 beds existed. Thus per 1,000 inhabitants there were 3.1 beds (as compared to 5.4 beds in general hospitals and 1.8 beds in mental hospitals). Ninety-seven percent of these beds were occupied throughout the entire year. At the end of 1978, there were 155 recognized nursing homes (18,600 beds) for the physically sick, 70 for the mentally sick (10,300 beds), and 72 combined homes (14,800 beds). Of the patients in nursing homes (in 1972), 17.4 percent were under 63 years old, and 42 percent were older than 78 years. In 1972, 57 percent of the inpatients had already spent more than a year in the nursing home.

A nursing home for physically ill old people is an institution for patients who do not need continuous medical specialist care but who do need expert medical treatment, continuous nursing, and general care, usually following examination and treatment in a general hospital.

The Netherlands clearly needs an institution that is between the hospital and the residential home in terms of care. According to extensive surveys undertaken by the author and in collaboration with others in the Netherlands, there exists a need for nursing home beds for the physically ill for 2 percent of the aged, and for about 1.5 percent who are somewhat less than moderately confused. Perhaps these percentages are on the high side, but it is clear that a good system of nursing homes of the three types will relieve general and mental hospitals of an important part of the burden of long-term care of chronic sick and disabled old people. Nursing homes also serve as final stations for those who remain chronically ill and disabled, cannot be cared for elsewhere, and stay until their death. Long-stay wings therefore form part of the nursing home.

Another absolute necessity is that nursing homes have strong formal functional relations with general and/or mental hospitals and also with a number of old people's homes. Unfortunately only in a minority of cases are these bonds already ensured. There is, however, a growing tendency in several cities to have or to create central referral systems so that each patient is referred to the appropriate institution. From an organizational point of view, hospitals, nursing homes, day hospitals, outpatient clinics, health and welfare clinics or service centers, and possibly residential homes and the whole array of extramural services should form one system of care. Such a system could very well serve other age groups, particularly the chronic sick and the disabled among them.

The term nursing home is not appropriate. A major function of this institution is to bring sick and disabled old people back to normal community life. Several nursing homes in Holland therefore are also called *geriatric clinics* or *reactivation centers*. The size of these institutions is on an average of 120 beds for the physically impaired, 135 for the mentally impaired, and 205 if they are combined homes.

In mental hospitals, of which about 30 percent of the inmates are older than 64, psychogeriatric departments often can be found. Community psychogeriatric and social services are gradually developing, and in a few provinces a complete service already exists.

Concerning the training and education of health personnel, in some professions more progress is made than in others. Medical education still offers very few specific subjects in gerontology and geriatrics; as indicated earlier. Often general practitioners are required to have worked for two months in a nursing home. The fact that geriatrics is not recognized as a proper medical specialty undoubtedly impedes the development and integration of more specific training in the fields of gerontology and geriatrics and of long-term care. There are two one-year postgraduate courses for nursing home physicians, of whom there are now about five hundred.

The education and training of registered nurses includes more topics in geriatrics and gerontology, and there are a few specific courses on gerontology for hospital and district nurses. Nurses in nursing homes have a regular inservice program.

Nurses' aides are specifically trained for working with the aged and long-term sick in a formal nearly 2½-year educational program in the nursing homes themselves. In 1977, the number of registered nursing personnel (nurses and nurses' aides) in nursing homes was nearly thirteen thousand, while another twelve thousand were in training. In somatic nursing homes in 1974, the ratio was one nursing person per 1.8 patients; in psychiatric nursing homes it was one per 1.7 patients. Fewer than half of these were registered nurses. This figure shows the very important position of the nurses' aides in the care of the aged sick and long-term ill.

In residential homes, in addition to an occasional registered nurse and a few registered nurses' aides, qualified care providers for the aged and helpers for the aged work. (They also often work in domiciliary care.) Before 1973 about 3,900 care providers (or care-rendering persons) and 7,600 old people's aides were qualified. At the end of 1973, about 9,200 qualified aides of both professions were working in residential homes. These figures illustrate the fact that much emphasis is laid on the formal education and training of these personnel for the care of the aged.

The domiciliary care-rendering persons and home helpers are important. Both have formal training, although for part-time helpers it is rather minimal. In 1979 about eighty thousand part-time home helpers were working in domiciliary care for the aged. Volunteers are also important; they receive five to ten half-days of information and lectures. In the period 1969–1973 about seven hundred courses for home helpers for the aged were organized, with about twenty-five people (almost always women) attending each course. In the education and training of other professionals such as physiotherapists, occupational therapists, and social workers, some specific attention is also given to the problems of old age.

As a whole, in certain fields of care of the aged (particularly intramural), it is expected that perhaps fewer personnel may be needed in the future (because the official policy is to reduce this type of care). Yet a serious problem may be expected with regard to those who fill these occupations since the number of women willing and able to do such work will probably not increase much, and in some instances it will even decrease. Men are still rather rare in these professions.

Mention should be made of the residential, or care-rendering homes. These old-age homes are intended for people who cannot cope on their own, particularly with regard to housekeeping. In the beginning of 1979 there were already more than 1,700 nonprofit homes with nearly 140,000 beds available, almost exclusively used by people 65 and over. Homes run for profit had about 8,000 beds. The former figure means that nearly 10 percent of old people in the Netherlands are living in this type of institution. This percentage is higher than in any other country and double that in Great Britain and the Federal Republic of Germany. The government's policy is to bring back this percentage to 7, allowing for certain areas (particularly the biggest cities) to have a higher percentage. To limit the influx to these homes, various scoring-systems have been introduced (for such indicators as physical disability and loneliness). Since 1977, each admission into each home (with the exception of the few that do not receive any public financing) must be considered by a small advisory committee, including a physician and a social worker. These so-called indication committes are not yet operational everywhere, however. The limitation enforced by the government is partly induced by the enormous costs involved.

More than 80 percent, and in some regions even 95 percent, of the inmates of residential homes receive general assistance support from local authorities because they cannot pay the full cost (on an average betwwen Dfls. 1800–2200 per month) out of their state old-age and other retirement pensions.

Medical care in the old-age homes (in which each person or couple has a private room and toilet) is provided by the family doctor, or, as is increasingly the case, by a general practitioner who acts part time as the house physician. These homes often provide some limited nursing care in addition.

Domiciliary Care

Both from the point of view that old people should stay in their own environment as long as medically and socially possible and that the soaring costs of care of the aged should be reduced, heavy emphasis is laid on community care. This means that various domiciliary services have to be expanded and in fact have been during the past ten years. But the government now seeks to reduce the costs in this area too. In the meantime, many services have been developed; the most important are homemaking assistance and the service centers. Both are not exclusively directed to the aged, but the majority of help is going to this population group. Homemaking assistance is available from home helpers who generally provide three or four hours of care a day for two or three days per week.

The development of service centers is strongly supported by the government through encouragement and financial contributions to the local authorities. The center provides social and recreational activities, meals, chiropody, gymnastics, and bathing, and it organizes home-help services. In 1979, there were about two hundred such centers and, in addition, two hundred so-called projects for coordinated work for the aged (small service centers). This number should be doubled in a few years.

Health care of the aged forms only part of the total care for many old people. The interrelationship of the various services to be provided is increasingly acknowledged, and this led in 1977 to the establishment of a so-called platform for integrated services for the aged. Although the emphasis is on extramural care, relations with intramural services are also taken into consideration.

Two other problems connected with health care will not be solved in the near future: changing the attitudes of many people toward the aged and toward long-term illness and overcoming the great lack of knowledge about processes of aging and diseases in old age. The mass media often devote attention to old-age problems, conferences and meetings are organized, and the societies of old people do their best to improve the situation, but clearly this process is very lengthy. More emphasis is gradually laid on drawing attention to the various aspects of aging beginning with children in schools.

The lack of knowledge is certainly not a unique Dutch problem, but geron-tological research in Holland is in general scarce and not well coordinated. Particularly research in clinical gerontology needs to be stimulated. Attempts are underway for more coordination, but financial and scientific support is often quite insufficient.

Nutrition

Large problems do not exist in nutrition. Financial problems in general are not the most important in this respect, although for those old people with the lowest income, the prices of certain food items (such as meat and fresh fruit) may be prohibitive. If special diets are considered necessary, the extra costs may be met by general assistance, although the situation can be improved. Nutrition programs include regular information through the Information Bureau on Nutrition, by the media, in lectures to old-age clubs, at service centers, and other organizations; and the provision of hot, nutritionally well-balanced meals in service centers, in day-nursing homes, or by meals-on-wheels services. The latter are used only by 2 or 3 percent of the aged population. Quite often home helps assist in or perform shopping and cooking. In addition certain fortified food components are provided to the elderly, as are dental care for teeth and dentures.

Housing

In 1963 the Old People's Homes Act came into force. It contains a large number of provisions to which residential homes have to conform and gives the provincial authority responsibility for supervising the implementation of these provisions. This work is done by special inspectors. The provisions not only concern the accommodational facilities and care but also the prices. The act also has a so-called notification duty. Everyone who runs an old people's home must notify the local authorities. This registration enables a higher standard of supervision. The Old People's Homes Act comes into force as soon as the building is in use and more than four elderly persons are housed in it.

Regulations for the actual building of old people's homes belong—as far as subsidized building is concerned—to the Ministry of Housing and Physical Planning. An old people's home is looked upon not merely as a form of housing but as a permanent replacement of the old person's living environment. The care thus should be geared to both material and nonmaterial needs. For this care, society bears a special responsibility. Therefore this kind of home, forming part of the social and welfare services, comes under the Ministry of Cultural Affairs, Recreation and Social Welfare.

In 1972 an important amendment to the act took place. The three major issues were the obligation for planning number, size, and distribution of these homes; rules for a greater voice for the aged residents themselves in the boards of the homes; the promotion of a general policy regulating supply and demand of placement (admission only on specified medical and/or social indication, checked by a small committee with as members at least a physician and a social worker); and the setting up of a Central Committee on Homes for the Aged, which provides a legal foundation for the consultations between government and the various organizations in this field.

Much attention is also paid to housing the aged in special small dwellings, often built in groups and with special equipment (for example, these dwellings are often connected with alarm systems to persons who may provide care in case of emergency and thus provide sort of sheltered housing). At the end of 1974 there were about 120,000 dwellings of this sort in which about 13 percent of all old people were living. The goal is for this percentage to be 25 by 1985. In addition many houses are adapted so that old people can remain in them. Financial support for adaptation is given by central and local authorities. Part of the specific dwellings are built as so-called service flats that include the services of a caretaker, hot meals, domiciliary care for cleaning, and communal meeting rooms. About 1 percent of the aged live in such service flats or service dwellings. Generally they have to be bought and are rather expensive.

Transportation

Rather much emphasis is laid on reducing impediments for the aged in transportation to keep them integrated in society as much as possible. One measure is the provision of cheap public transport. Passport 65+ entitles the bearer to travel for half-fare on local transport; the state railways (which handle also a great deal of interlocal bus services) also charge half-fare for bearers of a card, which can be obtained at a low price. Education (so far only in small numbers) is designed for groups of old people to help them walk safely; and attempts are being made to help younger people be more considerate of invalid and/or old traffic-participants. Other measures are to make certain streets, particularly cross-over places, safer; to provide more motorized wheelchairs; and to make public transport more accessible to old and invalid people.

Social Activities

With a view to keep the aged integrated in society, it is considered of great importance to keep old people physically, mentally, and socially active to prevent their isolation and loneliness. Particularly with regard to physical mobility, but also for mental activity and social contacts, much information is given for gymnastics by old people and in general to promote other motoric activities. An organizational structure, More Moving for the Elderly, is now in development. There are quite a few clubs (in or at service centers, health centers, and homes for the aged, among others) where certain gymnastic exercises are done under guidance and that promote folk dancing, walking, swimming, and other activities.

To promote mental and social activities, an important measure has been the introduction of Passport 65+. About a million old people (70 percent of the population) hold this card, which entitles them (besides reduced public transport fares) to participate at a reduced price in a variety of sociocultural activities—theater, cinema, folk dancing, study of nature, angling, general recreational activities, public libraries, holidays in special centers, and so on.

Activity is also promoted by various activities initiated and organized by the societies for old people in numerous centers and clubs for the aged (often these are also open to younger people) and by groups that organize short or longer holidays for the aged in Holland and abroad. An interesting example is the choir of old people. There exist many such choirs (more than forty), which have also annual competitions.

Finances

The social security program pays a basic old-age pension (equal to the official minimum wage and increasing with rising price indexes) to virtually all residents over the age of 65. Health insurance is available for about 80 percent of the aged (those under a certain level of income). The other 20 percent have private insurance, often at reduced prices.

RESEARCH

There exists in the Netherlands a great need for knowledge about natural and pathological processes in aging and old age and in the various aspects of being old. Relatively little has been done from a scientific approach. With the exception of a few specific research centers for gerontology, only scattered investigations are taking place.

In commission of the Minister of Science Policy and on behalf of the Planning Group for Gerontological Research, the Netherlands Institute for Gerontology made an inventory in 1977 of gerontological research (in the natural, behavioral, and the social sciences) in the Netherlands. The results were published in April 1978 (Nederlands Instituut voor Gerontologie, 1978). It appeared that about 71 man-years were devoted to ongoing research in gerontology: about 30 man-years in behavioral and social research, about 23 man-years in biological and biomedical research, and about 18 man-years in clinical research. In total about 160 different academic researchers were involved, most of them on a part-time basis. The medical faculties devoted 0.4 percent and the psychological and sociological faculties 1.0 percent of all their man-years for research to gerontological research.

Biomedical

Beginning in the 1950s, a few investigators in The Netherlands Cancer Institute (Amsterdam) were financially supported by the Organization for Applied Health Research TNO to undertake experimental research in aging and old rats and mice. In 1966 TNO financed the establishment of a special research unit for this type of research (under the leadership of Dr. C. F. Hollander), which entered into a relationship with the Radiobiological Institute TNO and the Primate Center at the same site in Rijswijk.

In 1971 the unit became the Institute for Experimental Gerontology TNO and since then has carried on the major part of biological research on aging in the Netherlands. Its scientific staff includes about twenty researchers from such disciplines as medicine, pathology, immunology, electron microscopy, biology, chemistry, and psychology. The research program of the institute includes the following main subjects:

1. Studies on phenomena of organ aging (particularly of the liver) in rats.
2. Research on the relationship between aging and disease. In this, a picture of the whole spectrum of bladder carcinoma in rats could be obtained, and it appeared to be identical to that observed in man.
3. Investigations on age-related changes in the immune system in man and animals (mice).
4. Studies on the late effects of various kinds of ionizing radiations, especially with regard to the induction of tumors and degenerative lesions, in particular breast cancer in rats.

Particularly in 1978 the Institute produced a number of important Ph.D. theses (Blankwater, 1978; Bezooijen, 1978; Burek, 1978; Kruisbeek, 1978—all in English).

Only one other major laboratory in the Netherlands is involved in this kind of research: the Laboratory for Physiology (directed by Prof. Dr. A. A. Knoop) of the Free University in Amsterdam. Its research program concerns investigations into the cardiovascular and respiratory systems, with emphasis on basic research, on pathophysiology, and on the influence of physical exercise. A special group of three scientists has been engaged in a study of the aging aspects of the cardiovascular system. These studies are performed on rats and human volunteers as well as on isolated blood vessels, which are obtained from animals or humans after necropsy. Important parameters studied are the distensibility of arteries and impedance.

In several other university and nonuniversity laboratories and institutes, studies on biological aging are also performed, but often on a minor scale, and they may be labeled atherosclerosis research or connective tissue research rather than gerontological research.

Medical

Medical gerontology in the Netherlands emphasizes a more scientific approach to the medical aspects of aging and as such is to be distinguished from geriatrics, which applies to the more practical activities with respect to health and disease in the aging and the aged. Medical gerontology is an underdeveloped field in this country. Only one handbook in Dutch (ed. van Zonneveld) is devoted to this topic, and few articles on clinical and biomedical research on aging appear in the relevant journals. There is also a Dutch handbook for nursing aides. This is another indication that in the biomedical and clinical institutes relatively little research is done in this scientific field. So far only one special chair in (medical) gerontology has been established (in the medical faculty of Utrecht University).

Medical gerontological and geriatric research is undertaken on a small scale in a number of hospitals (in general departments of general medicine and sometimes those of neurology or psychiatry) and somewhat more in the four or five hospitals with geriatric departments (such as the Slotervaart Ziekenhuis in Amsterdam and the Zonnestraal Ziekenhuis in Hilversum). These studies concern mainly practical clinical problems. About fifteen to twenty original books, monographs, and theses in Dutch are devoted to geriatrics, as are a number of articles in the quarterly *Nederlands Tijdschrift voor Gerontologie* ("Netherlands Journal of Gerontology"). In other medical journals, occasionally an article on research in the medical, clinical, or sociomedical field of aging and old age can be found. These articles rather often stem from observations or investigations in nursing homes.

In addition about ten books on geriatrics are available in Dutch, mostly translated from British or American texts.

Several sociomedical surveys, mostly of a small, local character but sometimes also of a regional or even nationwide character, have been undertaken in the past twenty years to provide insight into the demands of elderly sick people and the needs for care-rendering persons or organizations. Almost all of these have been described rather extensively in the two registers of social gerontological research in Holland.

Psychology

Psychological research is being undertaken at scattered psychological institutes of universities, in some psychogeriatric departments of mental hospitals, and in a few large nursing homes for mentally disordered old people. Emphasis is given to develop and evaluate tests to rate the mental, psychosocial, and psychophysical capacities of old people. Also various sorts of treatment are developed and evaluated.

The major psychogerontological research nucleus is found in the Institute of Psychology, which has its own unit for this kind of scientific studies, at the University of Nijmegen, and at the Gerontological Center and Guter Faculty Group associated with it. Various problems are studied there, such as attitudes toward old age and aged persons, isolation and disengagement of the elderly, stereotypes on aging, attitudes toward finitude of life and death, retirement, displacement of elderly people, psychosocial problems in nursing homes, family relations, and needs and demands of certain categories of old people. For some years a longitudinal study has been under way.

Sociology

Sociological studies are very scarce, unless one counts the many small studies of a purely local and descriptive character to measure needs and demands of the aged for certain services (mostly directed at obtaining figures for accommodation or services of various kinds). At the Gerontological Center and Guter Faculty Group, and the GITP Department of Social Gerontology in Nijmegen a relatively large amount of attention is paid to sociological and social research.

Economics

In the field of economics, research is very scarce on old people. There are some macroeconomic investigations as to the financial impact of various social security provisions and social services, as well as studies on the budget on which several socioeconomic classes of old people live.

International Research

In terms of international research, the center in Nijmegen has participated in a few cross-national investigations (one is on retirement problems in certain professions), as has the Institute for Experimental Gerontology at Rijswijk; a small number of foreign scientists have come to Holland to perform gerontological work (at the Institute of Experimental Gerontology and the Gerontological Center, for example); and Dutch experts are relatively often invited to participate in or to organize seminars, working groups, and study conferences of the World Health Organization, European Economic Community, Organization for Economic Co-operation and Development, and the IAG European Social Research Committee, among others. In 1961 the Netherlands organized the Third European Geriatrics Congress. At international gerontological congresses generally quite a number of Dutch people participate.

INFORMATION SOURCES

Information on gerontological activities and on care of the aged can be obtained at several places. Some follow.

- Experimental (biological) research: Institute for Experimental Gerontology TNO, Lange Kleiweg 151, Rijswijk.
- Social gerontology: Gerontological Center, Oude Kleefsebaan 10, Berg en Dal, Nijmegen; Institute of Psychology, Erasmuslaan 16, Nijmegen; and Department of Social Gerontology, GITP, Oude Kleefsebaan 10, Nijmegen.
- General information on research (in particular longitudinal research) and education of medical students and care of the aged and chronic sick: Dr. R. J. van Zonneveld, c/o Bureau Council for Health Research TNO, Juliana van Stolberglaan 148, The Hague.
- Policy on the aged, documentation of various sorts of care of the aged, and legal regulations: Netherlands Federation for Policy on the Aged, Eisenhowerlaan 142, The Hague (the federation brings together all private national bodies involved in care of the aged); Ministry of Culture, Recreation and Social Welfare (Department of Old Age Care), Steenvoordelaan 370, Rijswijk; Ministry of Public Health and Environmental Hygiene (with regard to medical provisions such as hospitals and nursing homes), Dokter Reijersstraat 12, Leidschendam; and Ministry of Social Affairs (on social security, pension systems, and employment), Zeestraat 73, The Hague.
- Netherlands Hospital Council (section on nursing homes), Oudlaan 4, Utrecht.
- Bouwcentrum (International Research Center on building, planning, designing, and constructing residential homes, nursing homes, sheltered housing, and similar residences), Weena 170, Rotterdam.
- Central Bureau of Statistics (the departments of Population Statistics and Health Statistics are relevant), Prinses Beatrixlaan 248, Voorburg.

SUMMARY

The Netherlands belongs to those countries that have a percentage of 10 or more of old people in their population. This means that various problems and programs regarding old age in this country are often not so different from those in other countries with similar conditions. Yet Holland has a number of somewhat unique features with respect to the so-called problems of old age—a relatively low percentage of old people (11.2); a centuries' old tradition of care for certain groups of old people; the very important role of private organizations; the expanded system of nursing homes for both physically and mentally impaired old people; the almost complete financial coverage of long-term disease treatment and care; the high rate of institutionalization; and the great variety and availability of extramural services in old-age homes.

Gerontological research is still rather underdeveloped. A few good exceptions are experimental gerontology and certain aspects of social gerontology.

In clinical gerontology great insufficiencies exist, though in sociomedical gerontology, many major surveys have been undertaken.

The role of the aged in society should be promoted and greatly expanded. Major problems of the aged concern their rather low status, their health, their social isolation, and a relative lack of sociocultural activities. To meet these problems, a great number of social security provisions and health and social care programs have been established.

REFERENCES

Beek, A., and Zonneveld, R. J. van. 1976. *Health in progressive old age.** The Hague: Gezondheidsorganisatie TNO.

———. 1973. Investigation on the longevity of old people with the use of the Longevity Quotient.* *Nederlands Tijdschrift voor Gerontologie* 4: 150.

———. Longitudinal research into the health status in an old-age home.* *Tijdschrift voor Sociale Geneeskunde* 46 (1968), 854, 996; 47 (1969) 22, 542, 566, 602, 634, 685, 722; 50 (1972), 306.

Bezooijen, C. F. A. van. 1978. Cellular basis of liver aging studied with isolated hepatocytes. Thesis, Utrecht.

Blankwater, M. J. 1978. Ageing and the humoral immune response in mice. Thesis, Utrecht.

Braadbaart, S., and Spruyt, O. 1977. *Reactivation of the aged.** 2d ed. Leiden: Stafleu.

Burek, J. D. 1978. Pathology of aging rats. Thesis, Utrecht.

Burger, A. K. C. 1971. A general somatic and electrocardiographic investigation in a group of aged people.* Thesis, Utrecht.

Cahn, L. 1964. Psychiatric problems of old age.* Thesis, Amsterdam.

Fennis, H. W. J. M. 1973. Medical demography of the aged.* Thesis, Leiden.

———. 1977. Developments in the pattern of provisions for the aged in The Netherlands.* State Committee on the Population Problems, report 13. The Hague: Staatsuitgeverij.

Fuldauer, A. 1966. Examination of the aged in a general practitioner's practice.* Thesis, Leiden.

Havighurst, R. J.; Munnichs, J. M. A.; Neugarten, B.; and Thomae, H. (1969). Adjustment to retirement, a cross-national study. Assen: Royal Van Gorcum.

Hollander, C. F. 1970. Functional and cellular aspects of organ aging. *Experimental Gerontology* 5: 313.

Kane, R. L., and Kane, R. A. 1977. *Long-term care in six countries (among others The Netherlands).* DHEW Publ. (NIH) 76-1207. Washington, D.C.: U.S. Government Printing Office.

Kruisbeek, A. M. 1978. Effects of ageing, thymus dependent immune competence. Thesis, Utrecht.

Leering, C. 1968. Disorders of human functions.* Thesis, Nijmegen.

---

*Titles given for asterisked publications are English translations of the Dutch titles. Often they include a summary in English.

Merkus, J. W. F. M. 1974. Patients in nursing-homes.* Thesis, Nijmegen.

Ministry of Public Health and Environmental Hygiene in The Netherlands. 1973. *Advice on gerontology.** The Hague: Staatsuitgeverij.

Munnichs, J. M. A. 1964. Old age and finitude.* (also published in English by Karger, Basel). Thesis, Nijmegen 1964. Assen: Royal Van Gorcum.

————. 1972. *Building elements for social gerontology.** Nijmegen: Dekker en Van der Vegt.

Nederlands Instituut voor Gerontologie. 1978. *Gerontologie, Inventaristatie van onderzoek in Nederland 1977.** Nijmegen.

Nota Bejaardenbeleid. 1975. *Memorandum on care for the aged 1975.* The Hague: Staatsuitgeverij.

Oostvogel, F. J. G. 1968. Care dependence in the aged.* Thesis, Nijmegen.

Sleeswijk, J. G., et al. 1948–1949. Old age from a medical point of view.* 2 vols. Amsterdam: Kosmos.

Social Sciences Council. 1966. *Register of social-gerontological research, 1945–1964.** Amsterdam: Noord-Hollandse Vitgevers Maatschappij.

Social-Gerontological Register 1965–1973, vol. II.* 1975. Amsterdam: Noord-Hollandse. Vitgevers Maatschappij.

Statistisch zakboek [statistical pocketbook] *1978.* 1978. Voorburg: Centraal Bureau voor de Statistiek.

Thung, P. J. 1958. Senile mouse ovaries.* Thesis, Amsterdam.

Tonino, F. J. M. 1969. Aged people at home.* Thesis, Nijmegen.

Verhage, F. 1964. Intelligence and age, in adults and old people.* Thesis, Groningen.

Welten, J. B. V. 1968. Old people in hospitals.* Thesis, Nijmegen.

Zonneveld, R. J. van. 1954. *Health problems of the aged.** Assen: Royal Van Gorcum.

————. 1961. *The health of the aged.* Assen: Royal Van Gorcum.

————. 1972. Medical gerontology.* Assen: Royal Van Gorcum.

————. 1975. Geriatric care in The Netherlands. In *Geriatric care in advanced societies*, ed. J. C. Brocklehurst. London: MTP.

————, ed. 1972. *Medical gerontology.** Assen: Royal Van Gorcum.

Zonneveld, R. J. van, and Fennis, H. W. J. M. 1966–1970. *Needs for intra- and extra-mural provisions for the aged.** 5 reports. Leiden: Nederlands Instituut voor Praeventieve Geneeskunde.

NEW ZEALAND

E. G. LOTEN

New Zealand is a small island community of some 103,740 square miles consisting of two major islands that are considerably different. The total population as of 1976 was nearly 3.4 million. The island's indigenous population (Maori) was small and of Polynesian extraction, most likely from Hawaii via the Cook Islands. European settlement of predominantly English stock began approximately 150 years ago.

Some interesting social legislation has been enacted in our short history, much of which has directly or indirectly affected the lives and health, mental and physical, of older people. There is nothing particularly new in New Zealand's social legislation; these experiments have been going on since the late 1800s. The most important acts are: universal vote for women (1893), pensioner schemes (from 1898); free education, 1877; forty-hour week (Factories Act of 1946); social security (contains comprehensive legislation offering free medical treatment by hospital, maternity, and family doctor, as well as free drugs; it also includes sickness benefit, home help, and domiciliary special services); state housing (an attempt at improving living conditions for certain groups); pensioner housing; school dental clinics; universal supannuation at the age of 65 (now adjusted to 80 percent of the average annual wage); unemployment benefits; and comprehensive accident compensation.

This list is not complete, but it shows that New Zealand is a highly socialized society. Some people believe that New Zealand's elderly do not necessarily benefit from this legislation. The present generation of elderly, and those approaching this socially discriminated against group, are well aware of their own contribution in thought and taxes. They are aware of what they were promised and, although now called consumers and noncontributors, are also aware that they continue to pay tax on superannuation benefits and that death duties await with the final levy on repeatedly taxed savings. This failure of legislation in a very vulnerable group does not help their quality of life and peace of mind.

Politicians and planners have problems in priorities, political expediency, moral values, and financial possibilities. As in most other countries, interested parties use what pressure they can for their own advancement. Integrated planning for the affairs of the elderly has not been conspicuous. The welfare state has openly claimed it will care for its citizens from the cradle to the grave (no funeral benefits). Perhaps such ideals have sapped individuality and self-reliance; many think so, yet it remains to be proved. One thing certain is that the health, happiness, and satisfaction of old people is only partly in their own hands, so all concerned with planning, administration, and care of this group should understand the background and the total environment.

DEMOGRAPHY

Geography

Geographic and climatic conditions partly influence the lives of elderly and retired people both in population distribution and by the scattering of family groups. New Zealand's two major islands lie in close proximity between latitudes 34° and 47° south and stretch mainly in a north-south direction for roughly a thousand miles. There are major climatic differences between the North and South islands. Population density also differs markedly, with a heavier distribution as one moves north. The age structure of the population also becomes older in the north, for people tend to retire to warmer, more developed, or, to them, more attractive parts. Their children, however, are more dependent on work locality, and so families separate. The distances in New Zealand may not seem great to people on continents, but the country is rugged and very hilly. Travel is becoming expensive, so family isolation is increasing. This nationwide trend is also reflected on the local scene; in large cities such as Auckland (population 700,000), elderly people are moving, when economically possible, to certain favored areas. Again, these moves tend to break up old homes, separate families and friends, and so create new problems for the people themselves and for planners. Necessary adjustments by elderly couples are often a challenge. To those who fail to adjust, stress is certain to cause problems for themselves, their distant families, and the services in that area. Planners believe that regional provision of services is the proper answer. The trend now seems to be that many elderly no longer remain in the district in which they spent their working life. Frequently the children have married and also moved away. Finally friends move off, become ill, or die, and an old person has no remaining roots in the area he grew up in.

This trend requires study of its significance and to establish the age structure in the various local areas of a city or its environs. Such a study was done for the city of Auckland when there was one large comprehensive geriatric hospital catering to all the Auckland Hospital board areas. The study, however, is no longer valid; the hospital has been demolished and five regional geriatric areas have been created in its stead. The relative requirements of services in these areas will need careful investigation. The future may contain some surprises in aging population distribution, for the city now covers a huge area, with expanding distant services and consequent cost.

Total Population

Tables 47-50 present data on the present state and trends of New Zealand's population. Table 49 shows the total population and areas of the two islands. In particular, the population is drifting to the north, causing a problem for local and central government in all matters, not just in care of old people. As in other Western countries, another significant population trend is the urban and rural disproportion and increase in shift (table 50).

The shift in European population shows a drop from 33 percent to 18.5 percent rural in forty-five years, but the Maori shift is colossal—some 55 percent. This represents a complete change in the way of life of the people and has produced problems in housing and work opportunities because many of these people were and are unskilled. However, because the Maori are a young population, no great problems yet appear among the older Maori, who represent only 2 or 3 percent of the total Maori population.

Age Distribution of Population

Such statistics are important to those studying facts related to the aged. The clinician's work is governed to some extent by them, and the planner has to understand the trends in order to gauge priorities or future political pressures. New Zealand, like many other places, has an aging population. Coupled with this is declining fertility, along with economic and the social conditions likely to maintain low fertility, so we need to know the extent of future demands created by this population aging. Table 51 shows the percentage of total population by age and sex, table 52 shows age by sex for the population over 65, and table 53 shows the projected population in five-year intervals from 1971 to 1991. New Zealand's population is expected to age progressively over the next twenty-five years, a projection based on the 1971 census. (The 1976 census is now becoming available, but many figures are not yet processed.) The projections in table 53 are based on 10,000 annual net gain by migration and medium fertility. The Census Department now questions whether these projections may be an underestimate; the actual rate of aging may be more rapid. This will require serious thought in some regional areas where the problem is certain to be greater than national projections suggest.

Marital Status

Data for marital status are shown in table 54. Some 72 percent of males 65 and over have a living spouse, while only 38 percent of females do. At age 65, 80 percent of males are married; the figure for females is 54 percent. The elderly widows now and in the future are a problem, one that lends itself to repeated illness or utilization by the patient of real disability to obtain security and company.

Table 47: TOTAL POPULATION AND ANNUAL INCREASE

Year	Male	Female	Total	Annual Increase
1970	1,425,435	1,426,702	2,852,137	1.7%
1975	1,573,900	1,574,500	3,148,400	1.7

Source: *New Zealand Official Yearbook* (1976), p. 57.

Table 48: MAORI POPULATION AND ANNUAL INCREASE

Year	Male	Female	Total	Annual Increase
1970	114,340	111,768	226,108	2.4%
1975	129,000	126,400	255,400	2.2

Source: *New Zealand Official Yearbook* (1976), p. 57.

Table 49: GEOGRAPHIC AND POPULATION VARIATIONS

Year	Population	Percentage of Total
North Island		
1971	2,051,363	71.7
1976	2,268,393	72.5
South Island		
1971	811,268	28.3
1976	860,990	27.5

Source: *New Zealand Official Year Book* (1976), p. 59.

Note: The area of North Island is 44,281 square miles; that of South Island is 58,093 square miles.

Table 50: URBAN-RURAL CONCENTRATION

Year	Urban		Rural	
	Number	Percent	Number	Percent
European population				
1926	937,304	66.9	464,370	33.1
1971	2,328,876	81.5	528,609	18.5
1976	2,592,680	83.0	532,443	17.0
Maori population				
1926	9,815	15.4	53,804	84.6
1971	159,497	70.2	67,801	29.8
1976	205,688	76.2	64,263	23.5

Source: *New Zealand Official Year Book* (1978), p. 66.

Vital Statistics

New Zealand figures include a very high Maori rate of increase and a lower European one. Life expectancy tables are presented in an abbreviated form for purposes of broad comparisons (tables 56–57). Prior to World War II, New Zealand's non-Maori population was probably the longest living of all national groups. This is not now so, although life expectancy is still high.

Table 51: AGE GROUPS AS PERCENTAGES OF TOTAL POPULATION

Year	Male			Female		
	Under 15	15–64	65 and Over	Under 15	15–64	65 and Over
1966	32.6	59.1	8.3	32.0	58.0	10.0
1971	31.8	59.7	8.5	31.0	59.0	10.0

Source: New Zealand Official Year Book (1970).

Table 52: SEX DISTRIBUTION BY AGE (IN PERCENT)

Sex	65–69	70–74	75–79	80 and over	Total of Population 65 and Over
Male	48	46	37	33	43
Female	52	54	63	67	57
Total population 65 and over	92,305	66,772	43,859	44,051	246,987

Source: G. Salmond, Accommodation and Service Needs of the Elderly, Department of Health Special Report Series 46 (1976), p. 20.

Table 53: ACTUAL AND PROJECTED POPULATION 65 YEARS AND OVER (IN PERCENT)

Age	1971	1976	1981	1986	1991
65–69	3.17	3.28	3.33	3.20	3.33
70–74	2.29	2.43	2.57	2.62	2.52
75–79	1.51	1.58	1.71	1.80	1.84
80 and over	1.56	1.44	1.46	1.55	1.65
Total population 65 and over	8.53	8.76	9.07	9.17	9.36
Total population of New Zealand	2,862,631	3,133,800	3,359,100	3,584,300	3,801,500

Source: G. Salmond, Accommodation and Service Needs of the Elderly, Department of Health Special Report Series 46 (1976), p. 20.

Note: The 1971 statistics are actual census figures. The others are as projected by the Department of Statistics.

Table 54: MARITAL STATUS OF THE ELDERLY POPULATION, 1971 (IN PERCENT)

Status	65–69	70–74	75–79	80 and Over	Total
Married	66	56	43	23	52
Unmarried[a]	34	44	57	77	48
Total population 65 and over	92,305	66,772	43,859	44,051	246,987

Source: G. Salmond, Accommodation and Service Needs of the Elderly, Department of Health Special Report Series 46 (1976), p. 21.

a. Includes never married, widowed, separated, and divorced.

Expectation of life for Maoris is shorter at all ages; it has been increasing in the past decades but is still not high. The average age at death of Maoris in 1972 was 47.14 and 46.08 years for males and females respectively (table 57). In 1972 less than 2 percent of Maoris as compared with 9.2 percent of Europeans were over 65 years (Salmond, 1976). For that year by the age of 65 years, 72.53 percent of Maoris of that birth group were dead compared with only 32.81 percent non-Maori. Statistically the problem for Maoris is not how to care for its elderly but how to become elderly.

Table 55: POPULATION INCREASE (BIRTHS OVER DEATHS)

Year	Number of Increase		Per 1,000 Mean Population	
	Total Population	*Maori*	*Total*	*Maori*
1976	31,525	5,445	10.21	21.55
1977	28,218	5,369	9.02	19.47

Source: New Zealand Official Year Book (1978), p. 86.

Table 56: NON-MAORI LIFE EXPECTANCY (ABBREVIATED TABLE)

	NUMBER OF YEARS REMAINING AT AGE					
Year	Male			Female		
	0	*20*	*60*	*0*	*20*	*60*
1901	58.09	46.74	15.40	60.55	48.23	16.64
1972	69.09	51.16	15.82	75.10	56.74	19.91

Source: New Zealand Year Book (1978), p. 97.

Table 57: MAORI LIFE EXPECTANCY

	NUMBER OF YEARS REMAINING AT AGE					
Year	Male			Female		
	0	*20*	*60*	*0*	*20*	*60*
1965–1967	61.44	45.13	12.89	64.78	42.48	15.09
1970–1972	60.96	43.97	12.96	64.96	47.54	14.60

Source: New Zealand Year Book (1978), p. 100.

Ages at Death

Among Maoris, the death rate per 10,000 population of both sexes is 35.2 for those between 25 and 44, 209.2 for those aged 45 to 64, and 935.2 for those 65 and over. The comparable figures for the non-Maori population are 16.3 for those aged 25 to 44, 100.4 for those aged 45 to 64, and 685.0 for those 65 and over. (These figures have been adjusted from crude death rates to allow for the age structure difference in the populations.) In both Maori and non-Maori populations, the death rate of males exceeds that of females considerably.

Causes of Death

In recent years, an autopsy was conducted in nearly a third of all deaths, which tends to improve the accuracy of cause-of-death statistics. The major killers in middle and late life are heart disease, neoplasms, cerebrovascular disease, and respiratory disease. Respiratory disease, of course, frequently is the terminal event in the older age group suffering from many degenerative diseases. There is no unusual major killer in New Zealand.

Until a few decades ago, tuberculosis was a serious problem among the Maori people, but it is now coming under control. Diabetes does not rate high on the list given, but in later life it contributes greatly to vascular disease. The Maori people do appear to be especially susceptible to infections, cancer, diabetes, hypertension, ischemic heart disease, gout, and rheumatic fever. Surveys indicate that overeating and a possible genetic predisposition to obesity may be an underlying factor. The *New Zealand Official Year Book* tables show an important contribution to fatal accidents under the heading of nontransport accidents, which occur at home and in hospitals, rest homes, work, and sports places. About 40 percent of these occur in or about the house and heavily involve the aged (*Year Book*). This fact is well understood by geriatric departments. Our medical social workers report any obvious hazards to the department. Before patients are discharged, rehabilitation teams visit the homes of the patient, study the situation, point out problems, and attempt to remove any danger. We need more knowledge of the etiology of these causes of death so we can better evaluate people's disability and associated pathology. Often such physical factors are not comparable for different individuals, a fact suggesting that the mental factors may play a role.

Living Arrangements

The majority of elderly males are married. In most cases the wife is in better health so the husband tends to be well cared. Many elderly women have lost their husbands, and although they are capable of good self-care, they do not always maintain it. Generally, however, the lone female is more capable of self-care than the male; hence their higher survival rate.

An important point is that 91.3 percent of the elderly live in private accommodations in the community. In the majority of cases, this accommodation is self-contained (that is, not shared). Table 58 illustrates the living arrangements of the elderly in relation to age, sex, and marital status. Of the aged groups, 65–69, 70–74, 75–79, and 80 years and over, some 96.7, 94.6, 88.3 and 77.7 percent, respectively, live in ordinary residences. The remaining 8 percent live in pensioner flats, residential homes, mental hospitals, or general hospitals of all types. The rates per thousand elderly living in hospitals in 1971 were 29.7 in public, 9.1 in private, 8.6 in mental hospitals, and 28.9 in residential homes. The total number of all people 65 years and over in such institutions was 16,005.

Table 58: LIVING ARRANGEMENTS BY AGE (IN PERCENT)

Living Arrangements	65–69		70–74		75–79		80 and Over	
	Male	Female	Male	Female	Male	Female	Male	Female
Alone	11.1	30.1	13.8	35.2	19.7	44.0	21.2	40.6
With spouse	62.1	47.3	62.7	38.1	63.6	27.6	44.6	11.5
With adults	20.6	19.0	19.1	21.3	13.0	24.5	28.6	43.0
With family	6.2	3.6	4.4	5.4	5.5	3.9	5.3	4.9
Total populations	43,344	45,918	29,276	33,920	14,641	24,100	12,151	22,095

Source: G. Salmond, Accommodation and Service Needs of the Elderly, Department of Health Special Report Series 46 (1976), p. 28.

PROGRAMS

Hospitals and Services

Public hospitals, both general and mental, are government's responsibility, administered through the Department of Health and by hospital boards elected at the local government level. They may administer a hospital group in large cities. They are financed by the government from general taxation and are free to patients. Doctors and staff are employed by the hospital boards on a salary and sessional basis. The hospitals are the major institutions responsible for postgraduate, medical, nursing, and paramedical training. They also set the medical standards. The overall standard is high.

Some private hospitals are purely private, and others are administered by church or welfare groups. Patients are free to make their choice. Private hospitals are responsible for their own finances but receive a government subsidy for each occupied bed-day. Those supplying long-term geriatric beds also receive a state contribution toward capital cost; the reason is that some hospital boards have fallen short of providing geriatric beds, and the government recognizes the contribution of welfare groups. There is supervision as to the type of geriatric admission. The doctor acts in a private capacity, although some institutions employ doctors on a sessional basis. Geriatric patients not able to find public beds can be placed in these beds, and hospital boards pay the difference. Limited means testing exists. A political move recently modified this means test, and as a result, it is now easier to place elderly patients outside public hospitals.

In general, there is provision for health care in the elderly, but it is not developed as well as existing knowledge could provide. A lack of personnel trained in and understanding the requirements of the aging still remains. In some communities, long-term geriatric beds are insufficient, with a consequent lack of acute medical and rehabilitation services. Public hospitals generally have not provided geriatric day hospital facilities, even though the need for and the value of these is well known.

New Zealand's position is thus similar to that of most Western countries, but its political structure differs, and its sparse population, geographic variations, and isolation create unique problems.

Nutrition

New Zealand is a primary producing country and nutrition is good. Experience from geriatric units shows that real malnutrition is rare. The few cases there are can be traced usually to fads, personal preference, ignorance, indifference, or depression. Those cases associated with loneliness or indifference or sometimes with disability have been solved by meals on wheels.

Health Care

With 92 percent of the elderly living at home in the community, the family doctor is the major supplier of services. Under general medical benefits, the old person's requirements are covered. Doctors are entitled to claim an additional benefit from the state for the pensioners they serve. Family doctors at their discretion can use private specialists, hospitals (general or mental), social workers, or nursing services. Pharmaceutical benefits cover the cost of prescribed drugs. Elderly people are heavy users of the services and time. In geriatric units, our opinion is that they are often too heavily supplied with medication, sometimes potent and expensive medication. This problem is not confined to New Zealand.

Community Involvement and Services

The number of elderly gainfully employed is hard to establish. Retirement benefits changed in 1977 to a new universal superannuation, which can be taken at 60 or 65 years. Figures for this will not be available for some time. In general, few people in good health and on good salary and wages retire at 60 because it does not make economic sense. At 65 years, all public servants and employees of businesses or institutions must retire. Politicians, judges, and owners of business are exceptions. In 1973, 276,000 people—about 9 percent of the population—were in receipt of age or superannuation benefits, so for the most part were removed from the work force (*Year Book*, 1974). Some between the ages of 60 and 65 were still working.

Many organizations and local bodies have services helping the aged. City councils, government, and private concerns give travel concessions. There are old people's clubs, budgetary advisory bureaus, and extensive Red Cross services, which also have a coordinating service for information on community services. There is also a National Council and Regional Old People's Welfare Councils. The former is a nationwide coordinating body, but the regional councils concern themselves at the personal level of seeking out problems. They help where they can and refer to other agencies when the need arises.

Several organizations are geared to help the disabled, both young and old. Generally the overall coverage is good, both by state and private sources. However, there are some deficiencies, which may be serious (Salmond, 1976). One of these is the identification of unfound problems, the social isolates, and those poorly advised. Many such cases exist that finally end in a hospital or institution. Conventional community medical effort is still primarily curative rather than preventive. Change will require a major alteration in medical thinking, but first some concrete evidence of the advantages of preventive medicine and some statistics on the size of the problem will have to be produced.

RESEARCH AND SOURCES OF INFORMATION

The discipline of geriatrics is now well established throughout New Zealand. Originally it was seriously studied at Cornwall Hospital and later spread widely. Some of the work was published: the excellent "Old Folk in Wet Beds" (Newman, 1962), "Some Aspects of Care of Old People" (Barker, 1965), "Housing and the Aged" (Barker, 1973), "The Day Ward" (Baskett and Loten, 1974), and "Man Was for Woman Made" (Evans and Loten, 1975).

Two societies are devoted to the elderly. The New Zealand Society for the Study of Aging is open to all people who are concerned with care of the elderly in any capacity. It has no research facilities or fixed headquarters. This society, with the Australian Gerontology Society, organized a successful conference in Auckland in 1974. The New Zealand Geriatric Society was recently organized; it is open to doctors only and is concerned with standards of geriatric medicine, dissemination of knowledge, and the training of geriatric physicians. Gerontology as a science has not yet begun in New Zealand. The universities have departments of sociology and of physiology, but as yet no concerted effort regarding gerontological research appears under way. New Zealand's Health Department has concerned itself with some wide-ranging surveys of the problems (social and medical) of the aged. A comprehensive list of available New Zealand literature is supplied in the Health Department Report No. 46 (Salmond, 1976). Finally, extensive information is contained in the *New Zealand Official Year Book*, much of which concerns social legislation, demographic data, and much up-to-date general information.

CONCLUSION

Psychogeriatrics was slower to develop an effective service. In recent years special efforts have been made by the Department of Health and some regional hospital boards in this field. As a result, several established psychogeriatric units are now operating. These units are developing a modern pattern of care as well as cooperating with specialized geriatric units in care and teaching. Considerable advances are under way. New Zealand is a welfare state supplying enlightened financial, accommodation, and working conditions for its people. Its medical care is extensive and excellent, but the wider aspects of health care seem to be neglected. Pride in self, pride in physical and mental health, individuality, initiative, and community involvement rather than self-indulgence, can become casualties in a welfare state. This is something we must watch, and there are signs that at least some of the younger generation are aware of this.

REFERENCES

Auckland Conference on Aging. March 1974.

Barker, R. A. 1965. Some aspects of care. *New Zealand Medical Journal* 64:626.

———. 1973. Housing and the aged. *Journal of Geriatrics* 42.

Baskett, J., and Loten, E. G. 1974. The Day ward, Cornwall Geriatric Hospital. *New Zealand Medical Journal* 79.

An Encyclopaedia of New Zealand. 1966. Vol. 2, p. 71.

Evans, B., and Loten, E. G. 1975. Man was for woman made. *New Zealand Medical Journal* 92:201.

Newman, J. 1962. Old folks in wet beds. B.M.J.: 1, p. 1824.

New Zealand Official Year Book. 1974.

———. 1976.

Salmond, G. 1976. *Accommodation and service needs of the elderly*. Department of Health Special Report Series 46.

NORWAY

EVA BEVERFELT

Norway is a prosperous country. It is a welfare state with an advanced social security system and highly developed social and medical services. Living conditions have been improved for all age groups. In principle, it is generally accepted as the responsibility of the society to organize the measures needed to prevent disease and social misery and to treat those suffering from poor health or who have personal adjustment problems.

These positive aspects of the welfare state are also reflected in the situation of elderly people. Anyone above 67 years of age is entitled to an old-age pension through the national insurance scheme. Substantial sums are appropriated over the state budget for various schemes of importance to the elderly. The participation of the central government in the care of the elderly over the last ten years has also made it possible to develop—or accelerate the development of—welfare measures in municipalities all over Norway.

DEMOGRAPHY

Since 1973 the lowest general retirement age has been 67, and the compulsory retirement age is 70. In statistics the elderly are usually defined as persons 67 years of age and more.

In 1975 nearly every eighth Norwegian was above 67 years of age. Table 59 provides data concerning population projections up to the year 2000. According to these projections the number and share of old people will increase up to the year 1990. This increase of elderly (98,000 persons) is almost the same as the increase of the total population (105,000 persons).

Table 59: POPULATION BY AGE (IN THOUSANDS)

Age	1975	1990	2000
0–66 years	3,544	3,551	3,622
67 and over	473	571	532
Total population	4,017	4,122	4,154

Source: *Population Projections: 1975–2000*. Central Bureau of Statistics of Norway, Oslo, 1976.

Note: Projections for 1990 and 2000 are based on lowest estimations of fertility.

When planning services for the aged, one has to bear in mind the proportions of the age groups involved because the need for assistance and care will increase with advancing age. Especially important is the number of those 80 years and over, which will continue to increase beyond 1990 (table 60). From constituting slightly over one-fifth of the elderly in 1975, the group of the very old toward the end of the century will account for between one-fourth and one-third of the aged population.

Table 60: SIZE OF ELDERLY POPULATION (IN PERCENT)

Age	1975	1990	2000
67 years and over	11.8	13.9	12.8
80 years and over[a]	2.5	3.3	3.6
	(21.4)	(23.8)	(28.3)

Source: Population Projections: 1975–2000. Central Bureau of Statistics, Oslo, 1976.

Note: Projections for 1990 and 2000 are based on lowest estimations of fertility.

a. Figures in parentheses show the percentage of those 80 years and over of the total elderly population.

In Norway, as in other industrial societies, women live longer than men. In 1974–1975 the life expectancy for women was 78.0 years and for men 71.7. The elderly population consists of 58 percent women and 42 percent men. Among those over 80 years, the figures are 62 percent women and 38 percent men (table 61).

Table 61: MARITAL STATUS OF THE ELDERLY POPULATION (IN PERCENT)

Age	Male	Female	Male		Female	
			Married	Single	Married	Single
67 and over	42	58	67	33	34	66
80 and over	38	62	46	54	13	87

Source: Population by Age and Marital Status, 31 December 1976. Central Bureau of Statistics of Norway, Oslo, 1977.

Among the conditions influencing the mortality rate are social class and geographical region of Norway. Low mortality rates appear in the following groups: technical and scientific work, pedagogical work, managers in farming and forestry, farm work, and forestry work. People belonging to these groups generally have regulated working hours, well-paid work, and jobs with few or no risks. In other occupational categories in this group, people are living outside the greater urbanized areas, and they are mostly working outdoors.

High mortality rates are found in hotel, restaurant, and service work; fishing; deck and machine crew work; mining; and work with explosives. A common feature of these vocational groups is that the workers often have irregular working hours and physically strenuous work. The last three groups also hold jobs with a high risk of accidents.

A comparison between geographical regions of Norway indicates that the mortality rate for men and for women is higher in Oslo and surrounding counties and in northern Norway than in other parts of the country.

STATUS AND ROLES OF THE AGED

Elderly People in Family and Society

Despite the positive aspects of the welfare state, its development has not been entirely in favor of the elderly. The disintegration of the multigenerational families and increased geographical and social mobility to some extent have separated younger and elder family members. The younger generation is leaving the farmland and the fishing villages in order to obtain education and jobs, while the elderly remain in the remote areas. Some coastal districts of the country therefore have a predominantly elderly population, and in some places only the elderly remain. Poor communications and long distances to neighbors and to shops are creating needs for specific health and welfare measures.

Along with the increasing geographical distance between younger and older family members is a growing psychological gap. This is mainly due to a more hectic and stressful life of the middle-aged generation, leaving less time available for being together with the elderly. Moreover because of rapid technological development, the knowledge of the older generation is often outdated and without interest for the younger ones. The elderly no longer hold a significant role as teachers for their children and grandchildren.

These circumstances have inspired laymen and researchers to dwell on nostalgic descriptions of the past although there is certainly no evidence on the full truth about old people in the old days. We do have knowledge about different groups of elderly in those days, such as the privileged and the underprivileged. The privileged elderly enjoyed life in supportive environments, and the underprivileged elderly passed their later years under most unfavorable and humiliating conditions. The latter group, which disturbs the image of the good old days, is somehow forgotten in spite of available information about poverty and social misery among old people.

The term *gammel* ("old") is often associated with negative traits, so old people describe themselves as *eldre* ("elderly"), which is also used in public documents and mass media. In the context of service and care, the elderly are those 67 years of age and more; an elderly worker is defined as a person between 45 and 67 years of age. Elderly people have been looked upon as more homogeneous than younger age groups. Stereotyped thinking about aging and the aged is reflected in terms like "the elderly want, wish, or are in need of." This judgment, wrong and unfair as it is, has hampered the planning and provision of adequate work and leisure time activities. To soften these attitudes, great efforts have been made in recent years by gerontologists, social workers, mass media, and, somewhat later, politicians and civil servants.

Some progress has been made, but much still remains to be done in order to raise the awareness of individual differences in old age.

The increase of the elderly in numbers and as part of the population has made them more visible and significant for the different political parties. Some of the elderly have answered this challenge by becoming more active in calling for their rights and thus have managed to strengthen their influence on matters concerning elderly citizens. Their demands to public committees and other policy-making bodies have been clearer and stronger over the last decade. Those active in pressure group movements constitute only a minority of the aged population, however, Norsk pensjonistforbund (the national association of pensioners), the main organizer of the elderly's actions, have about 70,000 members, about one-seventh of the elderly.

The remaining pensioners are not necessarily more passive. Some are gainfully employed. Hundreds of the ''young old'' participate as volunteers in social service, mainly for the elderly. Others have maintained their identity and prestige through various kinds of substitutes for paid work. Empirical findings show that some people extend their social contacts and activities after they retire. More and more of the aged enjoy traveling both in Norway and abroad. Visiting relatives in the United States is no longer a privilege for the very few. A better economy and numerous guided tours enable the aged to undertake travels that their parents would not have been able to consider.

On ther other hand, loneliness, isolation, and the feeling of being useless, a burden—even unwanted by family and society—are serious problems. Between 8 and 15 percent of the elderly say they want more social contact or are lonely. The proportion of elderly found through research to be lonely should be considered a minimum since loneliness may sometimes be difficult to reveal by an interview. Moreover, when it comes to the more severe cases of isolation, the old person is often shy and may be ashamed of the deterioration in his own appearance or that of his neglected home, and he therefore refuses to participate in a research project.

Work and Retirement

The development of the labor market is inclined to disfavor elderly citizens. Efficiency, competition, and demand for new methods and new knowledge are necessary for mass production. Faced with these aspects, the elderly are often at a loss, and persons over 50 years of age may have difficulties in getting new jobs. In a society that values work and productivity, the loss of work means a lowering of status and prestige.

Eight out of ten persons receiving disability benefits are in the age group 50–67 years, a fact indicating age-related health decline and job problems. But there is a relatively high disability rate in districts with a one-sided labor market indicating that when someone receives a disability pension, this may partly be due to lack of job opportunities. Thus an extensive part of the working population has left the labor force before they reach retirement age.

Arrangements implying possibilities for gradual retirement were introduced in the national insurance scheme in 1973. There is now a legal right to continue at work between 67 and 70 years of age. Persons in this age group may choose to take out a full or partial pension. The experience since 1973 shows that the option to draw part of the pension is used by less than 10 percent of the working population, while approximately 50 percent continue at work one to three years beyond 67 years of age.

The national insurance scheme covers virtually all persons domiciled in Norway. The old-age pension consists of a basic pension, which is equal for all, and an income-related supplementary pension. Of the 475,000 old-age pensioners today, only 98,600 enjoy supplementary pensions, which amount to Nkr. 6,700 annually. In other words, nearly four of five pensioners benefit only from the so-called minimum pension, which amounts at present to Nkr. 18,054 per year for single persons and Nkr. 28,890 for married couples. The old-age pension is cost-of-living related according to regular adjustments upward determined by the Storting (Parliament).

Some retired persons also draw pension from special occupational pension schemes, annuities, capital interest, or other income from self-owned trade or business. Elderly domiciled in rural areas usually have their own houses and can provide some of their own food, like vegetables, fish, or meat. Retired people with these benefits are fairly well situated economically, and for some of them even the minimum pension brings them more cash than they had when they were younger. On the other hand, the elderly living in the bigger cities—or other densely populated areas under rapid industrial development—may have a very strained budget if they draw only the minimum pension. This is particularly apparent in urbanized areas with high expenses as far as dwelling and heating are concerned.

PROBLEMS

In order to raise the economic level of pensioners with the lowest income, the government and Storting are faced with a serious dilemma: a substantial rise in the minimum pension would entail a considerable increase of expenses for the national insurance fund. Financing such an increase is probably not possible without lifting the member and employee contributions to the fund and/or increasing the contribution from the state. The government has decided to cope with these problems in several ways. Thus the pensioners in 1977 were included in the general income settlement for all gainfully employed people, thereby securing an increase of their income for the years 1977–1978, which is parallel to—and to some extent above—the average wage increase. According to the conception of supporting those especially in need, higher housing grants and new grants to compensate for higher fueling costs are reserved for pensioners burdened by their dwelling expenses* (Salvesen, 1977).

The interests of the elderly in the labor market appear for two groups: those active in the work force and those who have retired. Both categories are dealt with in a chapter of a white paper on future employment policies, presented to the Storting in 1977. In short, the white paper advocates increased information on the conditions of elderly in the labor market and the adoption of adult education schemes, increased possibilities to combine work and retirement pension, and more phased retirement programs.

The application of these aims is being considered with reference to the two groups in question: the elderly wage earners and the young retirees. Phased retirement in the sense of daily or weekly shortening of working hours is considered chiefly as the concern of employers. Except for one or two experiments, such programs have not yet been put into practice. Another effort introduced to phase retirement is to lengthen the annual holiday. Recent legislation entitles wage earners 60 years and over to a week of extra holiday (in addition to the four weeks already established). The expenses are paid through the national insurance scheme.

Retired people—from the age of 67 and up to 75—may often have the desire and the ability to carry out an ordinary job, but arrangements of this sort have been scarce and on a private basis only. The Employment Directorate has tried to stimulate the local employment offices to assist retired people seeking jobs—so far, without success. The main problem is that because of structural changes and the present recession, most work possibilities are found in districts with a shortage of retired manpower. When there is a shortage of jobs, the general idea is that old people drawing a pension should not take jobs from younger people, particularly not from family supporters. Recently governmental agencies have started studying whether public services that are understaffed could provide working opportunities for pensioners—for instance, at social welfare offices.

PROGRAMS

Public and Voluntary Agencies

According to the Social Care Act, the care of the aged is the responsibility of the municipalities, with the Social Welfare Board as the main organ. During the first twenty postwar years, the municipalities concentrated on providing supplementary pension and institutional care. The social service programs introduced during those years were initiated and operated mainly by voluntary

*The author is grateful to Kaare Salvesen, deputy director of the Royal Ministry of Social Affairs, for the access to his material and report, "Socio-Economic Policies for Elderly in Norway."

associations. Over the past decade, however, local public authorities have increasingly taken part in the organizing and financing of services, though the contribution by humanitarian, religious, and other voluntary associations is still important. A report on the care of the aged submitted by the Ministry of Social Affairs in 1976 states that the part of voluntary associations will remain significant in the years to come, mainly because of their efforts to find new ways of service delivery and their ability to incorporate otherwise inactive personnel resources. Whether this prediction by the ministry turns out to be correct remains to be seen. Voluntary associations need paid staff to organize the activity of the volunteers, and with the rapid wage increase in Norway, some of the associations already have financial problems. Moreover more and more women have paid jobs, so the group of women who formerly constituted the basis of voluntary manpower is diminishing. Still another problem is that the kind of community work especially needed is in the field of mental hygiene where professional skill is necessary.

Since the responsibility for the care of the aged has moved from the family to society, the state has become more active in policy making and in subsidizing services. In 1975, the government presented to the Storting a white paper, "The Elderly in the Society," which recommends a broad range of measures and services. The government also indicates guidelines for the future policy and condenses these aspirations in a code of action. The conclusions of the white paper were by and large endorsed by the Storting, but there is still a long way to go before the many valuable intentions and the procedures suggested are implemented.

Government programs for the elderly are provided by various ministries. Those most involved are the Ministry of Social Affairs (old-age pensions, nursing homes, and home nursing), the Ministry of Consumer and Administration Affairs (refund of expenses for home help), and the Ministry of Local Governments and Labor (the State Housing Bank and housing for the elderly).

The Division for the Care of the Aged in the Ministry of Social Affairs concentrates its activity on legislation, central planning, and preparation of guidelines and requirements in order to improve the standard and quality of provisions and services. In close cooperation with this division, three other units also operate on the national level. The National Council for the Care of the Aged, appointed by royal resolution, has an advisory function and is a common denominator for the interests concerning service for and care of the elderly in the community. The council coordinates state authorities, municipalities, and voluntary associations. The Norwegian Gerontological Institute was established by a private organization, and thus is a typical example of pioneer activity and significant contribution by a voluntary agency. Turning the institute into a state institution shows a recent trend: a readiness by the government to assume responsibility for gerontological research and dissemination of information. The primary task of the institute is research and education, but it also participates in planning, guidance, and advisory services. The third central unit in this field, the Joint Committee on Preparation for Retirement, was founded in 1969 on the initiative of the Ministry of Social Affairs and other public and private bodies. The aim of the committee is to stimulate the individual as well as society to engage in questions concerning the transition to retirement. The joint committee produces films, slides, and brochures, gives lectures, and conducts courses. Its expenses are financed mainly by the national budget. The daily activity of the joint committee is carried out by a secretariat and directed by a social psychologist. It is situated in the same building as the Norwegian Gerontological Institute, with which it has a close connection. A number of nationwide organizations and institutions are affiliated to the committee, among them the Norwegian Federation of Trade Unions and the Norwegian Employers Federation.

An ongoing pilot project introducing rural postmen as intermediaries of social services for the elderly may serve as an example of the close cooperation among the Ministry of Social Affairs, the National Council, and the Gerontological Institute. The council, which is concerned with service delivery in remote areas, studied various relevant systems in Sweden and concluded by suggesting to the ministry that a postmen service study should be initiated. The ministry approved the idea and invited the Gerontological Institute to carry out the project. The study aimed at ensuring the elderly greater security and information. The rural postmen participating took care of simple social services, such as delivering packages, giving information about municipal activities of interest, and, if needed, establishing contact with the Social Welfare Office. The project was financed by the Ministry of Social Affairs as an experiment for two years and was finished in 1978.

Social Services

The more vigorous engagement of the state over the past ten years has led to an improvement in the quantity and quality of services and care on the local level, but the impact of policy developed by the central authority also includes negative aspects. Although the municipalities are responsible for the care of the aged, their policy is partly directed by the availability of loans, subsidies, and other financial provisions from the state. Because of this system, ways and means chosen by local governments are not always adequate since decisions are based on financial considerations rather than on an assessment of the needs of the aged.

Another significant problem is whether the standard of living should be raised by increasing cash benefits or by developing services. The considerable increase of pensions has led to a stage where this problem must be discussed. There is a cross-political agreement as to the decisive importance of retirement income for the individual's freedom of choice. On the other hand, it seems obvious that even with a higher income, not all retired persons will be able to satisfy their needs because they will be buying services on the open market in competition with younger age groups. The problem is not a matter of either one procedure or the other but rather a question of priority.

As a starting point for information about social and health services for the elderly, the following is the distribution of the elderly according to living arrangements: 84 percent are in private households, 4 percent are in special housing projects, 4 percent are in residential homes, 4.5 percent are in nursing homes, and 3.5 percent are in general or psychiatric hospitals (Nygard, 1977).

Housing

The housing conditions of the elderly in Norway generally are poorer than those of younger age groups. The elderly more often have an outdoor toilet and more frequently lack bath facilities. In order to improve housing conditions and thereby enhance the possibility of the elderly's remaining in their own homes, the two main approaches are to adjust existing dwellings and to provide special housing. Loans for the purpose of modernizing and repairing flats and houses are granted by the State Housing Bank to private borrowers as well as to municipalities. During the first eight years, there is no repayment and the interest rate is 4.25 percent a year. After this period, repayment starts, and the interest is raised to 5 percent. Improvement loans from the State Housing Bank can be granted to persons seven to ten years before their retirement (while they still have work income). A positive attitude and initiative by the aging individual are needed in order to fill in application forms to various authorities and to deal with carpenters, plumbers, electricians, and other workmen. Experience has also shown that some elderly people are reluctant to raise loans on their property, even if they only have to pay the interest. The reason most frequently given is that they do not want to leave any debt to their heirs who would be responsible for the payment after their death.

Housing grants, another governmental scheme, aim to reduce the dwelling expenses for households with low income. Some municipalities also have their own projects for housing grants, which are subject to a means test and which vary in size.

Flats for the elderly are built in separate houses or as parts of buildings with family flats. Loans are granted on the same conditions as for building ordinary flats. In the rural areas, some of the housing projects are linked to institutions. Not until recently have the policy makers and planners realized that due consideration must be given not only to phyiscal design but also to the social environment as far as special housing is concerned.

A survey carried out in 1974 showed that between 3.25 and 4 percent of the elderly population lived in special flats for the old or frail. Of 444 municipalities, 247 provided special housing for the elderly and disabled and another 45 planned to provide this before the end of 1977 (Flaatten, 1976). The long waiting lists for such flats indicate an extensive unmet need for adequate housing. The pertinent question, however, is to what extent society should continue to meet this need by segregated housing provisions.

Social Services

Home-help service has been in operation for about twenty years and has been introduced in all municipalities. The service is free of charge or at a very low cost for the client. The state refunds 50 percent of the municipalities' home-help expenses.

About 15 percent of the elderly receive home help, on the average about three hours per week, but waiting lists indicate an unmet need. The main obstacle for a further development of home-help schemes is the lack of home helpers. Only 0.25 percent of the thirty thousand home helpers are employed full time. One might expect that this large proportion of part-time workers represents a resource that could be used to solve the problem of lack of personnel, but whether the part-time helpers want to extend their working hours is doubtful. Most likely some do not want to because they have their own chidren and households to attend to. In the remote areas with scattered population, home help often is the formalizing of previous family and neighbor help. The only difference is that the helper is now paid. In these cases, an extension of the help to include only one or two more families per helper implies a considerable increase of the working hours because of long distances and poor communications (Guntvedt, 1976).

Great emphasis is placed on enabling old people to remain in their own homes, and new approaches are appearing on the local level. For example, in a small community in the north of Norway, a couple has been employed full time by the municipality to provide care for seven retired persons. Difficult communications and lack of manpower made it impossible to organize help in the traditional way; the only alternative for the elderly would have been admission to an institution far from where they currently live.

A number of other kinds of measures and services have been introduced to meet the need for safety, as well as the need for independence. These services are financed partly by the state and partly by local authorities and/or voluntary associations. The state, for example, finances a subsidy arrangement for telephone installment and subscription expenses. These grants are subject to a means test, giving priority to frail elderly and those living alone. The organization Telefonkontakt ("Telephone Contact"), partly financed by the state, has calling services for elderly in several municipalities. Volunteers, known as telephone friends, call the elderly as often as the client decides. If there is no answer, the telephone friend finds out whether there is a problem. Another state-subsidized measure entitles everybody who has reached the age of 67 to obtain travel tickets at half-price when traveling by most of the country's means of communications. Legal aid is provided free according to a means test.

Several welfare measures, services, and recreational activities are financed by municipalities and/or voluntary agencies. Risk registers established by some municipalities ensure quick and efficient help for elderly persons likely to be particularly exposed to risk. Social counseling is provided by social workers, lawyers, and other professionals. The unmet need for this service is still great, partly due to a general lack of social workers and partly because work with the aged has not been considered an attractive field. Meals-on-wheels services started about twenty-five years ago, and different schemes are now in operation. The food is prepared either in institutions for the elderly or in restaurants and is distributed through voluntary action or by the municipal service.

In some municipalities, mobile domestic cleaning service is organized, and a number of municipalities offer transport service at a low cost or free of charge. Visiting schemes, physical exercise programs, hobby clubs, adult education courses, and library service are found in most of the local communities.

The idea of the service center for health and welfare is to assemble a wide range of measures under the same roof and thereby meet as far as possible the service needs of elderly people living in their own homes. The center also is intended to serve as a point of safety. It maintains contact with elderly in its immediate vicinity and offers them service and help at the center or in the home of the client. A center is available to all elderly people living within the geographical district of the center, and there is no means test for attendance. Eighty to ninety centers are now in operation, mainly located in the most densely populated areas of the country. The development of such centers has been rather slow and the need is far from being met. Loans for the construction of new centers and for modernizing old ones are granted by the State Housing Bank. The majority are operated on a voluntary basis, but in most cases the municipalities grant subsidies. The size of these subsidies varies from a few hundred to half a million Nkr. Ther are, however, subsidies from the government for operation costs, both for economic support and in order to apply certain standards for the operation of the center.

In order to meet the service needs of elderly who live at home and are too frail to use a health and welfare center, some municipalities offer care in day nursing homes. These institutions in most cases are affiliated with ordinary nursing homes, but some are independent. Day nursing homes, in existence since 1967, are considered an important link in domiciliary services. Recently it has been decided to let them profit from the financial system applicable to health institutions. Yet their appearance has been slow. In Oslo, the most developed municipality in this respect, there are about three hundred day nursing home accommodations available for a total population of seventy thousand.

Residential homes are designated for the elderly who can cope with their personal care but who need congregational living. The need for residential care and the role of residential homes in our health and social service system are issues now very much discussed by the government as well as by local authorities. The number of residential accommodations has diminished since the oldest and most inadequate institutions have been closed down. Other homes where residents had to share rooms have been rebuilt and now have only single-bed rooms.

Residential homes are administered under the Social Care Act and are consequently the responsibility of the municipality. The homes in most cases are municipal, but there are also private residential homes. The Social Welfare Board, however, is responsible for inspections of all homes, irrespective of ownership. Because loans for the building of residential homes are granted by the State Housing Bank, the bank in practice operates as an approval authority. Apart from this authority, there is no government system of approval of residential homes, either with regard to the standards or to the staff.

In principle, the pensioners themselves are supposed to pay for their stay in residential homes, but since very few of them have means above the minimum pension from the national insurance scheme, the payment is generally arranged by deducting part of the pension to cover the stay, whereas the municipality guarantees for the rest. The resident is guaranteed by law part of his old-age pension for personal use, and he also has the right to keep part of his own assets intact (up to 20,000 Nkr.).

Health Services

Health Conditions of the Elderly

The proportion of different age groups applying for disability benefits indicates a marked health decline with advancing years. Another indicator is the proportion of middle-aged and elderly patients in health institutions (table 62).In 1970, half of the elderly patients were in somatic nursing homes, 28 percent were in general hospitals, and the rest were patients in psychiatric hospitals (16 percent) or other health institutions. The greater need of the elderly for admission to health institutions is due not only to a high prevalence of disease. Elderly people have someone to provide nursing and care for them in their own homes to a far lesser extent than younger people, and the nursing of elderly is often more demanding than the nursing of younger people. This difference should be kept in mind when evaluating the health status of the elderly according to the relative number of younger and older persons in health institutions.

Table 62: AGE DISTRIBUTION OF PATIENTS IN HEALTH INSTITUTIONS

Age Groups	Patients in Health Institutions per 1,000
0–39 years	6.6
40–64 years	14.4
65–69 years	25.3
70–74 years	35.5
75–79 years	53.8
80–84 years	89.4
85–89 years	147.0
90 years and over	211.9
Percentage 65 years and over of all patients	44.4

Source: Committee for Gerontological Research. *Gerontologiens stilling i Norge*. Oslo: Norwegian Research Council for Science and Humanities, 1975.

Although the need for institutional care increases rapidly from the age of 70 to 80, evidence shows that the health condition of noninstitutionalized elderly 75 years or more is fairly good. In a study including a representative sample of 75 year olds in three municipalities, 59 percent were judged by the physician to be in good health, 39 percent had medium health, and only 8 percent were in poor health (Nygård, 1975).

Medical Service and Technical Equipment

For all Norwegian citizens, regardless of age, the national insurance scheme covers most hospital treatment and two-thirds of the doctor's fee for consultation at his surgery or for home calls. The rest is paid by the patient. Medicines are paid by the insurance scheme when they are of vital necessity for the patient. In some municipalities, the elderly may have free medical consultation and free medicine. These schemes are subject to a means test. Health control of elderly people has been discussed, and pilot schemes have been tried out, but so far the conclusion is that the most adequate system for the elderly would be a regular medical examination by their own doctors once a year.

Technical equipment (including hearing aids and spectacles) needed by handicapped retirees can be borrowed locally. If they have to be bought, the expenses will be paid entirely or partly through public schemes.

Home Nursing and Hospital Treatment

Home nursing schemes have been introduced in most of the municipalities in Norway. The aim of home nursing is to render sick care in the home when it is deemed medically acceptable to give the patient treatment outside ordinary health institutions (Salvesen, 1977). The service is not limited to elderly people, but in practice the great majority (about 85 percent) are more than 67 years old. The service is free of charge for the patients and is financed by the national insurance fund (75 percent) and by the municipalities (25 percent).

The first geriatric ward was established at the Municipality Hospital of Oslo in 1952, but very few such wards have been built since then. In fact those who still claim that geriatric wards are needed are now in a minority. The idea now is that all adult patients should be treated in the same way and on the same wards, regardless of age. Yet there are complaints from doctors and other health personnel that the wards are filled with old people. The high proportion of elderly in hospitals is partly due to the fact that their stay is unnecessarily prolonged because of a shortage of residential and nursing home accommodations. Therefore some hospitals are reluctant to admit elderly patients, who thus find themselves displaced by younger and more resourceful persons on the hospitals' waiting lists.

Nursing Homes and Psychiatric Care

Nursing homes are medical institutions, administered under the Hospitals Act. Building and operating nursing homes is the responsibility of the county, which also pays 50 percent of the operational cost; the other half is covered by the national insurance fund. Nursing homes are subject to approval by the Health Directorate, and insurance refunds are given only to approved homes. The estimated need for nursing home accommodations corresponds to 7 percent of the population 70 years of age and above, and the plans are aiming at reaching this on a country-wide basis in 1981 (Salvesen, 1977). Today a number of nursing homes, especially in the larger cities, have long waiting lists, and for the elderly themselves, as well as for their relatives, the waiting period can be a problem.

In nursing homes, as in residential homes, the patients cover part of the expenses through their old-age pension, and they receive the same amount of pocket money in the two institutions. The nursing homes also admit younger persons, but these constitute only about 10 percent of the patients. Policy makers and health planners emphasize the rehabilitation function of the nursing homes. The idea is that as far as possible, the health condition of the patients should be improved so that they can go back to their own homes or to a residential home. For many elderly, however, the nursing home becomes a permanent place to stay. Therefore it is important to have single-bed rooms in these institutions. New nursing homes are now required to have single-bed rooms for 75 percent of their accommodations, and financial support is arranged for building institutions with only single-bed rooms. Nevertheless most of the nursing home patients still have to share private rooms. This fact creates problems for those already in the homes, and it causes anxiety and a feeling of insecurity among those on the waiting lists.

In Norway, as in other industrial countries, the treatment and care of psychogeriatric patients is a serious problem. Some of these patients are admitted to mental hospitals, others to psychiatric nursing homes, and quite a number are in residential or somatic nursing homes. The number of psycho-geriatric patients in the different institutions and the number being taken care of by relatives are unknown.

Age-segregated Services

Few of these services and provisions are aimed at meeting the needs of elderly people exclusively. The majority are available to disabled or frail persons regardless of age who are unable to take care of their household or are in need of nursing care. This concerns, for example, home help and home nursing. Special flats are also provided for both the elderly and the disabled. The same is true as far as practically all other kinds of services subsidized by the state are concerned. On the other hand, the elderly constitute 90 percent or more of the consumers of the various services, a fact that explains and justifies the term *services for the aged*. The policy in Norway is based on the assumption that elderly would benefit from a service system under the label *for the aged*. Unless one does not emphasize the needs of the elderly in this way there is a risk that less interest and attention will be given to older than to younger age groups. Few social and health problems are unique to old age, but their appearance and symptoms may still differ from those of younger people. Appropriate means and services to meet a need may also vary from one age group to the other.

RESEARCH AND EDUCATION

Development

Most of the gerontological research done in Norway is social gerontology. The history of research in this field is only about twenty-five years old and started at the Institute of Social Medicine at the University of Oslo. The researchers, although recruited from the medical and paramedical professions, have always stressed the need of investigating aging from a psychological, sociological, and social point of view.

When the Norwegian Gerontological society was founded in 1954, the significance of a multidiciplinary approach was further underlined. Ever since this strategy has been demonstrated by the representation of the board of the society, which includes members from a variety of professions—general medicine, psychiatry, social medicine, psychology, sociology, and econom-ics. Another trend characterizing the development of gerontology in Norway is the part played by the voluntary associations concerning the care of the aged. In addition to providing different kinds of services, these organizations stress the need for research and actually provide opportunities for research projects and evaluation studies. This in turn promotes cooperation among different professional groups, like medicine, psychology, and social work. Since the voluntary associations have local branches all over the country, a nationwide effort was facilitated regarding both gaining and dissemination of knowledge.

In 1957 one of the greater voluntary agencies, the National Public Health Association, founded a national institute of gerontology. The institute was established in order to do research and function as a education and training center; it also included a multipurpose senior citizen center where practical measures could be evaluated. For fifteen years the institute was operated in cooperation with and partly financed by the municipality of Oslo. In 1973 the Institute of Gerontology became a state institute, Norsk gerontologisk institutt (NGI), under the auspicies of the Royal Ministry of Social Affairs. The service center had already been separated from the institute (in 1971), and evaluation studies had been undertaken in different parts of the country to an increasing extent.

Education and Training

The universities in Norway have shown little interest in gerontology. Of the four universities, only the Institute of Psychology at the University of Bergen has introduced the psychology of aging in the curriculum. For a few years, its teachers were provided by NGI. Now the Institute of Psychology at Bergen University has employed a psychologist to teach and conduct research in gerontology. The University of Oslo from time to time offers courses in social gerontology provided by cooperation between the university and the Geron-tological Institute. Students interested in writing theses within the field of gerontology are referred to the institute for guidance and supervision. Some of the NGI researchers have been temporarily employed by the Institute of Psychology as supervisors and teachers concerning psychological issues other than aging, but a more formal link between the two institutions is needed to promote the training of teachers on the academic level. Nevertheless the contact between the university and the NGI has been the basis for recruitment of researchers at the institute.

Students of psychology are showing a marked increase in interest for geron-tology. At the University of Oslo, an American expert on aging, Margaret Hellie Huyck, is teaching gerontology (1977). By offering this kind of train-ing, the university is indicating a growing interest in the field. Huyck's work at the NGI and at the university is of utmost importance for Norwegian research-ers and for the students of her seminars. The most significant impact of her expert contribution is the upgrading of prestige for gerontology in general.

There is no chair in gerontology or in geriatrics in Norway in spite of the fact that the latter has been acknowledged as a specialty since 1975. Postgraduate training is offered to physicians who plan to be geriatricians, but so far the new specialty has no impact on the curricula of the medical schools. Moreover, a chair in geriatrics, needed as it is, will not solve the problem of training social gerontologists.

The need for gaining more insight into all aspects of social gerontology is obvious. There is a need for the recruitment and training of sociologists, psychologists, economists, and anthropologists for research in gerontology. The problem is that because of the limited attention given to gerontology, there are practically no positions for teachers on the academic level. Perhaps even more serious than the shortage of research personnel is the unmet need concerning dissemination of knowledge to policy makers, administrators, various professional groups, and volunteers in the service of old age. Although there are a number of lectures, seminars, and courses provided (for example, matrons of residential homes and service center directors are offered a three-month training courses), not until 1977 was there nationwide action in the field of training. The government decided to appoint a council in order to promote education and training in gerontology. We hope that this approach will soon lead to a "gerontologizing" (Birren, 1971) of professional schools and increase the skills of existing personnel. The council is supposed to deal mainly with training in the applied field but necessarily has to consider training on an academic level as well, since dissemination of information requires research in order to extend and evaluate our knowledge. The council will act as a consultant to institutions offering in-service training; it will work in cooperation with the Council for the Care of the Aged and the Gerontological Institute in this regard.

Institutions and Professions Active in Gerontological Research

A few studies have been carried out by physicians, other health personnel, and social scientists associated with the universities. Training institutions like schools for social work and the district high schools (providing training on an academic level) have also done research in gerontology, although on a very small scale. Because of the increase in the proportion of elderly, especially in some communities, there is a growing interest among district medical officers to study the elderly from a sociomedical point of view. Another recent trend is the approach by a central group for health service research, financed by the Norwegian Council for Science and the Humanities. Among the problems this research group focuses on is cost-benefit analysis concerning different ways of providing care for the aged. A majority of these studies have been undertaken in cooperation with the NGI, which is functioning as the national center for social gerontological research.

In the broadest sense the institute is meant to gain and disseminate knowledge about the social and psychological aspects of aging and old age. The general goal of the activity is to contribute to optimum conditions for those growing and being old. Within this wide framework, the board and the staff of the institute are left with freedom and independence as to research, evaluation studies, and the organizing of education and training activities.

The social gerontological research undertaken at NGI could be classified as mainly psychological and sociomedical research. This is not the result of underestimating the need for research contribution from other social science fields but simply that psychology and medicine have been the professions where we have been able to motivate and recruit gerontologists.

Social gerontological research in Norway concentrated in the beginning on elderly people and those close to retirement. This approach was natural since the lack of knowledge about the later years was especially conspicuous. Over the past ten years, studies to a greater extent have also included the middle aged and, in a few instances, younger age groups. Research areas cover a spectrum, from more basic research like the impact of aging on mental capacity and sensory functions to broader health surveys. Depending on the problems to be investigated and on researchers and grants available, data have been collected through cross-sectional, follow-up, and longitudinal studies.

NGI Projects

The following examples of projects are presented in order to give a picture of the activity at the NGI. The various projects interlock in many ways, so it is difficult to undertake an exact grouping. Nevertheless the research activity can be classified within these main fields: elderly in working life, integration and housing conditions of the aged, the aged in their own homes and in institutions, and investigations of old-age institutions.

Attitudes toward work and retirement and coping behavior in the first retirement period were the main problems in a longitudinal study starting in 1966. Four hundred elderly were interviewed one year before retirement and one year after. A subsample was interviewed again four to five years after they passed the retirement age. In the late 1960s there was a strong motion to lower the retirement age in Norway. Yet the study showed that neary half of the original sample held some form of paid work the first year after they had passed the retirement age. Other areas studied through the project included paid work in retirement and the mortality rate, social participation before and after retiring, and the effect on social activity when being forced to quit the job compared to finishing off in accordance with one's own wish.

Another study of elderly wage earners was based on the assumption that the aged represent a vulnerable part of the work force because of the technical development and the constantly increasing demand for education and high speed. The investigation showed that the aged as a group have a less stressful working situation. A small number of the aged have shift work, they work less overtime, and a greater number of them than the young have jobs in which they themselves can set the working speed (their jobs are not controlled by machines). No difference was found between the age groups with reference to the perception of time pressure or physical and psychical stress. The aged experience risky jobs to a smaller degree than the middle-aged and younger workers. Apparently these findings are contradictory to the assumption that the aged have more problems than younger people in their work. But the main conclusion of the study is that the elderly who are active in the work force represent the survival of the fittest. Further research on problems of elderly workers therefore should concentrate on those most likely to have work-related difficulties. This refers to disabled persons, those in training workshops, the unemployed, and persons on long-range sick leave—wage earners who have left or about to drift away from the working life.

Integration of the aged has been studied by comparing social network and the intergenerational relationships of elderly in different local communities. Findings from these studies indicate that the degree of integration of the aged is higher in the rural municipality than in the small town, and higher in the small town than in the big town. This conclusion refers to all the activity variables that have been investigated. Regarding the contact between the generations, there are clear differences between the districts, varying with the degree of urbanization. There is thus a significantly higher frequency in rural districts than in Oslo (again, with a small city in the middle).

An analysis made on the basis of a nationwide registration of special flats and institutions for the elderly shows that municipalities with a good economy are well supplied with flats and nursing homes but are rather poorly supplied with residential homes. The latter are more often to be found in sparsely populated areas. In order to investigate how the different kinds of housing projects function, samples of tenants in cities and rural areas have been interviewed. Problems concerning moving from the previous flat to a new environment were often reported. With a few exceptions, the social and medical services provided do not meet the need of the tenants. A main concern of the elderly is the lack of safety provisions. Those living in integrated flats (blocks with ordinary family flats) have less neighbor contact than do the elderly in segregated housing projects.

The standards and personnel of residential and nursing homes have been studied through numerous projects. Comparative studies have dealt with elderly in institutions and in private households. Elderly on waiting lists for admission to institutions have been investigated by longitudinal studies. Findings from one of the institution projects indicate that many elderly (20 percent in nursing homes and 15 percent in residential homes) are cared for on a too high level. The consequence for the individual as well as for society is discussed in the research report, where the author claims that Norway is now on the point of building unneeded nursing homes.

The NGI has also been concerned with problems related to the organizing of service delivery, and through experiments and intervention research, it has tried to gain more knowledge in this field. One of these projects—a four-year study—was undertaken in a sparsely populated rural district. The project included upgrading existing services for the elderly, as well as introducing new measures. Training courses and group work were organized for personnel in domiciliary and institutional care. The theoretical part of the project focused on the functional capacity and the need for service among different subgroups of the elderly in the district. Valuable knowledge was gained about the life situation of elderly in a remote area, but the organizing of the various efforts did not always run as smoothly as might be desired. This fact, according to the researchers, was mainly due to insufficient planning of the applied part of the project.

For ten years the NGI has administrated a day center for elderly persons suffering from physical and/or mental decline. Follow-up studies in the center have given the NGI staff insight into the coping behavior of the clients and into the problems related to operating a day center of this kind. Group work in the center has demonstrated that even elderly suffering from serious health decline profit from group work; they become less self-concerned and more active and interested in social relationships.

This experience is supported by the findings from studies in residential and nursing homes. In one of these projects, the researchers, a psychiatrist and a psychologist, examined all residents and patients in an institution. The intervention part of the project focused on individual and milieu therapy for the residents. In addition to services and activities offered the elderly, in-service training and counseling for the staff was considered a significant tool of the treatment. Based on the findings from the theoretical and the applied part of the project, the researchers have suggested a plan for psychiatric-psychological services for elderly people in residential and nursing homes.

Knowledge gained through research can benefit the elderly only if it is available for personnel, administrators, and policy makers. Therefore dissemination of knowledge is a high priority at the NGI. A number of training courses are conducted for various professional groups and administrators. Lectures are given for students on academic and other levels, and the staff members also participate in broadcasting and television programs and in meetings arranged by the elderly themselves.

The NGI's staff of a dozen people often confronts a conflict between gaining knowledge on the one hand and education and information services on the other. Moreover its information service includes counseling and guidance provided on the request of ministries, local authorities, and private agencies. As an adviser to the Ministry of Social Affairs the NGI is represented on public committees and other policy-making bodies. To play the part of an expert is a demanding and time-consuming task. Trying to bridge the gap between theory and practice is a challenge to Norway's social gerontologists.

SUMMARY

Since World War II, living conditions in Norway have been improved for all age groups. Through the national insurance scheme, anyone above 67 years of age is entitled to an old-age pension. But despite the positive aspects of the welfare state, the development has not entirely been in favor of the elderly. The disintegration of multigenerational families and increased geographical and social mobility have separated younger and elder family members to some extent. A growing psychological gap between the old and the young family members is mainly due to the fact that a more hectic and stressful life leaves the middle aged less time for being with the elderly. Moreover the knowledge of old people is often outdated and of little interest to the younger ones. Thus the elderly are losing their former roles as teachers for children and grandchildren. The term *old* is often associated with negative aspects, and old people prefer to describe themselves as *elderly*. The increase of the elderly population has made the pensioners more visible and significant for the different political parties, and some of the elderly have become more active in claiming their rights. The National Retired Peoples' Association does not, however, cover more than a seventh of the elderly and has yet not appeared as a strong pressure group concerning policy development.

Approximately half of the group gainfully employed at the age of 67 continues to work one to three years beyond this age. Others have been able to find meaningful substitutes for paid work; for example, hundreds of elderly participate as volunteers in the social services. A good economy and guided tours enable more and more of the aged to travel in Norway and abroad.

Loneliness and isolation are serious problems, and neither the case finding nor the social therapeutic system is adequate to break the vicious circle of the lonely elderly people.

Problems of aging may be felt before retirement, especially on the labor market, which is inclined to disfavor the aging. Faced with the demand of new methods and new knowledge, the elderly are often at a loss, and persons over 50 years of age may have difficulties in getting new jobs. The government tries to solve these problems through various efforts. A white paper on future employment policies, presented to the Storting in 1977, deals with the interests of the elderly in the labor market. It advocates an increase in the information on the conditions of elderly wage earners and an adaptation of adult education schemes. Improved possibilities to combine work and pension income and more phased retirement programs are also recommended.

Retired people enjoying a supplementary and/or private pension usually manage quite well economically. Some of those drawing only the minimum pension complain about their lot. The majority, however, report that they have no serious economic problems. Evidence shows that even elderly on the minimum pension leave money in the bank upon their death (Erichsen, 1977). A significant problem for the policy makers is whether the standard of living should be further raised by increasing cash benefits to the elderly or by developing services. Retirement income is decisive for the pensioners' freedom of choice, but even with a higher income not all retired persons would be able to satisfy their needs through buying services on the open market in competition with younger age groups. The problem is not a matter of either one procedure or the other but the difficult question of priority.

The care of the elderly in Norway over the last decade has been characterized by an increasing involvement by the government and local authorities, but the contribution of private organizations is still important and most likely will remain significant in the years to come. The more vigorous engagement by the state has led to an improvement of the quantity and the quality of services and care on the local level. A wide range of domiciliary services has been introduced in order to help the aged to maintain themselves in their own homes. Housing conditions have been improved by modernizing dwellings and by providing new flats adequate to the needs of the elderly. The aim of day-care accommodation is also to avoid or to postpone institutionalization. As to residential and nursing homes, great effort has been made to enhance the well-being of the residents and the personnel. State subsidies and refunding systems have promoted the development of measures and services on the local level, but this state involvement may also include negative aspects if the local governments base their decisions on financial considerations rather than on an assessment of needs of the aged.

One of the serious problems in all kinds of services and care for the elderly is the shortage of personnel. Difficulties with the recruitment of personnel is partly due to the lack of an adequate education system in this field, which is a consequence of the limited attention given to gerontology on the academic level. Norway has no chair in gerontology or in geriatrics in spite of the fact that the latter is acknowledged as a medical specialty. By and large, the universities have shown little interest in gerontology. With a few exceptions, the gerontological studies undertaken in Norway come under the label of social gerontology. Since 1957, the Norwegian Gerontological Institute has been the center of research and training. The majority of studies undertaken have been done by this institute or in cooperation with it. In addition to research, the institute gives high priority to the dissemination of knowledge—for example, by conducting training courses and seminars for professional groups, administrators, and volunteers.

Services for the aged in Norway is far from perfect; and much remains in order to give training and research in gerontology the necessary attention and means. Communication and information between central and local authorities need to be further developed and strengthened. However, the gap between theory and practice, often dealt with by international gerontological conferences, is not a problem in Norway. Communication among policy makers, administrators, and researchers is rarely difficult. Gerontologists are often asked to act on various committees as members or consultants or to carry out special studies. Fruitful dialogues are also provided through conferences and seminars sponsored by the ministries.

REFERENCES

Beverfelt, E. 1973. Training within gerontology: Needs and organization. In *Recruitment and training of personnel*. Paris: International Center of Social Gerontology.

———. 1974a. The Norwegian Gerontological Institute: scope and methods. *Nordisk Psykologi* 26.

———. 1974b. Befolkningens struktur og alderssammensetning [Lecture for directors of old-age institutions.] Unpublished. Oslo.

———. 1977. Social services for the elderly. Paper presented to the Workshop on the Medical and Social Problems of Aging and Old People. European Economic Community. Luxembourg.

Birren, J. E. 1971. Methods for meeting the need for education on research training in the field of aging. In *Research and training in gerontology*. Washington, D.C.

Central Bureau of Statistics. 1974. *Population by age and marital status*. Oslo: NOS.

Committee on the Care of the Elderly. 1973. The health, activities, and well-being of elderly persons: Summary of the report *NOU 26*. Oslo.

Erichsen, O. 1977. Folketrygdens innvirkning på de eldresøkonomi. Paper presented to the Norwegian Gerontological Society, Oslo.

Flaatten, E. 1976. *Kommunenes utbygging av trygdeleiligheter og aldersinstitusjoner*. Rapport nr. 6. Oslo: NGI.

Guntvedt, O. H. 1975. *Arbeidstakere over 50 år*. Rapport nr. 4. Oslo: NGI.

———, et al. 1976. *Service, boligtiltak og institusjoner for eldre*. Rapport nr. 3. Oslo: NGI.

Helland, H., et al. 1974. Integration of the elderly in six local areas in Norway. Rapport nr. 2. Oslo: NGI.

National Insurance Institution. 1976. The national insurance scheme. Oslo.

Norwegian Gerontological Institute. 1977. *Report for the years 1973–1974–1975: Research, guidance, information, education and training*. Oslo.

Norwegian Research Council for Science and the Humanities. 1975. *Gerontologiens stilling i Norge*. Oslo.

Nygård, L. 1975. *Institusjon, helse og sosiale ressurser*. Rapport nr. 1. Oslo: 1975.

———. 1977. *Hedmarksprosjektet i lys av norsk eldreomsorg og sosialgerontologisk forskning*. Rapport nr. 1. Oslo: NGI.

Royal Norwegian Ministry of Social Affairs. 1976. *The elderly in the society*. White Paper presented to the Parliament. Oslo.

Salvesen, K. 1977. Socio-economic policies for the elderly in Norway. Draft working document submitted to the OECD. Oslo.

Vig, G., et al. 1976. Old people in institutions: Experiences from a Norwegian study. In *Research in Norway*. Oslo.

POLAND

L. DOBROWOLSKI

Since the earliest times, men have attempted to restore youth; alchemists searched for the elixir of youth, for example. And at the beginning of the scientific period of medicine, efforts were made to restore youth by means of transplanting the gonads (or their extract) of young apes. Although medicine has not yet discovered a way to restore youth, the improvement of general living conditions and the decrease of mortality as well as the development of medical science have decreased the risks that impair the health and life of middle-aged people so that more and more of them survive to old age. Consequently the number of aged continues to increase.

Both the medical and the economic sector have been overwhelmed by this problem. It is possible that the extension of life and the increase in the number of aged pose both to our generation and to the coming ones more difficult problems than the whole present and future technical development. The evolution of medicine will cause a future increase in the number of aged people suffering from multiple diseases and lingering afflictions, so the foremost problem will be not the impossible restoration of youth but the organization of protection, prophylaxis, and treatment of old people to prevent their premature failing.

Elderly people are characterized or stereotyped as ill, tired, not sexually interested, mentally slow, self-pitying, unhappy, and unproductive. The aging population of Poland comprises the largest group of consumers of traditional health services. In proportion to the rest of the population, the elderly occupy more hospital beds, take more drugs, and require more professional services than any other age group. They account for half of the chronically ill. Today the government and geriatric organizations are providing better care for the aged and are constantly doing research on the health and welfare needs of the aged. However, services for old people still need improvement in various areas, and there is room for further research and innovation.

DEMOGRAPHY

In 1970 Poland passed the threshold of demographic senility, which corresponds to 12 percent of persons 60 and over in the total population. At present, the proportion 60 and over is 13.5 percent of 35 million persons; by 1982, this proportion will decrease slightly. The decrease is a result of two factors: the aging of the generation born during World War I and the Nazi occupation and an increase in reproduction.

During the interval between the two world wars, the average life expectancy of men increased by nineteen years and that of women by about twenty-three years, to a life expectancy at birth of 67 and 74 years, respectively. By the year 2000 the average lifetime of men will probably increase to 72 and that of women to 77 years. It is unlikely that the probability of living will increase to 120 years of age, which seems to be the maximum limit of human life span.

Warsaw has always been called the City of Youth, but a systematic process of aging of the capital's population is proceeding. The percentage of citizens up to 17 years of age has declined by 4 percent. On the other hand, the percentage of population in the production ages increased by 3.6 percent, and the percentage of the retired (at present 18.8 percent in Warsaw) increased by 0.3 percent.

According to statistical data 350 persons of 100 years and over are living in Poland; 80 percent of them are women. Men live about five years less than women; their longevity is reduced by the following factors:

1. Wars, which cause the premature death of more men than women.
2. The kind of work men do.
3. Accidents, which occur primarily among men in connection with operating motor vehicles, trains, airplanes, and other vehicles.
4. Excessive smoking and alcoholism.
5. More stressful work.
6. Atherosclerosis, which develops in men earlier than in women, and, although the gonado pause lasts briefly, it nevertheless causes a predisposition toward cardiac infarctions, apoplexy, and other medical traumas.

According to demographic data, in 1976 there were 4.5 million persons who were 60 years or over. Four million were retired, and 416,000 were 80 or over. In the year 1985, these figures will increase to nearly 5.5 million aged 60 and over and over 0.5 million 80 and over.

It is foreseen that by 1990 the proportion of aged people in the total population will double. In Warsaw and in Lodz, every fourth citizen will be approaching the age of retirement or will have retired. In other cities very fifth will be retired.

PROBLEMS

The Polish population is aging quickly, and therefore researchers are searching for means of supporting physical and mental aptitude as long as possible. Old people are often depressed by feelings of loneliness, uselessness, and lack of interests. Inefficiency and passivity toward the benefits of free time of the retired are common. Mental age often shows stereotypic thinking and behavior. Many elderly people dreamed of having as much time as possible for themselves to be able to do justice to their manifold interests, but when the time came, they began feeling uneasy. Therefore the essential problem is to prepare people for accepting old age. The idea is to adjust gradually the social conscience from the point of view of how to live and what attitude to take toward old age. For this purpose I have written a popular scientific book, published in cooperation with Gustav Morf of Montreal and published in Canada under the title: *Let's Face It: We're All Growing Older—So Here's What to Do About It.*

PROGRAMS

Poland began investigations into the problems of aging and senility later than other countries because it had to devote the bulk of its resources to recovering from the damages caused by World War II. Nevertheless its progress has been fast. Poland now has 88 homes for retired people and 147 homes of social welfare for the chronically ill. The number of places in the latter has increased by 9,000 and will provde 64,800 places by 1980 and 100,000 by 1990.

Seventeen percent of the retired need help from their surroundings and 5 percent need hospital treatment. Recent years have also brought about an intense growth of the so-called clubs of the golden age; thirty-seven of them are functioning in Warsaw. Further, there exist forty day homes for the retired, ten of them in Warsaw, which are frequented by 340 persons who have their own homes but are lonely. In addition, a series of schools has been established to train social workers. Nearly four hundred of the Polish Red Cross attend sick persons in their homes.

Poland wants to keep old people in their usual surroundings as long as possible. The Health Service and Social Welfare has the supplementary and sustaining role of helping families. In the Supreme Board of the Polish Committee of Social Welfare, there is also a Commission of Friends of the Old, who provide fuel to old people, as well as helping them in cleaning, clothing, and other tasks. For thirty years, in my capacity as co-founder of the Polish Medical Society, I have trained physicians in twenty-one localities in geriatrics. In 1968 I organized a geriatrics section within the Polish Medical Association and through it have trained more than two hundred physicians in geriatrics for outpatient departments and clinical departments of geriatrics. The section now includes 462 members. In 1973 the Polish Gerontology Association was formed. It is open to anyone, though there are only about ninety members thus far. It is concerned mainly with social matters.

In Poland the retired and the disabled enjoy priority in shopping, and in cities they pay only half-fare for public transportation. Modern buildings are designed for aged people with flats in the lower floors, with bathtubs fitted with railings, and other special devices.

As some older people suffer from several illnesses simultaneously, which often take a different course than in young people, the physician meets great difficulties in diagnosis and treatment.

The main distinctions in illnesses by age are:

Type of Distinction	Young Patients	Old Patients
Cause of disease	External factors	Many, inside
Disease	Individual, known	Some disguised
Falling ill	Initial	Mostly relapses
Disclosure stage	Short	Long
Onset of illness	Mostly sudden	Insidious, indistinct
Course	Acute	Lingering with relapses
Rehabilitation	Speedy	Slow, incomplete
Immunity	Good	Little, predisposition to complications
Reactivity	Regular	Decreased
Individual differences	Insignificant	Dependent upon sex, age, constitution, previous illnesses, and so forth
Emotions	Stable	Increase
Mental ability	Stable	Decrease
Sudden death	Very Seldom	Often

Under my chairmanship, the geriatrics section of the Polish Medical Association organized in 1971 the First Symposium on Clinical Gerontology in Warsaw with the participation of foreign representatives. There were sixty papers delivered and its proceedings have been published. In 1976 I organized the Second Symposium on Geriatrics with the participation of foreign representatives. About five hundred persons, including eighteen foreign scientists, participated. Ninety papers were delivered. The symposiums have contributed to the popularization of modern views and the achievements reached in geriatrics so far. They will have an important influence on the further development of this problem and will contribute to a better understanding of how to treat old people adequately. In 1979 I organized the Third Symposium on Geriatrics.

Warsaw, Katowice, Lodz, Krakow, Bialystok, and Kodzko already have geriatric departments, and some also have special ambulances for geriatric patients.

We desire to have in all forty-nine voivodships an ambulance and at least a small hospital department on geriatrics with a geriatrician in attendance. We are hoping to create an institute of gerontology and geriatrics in Warsaw, which would facilitate larger scientific clincial investigations, as well as analyzing adequate data to make the lives of older people easier and secure them against premature aging. In the meantime, the so called Studium of Third Age came into being for people who are 65 or over. Its purpose is to offer them activities and to increase their interest in various areas.

REFERENCES

Dobrowolski, L. 1966. Zur Pathogenese und Prophylaxe arteriosklrotischer Varände-
rungen im Alter: Experimentelle Untersuchungen. Seventh International Congress of Gerontology, Wien.

————. 1971a. Arteriosclerosis and Calcification. *Giornale Geron.* 9:8.

————. 1971b. History of Geriatrics. *Geriatrics* (April).

————. 1971c. Zagadnienia problemowe geriatrii. *Zdrowie* Pub. 4.

————. 1973. Contribution to the prophylaxis and rehabilitation of coronary heart
insufficiency. *Europa Medicophysica* 9 Nr: 1, 1973

————. 1976. Lebensbedrohende Arteriosclerose Manifestatione. *Arztliche Praxis*
28:89.

————. 1977a. Neuere Möglichkeiten in der Therapie der Angina pectoris. *Therapie
Woche* 27.

————. 1977b. Danger of Dehydration in Geriatrics. *Medicina Geriatrica* 9:243.

————. 1978. Arteriosclerosis and Atherosclerosis and Atherogenic factors. Paper
presented at the Eleventh International Congress of Gerontology, Tokyo.

————. 1978. Nitroglycerin percutan eine neue Applikationsart für die Therapie der
Angina pectoris. *Deutsche Apotheker Zeitung* 118: 48.

————. 1979. Sexuality in the later years: Roles Behaviours. *Medicina Geriatrica.*
11:1

Dobrowolski, L., and Morf, G. 1977. *Let's Face It: We're all growing older—So
here's what to do about it.* Canada: PaperJacks Markham.

Gresham, G. A. 1976. Atherosclerosis: Its Causes and Potential Reversibility. *Triangle*
15:no. 2/3.

Szarugiewicz, G. 1975. Nursing aid as seen by the patient. *Annales Universitatis
Mariae Curie-Sklodowska Sectio D. Medicina* 30: 245-253.

RUMANIA

ANA ASLAN

DEVELOPMENT OF GERONTOLOGY

Research in the field of gerontology started as early as the nineteenth century. The outstanding neuropsychiatrist, Gh. Marinescu, was interested in the process of aging and the age pathology of the nervous system. He investigated particularly the colloid osmotic mechanism of aging and advanced an original theory on the subject (Marinescu, 1899, 1933).

C. I. Parhon, founder of the Rumanian school of endocrinology, investigated various aspects of the aging process, particularly the relationship between the endocrine glands and aging, other clinical and biological aspects of aging, and different prophylactic and therapeutic approaches to geriatrics (Parhon, 1955).

In 1949, C. I. Parhon chose me as co-worker in the field of gerontology and geriatrics. We both started a program of theoretical and clinical gerontological research in a home for the elderly. With a small number of collaborators, we achieved good results in the treatment of old age (Aslan, et al., 1950a, b). In 1952, the Institute of Geriatrics was founded at Budapest; its major objective was research on the problems of gerontology and geriatrics. I was appointed the director.

NATIONAL INSTITUTE OF GERONTOLOGY AND GERIATRICS

The institute was the first of its kind, so there was no organizational model available. Nevertheless, it was organized according to the three major directions of research in contemporary gerontology: clinical, experimental, and social. This structure has been recommended by the World Health Organization for similar institutes.

Because the achievements of the institute in the therapeutic, experimental, and medicosocial fields called for a more complex framework of organization and specialized and diversified research, it became the National Institute of Gerontology and Geriatrics (1973). The activity of the National Institute of Gerontology and Geriatrics has been directed toward the study of the aging of the human organism from the biological, clinical, therapeutic, psychological, and social points of view.

The better understanding of the mechanisms of aging of the human organism, the necessary steps for improving the health status of persons over 40 or 45, the maintenance of their work capacity, and the prolongation of the active life span have been major objectives of research at the institute.

For reaching these targets, the research activity at the institute has included biomedical and psychological fundamental and applied investigations on aging; geriatric curative and prophylactic steps; organization and guidance of other geriatric institutions of the sanitary network of our country; and appropriate gerontological training of the medical staff.

At present, the framework of organization of the institute contains various departments.

CLINICAL DEPARTMENTS

One department is for gerontological recovery where cross-sectional and longitudinal clinical and therapeutic studies have been carried out aiming at the development and improvement of the means of recovery and prolongation of the active life span. The target is to give a scientific basis to the improvement of the general health status to the maintenance and the prolongation of elderly's capacity. Research on the efficiency of eutrophic medication, age criteria, rhythm, and evolution of aging, as well as on the role of the genetic and endogenous determining factors, have been carried out.

In the clinical department for age pathology, the pathology of advanced age, as well as the clinical and therapeutic characteristics of chronic degenerative diseases, have been studied. Research on the interrelation of age-degenerative diseases and on the improvement of the prophylactic and curative steps in geriatrics has been carried out.

The clinical departments also include a number of specialized consulting rooms—cardiological, opthalmological, neuropsychiatric—and psychological and x-ray laboratories.

Research Departments

The department for the biology of aging includes laboratories specialized in clinical physiology, electrophysiology, hematology, biochemistry, bacteriology, immunology, cultures of cells, enzymology, drug conditioning, experimental biology, pathological anatomy, and medical electronics. This department has its own farm, which supplies animals for the experiments.

Research on subcellular, cellular, tissular, and systemic processes of aging have been carried out at this department through functional, morphological, and physiochemical explorations; pharmacological and pharmacokinetic studies; elaboration and conditioning of biotrophic products; findings of new methods of investigation and diagnosing; and studies of experimental gerontology. Research on the rhythms, pathogenesis, and pathology of aging, age criteria, and evaluation of therapeutic results have been carried out in close cooperation with the clinical departments.

The department of social gerontology includes gerohygiene, geropsychology, social biology, gerontology, methodology, social assistance, and gerodemography laboratories. The major objective of the activity at this department has been the study of the social, demographic, economic, medical, psychological, ecological, and cultural peculiarities of the process of aging, both of the individual as a member of a certain community or social stratum and of the social life as a whole.

From the methodological point of view, the department of social gerontology organizes and controls the research on old age prophylaxis and treatment, as well as providing the appropriate training of the medical staff.

Central Polyclinic

The elderly are attended by this polyclinic, which has specialized consulting rooms and laboratories. The polyclinic controls the geriatric, prophylactic, and curative assistance in different enterprises and other polyclinics in Bucharest, as well as the experimental centers for research and medical assistance. Prophylactic and therapeutic research on the efficiency of the biotrophic products on outpatients have been conducted. The central polyclinic also has consulting and treatment rooms for foreign outpatients.

Clinical Departments for Geriatric Treatment of Foreign Patients

Because a great number of foreigners have been interested in undergoing the treatment with "Aslan's method" (Gerovital H3), several clinical departments with specialized staff have been organized close to Bucharest and throughout the country. The Paro and Snagov departments of the Otopeniclinic function near Bucharest. Other clinics are located in Felix, Herculane, Eforie Nord, Neptun-Mangalia, Sinaia, and Caciulata.

RESEARCH

Therapy with Extracts and Procaine

Therapy of the aging has been considered with ever greater interest by both physicians and sociologists. The various treatments prescribed in the aging process are generally the result of conceptions regarding the pathogenetic mechanisms of aging. According to C. I. Parhon's conception, aging is a dystrophic state, which could be therapeutically influenced.

Aslan envisaged glandular treatments with thyroid extracts and, in certain cases, with thymus and epiphysis extracts, as well as treatments with extracts of ovaries or masculine hormones. Besides these therapeutic approaches, the procaine-based treatment Aslan started has been based on clinical and pharmacological investigations. The results obtained have pointed out the important part played by the nervous system in aging mechanisms.

Before 1946 this treatment was administered in trophic and circulation disorders, in asthma, arteritis, and syndromes for which it had already been mentioned in the literature (Leriche and Lafontaine, 1953; Visnevski and Visnevski, 1952).

From 1949 to 1951, Aslan experimented with intra-arterial therapy using procaine on young and old patients with circulatory and trophic disorders or with arthritis (Aslan et al., 1950a, b). The first reports mentioned the hair repigmentation, unknown at the time (Parhon and Aslan, 1953). Procaine-based therapy improved the memory and increased the muscular strength of elderly patients. This fact called for a systematic, long-term use of procaine-based treatment in old age.

Clinical long-term research started in May 1951 on 189 persons from the institute's home for the elderly. The patients were grouped for treatment with spleen and placenta tissue extracts, gland extracts of adrenal, pineal, and thyroid, vitamin E, yeast, and procaine. One group was used as control.

Procaine was administered in intramuscular injections three times weekly in a series of twelve injections a month with a ten-day interval between each series. Eight series were given annually, and the treatment was continued for a couple of years. After five years of comparative research, it was decided to continue only with procaine (Gerovital H3), vitamin E, and control groups. The elderly patients lived under similar environmental conditions and received the same food and care as the controls. The average age in the various experimental groups was 72 in the procaine-treated group, 75 in the vitamin E–treated group, and 73 in the control.

At first an ordinary solution of procaine was used. In 1951 Aslan elaborated the product; Gerovital H3 with procaine as the basic compound, the pH of which (3.3–3.5) provides a longer stabilization of the procaine molecule. Aslan, and later Gordon and Fudema (1965), pointed out that Gerovital H3 provides higher blood-procaine levels than procaine alone.

In order to evaluate the results of the procaine treatment in the old patients, Aslan has used a series of clinical and laboratory investigations in order to point out their biological and psychological age before and after the treatment. The following were the age criteria: the capacity to perform conditioned reflexes, the psychological reactivity, the velocity of the vascular reaction to various physical agents by plethysmographic and oscillometric tests, muscular strength shown by dynamometric tests, circulation time, and other biological aspects. The pattern of the patients' biological state was completed by biochemical investigations on the metabolic processes (concerning the proteins, fats, and hydrocarbonates) and hematological investigations (blood clotting, platelet aggregability, and blood morphological pattern among them). Life expectancy, morbidity, and morphopathological data were also studied.

After three years of treatment, the results obtained in the three groups were evaluated and compared. The best results were obtained in the group subjected to the procaine therapy; fewer improvements were noticed in the vitamin E group. A long-term treatment was then instituted for another thirteen years; mortality figures were recorded for the entire sixteen-year period. Mortality was 5.3 percent in the procaine-treated group, 10 percent in the vitamin E–treated group, and 16.5 percent in the control group.

From the beginning of the treatment with Gerovital H3, a favorable change in the patients' psychology appeared with regard to their life, activity, and family and social relations. Other changes were a diminution of the depressive state, a better mobility, and better articular elasticity (Aslan, 1956a, b, 1959a, b).

Gradually other scientific data have been added concerning the effects of Gerovital H3, including:

- Anabolic effect in 89.9 percent of the treated cases (Aslan, 1962; Aslan et al., 1965).
- Improvement of the psychic condition, memory, and time of fixation of conditioned reflexes, plus an increase in the number of sleeping hours (Aslan and Parhon, 1954; Parhon et al., 1955).
- Signs of reactivation of the regeneration process, noticeable in the skin and hair, and an acceleration of the consolidation time of accidental fractures (Crăuciun et al., 1959; Aslan et al., 1975).
- Improved circulation time (slowed in 81 percent of cases in 1952 but after eight years of treatment in only 23 percent of cases); increased vascular reactivity pointed out through oscillometric and plethysmographic tests; and increased muscular strength (Aslan, 1959a, b; Aslan, Vrăbiesou, 1955a, b, 1968).
- Modification of the proteinemy (the electrophoretic examination revealed a tendency of stabilization of the globulinic fractions) (Aslan and Parhon, 1954).
- Prevention of turning of micromolecules toward macromolecules, a general phenomenon in nontreated aged persons.
- Improved permeability of the capillary vessels for the various proteic fractions (electrophoretics) (Aslan et al., 1959).

The clinical results have been:

- Favorable effect in psychic and physical asthenia (Aslan and Parhon, 1954).
- Evident results in the ailments of the central nervous system induced by arteriosclerosis, in Parkinson's disease, pseudobulbar paralysis, cerebellar syndrome, and comitial crises (Aslan, 1956a, b; Aslan and Parhon, 1954; Aslan and David, 1960).

- Favorable effects in the treatment of sequela subsequent to cerebrovascular accidents and hemiplegia due to spasms, thromboses, or hemorrhages (Aslan and David, 1959).
- Improved motility, reflexes, trophic edema, and decreased spasticity (Aslan and David, 1957).
- Reappearance of estrogens and reactivation of androgens (Aslan, 1956a, b).
- Improvement in certain cases of the thyroid function and stimulation of cortico-suprarenal secretion (Thorn's test) (Parhon et al., 1956).
- Positive influences on all age-induced modifications of the skin, such as senile keratosis, cutis rhomboidelis and the troubles of hypothalamic origin, vitiligo, psoriasis, eczema, lichen planus, and alopecia (Aslan and Parhon, 1954; Aslan, 1957).
- Beneficial effects on scleroderma (investigations conducted on twenty cases for two to five years) and on collagenosis.
- Stimulation of hair growth and repigmentation (Parhon and Aslan, 1953).

The substance also proved to be quite active in the diseases of the circulatory system, particularly in peripheral and central atherosclerosis, in cerebrovascular disturbances, embolism, acrocyanosis, and trophic ulcers (Aslan and Parhon, 1954; Aslan and David, 1959; Aslan et al., 1970, 1971).

The influence of the substance on ulcers (gastroduodenal) was investigated in three hundred cases (Aslan et al., 1959). The diminution of disturbances was noticed after four or five injections (particularly when they were administered intravenously). There were also fewer digestive troubles such as hyperacidity and hypermotility, and the direct and indirect signs of ulcer were also influenced. Generally the results have been astonishing, particularly since they did not require any diet or a strict rest regime. Two old people ages 75 and 88 belonging to the group treated with procaine had bone fractures that were cured in a remarkably short time (forty days) with an endostal callus and complete functional recuperation.

Gerovital H3 is particularly effective in osteoarticular afflictions. More than seven thousand treated cases have proved the efficiency of the drug. The best results were noted in arthroses and spondyloses. The disappearance of the clinical subjective phenomena and the functional recovery were noticed in 28 percent of the cases, and general improvement was noticed in 61 percent. Only 11 percent of the cases were not significantly influenced (Aslan, 1956; Aslan et al., 1965; David et al., 1972).

The comparison of radiographies done before and after one to four years of treatment revealed the remineralization of the skeleton and the thickening of the bone bridges in 25 percent of the cases and the reestablishment of the subchondrial structures and the lessening of osteoporosis in 40 percent of the cases. Beneficial effects were also noticed in cases of rheumatoid arthritis, where small amounts of corticoids were added whenever necessary.

The stimulation of the defense reactions of the organism under Gerovital H3 treatment was described from a clinical and experimental point of view.

Aslan and colleagues (1965) noticed that during a severe influenza epidemic in the institute hostel in 1959, mortality in treated subjects was 2.7 percent whereas in nontreated ones it was 13.9 percent.

In research on rat peritoneal hystiomacrophage, Aslan et al. (1973) found the capacity of phagocytosis increased by 10.9 percent after treatment in vitro with Gerovital H3; and in the cells coming from treated animals, colloidopexy increased by 11.9 percent and phagocytosis by 14.4 percent as compared to the controls. They also followed the phagocytosis capacity of the human leukocytes of subjects submitted to a long treatment with Gerovital H3. The phagocytosis capacity was tested with inactivated Staphylococcus aureus. The average of the phagocytosis index for Staphylococcus aureus was 51.7 for the leukocytes from the controls and 68.4 in those treated with Gerovital H3, an increase of 16.7 percent.

Aslan et al (1977) directed research toward the possibility of controlling by Gerovital H3 the capacity of the lymphoid F_c receptors to bind immunoglobulin because of their importance in the mechanisms that concern the cell-mediated immune response. In rats treated with Gerovital H3, the percentage of F_c receptor bearing lymphocytes increased 44 percent in sixteen-month old rats, in comparison to the controls where the percentage was only 20. At the age of twenty-eight months, the percentages were 48 percent in the treated group and 13 percent in the controls.

Because the bonding capacity of lymphocytes decreases with age, our results show that treatment with Gerovital H3 leads to the maintenance of the lymphocytic reactivity that is the background of the cellular-mediated immune response. It is possible to assume, following these data, that long-term treatment with Gerovital H3 decreases the deterioration of structures, susceptible to becoming antigenic producers of autoantibodies. These data could explain the low level of autoantibodies in subjects treated with Gerovital H3, in comparison to the control group. Therefore Gerovital H3 appears to be a factor in the prevention of autoaggression in elderly subjects.

Investigations carried out at the Institute of Geriatrics on 150 elderly subjects treated with Gerovital H3 for nineteen years revealed a 36 percent increase of life expectancy (based on statistical tables for 1956–1957), but in controls, the calculated life expectancy exceeded the average life span 30 percent.

Mortality in the patients subjected to long-term treatment with Gerovital H3 was 4.1 percent; that in the control group was 16 percent. Crăciun and Tasoa conducted morphological studies particularly on tissues allowing the assessment of cellular metabolism; they pointed out the nuclear division in certain myocardial fibers. They concluded that this represents a reactivation at the level of the nucleus of the myocardic fibers correlated with the metabolic processes. The authors pointed out a morphological peculiarity: the absence of sclerosis consequent to atrophy of the liver, myocardium, brain, and endocrine glands.

Simultaneously with the clinical research, Aslan and her co-workers have conducted pharmacological investigations aimed at the mechanism of action of the procaine-based eutrophic medication. These investigations allowed a better understanding of the effect of this substance on the cellular biochemical activities, intermediate metabolisms, and integration systems of the organism. Stronger eutrophic effects have been noticed subsequent to the use of Gerovital H3.

The benefits derived from the regenerating effects of Gerovital H3 have been assessed based on experimental data. In one study the sciatic nerve was unilaterally crushed in rats. A group of rats received injections with Gerovital H3 (16mg/kg body weight) every two days, and the controls received only distilled water. Comparative studies were also carried out with Gerovital H3 and simple procaine (Aslan, 1962). The changes in the functional capacity of the triceps aural muscle were assessed through electromyographic determinations. Forty days after the pinching of the sciatic nerve, gravimetric determinations were made as well as the measurement of the transversal diameters of the muscular fibers of the injured area in comparison with the intact contralateral muscle.

A more rapid regression of the muscular atrophy was found in animals treated with Gerovital H3, the gravimetric difference between the muscle of the injured area and the intact muscle being 10.7 percent in treated animals and 22.6 percent in those belonging to the control group. Histologically the tranversal diameters of the muscular fibers of the injured area decreased by 2.3 percent in comparison with the normal condition in treated animals, whereas in the control group the decrease was 11.6 percent.

The effects of procaine with a pH of 7 on the regeneration processes has also been studied in comparative research. Thus the gravimetric difference between the muscle of the injured area and intact muscle were 19.6 percent, and the transversal diameters of the muscular fibers of the injured area decreased by 8.7 percent (in comparison with 10.7 percent and 2.3 percent in animals treated with procaine pH 3.3 Gerovital H3).

These investigations pointed out that Gerovital H3 has a stimulating action on the regeneration phenomenon at the level of peripheral nerves and of the striated muscles. Due to the synergism of procaine and that of potassium ions at the nervous and muscular level, it is understandable why Gerovital H3 (containing K) is more active than procaine alone.

In other studies experimental fractures at the level of the inferior third of the tibia and peroneum, without the mobilization of the respective limb, were used on forty female rats aged twelve to fourteen months, separated in two equal groups. The research aimed at studying bone regeneration. The study lasted sixty days. Radiographies performed every ten days revealed an earlier and a more intense periostal reaction in the Gerovital H3–treated animals (4 mg s.c. per day). Ten days later, the periostal reaction at the level of the fractured bones was present in 60 percent of the Gerovital H3–treated animals. The reaction was present in only 10 percent of the controls receiving distilled water. The precocity and intensity of the periostal reaction produced in those cases constitutes the essential stimulation for a more rapid consolidation of the two fractured bones. The results of the experimental investigations agree with the clinical pattern of the more rapid bone regeneration in Gerovital H3–treated elderly.

Stimulation of the tissues' regeneration by the biotrophic products based on procaine has been clearly shown in the research of Naum and Rusu (1973), who have established the quantitative variations of nucleic acids during hepatic regeneration. When it was shown that after twenty hours the rate of the DNA synthesis is much slower in old animals than in the young ones, it became obvious that in the treated old animals, the DNA synthesis is stimulated, and it approaches that of young animals. The stimulation of DNA synthesis determined by reduced doses of Gerovital H3 (0.4 percent) was also evidenced during research on secondary cultures of monkey kidney. The incorporation of labeled thymidine was 22.4 percent in treated cells and 6.2 percent in controls (Aslan et al., 1973).

Experimental research has also shown the anabolic effect of procaine, which was previously clinically observed. In Infusoria (Colpidium colpoda and Vorticella), we noted a stimulation of proliferation under the influence of procaine with low concentration solution, a fact indicating anabolic stimulation.

In 1950, investigations on rats drew attention to the anabolic influence of procaine, revealing weight increase and improved furry coat of the experimental animals (Aslan et al., 1950).

Aslan et al. (1965) have studied longevity in 1,840 rats. They pointed out a 21 percent increase of life span in Gerovital H3–treated animals. An improved general trophicity was also noticed, as well as an increased resistance to bronchial-pulmonary diseases. Fewer myocardial lesions were recorded on electrocardiograms (coronary irrigation disorders in 30 percent of the treated animals and 80 percent of the controls). Histological examination in the treated animals revealed a less important connective invasion in the myocardium and the striated muscle and less degenerative lesions in the renal tube.

Beside the anabolic action, a series of facts point to the vitamin-like biocatalytic role of procaine. Aslan has mentioned (Aslan, 1958, 1964, 1974; Aslan et al., 1965) Moeller and Schwartz's research (1948), which proves the stimulating action upon bacteria. This fact was also noticed by Kuhn (1948). They called the para-aminobenzoic acid a vitamin-like factor. Furthermore, the antisulphanylamide action of para-aminobenzoic acid has also been pointed out for hydroaminobenzoic acid, as well as for procaine (in the bacterial test, procaine can replace the para-aminobenzoic acid). The authors assert that carboxyl and amine groups are the prerequisites of the conservation of the vitamin-like effect.

Research we carried out (1960) in cooperation with Conniver upon the Staphylococcus aureus and Entamoeba coli have also confirmed the biocatalytic action of procaine.

The stimulation of the cellular proliferation under the influences of procaine and para-aminobenzoic acid has also been pointed out in research on Infusoria (Colpidium colpoda and Vorticella) by Parhon, Aslan, and Cosmovici (1957). Concentrations at which maximal stimulation had been obtained were 2 mg percent for APAB and 4 mg percent for Gerovital H3. The development of a certain yellow pigment in the Infusoria culture occurred in the presence of both substances, which proved their similar effects (Aslan, 1958). This yellow pigment has also been found by Mayer (1944) in experiments carried out with procaine and para-aminobenzoic acid on micobacterium tuberculosis.

Other research carried out on secondary cellular cultures from monkey kidneys showed that the concentration of 0.4 percent Gerovital H3 produced the stimulation of cellular proliferation. The average cellular density varied, depending on the age of the culture, between 218.9 cells/ml and 712.5 cells/ml in the Gerovital H3–treated group and between 163.5 and 480.3 cells/ml in the control group. The data point cut an intensification of cellular proliferation in the treated cultures. The average cell postmitotic life span was 72.4 days in cultures treated with Gerovital H3 having undergone fourteen passages and 62.3 days in nontreated cultures having undergone twelve passages.

Recent research carried out by Americans (Hrachovec, 1972; MacFarlane, 1974) supports the assertion that the effect of Gerovital H3 on the cellular biochemical activity has a much wider spectrum due to its capacity of inhibiting Monoaminoxidase (MAO). A correlation has been established between this effect and the procaine mechanisms of action.

The inhibition of monoaminoxidase was indirectly noticed by us in 1950, when we found that intravenous procaine injections administered to dogs produced an important increase of the blood pressure reaction toward epinephrine.

Procaine action at cellular level also involved restoring and maintaining the physiologic potential of the cellular membrane. The mechanism might be the densification of the cellular membrane—in Fleckenstein's opinion the "anelectronic repolarization" and the "stabilization" in Shanes'.

The same properties of the membrane have been pointed out by Teitel, Storesou, and Steflea (1965). Similar findings were pointed out in research on isolated organs of homeothermals and poikilothermals, the activity and reactivity of which toward certain substances are increased by procaine, thus providing a longer survival.

Considering the importance of activities on the organism as a whole, any improvements in its functional state brought about by the biotrophic treatment are particularly significant. The favorable influence upon depressive psychical states of the aged was also noticed (Aslan, 1956). The antidepressive effect of procaine has also been pointed out by Bucci and Saunders (1960), Siggelkov (1960), and other American researchers. Together with Parhon and colleagues (1955b), we found an improvement of memory, attention, and sleep in patients treated regularly with procaine.

Recently in a double-blind research using thirty elderly patients, Zung (1972) using placebo and imipramine, tried to evaluate the efficiency of Gerovital H3 therapy in depressive elderly patients. The clinical observations and psychometric tests performed before and after the four-week treatment pointed out the superiority of Gerovital H3 over imipramine.

Data recently published by American authors drew attention to the modification induced by aging and depressive states in the enzymatic activity of the nervous cell as well as upon the intervention of procaine at this level (Robinson et al., 1972; Hrachovec, 1972; MacFarlane, 1974). The increased MAO activity could play an important part in the biochemical modifications induced by aging and depressive states. As a matter of fact, depressive states have been correlated with the reduction of central amines (Bunney et al., 1967), which is due, as recently shown, to the increase of monoaminoxidase.

MacFarlane (1974) pointed out that the treatment of psychic depressive with irreversible MAO inhibitors (such as pargyline and phenelzine) is associated with severe adverse, sometimes lethal reactions. On the contrary, Gerovital H3, a reversible MAO inhibitor, may be safely used.

Although the mechanism through which procaine acts upon the nervous system is not known, the analysis of the effects it induces enables us to believe that it could play a part in the restoration of the electric potential and the biomedical substratum of the nervous cell.

Electroencephalographic research we carried out in 1963 with Brosteanu and Enachescu pointed out that people over 85 years subjected to long-term treatment with Gerovital H3 had, compared with the control group, a significantly higher (75 percent) alpha background activity, within normal limits for adults, a prompt reactivity to light, and no alternations to intermittent luminous stimuli. At the same time, the capacity for psychic effort increased, and the appearance of signs of fatigue was delayed.

Research has shown that procaine acts upon the nervous system not only at the whole molecule level but also through its hydrolysis products: diethylaminoethanol and para-aminobenzoic acid. The results obtained with the administration of procaine supports the assertion that diethylaminoethanol (resulting from the hydrolysis of procaine), through its transformation into diethylaminoethanol, is also a supplier of acetylcholine. In this way, procaine, through diethylaminoethanol, not only feeds the metabolic potential way, which determines the increased production of acetylcholine, but inhibits at the same time the hydrolytic action of acetylcholinesterasis; diethylaminoethanol is also a feeble antipsychotic.

In 1972, Hrachovec showed in research upon rat brain, liver, and heart that Gerovital H3 inhibited monoaminoxidase more intensely than hydrolytic procaine. According to MacFarlane (1972), the inhibition produced by Gerovital H3 is from 17.8 to 87.7 percent, the intensity depending on the dose.

All of these data, as well as the clinical studies pointing to the effects of Gerovital H3 on old people, support the assertion that the reduction of monoaminoxidase and its return to normal values affects positively the symptoms associated with aging. These are new proof of the action of procaine upon the central nervous system.

The research on clinical, biological, and social gerontology carried out at the institute have had direct applicability. The results obtained since 1950 in applying the biotrophic substances according to Aslan's method on two hundred thousand subjects proved its peculiar efficiency in the prophylaxis and therapy of premature aging. They aroused general interest and stimulated numerous studies, resulting in over six hundred published papers) both in our country and abroad. These achievements contributed to a large extent to the founding and development of the Rumanian school of gerontology, which has attracted hundreds of physicians and specialists from our country and from over eighty foreign countries to attend the specialized training at the institute.

Based on the results obtained, we started the prophylactic use of the biotrophic medication in 1954, when the first gerontological center was organized at an industrial enterprise in Ploiesti. Since then, the action has been extended within the numerous gerontological centers organized in the industrial and agricultural enterprises throughout the country. In collaboration with the department of social gerontology and the clinical departments, the gerontological center provide prophylactic assistance for persons aged 45 to 60.

The prophylactic orientation of the gerontological research, the main objective of which has been the prolongation of the active life span, is the characteristic of present and prospective activity at the institute.

SOCIAL GERONTOLOGY

The evolution of the demographic aging of the Rumanian population has been similar to that of the countries characterized by an intense economic-social development. Due to the rapid increase of the elderly population, the health care services have had to face new objectives, such as the founding of the department of social gerontology at the Institute of Geriatrics in 1958. The department has aimed at studying the medicosocial problems of the elderly and aged population. The main objectives of the multidisciplinary research carried out at this department have been studies on demography, anthropology, and social medicine; studies of applied medical and psychosocial sociology; medicosocial experiments; and methodological problems of the organization and functioning of new forms of geriatric assistance.

The research of social medicine had been focused on the main objectives in the present health care of the population: to decrease mortality and morbidity due to chronic degenerative diseases and to prevent premature and pathological aging through studies aimed at pointing out the causes of the peculiar rhythm of aging in certain geographical areas.

Longevity and environmental conditions have been studied based on medicosocial inquiries and psychological tests on fifteen thousand persons aged 85 and over (40 percent of the total of longevous persons in Rumania). The results of the study have pointed to the higher biological vigor and to the increased resistance to different diseases; 44 percent of the longevous persons had direct and collateral longevous ancestors.

The original contribution of the Rumanian research in social gerontology has been the assessment of the biological aging of certain groups of population; the criterion of average biological age has been used as a synthetic, positive indicator of the health status of the elderly population. This methodology has been applied in research conducted on the population suffering from endemic goiter in certain geographical areas in our country; it revealed the peculiarities of premature aging due to the thyroid endemic dystrophy specific to these groups of population. Research conducted on populations in those geographical areas with particularly increased frequency of longevity pointed out the peculiarities of the delayed process of aging in the population.

Both the theoretical and practical multidisciplinary research conducted by the department of social gerontology have enabled a better understanding as well as the solution of certain problems specific to the medicosocial assistance of the elderly population.

Medical care has been concerned with problems of prophylaxis, in centers specializing in the prevention of age pathology within the sanitary network including the gerontological centers and the dispensarization of the aged population, and with curative functions through outpatient and hospital care (geriatric departments in general hospitals, and homes for the chronically ill aged persons).

Social assistance has focused on services for those elderly living in the family environment and the institutionalization of the elderly (in homes for the elderly and for retired persons).

Medical units with prophylactic profile include the gerontological center, functioning within the medical units in enterprises, which provides prophylactic medical assistance for the working staff aged over 45. The center also provides medical supervision for elderly workers through semiannual medical check-ups; the use of the prophylactic therapy with biotrophic substances; the solution of social problems raised by changes in working place, labor protection, and conflicts; and the study of work and age interaction.

The main objective of the gerontological center has been prevention of ailments through periodic medical examinations, prolongation of the active life span, and the maintenance of working capacity. Also it assessed certain objective indicators concerning the evolution of health status, such as body weight, height, thoracic perimeter, pulse, blood pressure, and so on, as well as social indicators concerning the environmental conditions of the working staff, the age when they started to work, their occupational career, the characteristics of the working place and dwelling, nutrition, energetic and neuropsychic effort pointing out age-induced functional modifications, and the part played by one's occupation in the process of aging.

The analysis of the results obtained at the 144 gerontological centers between 1961 and 1970 point out the following:

- The necessity of specialized medicosocial assistance for retired persons.
- The necessity of preventing certain chronic diseases or detecting them at the onset.
- A 38 percent decrease in the number of sick leave days.
- A prolongation of the active life span pointed out by the fact that 24 percent of the persons served by the centers continued to work after reaching the retirement age.
- The maintenance or the increase of the work capacity in 41 percent of the working staff as a result of having to achieve a certain quota.

There are gerontological centers at present in 219 enterprises. By 1980 coverage of the active elderly persons by centers will be generalized throughout the country. Care for the elderly population has been differentiated by age subgroups. Biomedical peculiarities and the morphophysiological status of this group of population have been taken into consideration. Persons over 60 are cared for at the territorial polyclinics, where specialized consulting rooms such as internal medicine, cardiology, and neuropsychiatry have been at their disposal. They have been subjected to complete medical investigations every six months, and the results have been listed in the personal medical records.

Care for nearly 25,000 elderly persons achieved the following:

- Complex medical examinations, which pointed out the onset of chronic diseases of which the patient had no knowledge (such as cardiovascular diseases and diabetes).
- The active supervision of the patients, enabling the prevention of complications.
- The use of specialized therapy, as well as that of different geriatric recovery techniques and treatments with biotrophic substances.
- Certain social ergotherapeutic steps.

The action thus has a dynamic character, and the medical and social steps taken at the proper time ensure its quality and efficacy.

The dispensarization was applied also to persons aged 90 and over because of their high percentage of death from acute diseases. The main objective of the monthly supervision of these persons has been the prevention of the onset of the acute pathology, different complications, and worsening of certain chronic diseases. This step led to a 56 percent decrease in the number of deaths in longevous persons as compared to the year previous to the dispensarization by preventing acute diseases (influenza, bronchopneumopathies, acute afflictions of the digestive or renal apparatus). Research on this age group also includes a study on the interrelation between the environmental factors (physical and social) and longevity, and studies of data concerning life, dwelling and working conditions, peculiarities of nutrition, family life, the psychological aspects concerning personal nature, temper, affectivity, and so on.

Curative medical assistance includes outpatient care at the medical territorial units and polyclinics and geriatric units in polyclinics with specialized consulting rooms. Seventy geriatric consulting rooms function at present; by 1980 the number will increase to 130. Geriatric consulting rooms also provide outpatient treatment, including recovery and biotrophic therapy. The main aims of the geriatric consulting rooms have been specialized medical assistance, complex medical investigations specific to the age pathology, and geriatric training of the medical staff.

The medical dispensary with its gerontological profile functions within the retired people's associations. The retired medical and sanitary staff give consultations and treatments to members of the association. In cooperation with the territorial medical units, it provides treatments in different resorts and refers patients to specialized consulting rooms.

The organizers intend to provide medical assistance at home with the help of the dispensaries for patients unable to get around because of advanced age or chronic diease. Hospital assistance has been provided by the hospital for adults, but it has been inconvenient, particularly in cases of acute diseases. The pathology of the aged population, characterized by chronic degenerative diseases simultaneous with a deficient background, requires special units, apparatus, and conditions.

Hospital assistance within the units with geriatrics profile include geriatric departments, such as those functioning at the NIGG. Their main obejctives have been to diagnose disease, making use of the investigations required by the specific age pathology; to apply special treatments aimed at recovery (the physiotherapeutic, kinesiotherapeutic, and mechanotherapeutic techniques and medical gymnastics have been thus developed); to administer associated medications with biotrophic substances (Gerovital H3 and Aslavital); to develop appropriate diet required by the treatment; to supervise the convalescence of patients; and to meet the social needs of the aged through the social services.

Social assistance for elderly includes a series of social programs. NIGG has organized an experimental unit, referred to as the village for the elderly, for those from rural areas. This unit includes eighty rural houses with two or three adequately furnished rooms, vegetable gardens, and orchards, where the elderly can work according to their ability. The village is at the center of a rural community, so the elderly are in permanent contact with different age groups.

Among the multidisciplinary research conducted by the department of social gerontology, mention should be made of the study of the process of demographic aging and its medicosocial consequences; research on premature and pathological aging of the population living under environmental conditions with increased risk factors, such as geographical areas with endemic population or increased radioactivity; the study of the influence of the psychic factors on premature and pathological aging; research on the use of the elderly's working capacity; the study of the adaptive processes of the aged organism in relation to the changes of the main parameters of the environment, such as pollution, inappropriate diet, obesity, and working conditions; the study of modifications in the social status of the elderly due to retirement; studies of the mutations within the family structure and relations of the elderly; and studies of the dwelling, educational, and cultural needs of the elderly.

The results of the research conducted by the department of social gerontology have been published by specialized journals and in the *Treatise on Social Gerontology*.

REFERENCES

Abrams, A.; Gordon, P.; and Fudema, J. 1965. The effects of European procaine preparation in an aged population. I: Psychological effects. *Journal of Gerontology* 20:139.

Aslan, Ana. 1956a. Novokain als eutrophischer Faktor und die Möglichkeit einer Verlängerung der Lebensdauer. *Therapeutische Umschau* 9:167–172.

———. 1956b. Eine Neue Methode zur Prophylaxe und Behandlung der Alterns mit Novokain-Stoff H3—eutrophische und verjüngernde Wirkung. *Die Therapiewoche* 1:14–22.

———. 1957. Behandlung der Alterserscheinungen mit Novokain. *Der Praktische Arzt* 126:743–750.

———. 1958a. Zur Wirkung des Novokain. *Arztneimittelforschung* 8:11–14.

———. 1958b. La novocaïne, substance H3—dans la thérapeutique de la vieillesse. *Revue Française de Gérontologie* 4:321–330.

———. 1959a. A new method for the prophylaxis and treatment of aging with procaine. Eutrophic and rejuvenating effects. New York: Consultants Bureau.

———. 1959b. Recents experiments on the rejuvenating effect of novocain (H3) together with experimental, clinical and statistical finding. New York: Consultants Bureau.

———. 1962. The therapeutics of old age: The action of procaine—clinical and experimental conclusions. In *Medical and Clinical Aspects of Aging*, edited by H. T. Blumenthal, 4:272–292. New York: Columbia University Press.

———. 1964. The present stage of procaine therapy in geriatrics. Paper presented at the Fourth Congrès Médical International FIR, Bucharest.

Aslan, Ana, and Ciucă, A. 1972. Results of some practical researches in the field of gerontoprophylaxis. Paper presented at the International Symposium of Gerontology, Bucharest.

——. 1977, Recherches et actions de gérontoprophylaxie effectuées en Roumanie. Comunications to the Eighth European Congress of Clinical Gerontology, Neptun, Rumania.

Aslan, Ana; Ciucă, A.; Jucovschi, V.; and David, C. 1965. Le centre gérontologique. Paper presented at the International Conference of Gerontology, Akademiai Kiado, Budapest.

Aslan, Ana; Cosmovici, N.; Lalu, P.; and Bunescu, G. 1965. Development of the influenza virus epidemic in the Bucharest Institute of Geriatrics. Paper presented at the International Conference of Gerontology, Akademiai Kiado, Budapest.

Aslan, Ana, and David, C. 1957. Ergebnisse der Novokainbehandlung Stoff H3 bei dysmetabolischen Arthropathien. *Die Therapiewoche* 1:19–23.

——. 1959. Le traitment de l'ictus par la procaïne—subst. H3. *Rev. Fr. Géront.* 10:439–449.

——. 1960. Prophylaxe der Arteriosklerose. *Arztneimittelforschung* 11:869–876.

Aslan, Ana; David, C.; Chişoui, I.; Cîmpeanu, S. 1960. Study on the action of procaine (Gerovital H3) upon the dysproteinemia in some experimental nutritive deficiences in piglings. *Fiziologia Normală şi Patologică* 2:88–99.

Aslan, A.; David, C.; and Cipeanu, S. 1959. Der Einfluss der Dauerbehandlung mit Prokain auf die differenzierte Kapillarpermeabilität. *Arztneimittelforschung* 8: 480–482.

Aslan, Ana; David, C., and Enăchescu, G. 1971. Modifications du syndrome humoral chez les athéroscléreux agées sous l'influence du traitement biotrophique á l'Aslavital. Paper presented at the Sixth European Congress of Gerontology, Bern.

Aslan, Ana; David, C.; Hatmanu, D.; Nicolae, D.; Timand, A. 1965. Contribution to the study of involutional osteoporosis. A clinical-radiological-biochemical investigation. Paper presented at the International Conference of Gerontology, Akademiai Kiado, Budapest.

Aslan, Ana; David, C.; Nicolae, D.; and Ispas I. 1959. L'aspect de las maladie ulcéreuse et las résultats thérapeutique par décades d'âge. *Informations Médicales Roumaines* 2:94–95.

Aslan, Ana; Ieremia, G.; Bălan, L.; Bruchner, J.; and Tiţu H. 1973. Inclusion of methyl-thymidin H3 in culture of renal cells treated with Gerovital H3. *Fiziologia Normală şi Patologică* 3:277–281.

Aslan, Ana; Ionescu, Theodora; and Vrăbiescu, A. 1977. Studies concerning the immunological reactivity of the organism under Gerovital H3 treatment. Communications to the Eighth European Congress of Clinical Gerontology, Neptun, Rumania.

Aslan, Ana; Nicolae, D.; Jantea, F.; and Dumitrescu, Z. 1965. Deficiencies of procaine digestions and absorption in old age and their amendment. *Giornale di Gerontologia* 13:772.

Aslan, Ana, and Parhon, C. I. 1954. Novocain, eutrophic and rejuvenating factor in the preventive and curative treatment of old age. Bucharest: Rumanian Academic Editorship.

Aslan, Ana; Savu, S.; Brazdeš, L., and Vrăbiescu, A. 1975. Influence of chemotherapy with Aslavital in elderly patients with accidental fractures. Paper presented at the Tenth International Congress of the International Association of Gerontology, Jerusalem.

Aslan, Ana, and Vrăbiescu, A. 1950a. Treatment of acrocyanose with intra-arterially injected procaine. *Studii și Cercetări de Endocrinologie* 1:2.

———. 1950b. Intra-arterial treatment with procaine in arthritis and arthrosis. *Buletinul Stiințific al Academiei Republicii Socialiste România* 2:891.

———. 1955b. Oscillometric investigations in the aged by means of the effort test. *Studii și Cercetări de Endocrinologie* 6:215–221.

———. 1955c. Studies of the peripheric circulation by the plethysmographic method. In C. I. Parhon, ed., *Biologia vîrsterlor*, p. 257.

———. 1968. Contributions to the functional exploration of the cardio-vascular apparatus in the prophlaxis of precocious aging. Therapeutical results. Paper presented to the Fifth European Congress of Clinical Gerontology, Brussels.

Aslan, Ana; Vrăbiescu, A.; Domilescu, C.; Cîmpeanu, L.; Costiniu, M.; and Stănescu, St. 1965. Long-term treatment with procaine (Gerovital H₃) in albino rats. *Journal of Gerontology* 20:1–8.

Aslan, Ana; Vrăbiescu, A.; and Hartia, L. 1970. Clinical, physiopathological and therapeutical researches concerning leg arthritis in elderly patients. *Fiziologia Normală și Patologică*16:430–448.

Bucci, L., and Saunders, J. C. 1960. A psychopharmacological evaluation of 2-diethylaminoethanolparaaminobenzoat (Procaine). *Journal of Neuropsychiatry* 51:276–281.

Bunney, W. E.; Davis, J. M.; Weil, Malherbe H.; and Smith E. R. S. 1967. Biochemical changes in psychotic depression. *Archives Générales de Psychiatrie* 16:448.

Ciucă, A. 1964. Le réseau gérontologique, nécessité, organisation et fonctionnement. *La Semaine des Hôpitaux* 1:3–10.

———. 1966, A village for the elderly in Rumania. *Das Alternheim* 6:140–143.

———. 1967. Longevity and environmental conditions. *Gerontologist* 7:252–256.

———. 1969. Research of social gerontology in Rumania. Paper presented to the Thirteenth National Congress of Social Medicine, Trieste.

———. 1972. The planning of the social prorgammes in favour of the elderly population. *Tribune Medica*, no. 461.

Ciucă, A. and Jucovschi, V. 1965a. La vieillessement précoce de la population dans les zones de goitre éndemique. *La Semaine des Hôpitaux* 4:63–69.

Ciucă, A. and Jucovschi, V. 1965b. Appréciation de l'âge biologique dans las pratique du terrain. *Gazette Médicale de France* 8:1569–1570.

Ciucă, A. Sanda, Maria; Ghenciu, G.; and Bărbulescu, Theodora. 1977. Human longevity and some ecological factors. Communications to the Eighth European Congress on Clinical Gerontology, Neptun, Rumania.

Crăciun, E.; Aslan, Ana; and David, C. 1959. Sur la thanatogénése pathologique du vieillard. *Informations Médicales Roumaines* 3:16–17.

David, C.; Oancea, Tr.; Hatmanu, D.; Chira, Al.; König, V.; and Călinescu, M. 1972. L'efficience de la thérapie biotrophique au Gérovital H³ chez les personnes agées, dans le traitement des ostéoarthropathies. International Symposium on Gerontology. Bucharest.

Friedman, O. L. 1964. An investigation of Gerovital H₃ (procaine hydrochloride) in treatment of organic brain symdrome. *Gerontologist* 2.

Gordon, P.; Abrams, A.; and Fudema, J. 1965. The effects of a European procaine preparation in an aged population. II: Physiological effects. *Journal of Gerontology* 20:144.

Hrachovec, J. P. 1972. Inhibitory effect of Gerovital H₃ on monoaminoxidase of rat brain, liver and heart. *Physiologist* 15:3.

Jucovschi, V., and Ciucă A. 1977. Recherches concernant le vieillessement biologique differencié par rapport à certains facteurs de risque et aux conditions spécifiques de milieu. Communications to the Eighth European Congress of Clinical Gerontology, Neptun, Rumania.

Kuhn. 1948. quoted by R. Ammon and W. Discherl, in Fermenté, *Hormone, Vitamine*, II. *Auflage*. Leipzig: Georg Thieme, p. 935.

Leriche, R., and Lafontaine, R. 1953. De l'emploi des injections intra-arterielle de novocaine dans les formes douloureuses des artérites oblitérantes. *Presse Médicale* 17:327.

MacFarlane, M. D. 1974. Procaine (Gerovital H₃) therapy: Mechanism of inhibition of monoaminoxidase. *Journal of the American Geriatrics Society* 22:365–371.

Marinescu, G. 1899. Evolution et involution de la cellule nerveuse. *Revue de Neurologie* 7:715.

———. 1933. Studii asupra mecanismului biochimic al bătrîneţii şi al reîntinerinii *Buletinul Societăţii Române de Neurologie* 4:172.

Mayer, R. L. 1944. The influence of sulfanylamid upon the yellow pigment formed by Mycobacterium tuberculosis P-amino-benzoic acid. *Journal of Bacteriology* 1:93–96.

Moeller and Schwartz. 1948. Quoted by R. Ammon and W. Dirscher in Fermenté, *Hormone, Vitamine*, II. *Auflage* Leipzig: Georg Thieme, pp. 1936–1937.

Mustaţă, Ecaterina, and Ciucă, A. 1972. The social factors influencing work. Abstracts of the Ninth International Congress of Gerontology, Kiev.

Naum, M., and Rusu, Cornelia. 1973. Variation of nucleic acid and histones in hepatic regeneration of the Wistar white rat in relation to age and the biotrophic treatment with Aslavital. Paper presented at the Fourth International Symposium of Basic Research in Gerontology, Varberg, Sweden, September.

Parhon, C. I. 1947. *Bătrîneţea şi tratamentul ei*. Bucharest: Editura Medicală
———. 1955. *Biologia vîrstelor*. Bucharest: Rumanian Academic Editorship.

Parhon, C. I., and Aslan, Ana. 1953. Novocain, a factor against gray hair. *Buletinul Stiinţific al Academiei Republicii Socialiste România* 5:557–568.

Parhon, C. I.; Aslan, Ana; and Bojinescu, I. 1956. Studies about the influence of procaine (vitamin H³) on the thyroid function, made by I₁₃₁ radioactiv izotop. *Studii şi cercetări de Endocrinologie* 7: 161–166.

Parhon C. I.; Aslan, Ana; and Cosmovici, N. 1957. Action of vitamin H and H3 upon the proliferation of the animal cell (experiments on protozoa-infuzoria). *Scientific Bulletin of the Department for Medical Sciences* 9:135.

Parhon C. I.; Aslan, A; and Vrăbiescu, A. 1955. Superior nervous activity in young and old men, studied through the method of vascular conditioned reflexes. In C. I. Parhon, *Biologia vînstelor*. Bucharest: Rumanian Academic Editorship, p. 259.

Petolea, Rodica; Olteanu, Tatiana; and Ciucă, A. 1977. Some risk factors in accelerating the aging rate. Communications to the Eighth European Congress of Clinical Gerontology, Neptun, Rumania.

Robinson, D. S., et al. 1972. Aging, Monoamine and Monoaminoxidase levels. *Lancet*, 1:290–91.

Sanda, Maria. 1972. Social adjustment of the elderly after retirement. Abstracts of the Ninth International Congress of Gerontology, Kiev.

Siggelkov, H. 1965. Prokainbehandlung der hirnarterielle Mangelduchblutung im vortgeschrittenen Altern. Kongressberichte der Arbeitsgemeinschaft Alternsforschung der Deutchen Gesellschaft für Klinische Medizin, Leipzig, 1965. *Zeitschrift für Alternsforschung* 19:111.

Teitel, A.; Stroescu, V.; and Steflea, D. 1965. Investigations on the trophic and stimulating action of procaine upon isolated organs. *Fiziologia Normală și Patologică* 11:67–70.

Visnevski, A. V., and Visneski, A. A. 1952. Novocain blocking and oleoblastic antiseptics as a special type of pathological therapy. Moscow: Academy of Science.

Zdichynec, B. 1972. Unsere Erfolge mit der Novokaintherapie in der Vorbeugung Verfrühten Alterns. Paper presented at the International Symposium of Gerontology, Bucharest.

Zung, W. K., et al. 1974. Pharmacology of depression in the aged: Evaluation of Gerovital H^3. *Psychosomatics*, 15:127–131.

SOUTH AFRICA

S. P. CILLIERS

PLURAL SOCIETIES

The thesis that the "far-reaching and rapid changes of modern society have profoundly affected the position of old people and their ability to deal with their own problems" (Blau, 1973, p. 2) applies equally to developing societies, and in particular to developing plural societies such as the Republic of South Africa (RSA). Although no agreement exists on the exact meaning of the term *plural society* (cf. Smith and Kuper, 1969, p. 415), a plural society may be considered to be one that at its inception consists of a number of different population groups with different ethnic and cultural backgrounds all of which are incorporated into a common polity. In most of these societies, one of these groups tends to be dominant and to direct the nature and rate of modernization. The nature and format of formal institutions in such societies tend to be developed in accordance with the sociocultural heritage of the dominant group, which tends, furthermore, to be concentrated in and around major metropolitan areas.

These areas overwhelmingly serve also as the nuclei and growth points of development and modernization, and this process almost universally tends to involve a large-scale urbanization of increasing masses of the rest of the population. In this way, other racial and/or ethnic groups are increasingly involved in a social, economic, and political system evolved in accordance with the sociocultural heritage of the dominant population group.

In plural societies that have evolved from an earlier colonial situation that involved the formation of a settler element, the latter may well form the core of the dominant ethnic group after decolonization, as happened in the RSA. Even when this is not the case, the dominant ethnic group, though in itself of indigenous extraction, may well have been exposed to such a degree of acculturation by the colonial power that a formal societal system quite different from the original traditional system may have evolved.

This chapter is an extensively revised and enlarged version of an article entitled "Aging in a Plural Society," originally published in *SA Medical Journal*, July 3, 1976. Permission to use material published in this article is gratefully acknowledged.

Such societies tend overwhelmingly to aspire to modernization in the sense in which Eisenstadt (1966, p. 1) uses the term: as a process of change in the direction of the type of socioeconomic and political systems that emerged in Western Europe after the Middle Ages. Among many factors that have contributed to this tendency, the most important impetus today is probably population pressure caused by vastly increased natural population growth rates.

Because of these high rates of increase, a subsistence economy closely interwoven with other aspects of societal structure can no longer provide an adequate standard of living for the majority of such populations. Economic growth through modernization, and in particular through industrialization, tends to become a conscious goal. Virtually all such societies in recent times have therefore consciously adopted economic development programs in which central governments overwhelmingly play a strategic role in their planning, initiation, and implementation.

The result is that these modernizing plural societies tend to develop more and more structural aspects of social organization characteristic of modern societies. Most prominent among these are a high degree of differentiation and specialization with respect to individual activities and institutional structures (Eisenstadt, 1966, p. 2). Associated with this is a radical change from ascription as the basis of recruitment into these activities and institutions. These developments have major implications for the position of the aged in such societies, especially because in most traditional societies age and sex have served as most important ascriptive bases for the allocation of roles and statuses.

For the individual, the differentiation and specialization of roles involved in the process of modernization is the separation of different roles, in particular among occupational, familial, kinship, and political roles. This involves role differentiation in the sense of activities involved, the location of such activities, and the institutional structures in which such roles are embedded.

These processes of change usually do not occur evenly, and severe structural strains very often arise, giving rise to discontinuities and breakdowns (Eisenstadt, 1966; Parsons, 1958, 1977; Lerner, 1958). In plural societies a further complication arises because different ethnic or racial groups in the population are very often differentially involved in this whole process.

DEMOGRAPHY

Population Structure

The RSA presents a case study showing the process of aging and the problems of the aged in plural societies. It encompasses four major population groups with different ethnic and cultural backgrounds that are incorporated in a common polity. Descendants of Western European settlers form the dominant group and have successfully initiated a process of modernization in accordance with the pattern set by the leading Western nations. The other three major population groups are each at a different stage in the process of modernization, although considerable variation exists within each of the groups (table 63).

Table 63: ESTIMATED POPULATION STRUCTURE, 1975

	Number	Percent
Black African	18,173,000	71.4
Whites	4,233,000	16.6
Coloureds	2,333,000	9.2
Asians	727,000	2.8
Total	25,466,000	100

Source: Department of Statistics, R.S.A., Pretoria. *South African Statistics 1978*, p. 1.4.

None of these four major groups is completely homogeneous, but for our purposes, I will focus attention on differences between the groups. The Blacks are part of the southern Bantu of the African continent and have an African tribal cultural heritage. They are as yet only partly involved in the urban-industrial modernized sector of the broader South African society and are therefore categorized as a developing population. Approximately half of the total Black population still resides in rural tribal homelands, overwhelmingly sustained by an agriculturally based subsistence economy. Modernizing nuclei are only now taking root as growth points around industries being established through state initiative in these areas. While some degree of Westernization has affected virtually all of these people, their social patterns, life-style, and value orientation are still strongly traditional and tribal. Their contact with and exposure to the dominant Western culture of the broader South African society has always been and still is overwhelmingly through the formal religious, educational, economic, and governmental institutions rather than through informal interpersonal and associational processes of interaction. Those who do enter urban life as migrant workers in the modern sector of the economy or whose homelands are in close proximity to urban areas are, of course, exposed to a higher degree of Westernization.

The rest of the Black population consists of those domiciled relatively permanently in the urban and industrial centers and of farm workers who lead the life of a simple peasantry. Both have had a far greater amount of contact and association with the other population groups in the country and are therefore more Westernized than the majority of those living in the tribal homelands.

In contrast to that of the tribal homelands, the structure of contemporary Black urban society is socioeconomically and culturally complex. It is no longer a homogeneous traditional social unit and shows varying degrees of modernization. Increasing numbers of urban Blacks have become attuned to the market economy and value system that characterize the Western urban industrial society in contrast to the subsistence economy of traditional Black society.

The rest of the South African population consists of the dominant White group, which constitutes approximately 16.6 percent of the total population, the Coloureds (9.2 percent), and the Asians (2.8 percent), which may best be described as minority groups vis-à-vis the Whites. In terms of generally accepted economic and demographic criteria, the Whites may be regarded as an advanced and modernized people. The Coloureds are a community of mixed ethnic descent, deriving from a biogenetic contact situation, involving the remnants of nomadic Khoisan tribes, slaves from West Africa and the East Indies, and Europeans, over a period of more than three hundred years since the beginning of the White settlement at the Cape in 1652. In religion, language, and general way of life, they have always been closely associated with the Whites, and their culture, value orientations, and life-style are essentially Western. On the whole, the Coloureds reflect the demographic characteristics of an agricultural and industrial working class in modern Western society.

The Asians form a small minority of the total South African population. This group is mainly of Indian origin and owes its presence in South Africa primarily to the demand for farm labor on the sugar plantations in Natal during the latter half of the previous century under British colonial rule. Commercial and industrial development in Natal, where the overwhelming majority of Asians are still concentrated (83 percent of the total), have resulted in a rapid urbanization of this community. Today they occupy a position very similar to that of the Coloureds in the Cape. They have, however, retained many sociocultural traits derived from Muslim and Hindu origin. This is still most marked with respect to family life and kinship.

The Aged and Population Structure

Table 64, which presents data on the age structure of the different population groups, shows that the White population has the highest proportion of the aged: 6.6 percent. The age structure of a population is, of course, primarily a function of birthrates and specific mortality rates and thus that of the White population reflects a relatively low birthrate, a generally low death rate, and, in particular, a low infant mortality rate. In contrast, the age structure of the Black and Coloured populations reflects a very high birthrate combined with a high infant mortality rate. In the case of the Asian population, a relatively high but recently declining birthrate combined with a recently declining infant mortality rate is clearly reflected.

Unless unanticipated changes in the immediate future occur in either migration or birthrates, the proportion of the total population that includes the aged will rise even higher in the case of the Whites, will rapidly increase in the case

Table 64: AGE STRUCTURE OF POPULATION GROUPS, 1970 (IN PERCENT)

	15 and Under	15–64	65 and Over
Blacks	43.4	53.0	3.6
Whites	31.4	62.1	6.6
Coloureds	46.2	50.7	3.1
Asians	41.2	57.0	1.8

Source: Department of Statistics, Republic of South Africa, Pretoria. South African Statistics 1978, p 1.22.

of the Asians, and will remain around current levels in the case of the Coloureds and Blacks, at least until the turn of the century. This expectation is borne out by table 65, which is based on official population projections by the Department of Statistics. The table also shows a general demographic characteristic of modern societies: women live longer than men. The disparity in the sex ratio therefore tends to increase with age and tends to be greater for populations with a high life expectancy. Here, again, significant differences are apparent between the different population groups in South Africa.

Table 65: PROJECTED PERCENTAGES OF POPULATION 65 AND OVER, 1970-2020

	Blacks		Whites		Coloureds		Asians	
	Male	Female	Male	Female	Male	Female	Male	Female
1970	3.22	4.01	5.45	7.59	2.70	3.35	1.89	1.61
1980	2.65	3.59	6.93	9.04	2.72	3.22	2.19	2.18
1990	2.67	3.75	7.47	9.67	2.72	3.15	2.42	2.89
2000	2.97	4.17	7.71	9.90	2.99	3.62	2.76	3.87
2010	3.37	4.64	8.98	11.12	3.36	4.14	3.54	5.35
2020	3.98	5.37	10.29	12.65	4.34	5.18	4.60	7.39

Note: Excluding projected migration.

The various sex ratios reported for Whites in table 66 are in accordance with those for populations of advanced Western societies. While there is a preponderance of males at birth, an excess of females that becomes more marked for higher age groups is noticeable. In the age category of 75 and over, there were only 59.7 White males per 100 White females in 1970. This means that a high proportion of the White aged are single females. Although similar trends are also noticeable for Blacks and Coloureds, they are less marked. It is significant that Blacks approximate the position with regard to Whites more closely than either Coloureds or Asians. Because for a large sector of the Black population the traditional tribal social structure with its emphasis on the extended family and broad kinship system still provides the social basis, the

Table 66: SEX RATIOS FOR POPULATION GROUPS, 1970

	Blacks	Whites	Coloureds	Asians
At birth	99.0	105.2	100.7	103.5
Total population	96.6	99.2	96.8	99.4
Population 65 and over	74.7	70.6	83.7	108.1
Population 75 and over	65.6	59.7	70.4	109.7

Source: Department of Statistics, Republic of South Africa, Pretoria, 1976. *Population Census 1970, Report No. 02-05-10*, p. 2.
Note: The figures show the number of males per 100 females.

preponderance of aged females in the Black population takes on an entirely different significance from that of the preponderance of aged White females.

In the case of the Asian population, the position differs significantly: there is a preponderance of aged males over females. This pattern is a function of two factors: a sex-specific differential in immigration rates up to the late 1940s and high rates of maternal mortality until the mid-1940s. An analysis of younger age cohorts indicates a change in this pattern, so that the present preponderance of aged males over females is expected to be reversed within the next two decades. This means that in the Asian community at present, the aged have problems and needs entirely different from those of the aged in the White community.

Life Expectancy

Differences between sex ratios for different population groups may be a function of either sex-specific mortality rates or sex-specific migration patterns. In the case of the different South African population groups, the effect of sex-specific mortality rates is reflected by data pertaining to life expectancy.

Table 67: LIFE EXPECTANCY AT BIRTH, 1970–1975

	Males	Females
Blacks	52.05	59.39
Whites	65.08	72.96
Coloureds	50.54	57.22
Asians	60.32	64.91

Source: J. L. Sadie. "The Demographic Forces in South Africa." *Transactions of the Royal Society of South Africa* 43, Part 1, March 1978, p. 18.

The current life expectancy of Whites at birth closely approximates that of the populations of modern Western countries (table 67). Overall Asian life expectancy comes nearest to that of Whites, although the longer life expectancy of females is not as pronounced for Asians as would be expected.

The demographic features discussed thus far serve to illustrate that considerable differences exist between the various population groups. At the same time, demographic patterns for all groups tend increasingly to approximate those in advanced Western societies. In this process the major demographic differences between the White population group and the others will be diminished.

Marital Status

In a discussion of marital status, sociocultural differences with regard to sexual union, marriage, and kinship of different ethnic groups should be kept in mind. Two notable features are reflected in table 68. First, the proportion of aged males who are married is is significantly higher than that of females for all population groups. This is a function of patterns for remarriage and of differential mortality rates between the sexes. Second, the proportions of never-married aged females are significantly lower for Blacks and Asians than for Whites and Coloureds. This clearly links up with cultural differences between the kinship systems and marital practices of Western and non-Western population groups.

Table 68: MARITAL STATUS OF PERSONS 65 AND OVER, 1970

	Blacks		Whites		Coloureds		Asians	
	Males	Females	Males	Females	Males	Females	Males	Females
Never Married	3.60	2.14	5.03	8.02	9.35	8.61	3.58	2.58
Married	79.60	28.46	77.55	32.00	58.38	29.68	67.75	21.03
Widowed	14.99	68.52	14.78	57.32	25.22	58.02	26.62	74.72
Divorced	0.57	1.40	2.25	2.54	1.51	0.95	1.02	0.92
Cohabitation	1.24	0.48	0.39	0.12	5.54	2.74	1.02	0.74

Source: Department of Statistics, Republic of South Africa, Population Census, 1970, Reports Nos. 02-01-01, p. 9, and 02-01-02, pp. 9 and 21.

Economic Activities

The degree of economic activity of the aged is a function of a combination of such factors as the general standard of living and economic security and independence, the nature of involvement in economic life, and the level and nature of public provision for economic security for aged people. An analysis of data pertaining to the economic activity of aged persons in the RSA is presented in tables 69 and 70.

Table 69 shows that more of the Blacks above the age of 65 are economically active than is the case for any of the other population groups. The data for Coloured and Asian aged persons reflect the fact that these two groups occupy

Table 69: PROPORTION OF AGED ECONOMICALLY ACTIVE

	Percentage Economically Active
Blacks	24.15
Whites	19.63
Coloureds	16.14
Asians	16.33

Source: RSA, Department of Statistics, Population Census 1970, Report No. 02-01-05, pp. 11, 26, and 37; Population Census 1960, Sample Tabulation, Report No. 5, p.28.

Note: Data for Whites, Coloureds, and Asians are for 1970; those for Blacks, are for 1960.

comparable positions in the general economic structure of the South African society; both are overwhelmingly working- and lower-working-class strata. In order to understand the differences between population groups, it is necessary to make a more detailed analysis, presented in table 70.

Table 70: PROPORTION OF AGED ECONOMICALLY ACTIVE, BY SEX AND LOCATION

Population Group	Male		Female	
	Urban	Rural	Urban	Rural
Blacks	54	47	11	5
Whites	34	57	6	7
Coloureds	25	41	4	6
Asians	27	33	2	4

Source: RSA, Department of Statistics, Population Census 1970, Report No. 02-01-05, pp. 11, 26, and 37; Population Census 1960, Sample Tabulation, Report No. 5, p. 28.

Note: Date for Whites, Coloureds, and Asians are for 1970; those for Blacks are for 1960.

All rural groups except Blacks show a higher level of economic activity than urban groups, for both sexes. Since economic activity in rural areas primarily concerns agriculture, the pattern for a relatively high level of economic activity of aged persons is to be expected. The nature of the involvement of different population groups in agriculture explains differences in the frequency for Whites as against the other population groups. Approximately nine-tenths of all White males involved in agriculture are farmers or entrepreneurs and are not subject to compulsory retirement on reaching specified ages. Coloured and Asian workers in agriculture, on the other hand, are overwhelmingly employed as farm laborers who often cannot continue their strenuous work in old age.

The overall situation of a higher level of economic activity for the rural aged than for those in urban areas is a function of two sets of factors. First, the nature of agricultural activity is such that it is possible to provide some form of occupational opportunity in accordance with an individual's physical and mental ability to a greater extent than in the case of economic opportunities in industries in an urban location. Second, there is a clear tendency for the aged from rural areas to migrate to urban areas upon retirement, particularly in societies experiencing high rates of urbanization, as in the case of the RSA.

The divergent pattern for aged Blacks, reflected in table 68, is a function of their differential position and citizen status in the RSA. Blacks in urban areas outside the tribal homelands are subject to a complex and restrictive system of influx control. Two major categories may be distinguished: those who qualify for permanent residence in urban areas in terms of these influx control measures, and those who qualify for temporary residence in urban areas as migrant workers. With regard to the first category, one of the qualifying principles relates to employment. In terms of this qualification, the opportunity to migrate to urban areas after retirement, as in the case of Whites, Coloureds, and Asians, is excluded for Blacks. Furthermore, for some years it has been the policy of the state to resettle aged urban Blacks in need of institutional care in old-age settlements in rural tribal homelands.

This pattern provides the link with the second category of urban Blacks—migrant workers. In terms of the influx control measures applicable to Blacks, virtually only those who enter into contracts of employment are allowed to reside in urban areas. Thus only elderly persons from rural areas who are gainfully occupied as employees are entitled to migrate to urban areas for the duration of their contract of employment. The effect is that a disproportionately high percentage of urban aged Blacks are shown to be economically active.

Finally since Blacks form the poorest sector of the population of the country, with the lowest level of economic security, it is to be expected that this population will be least able to afford voluntary retirement from economic activity. In plural societies such as the RSA, one therefore finds a fairly high level of occupational involvement of the aged from both the most advanced group (Whites) and the least advanced group (Blacks), but for totally different reasons. In the case of the most advanced group, their privileged position and the scarcity value of their skills serve to boost the level of economic activity of the aged. By contrast, the level of economic insecurity, the involvement of a traditional subsistence economy, and the lack of privileges of the least advanced group (Blacks) serve equally to boost the level of economic activity of their aged.

ROLES AND STATUS OF THE AGED

In a discussion of the nature and pattern of involvement of the aged in each of the population groups, note should be taken of the family system and its relationship with other structural aspects of society. The Black population derives from a background of a traditional type of tribal social structure. Consanguinal bonds and the family play a very important role in the broad social organization of such African societies, in which the aged take on an important role. Writing about the Pondo people of the Eastern Cape, Hunter (1964) states:

Conservative tendencies in Bantu society are strong. Power is in the hands of the elders, and piety demands that there should be no departure from the ways of the ancestors, who by reason of their age must know better than their children. [p. 9]

She continues:

The ancestor cult is a sanction for the respect for seniors upon which the social and political system is based. . . . At a ritual killing, children see a beast, a thing of great value, slaughtered, and know that it is done that good relations with the *amathongo* [ancestors] may be maintained. Thus the power and importance of seniors is brought home to them. The ritual re-affirms the belief of all in the existence and power of ancesters. [p. 266]

The position of the aged in such societies is therefore one of relative security; they perform a meaningful role in social and cultural life.

Urbanization and industrialization bring dramatic changes to this situation. Contact with Western culture leads to a weakening of the role of consanguinal bonds and to the adoption of values and attitudes that differ significantly from those associated with traditional tribal life. Family life in accordance with the traditional system is weakened, in fact disrupted to a large degree, and changes toward the nuclear type of Western family occur. Research undertaken in urban areas in South Africa indicates that multigenerational families and matriarchal families are very common. Reviewing available empirical evidence on urban Black family life in South Africa, Steyn and Rip (1968) conclude that

the multigeneration type is considerably bigger than other types of families . . . . The data . . . also indicate that a large percentage . . . have a woman at the head. This, seen together with changes in the relative positions of authority of the husband and wife respectively and also in view of the fact that illegitimate children form part of the family structure of the wife, is an indication that the urbanised Bantu (Black) family is moving in the direction of a matrifocal family type. [p. 515]

Under such circumstances drastic changes occur with regard to the position of the aged. Age and sex as bases of status are being replaced by individual achievement, and the aged are becoming increasingly socially and economically insecure. Furthermore with urbanization and industrialization, a phenomenon of fairly recent origin for the Black population, a significant proportion of the aged in urban areas are still at least partly involved in the tribal social structure of the rural homelands. An increasing proportion of them are, however, second- and third-generation urbanites with hardly any tribal contact but often not yet involved in a stable urban social structure.

In the case of the White population, a social structure typical of modern Western societies prevails. This encompasses a typical nuclear family system, a high degree of structural differentiation between the family system and the economy and the polity, and achievement rather than ascription as a basis for the allocation of role and status. Under these circumstances, aging for a growing proportion of the aged group means an increasing exclusion from family life. Since aging furthermore tends to coincide with a high incidence of death of spouse and with retirement from work, social and psychological isolation from association with significant others tends to become fairly common. Furthermore the extension of life expectancy increases the extent of physical and mental infirmity among the aged.

Thus the problems and the needs of the aged in the White population tend to center increasingly on finding alternatives to replace the functions performed by the family system in this regard. There is a need to reestablish meaningful social relationships on other grounds than those of consanguinity and to be cared for physically on a formal institutional basis.

In the case of the Coloured minority, family life is much less stable. While middle- and upper-class Coloureds maintain a family system more or less identical with that of the Whites described above, the lower working classes in this group, which constitute the vast majority, differ significantly. A high incidence of matrifocal or mother-dominant families is found, and incomplete families consisting of mother and dependent children are fairly common. Especially in urban areas, there is a high rate of economic activity among adult females. Multigenerational families are therefore fairly common, and aged persons are overwhelmingly accommodated within the households of relatives, mostly those of their own children. The receipt of old-age pensions by a large section of this population under such circumstances serves the added function of providing a minimal degree of economic security in the otherwise relatively insecure circumstances of lower-working-class people.

In these circumstances the aged are therefore closely involved in the affairs of the household, very often with a large degree of responsibility for the supervising of day-to-day household chores. During the day the aged are often the sole adults present in the home together with preschool children. To a large degree, the care for and primary socialization of young children are the responsibility of the aged. Conversely the needs of the aged, especially of those physically and mentally infirm, are often tended to by young children with the assistance of neighbors.

Asians in the RSA have apparently been more successful in retaining many characteristics of the extended kinship system (*kutum*) of traditional Hindu and Muslim society under circumstances of urbanization and modernization than have the Blacks. In contrast to the Whites, aged Asians still overwhelmingly tend to be accommodated with and integrated into the extended family life of their children and relatives. The aged Asians therefore appear at present to be socially and psychologically reasonably secure.

LIVING CONDITIONS

In the case of the Whites, as is to be expected in terms of the preponderance of the nuclear family system, only a minority live with children, relatives, or other people. Approximately two-thirds of all persons above the age of 60 live on their own (with or without spouses), and only approximately 25 percent live with relatives. The degree of independence varies with socioeconomic status, so that, for instance, in the case of recipients of old-age pensions who are economically more insecure, the proportion living with relatives will be considerably higher. A recent survey of recipients of state old-age and war veterans' pensions in an urban community revealed that 47.7 percent were living with children or had children living with them and a further 10.4 percent were living with other persons (Van Tonder, 1972). It seems that aged Whites have accepted the ideal of the nuclear family, since hardly any of those not living with other people would prefer to do so. This conclusion confirms studies that have shown that elderly Whites generally prefer to retain their independence for as long as possible. Finally, approximately 6 percent of elderly Whites live in old-age homes. A degree of antipathy toward these homes seems to exist; they are generally viewed only as a last resort.

Since they form part of a predominantly working-class population group, aged Coloureds (in contrast to Whites) live mostly with their children. According to a recent national sample survey of aged Coloureds, 67.7 percent were living in multigeneration households with their children, and only 27.8 percent formed independent households with or without their spouses (Van der Walt, 1967, p. 39). According to the same source, only 14.7 percent indicated a willingness to be accommodated in homes for the aged.

Since the Coloureds overwhelmingly fall into the working- and lower-working-class strata of the total population, a very large proportion of them live in publicly controlled housing. In the provision of public housing, the general policy is to take the needs of the nuclear type of family as the basis for provision and control. As a result, accommodation in the homes of their children is often not available for the aged or can be provided only under conditions of overcrowding. Public authorities in control of such housing tend increasingly to exercise stricter control over overcrowding. The net effect is that the aged, and in particular the infirm aged, are increasingly forced out of the preferred arrangement of living with children or other relatives. While the physical need for shelter and accommodation for such aged persons is increasingly being met through the reservation of land for the erection of old-age homes for the infirm and through group housing for the independent, this whole development serves to illustrate the tendency in plural modernizing societies for the behavior patterns of the dominant (in this case, White) population group to be used as a model in terms of which approaches to the problems of caring for the needs of the aged for other population groups are made.

A recent sample survey on the socioeconomic position of aged Asians in the province of Natal, where 83 percent of all South African Asians reside, showed that only 3.8 percent were living alone or with spouses only. A further 24.0 percent were living with unmarried children, 53.6 percent with a married son, 13.1 percent with a married daughter, and 5.5 percent with other relatives and/or friends (Rip et al., 1974, p. 11). This finding clearly reflects the degree to which the extended family system still functions in the Asian community. The authors point out:

There is not even a word in any of the Indian languages used in South Africa for the English word ''family.'' The nearest to it are ''kutum'' (Gujarati, Hindustani and Urdu) and ''kudumbom'' or ''kuduma'' (Tamil and Telegu respectively). These terms refer to a kinship system of several nuclear families hierarchically arranged accordingly to a male seniority.

The nuclear units of the kutum usually contain an older parent(s) or relative(s). Irrespective of the composition of this unit most Indians are strongly attached to their kutum. This kutum consists of all those with whom he can trace consanguinity through a common paternal grandfather or grandfather's brother. The kutum is a restricted kinship group tracing descent through males. The relationship between members of a kutum is the same as between close relatives and the associated sentiments and role expectations also apply, the intensity of which depends on the closeness of the consanguinity. [p. 6]

The preferred pattern of living with a married son rather than with a married daughter stresses the fact that the kutum traces descent through the male in direct contrast to the pattern among the White Westerners, where aged persons living with married children predominantly share the household of their married daughters. Under these circumstances, relatively few aged Asians are in favor of residing in old-age homes. In view of the tendency toward Westernization, it may be expected that such attitudes may change with future generations of Asians in South Africa.

Empirical material concerning the living conditions of aged Blacks is not readily available. The general pattern, however, seems to be for aged Blacks living in the tribal homelands to be accommodated with relatives in accordance with the practices of the extended kinship system prevailing for each tribal group. The same pattern would also prevail for most of those living in the White-controlled rural areas. In the case of the urban Blacks, the tendency toward a matrifocal multigenerational type of family seems to indicate that the aged urban Black will, for the foreseeable future, be accommodated with relatives, although perhaps in a different role relationship from that now prevailing.

PROGRAMS

Statutory provision for a minimum degree of economic security for the aged through a system of state old-age and veterans' pensions has been available in the RSA for several decades. The system was first introduced in 1929 for White and Coloured aged persons and was extended to the other population groups in 1944. At present, males above the age of 65 and females above the age of 60 years may, subject to a means test, qualify for old-age pensions. Special allowances for the care of the infirm are also available. Both the means test and the pensions are adjusted from time to time in accordance with fluctuations in cost-of-living indexes. A comprehensive compulsory system of social security has been recommended by statutory commissions on at least two occasions, but no such system is as yet in operation. On the other hand, the state actively encourages personal and private efforts toward provision for old age through statutory control over pension schemes, income tax concessions on contributions to such schemes, and on life and other forms of insurance and related schemes. In general, a minimum level of economic security for the aged is provided for by the state, although this may not be much more than at a subsistence level.

The guiding principle in the state welfare services for the aged in the RSA is based on the assumption that the aged are an integral part of the community and that they must be given the opportunity to remain full members of the community as long as possible. This policy implies that services for the aged should meet three needs: services in the community, special housing, and institutional care. To achieve this policy, the state works in close liaison with voluntary organizations, which to a great extent are responsible for welfare services for the aged. The state assists by paying pensions and making monetary contributions to those bodies devoting their energies to the interests of the aged.

The provision of services in the community includes medical, social, and recreational services and a variety of other auxiliary services such as laundry services, home visits and help with the household, and meals on wheels. In its most elementary form, this service aims to see that the aged do not become lonely. One hundred percent building loans at an interest rate of 1 percent repayable over a period of forty years are obtainable from the state to local authorities, utility companies, and registered welfare organizations for the construction of service centers. In the case of a registered welfare organization maintaining a service center, the state also pays a subsidy amounting to 75 percent of the rental in respect of approved accommodation, a nonrecurrent subsidy of 75 percent of the actual purchase price of furniture and equipment, and a subsidy amounting to 50 percent of the approved running expenditure. The main object of these centers is to provide a variety of services to meet the primary needs of aged persons who wish to maintain an independent way of life as long as possible.

The state also administers a subsidy scheme with the object of granting registered welfare organizations financial assistance to enable them to establish and maintain clubs for the aged. The objects of these clubs are more or less the same as that of the service centers except that they are run on a much smaller scale.

Special housing for the aged implies providing individual aged couples or unattached aged persons with complete housing units (small flats) in which they can maintain their own household and live as independently as possible. One hundred percent building loans are made available by the state to enable local authorities, utility companies, and registered welfare organizations to construct such housing.

Except in exceptional circumstances, it is state policy not to establish homes for the aged but to assist welfare organizations financially in rendering this service. For this purpose the state provides one hundred percent subeconomic building loans for the establishment of approved new homes at an interest rate of 0.05 percent or 1 percent, depending on the economic group of residents the home plans to serve, repayable over forty years. The purchase of furniture and equipment is also subsidized. Monthly capitation grants are paid to these homes in respect of residents of the subeconomic income group. The amount of these grants depends on the grade of infirmity or dependency of the residents and the ratio of qualified nurses employed by the home. The state lays down standards for these old-age homes and inspects them regularly.

The Aged Persons Act (1967) provides for the protection and welfare of certain aged and debilitated persons, for the care of their interests, for the compulsory registration of all old-age homes, and for regulations as to the minimum standards with which all homes for the aged have to comply.

The salaries of social workers in the employ of registered welfare organizations that deal partly or exclusively with the aged who are living in the community are subsidized.

A few organizations assist prospective elderly people to prepare themselves (mentally, emotionally, financially, and in other ways) for retirement and are assisted financially for this purpose by the state.

Voluntary welfare organizations involved in work among the aged are coordinated by the South African National Council for the Aged. This council aims to coordinate the activities of and to make available advice to all organizations interested in this kind of work, to promote the interests and well-being of the aged, to promote and carry out services relating to the needs of the aged, to serve as a channel through which the problems, findings, or suggestions of member organizations can be conveyed to government departments, and to encourage the extension of the work among the aged throughout the RSA. The council, which cooperates with national and international organizations and is a member of the International Federation on Aging, supports, promotes, and watches over legislation that affects the interests of the welfare of the aged.

RESEARCH

No specialized research agencies concentrating exclusively on issues relating to the aged exist in the RSA; however, a considerable amount of both basic and applied research is being conducted at various institutes. According to the South African Medical Research Council, relatively few researchers in the RSA work specifically on problems in the field of gerontology, since most prefer to view it as part of broader projects and to concentrate on the process of aging throughout the life span. The plural character of the South African population offers unique opportunities for comparative research, particularly on diseases more prevalent among the aged, and biomedical researchers are increasingly turning to this field. Excellent examples of this kind of research are to be found in the work of Dr. A. R. P. Walker, director of the Medical Research Council's Human Biochemistry Research Unit at the South African Institute for Medical Research in Johannesburg, and his associates on subjects such as coronary heart disease in aged South African Blacks, on colon cancer and diet (Walker, 1976), and on minimum vascular sequelae of aging (Walker, 1966). A regular overview of progress in the field of biomedical research is provided in the *Annual Report of the South African Medical Council.*

Psychological, social, and economic research on the aged is undertaken by the Institute for Sociological, Demographic, and Criminological Research of the Human Sciences Research Council and by academic departments at South African universities. Subjects such as the general socioeconomic position of the aged of the various population groups, attitudes of the aged toward their living conditions and facilities at their disposal, and budget analyses of aged pensioners are dealt with in these studies; academic research tends to concentrate on the needs of the aged and the role of welfare agencies and service professions in meeting these needs. Finally evaluative and prescriptive research should be mentioned. In the RSA this kind of research is mostly undertaken or sponsored by the divisions for research and information of the various state departments responsible for social services for the aged. Thus, for instance, the extensive *Manual for the Care of the Aged in Homes*, based on an intensive study both in the RSA and in other countries and prepared by the Division for the Care of the Aged, was published in 1969 by the State Department of Social Welfare and Pensions. Similar publications deal with subjects such as the training of staff of homes for the aged, community services for the aged, and clubs for the aged.

SUMMARY

The analysis serves to illustrate the complexity of the problem of aging in the RSA as a plural modernizing society. Unlike advanced societies, no single dominant pattern can be isolated. Thus the problems and the needs of the aged in each of the different population groups in such a complex society differ.

A further complication arises from the fact that in such plural modernizing societies, the behavior patterns and institutional structures of the dominant population group often serve as the model in terms of which approaches to the problems of caring for the aged are made. Solutions to the problem therefore tend to be sought in terms of the needs of the aged in the advanced or dominant group in the society. At the same time, the need for democratization and equalization often leads to a situation in which any attempt to devise differential approaches to the needs of the aged from different groups may be viewed as an attempt to maintain or extend differentiation and/or discrimination. Such approaches therefore are often rejected on ideological grounds.

I have indicated that plural societies are characterized by the fact that population groups of different ethnic extractions are incorporated into a common polity. In the modern world, it has been generally accepted that the polity, and specifically the public sector as incorporated through the various local and central governmental institutions, should shoulder an increasing responsibility for the needs of the aged. In view of the fact that in plural societies one ethnic group usually tends to be dominant, it is to be expected that such a group will tend to set the pattern for public provision of the aged in accordance with the place of the aged in their own population group.

In such societies, there clearly exists a need for a flexible, nondogmatic approach to the needs of the aged. The social sciences in advanced societies with a comparative homogeneity have tended to concentrate on the problems of the aged in terms of the perspectives derived from the study of the societies. These perspectives may not necessarily suffice when approaching the problem of aging in plural societies undergoing processes of rapid modernizing change. Theoretical perspectives will have to be extended significantly, and a real need for much more empirical research on the situation in such societies is clearly required. This is particularly needed to form a basis for the development of public programs of care for the needs of the aged in such societies.

INFORMATION SOURCES

Publications and unpublished information on the subjects listed below may be obtained from the addresses listed, and should provide a general overview of most aspects of the position of the aged in the RSA. They can be used as sources from which more detailed information may be obtained on the aspects listed:

Demography

Department of Statistics, Private Bag, Pretoria, 0001, RSA.

Biomedical Asects

S.A. Medical Research Council, Box 70, Tygerberg, 7505, RSA.

Sociocultural Aspects

Human Sciences Research Council, Private Bag X41, Pretoria, 0001, RSA.

Programs

Department of Social Welfare and Pensions, Private Bag, Pretoria, 0001, RSA.
Department of Indian Affairs, Private Bag, Pretoria, 0001, RSA.
Administration of Coloured Affairs, Private Bag 9008, Cape Town, 8000, RSA.
Department of Bantu Administration and Development, Private Bag, Pretoria, 0001, RSA.

Voluntary Services

S.A. National Council for the Aged, Box 2335, Cape Town, 8000, RSA.

REFERENCES

Blau, Z. S. 1973. *Old age in a changing society*. New York: Watts.
Eisenstadt, S. N. 1966. *Modernization: Protest and change*. Englewood Cliffs, N.J.: Prentice-Hall.
Hunter, Monica. 1964. *Reaction to conquest*. London: Oxford University Press.
Lerner, D. 1958. *The passing of traditional society*. New York: Free Press.
Parsons, T. 1958. *Structure and process in modern society*. New York: Free Press.
————. 1977. *The evolution of societies*. Englewood Cliffs, N.J.: Prentice-Hall.
Rip, Colin M.; Verster, J. U.; and Groenewald, D. C. 1974. *Socio-economic position of aged Indians in Natal*. Pretoria: Human Sciences Research Council.
Seftel, H. C., et al. 1967. Coronary heart disease in aged South African Bantu. *Geriatrics* 20: 191-205.
Smith, M. G., and Kuper, L., eds. 1969. *Pluralism in Africa*. Los Angeles: University of California Press.

Steyn, A. F., and Rip, Colin M. 1968. The changing urban Bantu family. *Journal of Marriage and the Family*. 30.

Van der Walt, T. J. 1967. *Lewensomstandighede van Kleurlingbejaardes*. Department of Education, Arts and Science, National Bureau for Educational and Social Research.

Van Tonder, I. S. J. 1974. Lewensomstandighede van Blanke pensioentrekkers in 'n stedelike gemeenskap. *Humanitas* 1–4.

Walter, A. R. P. 1966. Minimum vascular sequela of aging. *Geriatrics* 21: 161-165.

———. 1976. Colon cancer and diet, with special reference to intake of fat fiber. *American Journal of Clinical Nutrition* 29: 1417–1426

SWITZERLAND

J. P. JUNOD

Switzerland is a confederation of twenty-two cantons, three of which are divided in half-cantons, thus making a total of twenty-five small states. The federal constitution guarantees these states great autonomy, especially in the areas of public health and education. There is no Swiss Ministry of Health, but the Federal Department of the Interior includes a Federal Service of Public Hygiene whose role is to make recommendations, to supervise the cantonal health authorities, and to coordinate their activities. This service also maintains a liaison between the cantons and the World Health Organization. It has no decision-making power for the cantons but does supervise the application and execution of any federal laws concerning public health.

Each canton has its own legislative body, the Grand Council, and its own governing body, the State Council. Health and social affairs are attributed in each canton to either one or two departments. Each canton makes its own policy and has its own budget.

For a long time the Helvetic Confederation limited itself to encouraging grants of financial aid. From 1929, this aid was first in the form of simple assistance, then later by means of insurance and the creation of the AVS (Assurance-Vieillesse et Survivants). This insurance for the aged and survivors dealt with the general problems of aging within the framework of a report that appeared in 1966 and is now in the process of being reissued (Saxer, 1966).

Private medicine is practiced in Switzerland. Although progress has been made in the area of social gerontology (Vischer, 1959), new tasks present themselves today. These tasks are physical and psychological care with the accompanying implications of financing and organization. It is also necessary to centralize the existing documentation, which is now being done by the Center for Information on Aging.

Various organizations cooperate in the development of gerontological action. The Swiss National Foundation for the Aged, shortly after World War II, encouraged the improvement of activities for the aged, including vacations, home meal service, information, and social services. The Swiss Gerontological Society, founded in 1953, consists of a medical section, a medicosocial section, and a biological section. Each year the society holds an assembly to discuss subjects of medical biology. Since 1958 this society has organized a second annual session devoted principally to medicosocial problems.

The Federal Council in 1973 appointed a Commission of Experts for the problems of the aged, which is under the auspices of the Federal Office of Social Insurance.

DEMOGRAPHY

According to generally accepted demographic criteria (Neury, 1975), in the 1930s Switzerland reached the condition of what is understood by the term *an aged population*. In the federal census of 1941, there were 8.6 aged persons 65 years or more for 100 individuals of all ages. In January 1971, this proportion reached 11.5 percent and at the beginning of 1976, 12.7 percent. These statistics place Switzerland among the most aged European countries.

The foreign resident population (16.5 percent of total residents at the beginning of 1976 due to massive immigration during the 1950s and 1960s) played a significant role in delaying the demographic aging of our country. On January 1, 1976, the proportion of aged persons was 14.5 percent among the Swiss population and only 3.9 percent among the foreign population. On January 1, 1971, the population aged 65 years and over was 710,700. The population aged 75 years and over was 242,500. Five years later the population figure for 65 and over was 807,000, an increase of 13.6 percent. For the figure for 75 and over was 291,400, an increase of 20.2 percent.

According to prospective calculations recently established by the Federal Bureau of Statistics, the number of individuals aged 65 years and over may reach 1,046,800 by the beginning of the year 2006 (an increase of 29.7 percent in thirty years), while the number of persons 75 years and over may reach 439,900 (an increase of 51.0 percent in thirty years). This demographic aging will probably continue its upward trend. It is estimated that by the beginning of the year 2006, the proportion of aged persons 65 years and over will reach 16.0 percent of all ages and that the old aged (75 years and more) will reach 6.7 percent. From these figures, we must conclude that the old aged may reach a proportion of 42.0 percent of all the aged in 2006 against 36.1 percent in 1976.

ROLE AND STATUS OF THE AGED

The Role of the Aged

Questions concerning the role of the aged vary from canton to canton and depend upon the particular character of the canton—whether it is industrial or agricultural. In certain cantons with both agricultural and industrial activity, we find the development of an industrial type ethic. In the cantons where there is a traditional agricultural activity, the aged continue to retain their place within the family, as well as activities suitable to their capacities. Where the industrial type of life predominates, the children leave the family very early, often even before establishing their own families. The role of the elderly parents or the grandparents is reduced to a minimum.

At the time of professional retirement, which occurs in a rigid manner for dependent salaried workers, especially since the beginning of the present recession, we witness certain problems of function linked to the importance given to the concept of the degree of usefulness of the individual based upon his socioeconomic worth.

We are now witnessing a collective awakening of serious concern (Ebersold, 1975 a & b; Satter, 1975; Scherler, 1970; Stücki, 1975). This sociological phenomenon is directed principally toward retired persons born after 1915. This concern, strongly encouraged in various ways in different areas of work but mainly by industry and commerce, is manifested by courses for those approaching retirement (Tournier, 1971), by the creation of clubs for the retired, by the stimulation of creativity and participation by the retired in associations directed by themselves, and by specialized publications.

Legal Status of the Aged

Those eligible for regular old-age pension (AVS) are entitled to collect such pension whether they continue to work or have other income. In addition, they are no longer required to make contributions to the old-age fund.

Created in 1948, the AVS allocates to those it insures an old-age pension granted from the age of 62 years for women and from 65 years for men. For wage earners the contributions to the AVS represent 10 percent of their salary (5 percent paid by the employer and 5 percent paid by the employee). For self-employed workers, the contributions represent 8.9 percent of their earnings. Married women who have no remunerated activity do not contribute to the AVS. At present, on an average yearly income of 18,000 Swiss francs, the basic monthly pension is 725 Swiss francs. The full pension is given whenever the contributions have been made by the insured without interruption since 1948. If contributions were not made in some years, only a partial pension is accorded. For women who have not made contributions during their marriage or their widowhood, these years are nonetheless counted as years of contributions. Those whose old-age pension does not reach certain minimums are entitled to additional compensation. Anyone can receive such additional compensation as long as their income and any other resources are not more than the limits fixed by the law. This law guarantees the solitary aged and couples a minimum income linked to the cost of living. As of January 1, 1977, this minimum for the canton of Geneva, for example, was fixed at 10,384 Swiss francs per year for single persons and 15,576 Swiss francs for couples.

PROBLEMS

Among the principal problems encountered at the present time are: the increase in the number of aged over 80 years with the responsibilities and questions this raises; the generation gap; a marked tendency toward a general protective attitude of the retired aged without consideration of their actual needs, which inevitably stimulates a rather unfavorable reaction from the adult population now confronting the present recession; and the traditional problems of health, lodging, and shelter.

PROPOSED PROGRAMS

General Considerations

The proposed programs are mostly suggested by the results of studies undertaken by the cantons. The solutions may vary considerably depending upon their locations. Thus the figures and facts can be used only as a kind of orientation, and they refer more to urban rather than rural regions.

The general outline that emerges from hospital and extramural plans (Feder and Junod, 1975; Gilliand, 1969, 1976; Junod and Simeone, 1975), may be defined as follows:

1. For routine hospitalizations without distinction of age (general, private, and psychiatric hospitals) the number of beds necessary represents about 5 percent of the total population. These establishments receive a significant proportion of the aged sick.

2. For geriatric and psychogeriatric hospitalization, the number of beds necessary represents about 1 percent of the aged population of 65 years or more.

3. For shelter of the sick and handicapped aged in institutions, the number of places necessary represents about 6 percent of the aged population of 65 or more.

4. For housing equipped with medicosocial services, the number of inhabitants represents about 5 percent of the aged population of 65 or more.

These needs are not all being satisfied at the present time (Gygy, 1976; Hoby, 1976). Establishing gerontological or geriatric programs requires great flexibility as well as constant attention to evolving requirements from both a qualitative and a quantitative point of view. Several cantons have found it advisable to form special commissions to counsel the authorities in different sectors on gerontological and geriatric action they may intend to take.

Information and Coordination

Maintaining an aged person at home requires the coordinated cooperation of private and public organizations. It is important that those concerned be informed of the facilities available to them. For this purpose centers and offices of social information have been created.

Gerontological action able to respond to all the medicosocial problems of the aged entails an efficient coordination of many different structures, as well as the systematic pursuit of anticipated studies that can supply information on the nature and importance of these needs. This does exist in some Swiss cantons where it permits close cooperation between private and public organizations that work with the aged.

Occupation and Leisure

It is not unusual that sudden inactivity exposes some retired persons to both physical and psychological health problems (Müller et al., 1969; Wertheimer, 1977). Courses in preparing for retirement give each individual the opportunity to consider some of the problems they may face.

In most cities and communities senior citizen clubs try to offer their members a place for contact and friendship. These clubs put at the disposition of their members various recreational activities, as well as cultural and creative activities.

For retired persons who wish to increase their intellectual knowledge, adult education courses are given at the university. These courses are varied and adapted from diverse disciplines. For those who are unable to move about easily, organizations that provide home visits guarantee some regular contact with the outside world. Gymnastic courses and other sports activities are increasingly popular. These programs help the participants escape from their solitude and have regular exercise adapted to their particular condition.

Traffic regulation courses are given with the help of the police and the Swiss Touring Club. We all know that traffic accidents take a heavy toll among the aged. Preventive action of this kind deserves to be pursued.

Vacations are no longer the exclusive domain of children and adults. The aged who benefit from vacations are more numerous than ever. It would seem especially useful to consider how to make vacations possible for the handicapped who cannot be accommodated by most hotels.

Care and Help at Home

Services that provide domestic help at home play an important role. They provide household helpers to perform tasks the aged are no longer able to do. The frequency of such help and the length of time required is determined for each case. Certain social organizations offer laundry services for the handicapped.

In some cases the aged are insufficiently nourished or have an unbalanced diet. A service that delivers hot meals at home has been created. It provides normal or dietary meals destined primarily for diabetics or cardiacs.

A great part of the ambulatory care for the aged is in the hands of practicing doctors who have a constantly growing clientele among the aged. Doctors are more and more often asked to advise the patient and his relatives when there is the question of placement. It is at such a time that collaboration with certain medicosocial organizations can be very helpful. The Geriatric Center of Geneva, for example, can advise on either medicosocial or psychogeriatric problems. This center complements the group of medical organizations devoted to the aged. Intended for ambulatory geriatrics, the center works in close collaboration with the group of hospital institutions or extramural orgnizations that care for the aged. In other cities, plans are being considered for the creation of multidisciplinary centers capable of satisfying the needs of the aged and their relatives. Polyclinics have many low-income aged among their clientele. Their services arrange for special consultations (for diabetics, for example).

Medical care taken at the present time is essentially curative. In the years to come, Switzerland should develop preventive care (Martin and Junod, 1977).

Ambulatory nursing care is carried out by services that, according to the importance of the area concerned, may function on a regional basis. The nurses attached to these services are customarily trained in public health, which enables them to take both curative and preventive action with the aged (Delachaux, 1977). When the question of maintaining the aged at home presents problems of physical hygiene, the public health nurses may be assisted in their work by nurses' aides who have been trained in these tasks.

Housing

In order to keep about 90 percent of the total of the aged population of 65 years or more in households of their own choice, it is necessary to call upon various household aid services, which must be well coordinated. The aged individual must have the possibility of remaining in his own home as long as possible. When this can no longer be done despite the services available, the solution may be an apartment within a medicosocial framework. It is estimated that in Switzerland about 5 percent of the population of 65 years of more should be able to be housed in this way. By grouping together in one building several apartments for the aged, it is possible to put at the disposition of everyone certain collective services such as a room reserved for ambulatory medical and nursing care, areas for general services (laundry in particular), and rooms for meetings, gatherings, and activities. Such buildings are usually supervised by a trained administrator. Special norms are considered in the plans for such construction and their equipment and activities. The confederation subsidizes part of these constructions. These apartments within such a medicosocial framework are always part of a regular apartment building in order to avoid segregating the aged.

Collective Shelter

Despite all efforts, the placing of an aged person in a collective shelter may be necessary, either temporarily or permanently. It is estimated that the number of places in a collective shelter milieu represents about 6 percent of the population 65 years or older.

These establishments can be roughly classified into three categories. Type A establishments are reserved for the aged who at the time of admission still enjoy an almost total independence in their general daily activities. These establishments are mainly for convalescent stays or are rest homes for the aged. According to general estimates, the number of places to be provided should not exceed 1 percent of the total population 65 years or older. As long as we do not have a sufficient number of apartments with a medicosocial environment available, we are forced to resort to this kind of establishment.

Type B establishments are for those who at the time of admission are somewhat handicapped either physically or psychologically. The number of places required is estimated at about 3 percent of the aged population. It would be advisable in the near future to provide these establishments with care-giving personnel and collaborators better able to stimulate the occupational, physical, and social therapies necessary. Continued efforts should also be made to improve the general environment in these establishments. The training of adminstrators for them should be further studied. Cantonal regulations do provide for their inspection.

Type C establishments are intended for patients who are seriously handicapped physically or psychologically at the time of admission. The number of beds needed can be estimated at 2 percent of the aged population. It is probable that the progressive increase in the number of old aged will require modification of this estimate. It is in this area that the shortage of beds is the most serious. Because the aged sick cannot be placed in establishments of this type, we find many who are seriously handicapped either physically or psychologically, living in hospitals.

Hospitalization

In geriatrics the rate of hospitalization is high, and the average stay is longer than in a traditional hospital. As a rule, the aged sick are hospitalized in a general hospital when somatic illness, surgery, or traditional medical specialist services are involved, or in the psychiatric hospital when it is a question of illness of a psychiatric nature (Ajuriaguerra et al., 1977).

Geriatric and psychogeriatric services or units are reserved for diagnosis and treatment of illnesses of the aged. These establishments provide traditional medical services along with special services whose purpose is to restore maximum independence to the patient within the shortest possible time. They often demonstrate what can be accomplished by an active multidisciplinary and therapeutic action for the aged. Priority is given to persons eligible for old-age insurance and whose state of health requires diagnostic and therapeutic action, together with functional readaptation measures, excluding, however, major surgery. These services usually have a day hospital, which may avoid hospitalization or shorten it. They are centers for treatment, research, and education (Gsell, 1964; Steinmann, 1963).

RESEARCH AND INSTRUCTION

Biological Research

In 1956 an experimental institute of gerontology was founded in Basel. Its research has contributed to the creation of an infrastructure for geriatrics that is indispensable (Verzàr, 1977). Diverse problems of biological gerontology are being researched in several university institutes in Switzerland.

Clinical Research

Clinical research is principally conducted within the framework of geriatric services and units. Traditional care services are increasingly more interested in this research. The questions being studied concern the somatic aspects, as well as the psychiatric or therapeutic aspects, of the illnesses of the aged.

Psychological, Sociological, and Medicosocial Research

Different groups are interested in the impact of age on human psychology and its sociological implications. Recently the Swiss National Fund for Scientific Research proposed a program for the social integration of aged individuals. These research projects are, for the most part, undertaken on a multidisciplinary basis and are designed to increase knowledge and comprehension of a question that has been neglected too long and whose fundamental aspects appear more and more evident.

In the medicosocial area additional research seeks to evaluate the usefulness, efficiency, and benefits of measures in operation both in hospitals and extramural organizations. It is to this task that the Swiss Society for the Study of the Problems of the Aged is now applying itself.

Medical Education

Neglected for a long time in our country, instruction in geriatrics was first integrated within the framework of general medical education. At the present time, the importance of geriatrics to medical students has gained the attention of some faculties. Such instruction is principally for fourth-year students. Where geriatric units or services exist, this instruction is completed by clinical training restricted to students of the third, fourth, and sixth years. Even though geriatrics is not usually a compulsory branch of medical education, because of its necessity, it now seems to be creating more and more interest among students and doctors (Martin and Junod, 1977; Müller and Ciompi, 1968; Müller, 1973; Von Hahn, 1975).

The teaching of geriatrics seeks first to improve the quality of treatment. It is based upon research and clinical study and includes, in addition to basic knowledge, a preventive as well as a curative approach. This instruction requires experience based upon the daily practice of this medical discipline (Junod and Simeone, 1975; Schaefer, 1977). The students must be helped to rethink present norms of medical efficiency in a dynamic perspective, always bearing in mind that the aged of tomorrow will not live through their old age as those of today.

Postgraduate instruction of interns is generally given in geriatric services. It includes clinical observations, anatomic clinical discussions, and multidisciplinary seminars or lectures. The teachers aim to train the newly graduated doctors for the tasks that await them. Five services in our country now meet this need.

The specialty of geriatrics is not recognized in Switzerland. In the near future it will be necessary to provide training for doctors who are attached to geriatric institutions or to hospital or extramural geriatric institutions or are involved in the planning of health, research, and education programs. It is important that the geriatric services permit practicing doctors to familiarize themselves with these tasks.

Continuing education courses are organized from time to time under the auspices of medical faculties, certain hospital services, professional organizations, or the Swiss Society of Gerontology. These activities are not yet well enough organized and must be reinforced in the years to come.

Instruction for Paramedical and Care-giving Professions

The nature and importance of this instruction varies from one canton to another. The Swiss Red Cross, responsible for training nurses, gives this instruction particular attention. It seeks to improve the knowledge of those who are to work with the aged sick, as well as to motivate them for an action at times difficult to perform.

Instruction for Volunteers

In certain places, instruction is given to voluntary workers. This includes especially group discussions to define the means and the areas that lend themselves to such activity, as well as the question of what compensation the services should offer volunteers.

Instruction for the Aged

This instruction is available through different activities such as the university adult education courses or through special courses that prepare for retirement. In this area we should approach the aged in a more positive way in order to attempt to make them less passive and more active participants from whom we may be able to understand better criticism and suggestions.

Geriatrics must always remain multidisciplinary but also coherent, unified, and, if possible, attractive. We must hope that teachers of this still new and long neglected branch of medicine will be able to communicate both its interest and identity.

SUMMARY

According to criteria adopted by demographic studies, Switzerland has crossed the threshold that defines aged populations. The decentralization of public health and social action to some degree has provided solutions for various needs. However, the question has taken on such importance that there must be a better coordination and a better rationalization of proposed action. Numerous gerontological and geriatric programs are now in progress. Their success will depend upon what society is prepared to do for its aged.

INFORMATION SOURCES

Bureau fédéral de statistique
Halwylstrasse 15, 3003 Berne.

Centrale Information Vieillesse
Rue Saint-Martin 26. 1005 Lausanne.

Communauté suisse pour l'étude des problèmes de la vieillesse
(C.E.V.) Boïte postale 3158. 8023 Zurich.

Croix-Rouge Suisse
Secrétariat central
Taubenstrasse 8. 3001 Berne.

Fonds national suisse de la recherche scientifique
Wildhainweg 20. 3000 Berne.

Office fédéral des assurances sociales
Effingerstrasse 33
3003 Berne.

Pro Senectute, Fondation suisse pour la vieillesse
Secrétariat central. Witikonerstrasse 56. Böite postale
8030 Zurich.

Schweizerische Vereinigung fur Altersturnen
Taubenstrasse 12. 3001 Berne.

Service fédéral de l'hygiene publique
Bollwerk 27. 3011 Berne.

Société suisse de gérontologie
President: Professeur B. Steinmann. Inselspital. 3010 Berne.

REFERENCES

Ajuriaguerra J. D.; Richard, J.; and Tissot, R. 1977. Maladies psychiatriques. In *Abrégé de gérontologie*, pp. 268-291. Berne and Paris: Huber-Masson.

Delachaux, A. Principes de traitement et nursing. In *Abrégé de gérontologie*, pp. 434-442. Berne and Paris: Huber-Masson.

Ebersold, W. 1975a. *Nicht-materielle Aspekte der Betreuung von Betagten.* Zürich: FAS.

———. 1975b. *Problèmes du troisième âge en Suisse.* Zurich: CEV.

Feder, M., and Junod, J. P. 1975. Psychiatry in the geriatric hospital: Its goals and limitations. *Gerontologia Clinica* 17:58–60.

Froidevaux, C. 1978. *Services for the elderly in Geneva.* Geneva: Sardot Institute for Health and Socio-economic studies, March.

Gilliand, P. 1969. *Vieillissement démographique et planification hospitalière.* Lausanne: Payot.

———. 1976. *Démographie médicale en Suisse.* Lausanne: Office de statistiques de l'Etat de Vaud.

Gsell, O., ed. 1964. *Krankheiten der Über Siebzig Jährigen.* Berne: Huber.

Gygi, P., and Heiner, H. 1976. *Das schweizerische Gesundheitswesen.* Berne: Huber.

Hoby, G. 1976. *Politique générale et politique de santé publique en Suisse.* Aarau: Institut Suisse des Hôpitaux.

Junod, J. P. 1979. *Gerontology and geriatrics in medical practice and medical education.* Geneva. Single copies available from J.P.J. Geriatric Hospital of Geneva, 1226 Thönex, Geneva.

Junod, J. P., and Simeone, I. 1975. La geriatria. *Publicazioni Mediche Ticinesi* 33:9–16.

Martin, E., and Junod J. P. 1977. *Abrégé de gérontologie.* 1977. Berne and Paris: Huber-Masson.

Müller, C. 1973. *Bibliographie Geronto-psychiatrica.* Berne: Huber.

———. 1969. *Manuel de géronto-psychiatrie.* Paris: Masson.

Müller, C., and Ciompi, L., eds. 1968. *Senile dementia.* Berne: Huber.

Neury, J. E. 1975. Vieillissement démographique et modèles de populations stables. *Forum Statisticum* 1:47–62.

Satter, H. 1975. *Das Leben beginnt mit sechzig*. Berne: Hallwag.

Saxer, A. 1966. *Les problèmes de la vieillesse en Suisse*. Berne: Centrale fédérale des imprimés. (English edition forthcoming.)

Schaefer, R. K. 1977. Rhumatismes dégéneratifs. In *Abrégé de gérontologie*, pp. 338-345. Berne and Paris: Huber-Masson.

Scherler, A. 1970. *Demain, la viellesse*. Lausanne: Payot.

Steinmann, B. ed. 1963. *Die Pflege des Betagten und chronisch Kranken*. Berne: Huber.

Stücki, L. 1975. *Alt werden mit uns*. Winterthur: Winterthur-Versicherungen.

Tournier, P. 1971. *Apprendre a vieillir*. Neuchatel: Delachaux et Niestle.

Verzàr, F. 1977. Aspect biologique de la sénescence. In *Abrégé de gerontologie*, pp. 30-33. Berne and Paris: Huber-Masson.

Vischer, A. L. 1959. *La vieillesse, destiné et accomplissement*. Paris: Flammarion.

Von Hahn, H. P. 1975. *Gériatrie pratique*. Bale: Karger.

Wertheimer, J. 1977. La confusion mentale du vieillard. In *Abrégé de gérontologie*, pp. 292-301. Berne and Paris: Huber-Masson.

Zeitlupe. 1922. *Das Senioren-Magazin*. Zurich: ProSenectute.

UNION OF SOVIET SOCIALIST REPUBLICS

DMITRI F. CHEBOTAREV
and NINA N. SACHUK

The interest in problems of gerontology and its rapid development throughout the world is related mainly to two factors: an ever-growing demographic aging, and significant success in biology, medicine, health care, and other research and practical fields of human endeavor, such as demography, sociology, social psychology, and economy.

These factors were decisive for the intensive development of gerontology in the Soviet Union. Because of the radical social, economic, and cultural transformations that have occurred in this country during the last sixty years, the structure of the economy has changed considerably, and much success has been achieved in the development of science, engineering, medical care, level of culture, and well-being of the population. All this resulted in the improvement of health, a decreased mortality rate, and an increased number of persons living through old age. In the Soviet Union, as in other industrial countries, there is a tendency toward increases in both the absolute and relative numbers of the elderly population, resulting from the drop in the birthrate.

In recent decades, significant demographic shifts and increased needs of the population in the U.S.S.R. for specialized social and medical services have determined the concentration of attention on problems of gerontology and geriatrics.

Here we should probably add one more factor that has contributed to a more rapid formation of positive public attitude to ideas of gerontology: the presence of certain traditions in the study of old age. As early as the end of the 1800s, prominent theorists and clinicians referred to the mechanisms of aging and causes of premature pathological aging. Since 1950 a number of prominent Soviet scientists have laid the basis for contemporary clinical, experimental, and social gerontology in the country.

DEMOGRAPHY

The aging of the population in the U.S.S.R. became especially marked after World War II. In 1939 the share of persons aged 60 and over was 6.8 percent; in 1959 it was 9.4 percent. According to the 1970 census, this percentage increased by one-fourth to 11.8. The absolute number of persons 60 and over in 1959 was 19.7 million, and in 1970 it was 28.5 million.

The process of demographic aging in different areas of the country is irregular. Aging of the population is the most marked in the Baltic region in the Latvian, Estonian and Lithuanian union republics, in which the share of the aged population is still growing (table 71). High rates of aging were registered from 1959 to 1970 in the vast territory of the European part of the U.S.S.R. (the Ukrainian, Belorussian, and Moldavian Republics and some regions of the Russian Federation). The areas with low levels of population aging include almost all the republics of Central Asia and Transcaucasus.

Table 71: AGING OF POPULATION IN THE REPUBLICS

Union Republics	Persons Aged 60 and Over per 100 Population			1959 (as percent of 1939)	1970 (as percent of 1939)
	1939	1959	1970		
Latvian	14.4	15.0	17.3	104	120
Estonian	13.9	15.1	16.8	109	121
Lithuanian	10.3	11.9	14.9	116	145
Ukrainian	6.2	10.5	13.8	169	223
Belorussian	7.4	10.7	13.1	145	177
Russian Federation	6.7	9.0	11.9	134	178
Georgian	8.8	10.9	11.8	124	134
Moldavian	6.1	7.7	9.7	126	159
Kirghiz	7.3	9.7	8.9	133	122
Uzbek	7.1	8.4	8.7	132	123
Armenian	6.9	8.0	8.2	116	119
Kazakh	5.0	7.8	8.2	156	164
Azerbaijan	7.4	8.4	8.0	114	108
Tajik	5.9	7.9	7.5	134	127
Turkmenian	6.4	7.9	7.2	123	113
Total	6.8	9.4	11.8	138	174

Sources: U.S.S.R. 1959 Census (Moscow: Gosstatizdat, 1962, 1963), table 12; U.S.S.R. 1970 Census (Moscow: Statistika, 1972), vol. 2, table 3.

General demographic aging and its regional peculiarities depend first upon the degree of decline in birthrate. The more marked shifts in age structure of women (as compared with men) are conditioned by lower female mortality and therefore by the greater survival of women through old age (table 72). Along with the higher accidents and harmful effects of alcohol and smoking, the causes of men's earlier deaths include the aftermaths of war, which manifest

Table 72: LIFE EXPECTANCY AND SURVIVAL

Census Periods (years)	Life Expectancy of Men			Life Expectancy of Women		
	At Birth	At 65	Percentage Surviving to Age 65	At Birth	At 65	Percentage Surviving to Age 65
1896–1897[a]	31.43	11.50	23.4	32.37	11.54	24.3
1926–1927[b]	41.93	12.07	34.1	44.35	13.59	39.0
1958–1959	64.42	14.01	61.1	71.68	16.79	76.9
1968–1971	64.56	12.97	59.8	73.53	16.13	79.9

Source: For 1896–1897 and 1926–1927: Plankhozgiz, Moscow-Leningrad, 1930, tables 1, 55. For 1958–1959: Results of the U.S.S.R 1959 Census (Moscow, Gosstatizdat, 1962), pp. 264–267. For 1968–1971: Vestnik statistiki, 1974, No. 2, pp. 94–95.

a. European Russia in boundaries of the European part of the U.S.S.R.
b. European part of the U.S.S.R.

themselves in more premature and pathological aging of men. These differences resulted in a sex disproportion in the older age group of the population: there are 2,096 women per 1,000 men among those 60 years and over (1970), which is more than among the whole population (1,170 women per 1,000 men).

Age redistribution between rural and urban areas caused by a migration of the population within the U.S.S.R. is marked. In view of the development of industry, urbanization, and the rise of cultural and educational levels, a significant part of the rural population, particularly youth, move to towns. This is the most essential cause of the more marked aging of the rural population. Despite higher birthrates in the villages, the proportion of persons aged 60 and over among rural residents in the U.S.S.R. in 1970 was, for example, 13.6 percent; among the urban population, it was 10.4 percent.

Before 1970 almost 770,000 older persons or 20 per 1,000 persons of retirement age (men 60 years and over and women 55 years and over) changed their place of residence. In a number of cases, the migration was linked with the move of the elderly parents from villages to live with their adult children in towns. The incidence of moves of this kind was approximately 1.5 times as high among elderly women as among elderly men. Moves in the opposite direction (from town to village) were one-half to one-third as frequent. The aged in such republics as the Kazakh SSR. (about 42 percent of men and 28 percent of women) and the Estonian SSR, Latvian SSR, Lithuanian SSR, and Russian SFSR (about 25 percent of men and 15 to 20 percent of women) were found especially mobile (U.S.S.R. Census, 1970). No wish to change the place of residence was noted among older women in Uzbekistan, Azerbaijan, Armenia, Georgia, and Turkmenia, which is probably related to features of family structure and family interrelations in these republics.

Modern urbanization has had a noticeable impact on the older generation. The process of population concentration in towns resulted in an increased proportion of older town residents: in 1959 they were 34.3 percent of the aged, and in 1970, 49.5 percent (U.S.S.R. Census). Living in town facilitated the rise in education and sanitary knowledge. Along with such negative factors as air pollution, excessive noise, and population density, there has been a considerable improvement of sanitary and domestic conditions of the majority of the older population. It became easier, therefore, for medical workers to improve the mode of life, behavior, nutrition, and everyday life of the people.

An analysis of the tendencies in the development of the aging population suggests that the future generation of the aged will not only be great in number but will be more educated, more knowledgeable about health, and more critical and will have a wider scope and variety of interests.

Longevity is one of the important indexes of age-related characteristics of the population and its health status. In the Soviet Union in 1970, 2,894,000 persons were aged 80 years and over; of them 297,000 were aged 90 and over. Of particular interest are the 19,304 centenarians. The distribution of longevous persons in the main categories of the population is shown in table 73. The most marked areas of longevity with 30 to 60 persons aged 90 and over per 1,000 older people were registered in a number of autonomous republics and regions of northern Caucasus and Transcaucasus.

Table 73: LONGEVOUS PERSONS BY SEX AND LOCATION (U.S.S.R.)

	Urban Population		Rural Population	
Age Group	*Men*	*Women*	*Men*	*Women*
80 and over	297,657	924,757	485,101	1,186,854
90 and over	22,460	87,384	48,456	138,803
100 and over	955	4,413	3,297	10,639

Source: U.S.S.R. 1970 Census (Moscow: Statistika, 1972), vol. 2, table 3.

The division of complex families into smaller families continues. Increasingly, elder couples and single elderly people live alone. According to the estimates based on the 1970 census, 45 percent of men in cities and 49 percent of men in villages are aged 55 years and over, and about 20 percent of women aged 50 years and over in cities and villages live with only a spouse. The proportion of persons aged 60 years and over living alone was 18.5 percent. The territorial deviations in the Soviet republics were rather high; they ranged from 8 percent (Tajik SSR) to 32.9 percent (Estonian SSR). Many more women than men live alone. Of the total number of aged living alone, there were 4.8 million women, or more than 90 percent of the aged living alone. The reason is accounted for primarily by the higher survival rate of women and their greater frequency of widowhood (table 74). The proportions of married men within the same age groups is up to four times as high as that of women.

Table 74: MARITAL STATUS OF THE OLDER POPULATION

Sex	Married Persons per 1,000 Persons			
	50–54	55–59	60–60	70 and Over
Men	952	948	920	778
Women	603	501	371	198

Source: U.S.S.R. 1970 Census (Moscow: Statistika, 1972), 2:263.

This situation is accounted for not only by the higher longevity of women as compared with men but also by the fact that men remarry more easily and as a rule marry younger women. Elderly women have a poorer chance of a second marriage than men do.

The progressive increase in the absolute and relative number of the aged in the U.S.S.R., which is especially marked in a number of rural regions, the intensification of the division of complex families, and the rise in the proportion of older persons living alone necessitate the solution of many complex socioeconomic, medical, and psychological problems.

STATUS OF THE AGED

The status of the aged depends greatly on the level of society's evolution. This is therefore one of the principal indexes of society's social maturity. This problem became especially urgent in the epoch of revolution in science and technology, which is accompanied by an intensive aging of the population. The measure of the status of the aged in society is not only the level of the state's care about their material well-being but the satisfaction of their spiritual demands and involvement in the interests and life of the whole society.

Relations between the aged and society are formed by a complex combination of a number of factors: political structure, level of economic and cultural development, familial structure, mode and conditions of life, and national traditions. These relations are determined by the place and role of various categories of people in the labor process during the active years and the process of aging.

The public status of the elderly population depends on their contribution to the promotion of the general development of the country's economy and culture and on the volume and quality of results of their work. The lack of any legislative limitations with regard to age, the access to free occupational training and retraining, as well as the adequate choice of occupations and working places related to the constant increase of production and the deficit of manpower in the country create favorable conditions for the participation of the aged workers in production.

Since the objective social and economic prerequisites for conflict between generations are lacking, the overwhelming majority of the aged live and work in an atmosphere of mutual understanding and support of the younger generation. According to economists, labor veterans in both cities and the countryside not only promoted the rise of national income and successful development of the country's national economy, but the value of the gross product of their labor was quite sufficient to cover their pensioning. The Soviet society considers the material provision for labor veterans as a return of debt to the older generation.

Social welfare for the aged is an integral part of the general social and economic program aimed at the increase of well-being of the whole population. The major principles of social welfare for the aged are specified in the U.S.S.R. constitution. They include universal welfare services for different kinds of loss of working ability (in this case due to old age), state guarantees of these services without any deductions from citizens' income, constant rise of standards, and the realization of various forms of social welfare by state bodies and public organizations.

The following data testify to the systematic rise of the state's expenditures for social welfare: in 1940 they equaled 0.3 billion rubles; in 1950, 2.2 billion; and in 1974, more than 16 billion (Statistical Yearbook, 1975).

Because of recent changes in pension legislation, new contingents of the aged began to receive state pensions. These were added to the several million aged persons receiving pensions for long service, disability, loss of breadwinner, as well as veterans of the Great Patriotic War (1941–1945) and their family members. This results in the rise of the material well-being of the aged population and an expansion of possibilities for satisfying their needs.

The economic position of the aged in the U.S.S.R. is determined not only by the amount of pensions, which are not taxable, but also by a number of other privileges from the so-called public consumption fund, which help many pensioners to maintain their prepension level of life. These privileges include low rent, capital repair of state-owned houses, inexpensive public transportation services, and easy access to free medical services at clinics and hospitals, as well as to many cultural facilities (inexpensive or free tickets to museums, exhibitions, and daytime theater and cinema performances, for example). Each year hundreds of thousands of pensioners and invalids can obtain three- to four-week passes (free or at a low cost) to sanatoriums, rest homes, and resorts.

Since there is no system of forced retirement, an elderly person can decide by himself whether to continue or cease his working activity. The Soviet government encourages the labor and public activity of older people. Thus within recent decades, a number of decrees have been passed providing for the material incentive of working pensioners (the right to receive both pension and salary) and more appropriate working conditions. The continuation of work in industry is an additional source of income for the pensioner and his family and the means to maintain his public role and prestige in his family. Realization of these arrangements raised the employment level of the aged almost 2.5 times;

more than 20 percent of pensioners found useful jobs, which raised their well-being. The range of occupations of working pensioners who receive full pension in addition to their wages has greatly widened to include industrial enterprises employees, junior service personnel, foremen, communications workers, public nutritionists, trading and communal establishments employees, builders, insurance agents, accountants, physicians, paramedical personnel of public health and children's preschool institutions, and teachers. These measures are of special value in view of significant shifts occurring in the population age composition toward aging, the increase of average life span, and the growing demand for experienced and skilled workers.

The employment level of pensioners varies from one area to another. According to the 1970 census, the greater proportion of pensioners working in public production during the first five-year period following retirement was 50–60 percent (Baltic republics), while the lowest was 15–20 percent (republics of Central Asia). These differences are caused by many factors, including the character of the economic structure of industry, the state of manpower resources in a given territory, the availability of working places and adequate working conditions, and peculiarities of regional and familial traditions.

Very often the pensioner works to increase his contribution to family budget. Morale considerations—the wish to perform an enjoyable job—take second place.

Nonemployment of the majority of pensioners under the present favorable conditions is explained by the fact that many pensioners cannot or do not wish to work. Deterioration of health is the major limitation; many of them suffer from chronic diseases that affect their working capacity. In addition, increases in the size of the pension reduce the desire to work.

A limited employment level of women pensioners is due to a change in their roles within the family: becoming grandmothers and having active participation in household and baby care, thereby providing the younger family members additional time for work, education, and recreation.

When an elderly person discontinues activities, he often looks for and finds an interesting and useful role within his limited capacities. According to numerous publications and information disseminated by the social organizations, a significant number of pensioners continue to participate actively in voluntary social work. Many of them maintain contacts with their former work community and transfer their experience and skills to younger workers. They are the so-called instructors and work as members of Councils of Labor Veterans at enterprises and institutions. They help fulfill production quotas and solve work and professional problems.

Pensioners' Block and House Committees carry on extensive work in the organization of settlements and the arrangement of leisure time of the aged, as well as of the children whose parents are at work. They also help the disabled and single aged persons in their households.

Public ticket inspectors in the transport and trading controllers, nonstaff newspaper correspondents, and voluntary librarians are a few of the characteristic forms of activity that pensioners engage in. Participation in the life of society and community and a perception of the usefulness and significance of the work they do give old people moral satisfaction, stave off depressive moods, and counteract progressive health impairment.

With advancing age the role of the family in the life of the aged is increased. Cessation of work after reaching retirement age, deterioration of health, and progressive decrease of mobility often determine the restriction of interests and kinds of activity. Often attention is transferred to family affairs. Contacts within a family serve as substitutes for lost contacts. Weakening of health and progressive physical disability make the aged more dependent upon the other family members for care and assistance. This need is especially pronounced during exacerbation of chronic diseases in the aged. Living in a family, the elderly can rely on the family for security and care. At the same time, the aged can help the rest of the family with the household and child care; they thus feel useful.

The position of the aged both in the family and society is determined by general social, economic, and cultural development, by material and economic relationships, and by local and national traditions. This explains marked territorial peculiarities in the position of the aged in the family in some areas of the Soviet Union.

In the past, patriarchal families in which the three generations (aged parents, their adult children, and and their grandchildren) lived together were the rule. More often now, however, adult children live separately from their aged parents. This tendency toward separation of generations varies among different areas of the country. It is more distinct in the republics with a high degree of demographic aging (in the Baltic republics, as well as in some regions of the European part of the U.S.S.R.) and is significantly less in the territories with a low degree of population aging (republics of Central Asia and Transcaucasus). The latter are characterized by the two inhibiting factors of many children and other patriarchal traditions related to regional and religious background.

A relatively high frequency of the aged living with other relatives determines a special psychological climate and interrelations within their family. Both the character of interrelations between members of the family and its structure are influenced by a number of objective and subjective factors. These factors are not transient situations; they are an outcome of the long-term process of life.

Considering the modern tendency toward the separation of adult chidlren and their aged parents, one should take into account both further possible contacts between them and certain difficulties related to distance. Still it should be noted that warm relations, which are so important for the elderly, can show themselves irrespective of whether the aged live with or apart from the rest of the family.

PROBLEMS AND PROGRAMS

Along with the provisions for an adequate income, medical care of the aged is one of the central programs; it is considered to be a social task with both medical and economic aspects. Maintenance of physical and psychic abilities of the aged provides for their wider employment, reduction of expenditures for public health and social welfare services, and reduction of time losses by the working members of the family for care of the sick and the old.

The system of free medical care in the Soviet Union ensures easy access by the aged to inpatient and outpatient medical aid, as well as home visits by a physician. An increase in general expenditures for medical care of the population, involvement of additional medical personnel, and growing bed capacity make a favorable basis for improvement of this system. Within the 1971–1976 period, the number of physicians per 10,000 people increased on the average from 27.4 to 32.6, and the number of physicians' calls per town resident per year increased from 10.7 to 11.19 (Golovteev, 1976).

According to numerous studies, however, the available medical care system cannot as yet fully meet the ever-growing demands of the older population. The population aged 50 and over make about 25 percent of all visits to physicians and more than 50 percent of all visits by physicians to homes.

In view of the peculiarities of old-age pathology, needs in short- and long-term hospitalization among the population aged 60 and over are almost three times as high as for the whole population (240–350 cases per 1,000 people). Most geriatric patients are hospitalized in general hospitals. At the same time, a number of specialized institutions render medical assistance to older patients. More than 150 geriatricians now consulting at the outpatient departments were trained at the chair of geriatrics (Kiev Institute of Advanced Training for Physicians) organized in 1970.

There are plans for a further expansion of hospital facilities for patients with chronic diseases, including the construction of large rehabilitation centers for patients with cardiovascular, nervous, and other diseases. Special attention should be given to adequate provisions of differential medical services of the aged with consideration of their pathology and with special requirements regarding pharmacotherapy, prevention, and treatment. To perfect the knowledge and skills of physicians who deal with older patients, a variety of comprehensive programs for training in gerontology and geriatrics are to be elaborated for medical students and physicians. Therefore special courses and manuals in gerosurgery, geroneurology, and other areas need to be available. Some additional training of both students and teachers will be required.

Special attention must be given to the training of paramedical personnel and social workers in terms of medical and social care and social and domestic services of the aged. All this is facilitated by the 1977 order of the health minister on geriatric care.

The Institute of Gerontology A.M.S. U.S.S.R. has elaborated the principles of medical and social care of the aged. This care should be large scale, close to the population, and with special emphasis on services at home. The care should be aimed at psychic rehabilitation, stimulation of patients' mobility, ability to take care of themselves, and, if possible, maintenance of working and public activity. The assessment of organizational forms and volume of medical and social care should be differential, account being taken of population age composition in various regions of the country, the peculiarities of the setting, health status, and other factors.

In view of the growing division of complex families, the problem of loneliness of the aged, especially in the rural areas, is very urgent. After the age of 70, many of them show limited mobility and loss of ability for self-service; they need constant care and help in their households. Sometimes such help cannot be rendered by the relatives, particularly by those living far way.

In many towns and villages (North Osetia, Rostov-on-the Don, Moscow, Kuibyshev, and many other regions) some of the older persons living alone in their houses are supervised by nearby boardinghouses. This form of care, however, cannot cover all those in need. In most cases, therefore, delivery of food and hot meals at home, assistance in households, cultural therapy, and other help are provided by the Red Cross nurses, volunteers, and domestic and training institutions. The pensioners-to-pensioners movement is becoming more popular. At the present time, this important aspect of organization of geriatric care is not yet widely spread and cannot meet all needs of this kind.

The local social welfare boards are facing the problem of assessing and meeting the specific conditions and needs of pensioners, elaborating individual and general programs for social and domestic care of pensioners living alone, stimulating their participation in various public voluntary organizations, and coordinating these programs with public health organs and institutions.

In the U.S.S.R., as in many other countries, there is a clear-cut desire for aging persons to remain in their own homes as long as possible. Sometimes, though not often, the aged person cannot or does not wish to live in his home. Then he is accommodated in a special institution. Such boardinghouses and homes for the aged have become common in the U.S.S.R. During the last two decades their total capacity has doubled. From 1960 to 1975 the number of places in boardinghouses for the aged increased more than two times from 156,300 to 330,000 places (Pritaljuk, 1970). The national economy plans provide for a further significant expansion of the network of boardinghouses during the next five to ten years. It is quite obvious that differences in the family structure in different regions of the Soviet Union should be thoroughly considered.

Apart from the quantitative aspect, much attention is being given to raising the living standards as well as medical and cultural services of the aged in these institutions. Creating the favorable atmosphere and environment that would alleviate the consequences of admittance still awaits solution.

There are also many other important problems of the aged population that require constant care and elaboration of measures necessary for their solution, not only on the part of gerontologists and the medical community, but also on the part of official bodies responsible for the planning of public health, social welfare, and domestic services. In addition to measures aimed at improving and maintaining health in old age, there must be ways for the aged to maintain their cheerfulness and interest in life. It is essential, therefore, to have the nonworking pensioners involved in socially useful activity.

Both the state and the aged are interested in extending their working capacity to more advanced ages, in involving healthy pensioners in socially useful work, and in utilizing their skills and knowledge. In this respect, wide-scale medical and hygienic arrangements aimed at preventing premature aging and maintaining active longevity play a special role. The need for the elaboration of hygienic standards, rational norms of nutrition, optimal regimens of work and rest, and the introduction of physical exercises into health-restoring measures while taking into account the physical and psychic health of the aged is important.

For persons approaching retirement age, the measures aimed at preparing them for retirement, breaking the stereotype, and adapting to new living conditions are of great value. The problem of choice of new activities and retraining of persons of retirement and even preretirement age requires a thorough consideration.

People need to be educated in such a way that they themselves help prevent their premature aging and prolong their active life.

One of the special problems of the aging population is living arrangement, which is determined not only by the existing level of housing provisions but also by some specific requirements in the construction, design, and equipment of houses for the aged, with consideration of their social and family status and health and age peculiarities. In recent years these problems have been tackled seriously, and some practical steps have been made, especially in the construction of boardinghouses.

At present much attention is paid to the study of the relationship between the family structure and the birthrate. A high degree of positive correlation has been found between the availability of a grandmother in a family and the birthrate. Therefore this fact should be taken into consideration in the demographic policy as a social measure stimulating childbirth. There must be a system of uniting divided families to allow the grandmother to be near her adult children.

Manpower reserves will be significantly increased with the reduction of the mortality rate in preretirement and early retirement ages. The public health bodies and labor protection systems at enterprises are confronted with the tasks of elaborating and applying preventive measures aimed at reducing premature deaths.

Increased leisure time for pensioners necessitates the creation of forms of rest and recreation and ways to use their energy and hobbies in various public activities. Retirement should not be a transition to doing nothing. In this respect various clubs and circles may become very useful. The elaboration and organization of various forms of collective rest and recreation, an expansion of club activities, and the organization of day centers for the aged are problems requiring solution.

The study of problems linked with demographic aging and the elaboration of definite measures, which are necessary for the realization of proposals in the field of population policies, require time, money, and the efforts of many specialists—theorists and practitioners—practicing in economics, demography, hygiene, and gerontology. The importance of further complex investigation in social gerontology and gerohygiene is determined by the need for a scientific substantiation of state and individual programs of care of the aged in the U.S.S.R.

RESEARCH

The success of gerontology in the solution of many important theoretical and practical problems has always depended upon achievements in biology and medicine. Therefore the rapid development of fundamental research in this country at the beginning of this century laid a firm basis for the development of major gerontological fields: biology of aging, geriatrics, and social gerontology.

The works of biologists such as I. I. Mechnikov, I. P. Pavlov, A. A. Bogomlets, and A. V. Nagorny and their schools determined the three major features of gerontology in this country. One of them was the special attention paid to theoretical problems in the biology of aging. This feature was determined in great measure by I. I. Mechnikov's work from 1899 to 1912.

In the study of age-related changes, of great importance were the works of I. P. Pavlov's school (1913–1938), which laid the basis for the present work on the higher nervous system, revealed the most mobile and modern forms of regulation of the organism's adaptation to the environment, and established the most essential interrelations between the cerebrum and thyroid glands. These studies determined another feature in the development of gerontology in this country: special interest in the study of mechanisms of neurohumoral regulation of metabolism and the function of an aging organism—his psychic activity.

The third trend in the development of the biology of aging was conditioned largely by the work of schools headed by A. A. Bogomolets (1926–1940) and A. V. Nagorny (1940–1958), who studied age-related changes in general ontogenetic aspects and searched for such changes at molecular, cellular, and tissular levels. A. A. Bogomolets was the first to point to the possible role of age-related changes of connective tissue in the genesis of aging.

Modern Soviet gerontology unites these different approaches to the studies of the biology of aging. It is characterized by the comprehensive analysis of age changes occurring at molecular, cellular, and systemic levels on the one hand and by the attempt to establish a relationship between these different levels of aging and by the determination of the whole mechanism of aging of the whole organism.

The development of problems of geriatrics are closely linked with the name of S. P. Botkin, who worked out a program and headed a health examination study of 2,240 elderly and old persons (Petersburg, 1899). Botkin's ideas were implemented in the works of his disciples (A. A. Kadarjan, 1890, A. N. Alelekov, 1892, and others). Among the conclusions, which are still quite valid, Botkin's concept of physiological and pathological aging, which dismissed the definition of aging as a disease, was of special importance.

In 1938, A. A. Bogomolets and N. D. Strazhesko organized a conference in Kiev on the problems of aging and the prevention of premature aging. This conference, which dealt mainly with the results of study of the longevity of Abkhasians and peculiarities of diseases of the aged, was an important step in the development of the biology of aging and geriatrics. That was a powerful stimulus for further development of research in this field in the U.S.S.R. During recent years a number of research centers have been organized in Kiev, Moscow, Kharkov, Minsk, Leningrad, Tbilissi, Gorky, and Baku, which concentrate their efforts on the study of gerontological problems.

The study of social and health problems of gerontology in the Soviet Union is closely linked with the Soviet social and health sciences in general. F. F. Erisman (1870, 1878), I. V. Klimenko (1906), and many others are known for their studies of the effect of industrial and domestic factors upon the health of workers of various age groups.

A study of forty-seven thousand labor pensioners, carried out by the Leningrad Institute for Evaluation of Working Capacity (Z. E. Grigorjev et al.) in 1934–1935, was important. In 1945 Z. G. Frenkel published *Prolongation of Life and Continuous Old Age*, a fundamental contribution to social gerontology.

The organization in 1958 of the large national Institute of Gerontology (Kiev) with the U.S.S.R. Academy of Medical Sciences provided for further studies of various gerontological problems. As a next step, the U.S.S.R. Academy of Medical Sciences set up the Scientific Council on Gerontology and Geriatrics and made the Institute of Gerontology responsible for the coordination of research of these problems in this country. At present, a variety of research institutes (both of biological and medical orientation), chairs of many universities, and health care institutions are engaged in the investigation of these problems.

In its research activities, the Institute of Gerontology A.M.S. U.S.S.R. has close links with the gerontological research centers of many other countries. In 1963, the institute served as the basis for the WHO-sponsored Seminar on Health Protection of the Aged and Prevention of Premature Aging and, later, the WHO-sponsored International Course on Advanced Training in Gerontology.

The major purpose of Soviet gerontology is to reveal the leading mechanisms of aging, to search for means of prolonging the life span, to elaborate methods for preventing and treating pathological processes common among the aged, to study the effect of social environment and mode of life upon human aging, and to elaborate measures extending the period of active working ability.

In the biology of aging, important clinical experimental data have been obtained during recent years in the leading mechanisms of aging and adaptive possibilities of an aging organism. Special emphasis has been laid on neurohumoral mechanisms of aging. It was shown that neurohumoral shifts may lead to secondary age changes in other organs and tissues, including the alterations in cell genetic apparatus. This direction is being successfully developed in the U.S.S.R. Further research in this field is essential since it can help to explain the peculiarities of the onset and course of many diseases of an aging organism, such as cardiovascular diseases and diabetes.

In the study of mechanisms of aging, special attention is devoted to age changes in cell genetic apparatus (Kiev and Kharkov Universities, Institute of Biophysics U.S.S.R. Academy of Sciences, and others). Significant changes were revealed in DNA physical and chemical properties with aging and in DNA structure and strength of bonds between histones and DNA. Of principal importance is a series of studies by the Institute of Gerontology A.M.S. U.S.S.R. on the relationship between the activity of cell genetic apparatus and the state of its membranes during aging, which enabled the elucidation of some mechanism at the cellular level. At present, extensive research is being carried on in both the U.S.S.R. and some other countries on the peculiarities of human aging. Much information has been accumulated on the age changes of the cardiovascular and respiratory systems (by the Institute of Gerontology A.M.S. U.S.S.R., Institute of Cardiology, Academy of Science, Georgian S.S.R., and others), hormonal regulation (by the Gerontology Section of the Academy of Science, Belorussian S.S.R., and others), and locomotor apparatus. Studies of the psychology and changes in the human nervous system during aging are underway at the Institute of Gerontology A.M.S. U.S.S.R. However, there are disputable questions dealing with the criteria of human aging and the biological age of man. Their solution has great implications for the prophylaxis of aging, health prognosis, professional arrangement, and understanding of many questions of pathogenesis of human diseases.

At the Institute of Gerontology A.M.S. U.S.S.R. and many other scientific institutes, considerable research has been carried on in the areas of geriatric pharmacology and pharmacotherapy aimed at studying the effects of various drugs on an aging organism, studying the efficacy of different biological agents in combating premature aging, and in the maintenance and normalization of the body functional systems and metabolism.

Extensive work has been done in statistical verification of the sociohygienic aspects of gerontology in the U.S.S.R. using the 1959 and 1970 censuses. Within recent years such investigations have been conducted in the Ukraine, Belorussia, Georgia, Uzbekistan, Estonia, Siberia, and Dagestan.

Between 1960 and 1963, under the auspices of the Institute of Gerontology A.M.S. U.S.S.R. and using the methods elaborated by it, a mass survey of about forty thousand people aged 80 and over was conducted in seven Soviet republics. This unique survey based on a new system of indexes made it possible to reveal some significant sex differences in the health of longevous subjects and to study the dependence of the better health status of longevous men on the higher mortality rates in younger age groups (Sachuk, 1964, 1965). These higher mortality rates were caused by the more severe forms of pathological processes characteristic of premature aging from the ages of 50 to 70. The relationship between the health status of longevous persons and their mode of life has been established, and their needs for inpatient and outpatient care, prosthetics, institutionalization, and other help have been assessed. As a result of the analysis of the data on the professional and working background and health of longevous persons, it was found that longevity accompanied persons who were continuously engaged in work; physical rather than intellectual work contributed to a healthy and active longevity; and social, professional, and industrial factors counteracted the genetically conditioned predisposition to longevity.

It was concluded, therefore, that the aging of residents of separate economic areas of the U.S.S.R. is an irregular process regarding both its rate and degree. In this view, the main sociohygienic problems waiting for their solution have been outlined (Chebotarev and Sachuk, 1964).

In recent years one of the most important trends in gerontology has been formed. Within its framework a complex study of health, working capacity, working conditions, and regimens for persons of retirement age who work under usual conditions has been conducted by the Institutes for Evaluation of Working Capacity); the hygienic requirements for industries that employ mainly elderly persons have been elaborated (by the Institutes of Hygiene of Labor and others; the problems of age-related occupational ability and ways of delaying early occupational aging are being developed by the Institute of Gerontology A.M.S. U.S.S.R. and the Institutes of Hygiene of Labor; and the data of the censuses dealing with the utilization of manpower resources of the country under conditions of the scientific and technological revolution have been analyzed. The sociodemographic problems of gerontology, geography, and epidemiology of population longevity are being investigated further by the Institute of Gerontology A.M.S. U.S.S.R. and the laboratories of hygiene of some research institutes in Georgian and Belorussian S.S.R.

Much attention has also been attached to studies of nutrition, its relation to health, and regularities of food assimilation with a consideration of age differences by the Institute of Nutrition A.M.S. U.S.S.R., the Institute of Gerontology A.M.S. U.S.S.R., and the Institute of Cardiology A.S. Georgian S.S.R.

Relatively new problems that have been recently investigated by the Institute of Gerontology A.M.S. U.S.S.R. are questions of social gerontology dealing with mode of life and leisure of persons of retirement age and their relationship to health. The complex elaboration of the position of the aged in family and society based on a wide use of modern sociological and sociopsychological methods has yielded some interesting data.

A distinctive feature of the studies in social gerontology and gerohygiene is their complexity and their involvement of specialists of different backgrounds, as well as a close interrelationship of various aspects dealing with hygiene and the physiology of labor, the hygiene of nutrition, social hygiene, the organization of medical care, and some other aspects of life of the older population. The results of hygienic and social studies of gerontology are widely used in practice. The reference material, methods, and recommendations are systematically provided to the state, planning, and public organizations and institutions, and the recommendations in hygiene are applied in practical public health, social welfare, and other areas. Provisions are being made for raising the skills of practical workers of the respective branches.

The versatile character of social gerontology requires its further development in several main directions:

1. Study of occupational aging and elaboration of the necessary conditions and labor regime for maximal prolongation of high working ability.

2. Elaboration of measures promoting higher social activity, social adaptation, and rational mode of life during the retirement period to ensure active longevity.

3. Elaboration of optimal norms of needs of the aged in nutrients and energy, account being taken of their mode of life in different geographic regions of the country.

4. Scientific verification of the demographic prognosis of population aging and longevity in different economic and geographic regions of the country.

5. Elaboration of recommendations in the area of sociodemographic policy aimed at decreasing the rate of population aging and increasing birthrates, especially in the western part of the U.S.S.R.

6. Elaboration of forms and methods of organization of the medical care for the aged.

7. Elaboration of standards and measures for improving sanitary and everyday services for the aged.

The problems of elaboration of the hygienic bases for a rational mode of life, as well as the social environment and the needs of the aged, which undergo constant changes due to socioeconomic transformation in this country, are complex, and a simultaneous solution of all main problems is required in the first stage, followed by the correction at the next stages.

The development of gerontology in the U.S.S.R. in the past two decades has acquired an international reputation. There is an exchange of publications with many research centers of the world. The Ninth International Congress of Gerontology, attended by more than three thousand scientists and practitioners from forty-one countries, was held in Kiev in 1972.

Since 1972, over a thousand scientific papers dealing with gerontology and geriatrics have been published annually in scientific journals. The results of studies of various aspects of gerontology have been summed up, and plans for future development have been outlined at nationwide and republic conferences.

REFERENCES*

Acharkan, V. A. 1965. *Provision for labor veterans in the U.S.S.R.* Moscow: Nauka.

Acharkan, V. A.; and Solovjev, A. G. 1975. *Working pensioners*. Moscow: Juridicheskaya Literatura.

Bedny, M. S. 1967. *Lifespan*. Moscow: Statistika.

Bedny, M. S. 1972. *Demographic processes and forecasts of population health*. Moscow: Statistika.

Berdyshev, G. D. 1968. *Ecologic and genetic factors of aging and longevity*. Leningrad: Nauka.

Bogomolets, A. A. 1939. *Prolongation of life*. Kiev: Izdatelstvo A.N. Ukr.S.S.R.

Chebotarev, D. F. 1969. Development of gerontology in the U.S.S.R. *Vestnik A.M.N. S.S.S.R.* 1:142–148.

———. 1977. *Geriatrics in the clinic of internal disease*. Kiev: Zdorovja.

Chebotarev, D. F., and Boiko, V. I. 1975. *Care of the aged patients*. Kiev: Zdorovja.

Chebotarev, D. F., and Frolkis, V. V. 1975. Research in experimental gerontology in the U.S.S.R. *Journal of Gerontology* 30:441–447. (In English.)

Chebotarev, D. F., and Sachuk, N. N. 1964. Socio-medical examination of longevous people in the U.S.S.R. *Journal of Gerontology* 19:435–439. (In English.)

Chebotarev, D. F.; Mankovsky, N. B.; and Frolkis, V. V., eds. 1969. *Fundamentals of Gerontology*. Moscow: Meditsina.

Davydovsky, I. V. 1966. *Gerontology*. Moscow: Meditsina.

Dilman, V. M. 1968. *Aging, climacteric and cancer*. Leningrad: Meditsina.

Frenkel, Z. G. 1949. *Prolongation of life and active old age*. Moscow: Izdatelstvo A.M.N. S.S.S.R.

Frolkis, V. V. 1970. *Regulation, adaptation and aging*. Leningrad: Nauka.

Gatsko, G. G. 1969. *Endocrine system in aging*. Minsk: Nauka i tekhnika.

Golovteev, V. V. 1976. Main results of development of public health within a five-year period (1971–1975). *Sovetskoye Zdravockhranenie* 1:4.

*All titles are in Russian unless otherwise noted.

*Intellectual work and active longevity. 1976. *Gerontology and geriatrics, Year-Book 1976*. Kiev.

Jubilee statistical guide. 1972. *National economy of the U.S.S.R. 1922–1972*. Moscow: Statistika.

Maikova A. Z., and Novitsky, A. G., eds. 1975. *Problems of part-time working day and employment of population*. Moscow; Sovetskaya Rossija.

Main problems of Soviet gerontology. 1972. Paper presented at the Ninth International Congress of Gerontology, Kiev.

Mankovsky, N. B., and Mints, A. Ya. 1972. *Aging and the nervous system (essays in clinical neurogerontology)*. Kiev: Adorovja.

Mechnikov, I. I. 1904. *Studies on human nature*. Moscow: Izdatelstov A.N. S.S.R.

———. 1964. *Etude of optimism*. Moscow: Nauka.

Mints, A. Ya. 1970. *Atherosclerosis of cerebral vessels*. Kiev: Zdorovja.

Mode of life and human aging. 1966. *Symposium proceedings*. Kiev: Zdorovja.

Nagorny, A. V.; Nikitin, V. N.; and Bulankin, I. I. 1963. *Problems of aging and longevity*. Moscow: Medgiz.

Podrushnyak, E. P. 1972. *Age-related changes in human joints*. Kiev: Zdorovja.

Pritaljuk, M. S. 1970. In *Social environment, mode of life and aging*, pp. 277–284. Kiev.

Proceedings of conference on problems of genesis of aging, old age. 1939. Kiev; Izdatelstvo A.N. Ukr.S.S.R.

Rubakin, A. N. *Praises to old age*. Moscow: Sovetskaya Rossija.

Sachuk, N. N. 1974. Aging of population and problems of demographic policy. In *Demographic policy*, pp. 146–154. Moscow: Statistika.

Sachuk, N. N., and Stakhovich, V. A. 1968. On the characteristics of migration of longevous people during life. In *Problems of demography*, pp. 158–162. Kiev: Statistika.

Social environment, mode of life and aging: Gerontology and geriatrics year-book 1969–1970. 1970. Kiev.

Spasokukotsky, Yu. A.; Barchenko, L. I.; and Genis E. D. 1963. *Longevity and physiological aging*. Kiev: Gosmedizdat.

Statistical Yearbook: National Economy of the U.S.S.R. in 1974. 1975. Moscow: Statistika.

Urlanis, B. Ts. 1963. *Birthrate and lifespan in the U.S.S.R*. Moscow: Gosstatizdat.

UNITED KINGDOM

W. R. BYTHEWAY

The birthrate in the United Kingdom has fallen consistently since 1871 when it stood at 35.5 per thousand, with three exceptions: following World Wars I and II and during the 1960s. It is currently 11.9 per thousand. Death rates over the same period have fallen from 22.3 to 12.2 per thousand. Death rates in the 55 to 64 year age group have dropped to 61.6 percent for men and 35.5 percent for women of the 1871 rates. However the equivalent drop for those aged over 85 years is only 76.9 percent and 66.1 percent respectively. Thus the major trend over the last one hundred years has been for death to occur within an increasingly narrow age period—in fact, that period generally referred to as old age.

The registrar general for England and Wales has predicted increases of 34 percent and 24 percent in the number of men and women over 75 years between 1976 and 1991. In the context of a falling or stationary birthrate, there will be a massive increase in the ratio of nonworkers to workers as a consequence of this rise in the number of old people. Armed with these predictions the Department of Health and Social Security has named the elderly as their first priority client group.

One frequently sees rather uncritical references to the problems of adult children being caught between the needs of increasing numbers of elderly relatives and their own demanding schoolchildren. In fact this will increasingly become a phenomenon of the past because the ages of the parents at childbirth has dropped markedly. The average age at first marriage has dropped between 1901 and 1975 from 27.2 to 24.9 for men and 25.6 to 22.7 for women. In addition to this decline, fewer children have been born and at shorter intervals immediately following marriage. Consequently the average difference in age between parent and child has fallen by perhaps as much as five years. This will make the four-generational family increasingly common over the coming decades: people in their seventies will have children straddling the age of 50 who in turn will have children in their teens, twenties, and thirties. If the low average age of parenthood is maintained over the next two or three decades, then it is reasonable to anticipate growing numbers of five-generational families.

Trends in familial relationships have been subjected to a much more dramatic complicating factor: divorce. In 1971, the laws on divorce were amended in such a way that there was an immediate doubling in the number of divorces. In 1970 there were 50,239; two years later there were 119,025. Looking at the age-sex specific divorce rates of 1968 and 1973, the increase has been greatest in the older age groups (although the absolute rates still reduce with age): men in their fifties are three times as likely to experience divorce and women four times as likely in 1973 relative to 1968. This development may promote an increase in remarriage rates in the older age groups, but the safest prediction is that it will lead to increased numbers of old people living on their own. David Hobman in his address to the 1979 AGM of Age Concern anticipated that increases in divorce and mobility will lead to changes in the grandparent role and in particular to the development of surrogate grandparents for one-parent families.

Turning to old people in nonprivate households and contrasting the census of 1961 (equals 100) with that of 1971, we find there has been virtually no change in the number residing in psychiatric hospitals, except among those over 80 years (ratios for 1971 to 1961 of 123 for men and 138 for women). Similarly there has been virtually no change in other hospitals (despite talk of the "silting up" of hospitals by the elderly): ratios range from 88 (75- to 79-year-old men) to 105 (65- to 69-year-old men), with the notable exception of 125 for women over 80 years. The most dramatic increase has been in the number in homes for the old (predominantly administered by local authority social services departments). The ratios here range from 139 in men aged 75 to 79 years to 240 in women over 80 years.

Thus the national statistical picture is ominous indeed. Many of those concerned with the aging of the population have been anxiously looking for ways to change attitudes and for solutions to problems that are both cheaper and more effective. But they have found that achieving these objectives is extremely difficult, if not impossible. Despite this, optimism, like Queen Elizabeth II, reigns supreme and every so often something works gloriously successfully.

ATTITUDES

One element of the British character is commonly thought to be a respect for—if not a knowledge of—the nation's history. This, together with the deep involvement of all the population in the experience of World Wars I and II, places those generations who fought in these wars in a special position in regard to commonly held attitudes toward the aged. There is a widespread belief that more recent generations owe them a debt of gratitude. This has, of course, been disputed by some who have been impressed by arguments disputing the effectiveness or morality of British wartime efforts. The children of those who fought in World War II, however, are now no longer skeptical teenagers themselves, and consequently the war as a subject of conversation and argument is less common than it was ten to twenty years ago. Nevertheless the feelings of indebtedness are now increasingly being revived in respect to the debate concerning the position of the retired and elderly. The soldier of 28 in 1940 is now 67 years of age and at the point of retirement. He was 33 years old when the Labour government of 1945 was voted in and 36 when it established the National Health Service and the related components of the welfare state. On these grounds it is reasonable to suppose that the attitudes of those over 65 years—those of pensionable age—will change considerably over the coming decade.

Most of the retired of 1979 were educated before, during, and shortly after World War I, and it is widely felt that their ready acceptance of the relative deprivation of their present circumstances is due to the attitudes inculcated in them during their early education. Thus a recent survey found that 35 percent of 1,959 persons over the age of 65 years who thought that their health was "good for someone of your age" still answered positively to the question, "Is there any physical condition, illness or health problem that bothers you now?"

There is widespread uncertainty about whether adult children fulfill their responsibilities to their parents. There is recognition of the fact that modern industrialism has forced workers to be mobile, frequently to the extent of their being free to work in any part of the country—and increasingly in other countries of the European Economic Community—but the question of whether the family or the new system of social services (comprehensively reorganized in 1974) bears the ultimate responsibility for dependent parents remains unresolved. As the issue is debated year after year and as the many interested parties seek to build an appropriate and reliable system of care based upon liaison, coordination, and partnership, so attention is regularly drawn by those who have been abroad to the laudatory ways by which other countries have been able to retain a so-called old-fashioned role for their elderly, bestowing upon them respect, wealth, and comfort.

Regardless of this debate, within the course of everyday life in modern Britain, there is a range of attitudes about age, which, it can be argued, includes bigotry and prejudice of an extent that rivals that associated with color or gender. But the power of such forces is tempered by tolerant dry humor, fostered by the knowledge that age comes to all with time.

ROLES

The coming of the welfare state brought not only statutory pension schemes but also a wide range of provisions covering housing, health, employment, financial support, transport, and domestic help, which collectively have created a statutory role of being elderly. This above all else dominates the age-specific role system of later life in modern Britain. People as they approach and pass certain key ages—60 years, 70 years, and most frequently 65 years—find themselves being continually reminded of their age and consequent status. Public transport is one instance in which age status is declared (or denied) in a public rather than private milieu. There is much debate and concern centered upon the propriety of such administrative systems that work only if the recipient publicly displays his age status. However most reminders come in less obvious ways. Because of the enormous complexity of the welfare services, the elderly have become the recipients of advertising campaigns and the clients of advice centers. People are increasingly faced with the question: "Are you over 65? If so, read on or listen to me."

There is little ambiguity about the overall administrative role of being elderly. It is universally recognized, and the experience and consequences of the transition into it have been the subject of a number of studies. These have demonstrated that this status passage is statistically associated with a variety of problems of adjustment. The problem is compounded in most instances by an instantaneous and complete cessation of paid employment.

Perhaps the second major role that older people are called upon to play is that of widowhood. Marital status is all too frequently a grossly oversimplified dimension both in age research and in popular mythology. Although it is undoubtedly true that widowhood is predominantly a characteristic of women in later life, it does not follow that the role is simply that of the older woman following the termination of her marriage. Many widows, and particularly widowers, proceed to remarry, and this trend, perhaps stimulated by the greater mobility within the population, has increased markedly over the last twenty years. Certainly many older people find themselves during their sixties and seventies being bereaved of their spouse and thereby left to continue life in a one-person household. However this presents them with a decision rather than a role: whether to combine households through marriage or with a relative (such as a widowed sister), whether to move to a grouped housing scheme in which they can participate in a small community of contemporaries sharing a number of domestic facilities, or whether to stay where they are. Despite the trend, the elderly one-person household remains a particularly common feature of present-day Britain, a feature that is maintained and supported by the well-developed domiciliary services, which cover meals, cleaning, health care, chiropody, and alarm systems. The national survey "The elderly at home" (Hunt, 1978) carried out in 1976 found that 30 percent of the sample of 3,869 people over 65 were living alone. Of those living alone, 28 percent had received a visit from their doctor in the last six months, and 19 percent receive a visit at least once a week from a home help employed by the local authority's social services department. A potentially important recent development in these services has been the good neighbor or street warden scheme, which uses volunteers to maintain regular friendly contact. It is perhaps more appropriate to speak of the elderly one-person-household role rather than the widow role.

An increasingly common and important role that the retired are filling is that of the volunteer worker. Paid work is financially discouraged (through the infamous earnings rule, which reduces pensions for those with substantial earnings), but the work ethic survives even in the absence of monetary inducements. There are two kinds of volunteer work. One is the informal work involved in offering time or assistance to others, or in responding to calls for help: work that is generally acknowledged although rarely documented or fully recognized. The other is organized volunteer work, and this is generally distinguished by the volunteer's having a position within an organization. Typically he is a member of or on the committee of the local branch of a national organization. There can be little doubt that the acquisition of such a position gives the individual a role that is very similar to that of being employed: it becomes his or her work. In Britain today, voluntary organizations are flourishing—at least in terms of interest and membership, if not financially—and in response to this the Pre-Retirement Association (a body concerned with preparation for retirement), for example, organizes social evenings to which the local organizers of voluntary bodies are invited and at which the preretirees are frequently recruited.

In contrast to this positive role of the elderly, a negative role of dependency is frequently associated with age. Old age, if nothing else, is that period of life within which death most commonly occurs, and death at such ages is usually preceded by a period of dependency. It is perhaps the role of terminal dependency that people in Britain fear most. High value is placed upon provisions that maintain independence within the community for as long as possible, and little attention is given to the implication within this objective that, following either success or failure, a period of dependency may unavoidably follow. In such circumstances, dependency is administratively recognized by the transfer of the person into either a hospital or a home for the old. Contact with previous supporters of his or her independence is frequently administratively severed, and in the case of volunteers of whatever kind, contact is usually greatly reduced. Transfer into such settings is all too commonly a form of social death.

PROBLEMS

The major problem with the elderly is the word *problem*. Although it is generally accepted in Britain—disputed by some—that the elderly form a section of the population who can be discussed in the context of problems, it is only done so with a feeling of dissatisfaction. Sometimes this dissatisfaction is manifested in a reference to the heterogeneity of the elderly. There is as much variation within the elderly as within the entire population. Sometimes there is reference to the fact that the vast majority are not a problem. Sometimes dissatisfaction is directed at chronological age (some are still young at 80 while others are old at 53). Sometimes it is suggested that the elderly who have problems have always been problem people. Sometimes our attention is directed toward the problems of the very old.

Perhaps the most effective way of representing the major problems that are seen to be associated with later life is to quote from the Age Concern Manifesto. Under the heading ''Income,'' it is claimed that ''providing a minimum basic pension for all, and assessing the needs and resources of individuals and then providing extra benefit to bring each individual's income up to a fixed level, is no real solution because the necessary enquiries are often upsetting to old people, who feel humiliated at having to disclose personal details. Similarly, it is no more than a temporary measure to provide rebates of rent or other housing costs to those with incomes below a certain level, and it should be recognized that housing costs are probably the most variable circumstance, with the least opportunity for change.'' Given that the income of the retired is not based upon current earning through work, there is a very real administrative problem of establishing a system that meets legitimate financial needs in a way that does not offend. The primary problem of income, which the manifesto sidesteps, is that the pension has to be paid out of the national exchequer, which in turn draws upon the current national economy. The enormous size of the pensionable population and the consequent national cost of maintaining and increasing pension levels is the major obstacle to providing more widely acceptable levels of income. Nevertheless as David Hobman has pointed out, recent surveys of the working population have found a readiness to pay more in tax if this could lead directly to increased pensions. It may be that additional arguments based upon the unpaid productive or supportive work that the retired carry out may lead to new assaults upon this problem.

Under ''Health,'' the manifesto notes that old people may suffer from several conditions at the same time and that they may need extra services such as nutritional advice, rehabilitation, domiciliary services, and support following bereavement. The manifesto notes that the National Health Service does not take their special needs sufficiently into account. The problem with changing this situation is not simply that of getting the Department of Health and Social Security to start taking account of such special needs—indeed the department has recently published a document on priorities that places the elderly as being the top priority client group. The real problem is that the medical profession, which still enjoys considerable autonomy, is continually deciding within itself both the priority that should be accorded to the old and more particularly how the needs of the elderly should be organizationally met. Thus we find that Age Action Year in 1976 was primarily directed toward the establishment of professional chairs in geriatric medicine. While in reality this may well be the best way of changing the health service so that the special needs of the elderly are taken into account, it does suggest that it is the special needs of certain branches of the medical profession that gain first priority when it comes to action.

The manifesto next points out that "several million elderly people live in substandard, inconvenient, unsuitable accommodation." It is my opinion that the most appalling aspect of the British situation is the unbelievable tolerance of the circumstances in which the elderly are sometimes forced to live. I have seen a street of terraced housing, adjacent to a large development site for central city offices and shopping, being demolished house by house with people of considerable age still living in upstanding housing. The officials blandly say that any house adjacent to an occupied house will be left standing so that the weather will not get in through the exposed roof, yet the adjacent house is full of the refuse of demolition: dust, smells, vermin, and rotting timber. Nowhere can one see the ideal of "maintained independence" go more terribly wrong.

Other areas that the manifesto discusses are occupation and mobility. The work ethos dominating Britain's view of itself is such that work is confined to set times. At weekends, on holidays, and following retirement, one does not work, and as a result of this simple conception, the sixty-fifth birthday is accorded the same status as Friday teatime: "time to knock off." The situation is complicated by current rising unemployment levels. A scheme has come into operation offering retirement and a pension a year early in order to release jobs for the younger unemployed. Miners have succeeded in obtaining a special system of early retirement, and it is anticipated that other industries may follow. There has, however, been little sign of phased or graded retirement, and it seems probable that the way retirement is effected will continue to be dominated by economics and industrial relations rather than by a gerontological perspective. When transport is discussed, it tends to be limited to schemes for subsidizing public transport fares. In this field, British Rail appears to have been particularly active, and it would be interesting to research the question of how effective their senior citizens' railcard has been in facilitating links within families (and in particular, support by the elderly). Physical handicap is a problem area that has not become age specific, even though it is widely recognized that the problem is strongly related to age. In general, however, the problems of mobility have received little more than symbolic attention. In the 1976 survey "The Elderly at Home" 24 percent of the sample over 65 reported that they were only able to get out of doors with difficulty or help. We know very little about the nature of such difficulty and which kinds of obstacles or inconveniences hinder them in the course of their daily affairs.

The manifesto ends: "The loneliness of many elderly people could be eased by persuading them to take part in informal systems of neighbourhood help, encouraging their participation in the planning and activities of day-centres and clubs of all kinds, and making sure that they are involved in any community activity they want." This encapsulates the problem of loneliness, the problem most commonly ascribed to the elderly. The solution to loneliness does not cost money or require buildings or expensive, highly trained specialists. It just requires "us to go out there and help them, encourage them and persuade them." If nothing else, this is one problem that can and should be solved. Unfortunately the image of a solved problem is a mirage. As we help, encourage, and persuade one reluctant old person, we see another over her shoulder.

PROGRAMS

The following programs, schemes, or issues concerning the elderly have been publicized recently. Many others have been continuing without publicity so that the following is no more than indicative of the range of current concerns in Britain in 1979. Authorities known to be active have been named only as examples. Further information about these schemes and about other programs not listed can be obtained from the addresses given at the end of this section.

Fuel. A major concern is that of ensuring that the elderly can afford an adequate level of heat in their homes. During the 1976–77 winter a scheme was established by the Department of Energy which offered a 25 percent discount to people on supplementary pensions. This covered half a million pensioners. Age Concern has highlighted an anomaly whereby persons who pay a landlord for their fuel are excluded. It has not been decided, since the change of government in 1979, whether the scheme will be continued. Fuel remains a primary concern of the all-party Parliamentary committee on pensions.

Job Creation Programme. In response to the rising numbers of the unemployed, in particular the unemployed school leavers, the Manpower Services Commission has established a scheme to create jobs to carry out work that would not otherwise be done. This opportunity has been actively taken up by organizations concerned with the elderly, such as Age Concern, and as a result many young workers are currently employed on jobs such as insulating the houses of old people.

Pensions. A 19.6 percent increase came into effect in November 1979, bringing the married couples' pension to £37.30 and the single person's pension to £23.30. Men are pensioned at age 65 years and women at 60. This anomaly and that of different financial provisions for widowed persons are the only two exceptions in the new bill legislating against discrimination on the grounds of sex. The Equal Opportunities Commission has recently reported on this subject.

Supplementary Benefits Commission. This replaced the National Assistance Board in 1966. Sixty percent of all claims are from people of pensionable age—23 percent of all pensioners. The average benefit for pensioners in late 1975 was £5 per week. The commission is reviewing the large increase in discretionary payments (53 percent of supplemented pensioners receive an additional payment for exceptional circumstances and the low take-up rate (about a quarter of all eligible pensioners fail to claim benefits).

Means tested benefits. Many income benefits are based upon a means test. The National Consumer Council and the Welsh Consumer Council have called for these to be abandoned since about £600m was unclaimed in 1975. In particular over 500,000 pensioners failed to claim £150m due to them.

Death. The Death in Dignity Alliance is campaigning for an increase in the death grant. The death grant has remained at £30 since 1949, and is now less than one quarter of its original value. In many parts of the country it is felt that the cost of funerals is causing many of the very old and frail serious anxiety.

Mass media. A new course being developed by the Open University Post-Experience Unit, supported by the Department of Health and Social Security, entitled "An Ageing Population," is followed by a thousand enrolled students. These may be predominantly drawn from paid workers in the health and social services, but it is also anticipated that the television and radio programs will be followed by many more people, including pensioners.

Good Neighbour Schemes. At the beginning of winter 1976–1977, the minister for social services launched a heavily publicized Good Neighbour Campaign. This was directed at the general public and has been fostered by many local authority social services departments (Berkshire, West Glamorgan, Tower Hamlets, for example) and Age Concern groups (Leicestershire, Devon, South Humberside, Brighton) as well as the BBC.

Street Warden Schemes. Whereas Good Neighbour Schemes have tended to be based upon referral systems or on an initial blanket survey (frequently under the auspices of the Job Creation Programme), Street Warden Schemes have been more firmly rooted in the street or small local area. They enable the central organization (social services departments usually) to establish a more effective cover.

Neighborhood care. Somerset Social Services Department has launched a campaign program to recruit families who will "foster" old people who would otherwise be placed in old people's homes. The families will be offered £30 per week. Cornwall has experimented with payments to neighbors to cook meals or clean the homes of elderly people. Kent is setting up an ambitious program of community care with the objective of preventing otherwise unavoidable admission to old people's homes.

The action research program pioneered by David Cheesman in Nottingham in 1965 created twelve neighborhood groups. There are now twenty-two, and they engage in a wide range of activities. A similar program of thirty-two neighborhoods is planned by the Leicester Social Services Department. A basic objective of such schemes is to the provide local community support to elderly persons.

Perhaps the most important arm of the statutory services directed at helping old people remain in their own homes is the home help. In September 1975, there were 42,500 home helpers (6.5 per 1,000 persons over 65) cleaning, washing, and lighting fires for elderly people.

Transport. Outside London, local public transport is based primarily upon buses. These are heavily subsidized by local authorities, and recent expenditure cuts and general transport trends have led to a crisis characterized by high fares and less frequent services. These changes have affected the elderly considerably, particularly in rural areas. In response, Age Concern Somerset has set up a voluntary scheme centered upon referrals to a volunteer controller. Norfolk County Council, in association with the National Bus Company, has established a community bus service; the bus is supplied by the company and driven by volunteers.

Mobility allowance. Disabled people are able to claim a £12 a week mobility allowance. About 150,000 people qualify. An upper age limit applies, however. This was increased from 60 to 64 in the autumn of 1979.

Housing. There are more people now in purpose-built housing linked to a residential warden by an alarm system than there are in local authority homes for the old. However, success and the aging of the tenants has led to increasing demands for extra support. Some authorities (Oldham, Newcastle-upon-Tyne, and Lancashire, for example) have been experimenting with mobile staffing arrangements. Others have been experimenting with linking sheltered housing administratively with old people's homes (Cheshire) or with day centers for elderly people in the adjacent community (Birmingham Council for Old People, Anchor Housing Association). Housing Associations have developed rapidly over the last few years as a government-backed source of rented accommodation. Forty-nine percent of their tenants are over 60 years.

The idea of "granny annexes" was to provide linked accommodation for families and their elderly relatives. A recent report by Anthea Tinker for the Department of the Environment has demonstrated that such housing works well in promoting neighborliness but that it is rarely possible to fill vacancies by relatives in the manner intended.

Meals on wheels. One of the main components of local authority domiciliary services is the provision of meals to the elderly in their own homes. For example, Northamptonshire Social Services Department is experimenting with a system based upon frozen food stored in sheltered housing schemes.

Home from hospital. A number of programs are concerned with the problem of discharge from hospital. The British Geriatrics Society has recognized its importance, and a number of action studies (Age Concern Liverpool: Care Is Rare; National Association for Mental Health—MIND: Home from Hospital), and local schemes (Age Concern Calderdale, Age Concern West Glamorgan) have responded.

Geriatric day hospitals. Not only is hospital care at night expensive for those receiving little treatment, but uninterrupted removal from the home tends to lead to problems of adjustment and discharge, which can be avoided through the use of day hospitals. Increasing numbers of health authorities are creating day hospitals or day wards. Medway Health Authority is introducing a hospital-at-home scheme for postoperative nursing care. A major Hospital-at-Home scheme, modeled upon medical provision in France, has been established by the Department of Health in Peterborough.

A Happier Old Age. In 1978 the Department of Health and Social Security issued a major discussion document entitled *A Happier Old Age.* This generated over 1,100 submissions of evidence from a wide range of different national and local bodies. Although the document concerns the prospective requirements of elderly people over the remainder of this century, the main focus tends to be upon their present circumstances and needs. It draws upon a large survey of elderly people living in their own homes in England (Hunt, 1978). A White Paper on the elderly was promised for 1979, but has been held up by the change in government.

Incontinence. The Disabled Living Foundation has set up a program of conferences and reports aimed at changing attitudes and practices concerning incontinence.

Rheumatism. This is only one of a wide range of health problems that are the subject of special campaigns or programs. The British League against Rheumatism produced a detailed report as a contribution to World Rheumatism Year 1977.

RESEARCH

Gerontology has suffered as a scientific discipline in Britain as a consequence of a number of historical circumstances. Like geriatrics within medicine, it cuts across a number of other well-established disciplines. For this reason gerontological research is published in a wide range of journals and under a number of different guises. Unlike other countries, gerontology in Britain has failed to find a home in one university or specialist institute. Added to this, the plight of the elderly following the industrial revolution led the great social reformers at the turn of the century to define the elderly as a welfare problem (see MacIntyre, 1977). As a result, gerontological research in the United Kingdom has almost always been orientated toward the study and solution of perceived problems rather than directly to the study of the process of aging. Further, the physiological manifestations of aging have served to direct much research toward the biological base and the medical response.

As a consequence of these difficulties, gerontologists have tended to find that their time is spent arguing the case for gerontology rather than on carrying out research. Nevertheless much research has been undertaken that reflects the aging process. This is particularly true of recent years.

The British Society of Social and Behavioural Gerontology (established in 1971) serves as a focus for all branches of gerontology outside medicine and biology. It has organized or taken part in two or more conferences each year, and it produces a regular newsletter. Professor Alan Lipman of the University of Wales has recently succeeded Professor Denis Bromley as chairman. The BSSBG has strong links with the British Geriatrics Society and the British Society for Research on Aging (predominantly serving biologists).

Following the success of the manifesto operation, Age Concern has established a research unit under the direction of Professor Mark Abrams. This unit is involved in the commissioning and collating of research and is currently publishing a series of profiles of the elderly in Britain.

The Department of Health and Social Security is perhaps the largest source of research funding, and a recent revision of its organization in this area has led to the creation of the Research Liaison Group for the Elderly. The Scottish Home and Health Department carries out a similar function in Scotland, and the Welsh Office has recently commissioned two large studies in Wales concerning geriatric services and social needs in rural areas. The Social Science Research Council is the primary source of government funds for scientific studies of social science aspects of aging.

Peter Coleman (1975) has produced an admirable review of contemporary gerontology in Britain. It would be inappropriate to duplicate that and so this section is primarily concerned to update his review. The main source used is the register of social research on old age produced and regularly updated by the National Corporation for the Care of Old People.

Coleman begins with reference to the uneven distribution of the elderly population and refers to Mellor's review of coastal migration and Karn's research on this issue. Geographers have been particularly active in this field recently. Kate Barnard (University of Southampton) has analyzed in detail the national distribution, and Tony Warnes (King's College London) and Chris Law (University of Salford) have completed a study corroborating and extending the results of Karn's study. Yvonne Neville (Age Concern Scotland) has carried out a study of migrants in the Scottish resort of Largs. Helen Whittington (University of Lancaster) has undertaken a study of widows in the resort of Morecambe. Local authorities in such coastal areas have also been active in research. For example, East Sussex Social Services Department has completed an analysis of the allocation of resources to the elderly.

Studies of poverty and the financial circumstances of the elderly are centered in the University of Essex under the direction of Professors Townsend and Atkinson. Economists involved in research and the elderly have tended to be found in the area of cost-effectiveness of service provision. The major study in this area is that of Ken Wright of the Institute of Social and Economic Research at the University of York. Closely related is research into the planning of service provision (R. W. Canvin, Institute of Biometry and Community Medicine, University of Exeter, and B. T. Williams, Medical Care Research Unit, University of Sheffield).

Coleman includes a detailed and valuable account of the development of studies of the older worker. With the rise of unemployment, this area of research has declined, and researchers have moved into other areas. Some psychologists, such as Bromley and Griew, have become influential in directing and promoting gerontological research. Studies such as that of Michael Fogarty (Centre for Studies in Social Policy) on aging and leisure between 40 and 60 years and that of Colin Phillipson (University of Keele) on the experience of retirement continue work in this area.

Kushlick's program of research on health care evaluation, reviewed by Coleman, has pioneered a wide range of studies on medical care for the elderly. Many of these have been carried out by research officers in the area health authorities (for example, Colin Rees at South Glamorgan). Others have been carried out by medical sociologists such as Charlotte Kratz (Department of Nursing, University of Manchester) studying the long-term care of stroke patients, Audrey Sutherland's project on long-stay admissions (Scottish Home and Health Department), Vera Carstairs well-known surveys of the elderly and their receipt of health services (Scottish Health Service Common Services Agency), David Hall's study of length of stay and decisions to discharge (Medical Sociology Research Centre, Swansea), and Jonathan Barker's study of discharge experiences in London (Medical College of the University of London). We should also not forget the action research of Geraldine Amos concerning care following hospital discharge in Liverpool (Age Concern), currently being extended to Birmingham, and of David Kettle who explored and promoted community-based health care for the elderly in Newcastle (Young Volunteer Force Foundation).

A proliferation of research has also occurred in the social services area. The Clearing House for Local Authority Social Services Research at Birmingham is the main source of information in this field. In addition are studies by the National Institute of Social Work on day care centers (Jan Carter) and Kathleen Jones on voluntary visiting in York.

Coleman's review moves on to housing. A study that should be added is that of Anthea Tinker concerning mixed housing schemes and referred to as "granny annexes." She has recently moved on to a study of the problems of housing old people near their relatives. In addition I have carried out a series of studies on the trends and implications of sheltered housing for the health care of tenants.

Coleman concludes with a short but detailed review of old age and the social sciences: "Neither psychology nor sociology have provided very far reaching or meaningful theoretical frameworks which applied social gerontology can readily make use of." A hint of the reasons for this rather depressing conclusion can be found in both his review and the research abstracts in the register of the National Corporation for the Care of Old People. There is a near-universal uncritical acceptance of the concept of old age. This is highlighted by two abstracts in the register that are the exceptions to this rule: Eileen Fairhurst's study on definitions of aging, which examines the consequences of these for social action, and H. Hazan's project, "The Limbo People: A Study of the Management of Time amongst the Elderly." This concern with the awareness of aging and with the appreciation that aging is the passage of time as much as it is the passage between stages, or the being in a stage, points to an approach to gerontological research that could be particularly valuable. It is reflected in Malcolm Johnson's decision to study the careers of doctors; his gerontological study makes no reference to old age or being elderly.

It may be that the aging of the great child cohort studies, which were established during the 1950s (the Aberdeen 1950–1955 birth cohort, the National Children's Bureau study, and the National Birthday Trust cohort), will prove to be a new focus for gerontological research. The members of these cohorts are now well into parenthood. Nevertheless cohort studies are only one of many approaches to gerontological research. A more general concern among British gerontologists is with the need for more detailed and critical studies of aging in Britain in the 1970s.

SOURCES OF INFORMATION

The three main national charitable organizations concerned with the elderly are Age Concern, the National Corporation for the Care of Old People, and Help the Aged. They have recently jointly issued a leaflet, *One Cause*, describing their different origins and objectives. Very briefly, Age Concern is the cover title for four National Old People's Welfare Councils (England, Northern Ireland, Scotland, and Wales) and a large number of local voluntary groups. It produces a journal, *New Age*, and a monthly information circular (available from Bernard Sunley House, 60 Pitcairn Road, Mitcham, Surrey, CR4 3LL). The NCCOP is a smaller central organization concerned with promoting experimental programs and discussion of national issues. It publishes a regularly updated register of social research on old age (available from Nuffield Lodge, Regent's Park, London, NW1 4RS). Help the Aged is primarily concerned with fund raising for schemes to aid the elderly in both Britain and in other countries. In addition it produces a monthly newspaper for pensioners in Britain, *Yours* (32 Dover Street, London, W1A 2AP).

All the government departments concerned with the elderly (Health and Social Security, Environment, and Energy) maintain valuable information services. The professional bodies specifically concerned with gerontological research are: the British Society of Gerontology, which publishes *Ageing Times* (Secretary: Personal Social Services Council, Brook House, Torrington Place, London WC1), the British Geriatrics Society, which publishes *Age and Ageing* (60 Pitcairn Road, Mitcham, Surry, CR4 3LL), and the British Society for Research into Aging (Department of Medicine, University of Leeds). These bodies supply information about gerontology programs and research. Other relevant organizations are:

Age Action Year 1976, Room 404, 101 Queen Victoria Street, London EC4P 4EP.

Association of Directors of Social Services, Kent County Council, Social Services Department, Springfield, Maidstone, Kent, ME14 2LW.

British Association of Social Workers, 16 Kent Street, Birmingham B5 6RG

British Association for Service to the Elderly, 60 Pitcairn Road, Mitcham, Surrey.

British Council for Aging, c/o NCCOP.

Central Council for the Disabled, 34 Eccleston Square, London SW1V 1PE.

The Clearing House for Local Authority Social Services Research, Department of Social Administration, University of Birmingham, P. O. Box 363, Birmingham, B15 2TT.

Kings Fund Centre, 24 Knutford Place, London W1H 6AN.

MIND (National Association for Mental Health), 22 Harley Street, London W1N 2ED.

The National Council for the Single Woman and Her Dependents, 166 Victoria Street, London SW1.

National Council for Social Service, 26 Bedford Square, London WC1.

The Pre-Retirement Association, 69/73 Manor Road, Wallington, Surrey.

The Royal College of General Practitioners, 14 Princes Gate, Hyde Park, London SW7.

SSRC Survey Archive, University of Essex, Wivenhoe Park, Colchester, Essex CO4 35 Q.

The Young Volunteer Force Foundation, 7 Leonard Street, London EC2.

REFERENCES

Abrams, M. 1977. *Beyond three-score and ten*. Age Concern.
———. 1978. *The elderly: an overview of current British social research*. Age Concern.
Age Concern. 1974a. *The manifesto*.
———. 1974b. *The attitudes of the retired and elderly*.
Amos, G. 1973. *Care is rare*. Age Concern Liverpool.
Bosanquet, N. 1978. *A future for old age*. Temple Smith/New Society.
Brearley, C. P. 1975. *Social work, ageing and society*. Routledge and Kegan Paul.
———. 1977. *Residential work with the elderly*. Routledge and Kegan Paul.
Bromley, D. B. 1974. *The psychology of human ageing*. Penguin.
Butler, A.; Oldman, C.; and Wright, R. 1979. *Sheltered housing for the elderly: A critical review*. University of Leeds.
Bytheway, B. 1979. "Ageing and sociological studies of the family." In *Family Life in old age*. edited by G. Dooghe and J. Helander. The Hague: Nijhoff.
Bytheway, B., and James, L. 1978. *The allocation of sheltered housing*. M.S.R.C. University College Swansea.
Cang, S. 1976–1977. "Why not hospital at home here? *Age Concern Today* (Winter).

Canvin, R. W., and Pearson, N. G., eds. 1973. *The needs of the elderly for health and welfare services*. University of Exeter.

Carver, V., and Liddiard, P. 1978. *An ageing population*. Holder and Stoughton.

Cheeseman, D., et al. 1972. *Neighbourhood care and old people*. Bedford Square Press.

Chown, S. M. 1972. *Human ageing*. Penguin.

Coleman, P. 1975. "Social gerontology in England, Scotland and Wales," *Gerontologist* 15:2.

Crawford, M. 1971. "Retirement and disengagement," *Human Relations*.

Department of Health and Social Security/Welsh Office. 1978. *A happier old age*. Her Majesty's Stationery Office.

Elder, G. 1977. *The alienated—growing old today*. Writers and Readers Publishing Cooperative.

Fairhurst, E. 1976. "Sociology and ageing: an alternative view" *Concorde*, No. 6.

Hadley, R., et al. 1975. *Across the generations, old people and young volunteers*. Allen and Unwin.

Hobman, D. 1978. *The social challenge of ageing*. Croom Helm.

Hunt, A. 1978. "The elderly at home," Office of Population, Censuses and Surveys. Her Majesty's Stationery Office.

Isaacs, B.; Neville, Y.; and Livingstone, M. 1972. *Survival of the unfittest*. Routledge and Kegan Paul.

Johnson, M. 1976. "That was your life." In *Dependency or interdependency in old age*, edited by J. M. A. Munnichs and W. J. A. Van Den Heuval. The Hague: Nijhoff.

Karn, V. 1977. *Retiring to the seaside.*. Routledge and Kegan Paul.

Law, E. M., and Warnes, A. M. 1976. *The changing geography of the elderly in England and Wales*, Institute of British Geographers Transactions New Series, 1 (4).

MacIntyre, S. 1977. "Old age as a social problem." In *Health care and health knowledge*, edited by R. Dingwall et al. Croom Helm.

Meacher, M. 1972. *Taken for a ride*. Longman.

Muir Gray, J. A. 1977. "A policy for warmth," Fabian pamphlet.

National Corporation for the Care of Old People. 1977. *Old age: a register of social research*.

Personal Social Services Council. 1978. *Residential Care Reviewed*.

Phillipson, C. 1977. "The Emergence of Retirement," Working Papers in Sociology, No. 14, University of Durham.

Sumner, G., and Smith, R. 1970. *Planning local authority services for the elderly*. Allen and Unwin.

Tinker, A. 1976. *How successful are granny annexes?* Department of the Environment.

Townsend, P. 1977. "The failure to house Britain's aged," *Help the Aged*.

Wicks, M. 1978. *Old and cold: Hypothermia and social policy*. Heinemann.

Wright, K. G. 1979. "Economics and planning the care of the elderly." In *Economics and health planning* edited by K. Lee. Croom Helm.

UNITED STATES OF AMERICA

ERDMAN PALMORE

When the United States is compared with other countries in regard to its resources, research, problems, and programs for its elders, several anomalies appear. The United States undoubtedly is one of the richest countries in the world in terms of natural resources, technical and scientific resources, and per-capita gross national product. With one of the largest proportions of aged in the world, it was one of the first countries to develop substantial gerontological research in all related scientific and applied disciplines, and it probably has more professional gerontologists and produces more gerontological research than any other country. It spends more per capita on health care for its elders—$1,521 in 1976—than perhaps any other country (Gibson, Mueller, and Fisher, 1977).

Yet despite all these laudable facts, it apparently has not solved its problems of health, integration, and status of its elders as well as many other countries have. Some of the most important problems are indicated by the following facts. Life expectancy of males born in 1970 in the United States was lower than that of twenty-five other countries (United Nations, 1976). Over 15 percent of persons over age 65 had incomes below the official poverty levels in 1975, and another 10 percent were below the near-poverty level (Fowles, 1977). Compulsory retirement affects perhaps half of those retiring at are 65 or older (Palmore, 1972a). As a result, millions of elders are willing and able to work but cannot find employment because of age discrimination (Harris, 1975). Few elders participate in senior citizens' clubs or centers (probably less than 5 percent), and many find themselves isolated from the mainstream of family and community life. About one-fifth of the elders live in substandard housing, and more than half live in units built over thirty-five years ago (Binstock and Shanas, 1976). Despite many new programs for the aged, the United States tends to lag behind many European countries in offering a full spectrum of social services. Other evidence of "ageism" (prejudice and discrimination against the aged) is widespread (Butler, 1969; Palmore and Manton, 1973). Thus, our rich resources and gerontological knowledge do not seem to be matched by our attitudes and actual treatment of our elders.

There may be several extenuating circumstances for this discrepancy. The United States has one of the most heterogeneous aged populations in the world in terms of race, national origin, religion, socioeconomic status, and regional variations. These variations may have hampered attempts to deliver adequate programs and services. Also, until the twentieth century, the United States has been largely a frontier society with a corresponding emphasis on the new and the young. This youth cult may have retarded recognition and concern for its elders. On the positive side, it does appear that recognition and concern for elders is growing at an unprecedented rate. Finally, while the United States has one of the more democratic forms of government, it has an unusually elaborate system of checks and balances, which often frustrates attempts to develop needed programs.

GROWTH IN GERONTOLOGY

The growth in gerontology and programs for the aged since the late 1940s has been dramatic. A generation ago there were hardly any gerontologists identified as such. Now there are about four thousand professional members of the Gerontological Society. A generation ago there were almost no courses offered in gerontology. Now there are literally thousands of such courses in over eight hundred colleges and universities and in more than four hundred community and junior colleges across the nation (Sprouse, 1976). A generation ago there were no centers for the study of aging. Now there are about two dozen major ones primarily devoted to research and teaching gerontology and about thirteen hundred other programs in gerontology. A generation ago there were no journals in gerontology. Now there are at least six professional journals and a couple of dozen popular journals and newsletters in aging. The federal government recently established the National Institute on Aging devoted primarily to research. The Administration on Aging spends over $27 million annually on research and training.

A generation ago there were almost no special programs for the aged, except for the Social Security Administration, which provided minimal retirement income. In 1977 the Administration on Aging alone spent about $500 million on a dozen different programs. Public programs such as Medicare and Medicaid spent about $24 billion on health care for the aged (Gibson et al., 1977). Many other federal agencies, such as the Department of Housing and Urban Development, Department of Labor, and the Veterans Administration, have special programs for elders.

The phenomenal growth of gerontology on the one hand and programs for elders on the other have been mutually reinforcing, and both are related to the increasing numbers of elders, as well as to the general expansion of governmental support for welfare and social services and for research.

DEMOGRAPHY

The number of persons over 65 in the United States has increased and will continue to increase by about 3 to 5 million every ten years (table 75). Furthermore the percentage of the total population over 65 has increased by about one point every decade and will probably continue to do so until 1990. These increases are due to the combination of decreasing mortality and decreasing fertility. If either or both of these should decrease more than expected, the resulting percentage over 65 will increase even more. Of equal importance to planning programs and services for the aged is the fact that the numbers and percentages of persons over age 75 have been increasing even more rapidly; those over 75 tend to need substantially more services than those aged 65 to 75.

Table 75: ESTIMATES AND PROJECTIONS OF PERSONS 65 AND OVER (IN THOUSANDS)

Year	Number	Percentage of Total
1900	3,100	4.1
1940	9,036	6.8
1950	12,397	8.2
1960	16,675	9.0
1970	20,087	9.8
1980	24,927	11.2
1990	29,824	12.2
2000	31,822	12.2

Source: U.S. Bureau of the Census, Current Population Reports, Series P-25, No. 704, *Projections of the Population of the U.S.* (Washington, D.C.: Government Printing Office, 1977).

Another demographic fact relating to programs for elders is the increasing sex ratio. Because women enjoy greater longevity than men, there are progressively more women than men in the older age groups. There are now about 145 women over 65 for every 100 men. This ratio is expected to increase to 155 by the year 2000 (Brotman, 1977). When this greater longevity of women is combined with the practice of women marrying older men, the result is a much larger number of widows than widowers. There are about three unmarried women over 65 for each unmarried man, so even if every unmarried man over 65 married a woman over 65, two-thirds of the unmarried women would remain unmarried. Unmarried elders in general have lower incomes, poorer health, and require more services than the married do.

PROBLEMS AND PROGRAMS

In 1976, the Federal Council on the Aging published a Bicentennial Charter for Older Americans, which contained nine "basic human rights for older

Americans.'' (This is similar to the Declaration of Objectives in the 1965 Older Americans Act.) We will examine each of these ideals in terms of the needs they represent and the extent to which these needs are or are not being met.

The Right to Freedom, Independence and the Free Exercise of Individual Initiative. This should encompass not only opportunities and resources for personal planning and managing one's life style, but support systems for maximum growth and contributions by older persons to their community.

This reflects the American ideal of individual freedom and independence from governmental or other control. However this ideal often interferes with the effective delivery of services. Most programs for the aged are voluntary, and so millions who could benefit from them are not served because of ignorance that they exist, pride that prevents them from accepting "charity" or "welfare", misconceptions about the nature of the programs, inability or unwillingness to pay the minimum fees necessary, or even inability to fill out complicated application forms. In order to overcome some of these problems, information and referral services have become one of the most common (and perhaps most important) of all services to elders. Many agencies are putting more emphasis on outreach activities: attempts to find eligible participants and to motivate and facilitate their participation.

One exception to the generally voluntary nature of programs for elders is the social security program, which includes retirement, disability, and medical care insurance. Taxes for these programs are compulsory for most wage and salary workers. Unless these programs were compulsory, it is probable that those who need them most would be least likely to participate voluntarily.

The emphasis on personal planning in this ideal is reflected in the growth of preretirement planning programs offered by various corporations and educational institutions. Several studies have shown that those who participate in such courses report better adjustment after retirement, yet few corporations have comprehensive preretirement planning programs and few elders have participated in them (O'Meara, 1977).

The Right to an Income in Retirement Which Would Provide an Adequate Standard of Living. Such income must be sufficiently adequate to assure maintenance of mental and physical activities which delay deterioration and maximize individual potential for self-help and support. This right should be assured regardless of employment capability.

It is probable that the retired in the United States enjoy one of the highest standards of living of retired period in the world. In 1975 families with a head 65 or over (usually just a couple) had a median income of $8,057, and unrelated elders had a median income of $3,311 (Fowles, 1977). Furthermore, it appears that elders receive a share of the national personal income that is about equal to their proportion in the population (Binstock and Shanas, 1976). The Supplementary Security Income (SSI) program now guarantees a minimum income to all persons over 65, even though this minimum is usually not enough to raise them above the official poverty level. Most workers and their dependents are covered by social security (Old Age Survivors and Disability Insurance) so that in 1977 over 33 million persons were receiving a total of $78 billion a year in benefits.

Yet median incomes of the elders remain at about one-half that of younger persons, and poverty is substantially more frequent among the elders than others: 15.3 percent for those 65 and over compared to 12 percent for those under 65 (Fowles, 1977). Another 10 percent had incomes below the near-poor level. Thus at least one-quarter of our elders do not have adequate incomes by American standards.

The Right to an Opportunity for Employment Free from Discriminatory Practices Because of Age. Such employment when desired should not exploit individuals because of age and should permit utilization of talents, skills, and experience of older persons for the good of self and community. Compensation should be based on the prevailing wage scales of the community for comparable work.

This is one of the most frequently violated rights. This violation takes two forms: compulsory retirement because of age and individual discrimination because of age. Most large businesses as well as most private and public institutions (including the federal government) force their employees to retire at a certain age (usually 65) regardless of their ability or desire to continue working (Palmore, 1972a). In addition, millions of older workers (some as young as 40) face individual employment discrimination because of their age. This is despite the fact that there has been a law (since 1967) prohibiting discrimination on the basis of age for persons aged 40 to 65. This law was extended in 1979 to cover most workers up to age 70. It remains to be seen how effectively it will be enforced.

As a result of these two kinds of age discrimination (compulsory retirement policies and individual discrimination), about 10 percent of persons over 65 (over 2 million elders) say they are willing and able to work but cannot find employment (Harris, 1975). There are many arguments for and against such age discrimination (Palmore, 1972a), and the issues are currently being tested in the courts and debated in Congress. It is relevant to note that several other countries (notably the communist ones) not only have no compulsory retirement but have the opposite problem: how to motivate older workers to continue working.

Several federal programs attempt to provide more employment opportunities to elders. The Senior Community Service Employment Program (Title IX of the Older Americans Act) pays for part-time community service jobs for low-income persons 55 years old and older. In 1976 about twenty thousand individuals participated at a cost of $85 million. (Information on this and the following federal programs are derived from Office of Management and Budget, 1977). The Senior Opportunities and Service Program funds projects that serve or employ older persons. In 1976 about a million persons were served at a cost of $10 million. The Department of Labor also provides special job placement services for older workers.

The Right to an Opportunity to Participate in the Widest Range of Meaningful Civic, Educational, Recreational and Cultural Activities. The varying interests and needs of older Americans require programs and activities sensitive to their rich and diverse heritage. There should be opportunities for involvement with persons of all ages in programs which are affordable and accessible.

Several barriers interfere with this right. First is the cost barrier: many elders are not able to afford participation in such activities because of reduced income. Second are transportation barriers: many elders do not have private transportation, and public transportation is often inadequate or inconvenient. More subtle is the barrier of age prejudice: many persons (even older ones) discourage the participation of elders in these activities because they believe older persons have little or no ability to contribute or benefit from such activities.

One attempt to overcome these barriers is the Model Projects on Aging Program (Title III of the Older Americans Act), which funds a wide range of projects "contributing toward wholesome and meaningful living for older persons." In 1977, $12 million was spent on these projects. Another attempt is the Senior Citizens Program (Title V of the Older Americans Act), which helps community senior centers develop and deliver social and nutritional services for older persons. In 1977 $20 million was devoted to this program. The Retired Senior Volunteer Program (RSVP) develops community volunteer service opportunities. In 1977 about two hundred fifty thousand older volunteers were serving in these projects, and $19 million was devoted to them. Over five hundred Area Agencies on Aging provide development and coordination of these and other programs for elders. Over $150 million was appropriated for these agencies in 1977.

The Right to Suitable Housing. The widest choices of living arrangements should be available, designed and located with reference to special needs at costs which older persons can afford.

Elders often have special needs or preferences in housing that make much of existing housing unsuitable. Their disabilities may make stairs and heavy doors difficult or impossible to manage. Their lack of private transportation may make certain locations inaccessible. Noisy children or neighborhoods make certain apartments undesirable. Vulnerability to crime makes certain neighborhoods undesirable. And of course low incomes place much desirable housing out of reach. Poor housing is concentrated among low-income and minority elders. Yet only 4 percent of all persons over 65 list poor housing as a "very serious" problem, which is somewhat less than for persons under 65 (Harris, 1975).

In addition to regular public housing for which low-income elders are eligible, the Housing for the Elderly and Handicapped Program provides low-interest loans for housing projects for persons 62 and over. In 1976 about twenty-five thousand units were funded under this program.

The Right to the Best Level of Physical and Mental Health Services Needed. Such services should include the latest knowledge and techniques science can make available without regard to economic status.

It is well known that elders tend to suffer from more illness and disability than younger persons. Yet many believe that most elders receive adequate medical care because they are the only age group covered by a national health insurance program (Medicare). It is true that this program spent about $21 billion for the health care of about 20 million persons. Nevertheless Medicare and other public programs pay for just two-thirds of the total health care of elders. The other third must come out of personal funds or from private insurance. Because of increased costs and services, elders now pay more than double the actual dollars out of pocket for their health care than before Medicare went into effect in 1967.

There are many barriers to more adequate health care for elders, including financial, transportation, ignorance and denial among the elders, and attitudes of health care providers (Palmore, 1972b). As a result, 10 percent of elders state that not enough medical care is "a serious problem" for them (Harris, 1975).

The Right to Ready Access to Effective Social Services. These services should enhance independence and well-being, yet provide protection and care as needed.

It is clear that millions of elders need a variety of social services because of the biological, psychological, and social processes of aging. It is not clear how many need which kinds of services and how much they need. Numerous surveys have been carried out to attempt to answer these questions, but there are many limitations to the answers these surveys provide. Many are not even representative of the aged population in the locality in which they were conducted, much less representative of the nation as a whole. There are a few nationally representative surveys of elders' needs (Harris, 1975; Shanas et al., 1968), but these provide little or no information on regional or local variation.

Furthermore many elders have a vague awareness that they need some kind of help but may not know just what kinds of social services could help them. Finally, some elders deny their needs, while others exaggerate them, so that accurate objective estimates are difficult.

However, in attempting to provide needed social services, the government and private agencies have developed a bewildering variety of services. Some of the major ones follow.

Home-help services include a broad range of supportive help for the elder and his family, including personal care. These services are provided by paid homemakers or home-health aides. In 1975 over eighteen hundred agencies provided over twenty thousand homemakers (Binstock and Shanas, 1976). The United States has many fewer home helps per hundred thousand population than most European countries.

Friendly visitors are volunteers who are trained and supervised by professionals to provide social services in the home and especially to recognize situations or problems for referral.

Meal services provide both meals to homes of those with limited mobility and congregate dining in central locations. This latter service also stimulates socialization and participation in other programs for elders. In 1977 the Nutrition Program for the Elderly (Title VII of the OAA) served about 435,000 meals at approximately 8,500 sites, at a cost of $225 million.

Home repair services employ older persons to provide minor repair and household maintenance services for other older persons who cannot purchase such services on the open market. This is a widespread need both because elders are more likely to live in deteriorating housing and because many elders have become so frail that they can no longer perform the repairs that they once did themselves.

Day care or geriatric day hospitals are centers that usually provide a full range of medical, nutritional, psychiatric, and rehabilitative and recreational services for those who need such care during the day but can be taken care of at home during the night. Such services often relieve family members throughout the day and prevent premature institutionalization of frail elders.

Respite services relieve primary caretakers, such as adult children, of their continuing responsibilities for older persons over weekends and vacations. This service is often offered through the geriatric centers.

Registrant service is a program by which elders living in their homes register with a geriatric center to have available to them the various services provided by that center on a continuing basis.

Social group activity programs provide recreational and therapeutic activities in a variety of settings, including senior centers, neighborhood and settlement houses, parks and recreation departments, hospitals, and institutions for elders. This is an important service for those who have not found adequate substitutes for lost roles as parents, workers, and family members.

Legal services are provided in the areas of wills, consumer rights and protection, guardianship, conservatorship, and protective services. Many elders are unaware of their legal rights or of how to get what they need because of complicated regulations.

Protective services focus on the mentally impaired older persons who have no one to provide help and support.

Of course, along with all other citizens, needy elders are eligible for many other services such as food stamps, public welfare, vocational rehabilitation, and educational programs.

The Right to Appropriate Institutional Care When Required. Care should provide full restorative services in a safe environment. This care should also promote and protect the dignity and rights of the individual along with family and community ties.

About 5 percent of all persons over 65 are in some kind of long-term institution such as nursing homes, retirement homes, and mental hospitals. The total chance of an elder's being institutionalized at some time before death has been estimated by two studies at about 25 percent (Palmore, 1976a). Some argue that we could substantially reduce this figure if we provided more adequate alternatives to institutionalization such as more foster homes, day-care centers, and home services. Others argue that many elders in need of institutionalization cannot get it because of financial and other barriers. It may be that the two groups just about balance each other; that is, if we removed all elders from institutions who could get along in the community and put into institutions all those who need it, we might end up with about the same percentage as we have now.

Regardless of how many should be in institutions, it is generally agreed that many, if not a majority of, present institutions are inadequate in their facilities, treatment, and personnel. Most do little or nothing toward restorative services and provide little more than custodial services while their patients await death.

The Right to a Life and Death with Dignity. Regardless of age, society must assure individual citizens of the protection of their constitutional rights and opportunities for self-respect, respect and acceptance from others, a sense of enrichment and contribution, and freedom from dependency. Dignity in dying includes the right of the individual to permit or deny the use of extraordinary life support systems.

While it is difficult to quantify the extent of this problem, it is probably safe to say that millions of elders are robbed of their self-respect and denied respect from others by the widespread age prejudice in our society. Probably a majority of Americans believe the false stereotypes that many, if not most, aged are senile, sick, disabled, helpless, useless, unable to change or learn, miserable, or poverty stricken (Palmore, 1977b). As a result, many elders are denied "opportunities for self-respect, respect and acceptance from others, a sense of enrichment and contribution." Certainly American elders are given less respect than in many other countries (Palmore, 1975).

On the positive side, many Americans are becoming aware of the problems and injustices caused by age prejudice, programs are being accelerated to solve these problems, and age prejudice may be declining. Age prejudice should decline as a result both of growing knowledge about the facts of aging and as a result of actual improvements in the relative status of the aged (Palmore, 1976b).

The right to dignity in death, including the right of the individual to deny the use of extraordinary life support systems, appears to be gaining support. Several states have passed laws making it legal for doctors to withdraw extraordinary life support systems upon request of the patient and/or relatives. The issues of various kinds of euthanasia under various conditions are being widely debated. In addition to reducing the suffering of dying, such trends should reduce the escalating cost of dying in our society.

BIOLOGICAL RESEARCH*

Molecular Level

Extensive research in the United States supports the theory that aging results when inappropriate information is provided for normal cell function from the cell nucleus. Genetic information provided by an aging cell may become altered in at least four ways.

1. Through changes in the base pairs of coding of the DNA, the result of coding errors in replication, point mutation, or chromosome aberrations.
2. Through increasing levels of error in RNA synthesis, charging of transfer RNA, or protein synthesis.
3. Through deteriorative alterations in the arrangement of fundamental control elements in chromatin such as histone and nonhistone protein and RNA.
4. Through expression of a normal program of differentiation that includes aging as the final step.

There has also been extensive research showing substantial increases or decreases with age in enzyme activity, which could produce the symptoms of senescence.

*Much of the material in this section is based on Finch and Hayflick (1977).

Cellular Level

Research has shown that aging usually causes an increase in the length of the cell cycle and the length of the prereplicative phase in stimulated G₀ cells, as well as changes in the template activity of chromatin, and changes in the synthesis and storage of nonhistone chromosomal proteins. This research has led to the tentative conclusion that aging cells are those that go into deeper states of G₀ from which it becomes increasingly difficult to rescue them. This could be due to changes in chromatin and its components in aging cells.

In 1961 Hayflick and Moorhead found for the first time that cultured normal human cells (fibroblasts) underwent a finite number of doublings (about fifty) and then died. Although this Hayflick phenomenon was at first met with considerable skepticism, the occurrence of alterations in cell functions after a finite number of doublings (phase III) is now generally accepted; however, the bearing of this phenomenon on biological aging is still controversial.

Tissue and Organ Level

Most research on age differences in anatomy and body composition have been based on cross-sectional studies: those that compare different age groups at one point in time. Attribution of these cross-sectional age differences to age changes over time are complicated by two factors. There may be cohort (or generation) differences between age groups that account for the cross-sectional differences. An example would be that in the United States succeeding generations have tended to be taller, which may explain much of the shorter stature of older persons in cross-sectional studies. A second factor is differential survivorship. Thus, if obesity tends to shorten life, a selective survivorship of thin persons would tend to exaggerate the apparent weight loss in late life observed from cross-sectional studies. Despite these difficulties, the following appear to be the main anatomical changes with age that are supported both by cross-sectional studies and the few longitudinal studies of these changes.

1. Height tends to decline after about age 50.
2. Span (distance from fingertip to fingertip with arms outstretched) tends to decline after age 40.
3. Weight tends to increase in middle age, except where energy expenditures are high and food supply is restricted, and then decline after age 55 for men and after age 65 for women.
4. Similarly skin folds (a measure of fatty deposits) tend to thicken in middle age in Western society (but not in the primitive cultures studied) and then begin to shrink in the seventh decade.
5. The skull tends to thicken from early adulthood onward.
6. The nose and ears tend to grow longer and thicker with age.
7. Joints, particularly knee joints, tend to deteriorate with age.

8. Total body potassium tends to decline with age.

9. Skin tends to wrinkle with age, especially when exposed to sunlight.

10. Hair tends to thin and become gray.

11. Osteoarthritis, the "wear and tear disorder," tends to increase in the vertebral column and joints.

12. The lens of the eye tends to thicken with age.

As for anatomical changes in the nervous system, it was thought for many years that aging is accompanied by a reduction in brain weight, narrowing of the gyri, meningeal thickening, and ventricular enlargement. However, recent research in the United States and elsewhere has questioned all these assumptions.

In terms of immunology and aging, recent research shows considerable evidence for the following.

1. Normal immune function tends to begin to decline shortly after sexual maturity when the thymus begins to involute.

2. This decline is due to selective changes in T cell functions, including their inability to proliferate and to promote B cell differentiation.

3. Age-related immune dysfunction predisposes one to autoimmunity, immune complex diseases, and cancer.

4. Immunoengineering may offer an effective approach to minimize diseases of aging.

Kidney function also appears to decline with age, but the question of whether this is due to an intrinsic and universal aging process or to selective disease processes is unresolved.

Lung capacity and respiratory functions also tend to decline with age, but there is considerable variation dependent on exercise and on presence or absence of disease.

Whole Animal Level

All research in the United States and elsewhere agrees that mortality increases logarithmically with age, with the probability of dying doubling about once every eight years beyond age 30. This concept was first described mathematically by Gompertz in 1825 and has since become known as Gompertz's law. There are, of course, considerable variations among sex, race, socioeconomic, and nationality groups in the exact levels of these mortality rates, but the general shape seems to hold among all humans studied (and even among other mammals protected from malnutrition, predation, and infection).

Considerable research indicates that there are many factors other than age and sex that influence or predict mortality rates (Palmore, 1971). In the United States many studies have found that cigarette smoking, obesity, lack of exercise, poor nutrition, and poor medical care increase mortality rates among the aged, as well as among younger groups. Rapid declines in certain kinds of cognitive functioning also predict shorter longevity. Several studies show that certain social factors such as isolation or lack of social interaction, lower education and occupation, lower work satisfaction, and lower life satisfaction predict shorter longevity.

Shock has summarized the convincing evidence (primarily from research in the United States but supported by research elsewhere) that aging is more than a summation of changes that take place at the cellular, tissue, or organ level (Finch and Hayflick, 1977). Continued effective functioning requires the integrated activity of all the organ systems to meet the stresses of living. Regulatory mechanisms that control adaptation of body temperature to environmental changes and those that affect the ability to perform muscular work are two clear examples of systems integration that tend to decline with age, although these too are influenced by exercise, stress, and other environmental factors.

PSYCHOLOGICAL RESEARCH*

As in biological research, firm conclusions about psychological processes of aging have been hampered by the predominance of cross-sectional data with their twin problems of cohort effects and selective survival. However, gerontologists in the United States have pioneered in developing longitudinal, cross-sequential, and experimental methods to supplement data from cross-sectional studies. The following summarizes the main conclusions about aging and behavioral processes that can be drawn by comparing cross-sectional, longitudinal, cross-sequential, and animal research in the United States.

Motivation and Activity

1. Locomotor activity tends to decrease with advancing age after sexual maturity, but a significant decrement does not usually occur until senility.

2. It is not yet clear as to whether aversive stimuli are equally motivating for all age groups.

3. Overinvolvement or overarousal resulting in a heightened drive state may impair performance for the elderly relative to the young.

4. Sexual activity continues among a majority of healthy men in their seventies.

5. Sexual competence and interest continues for many older persons long after sexual activity ceases. Loss of spouse or willingness or ability of spouse to perform sexually is the major reason given for cessation of sexual activity, especially among women.

6. Age differences in a variety of activities may be more related to changes in motivation than to intellectual or physical competence.

---

*Much of the material in this section is based on Birren and Schaie (1977).

Memory

1. Age differences in short-term memory are minimal, provided that the items have been fully perceived and that no reorganization is required.

2. Long-term memory tends to decline with age. This is contrary to the previous general belief (based entirely on anecdotal evidence) that memory for remote events is unimpaired by aging.

3. Recognition memory (recognizing items when they are presented) shows less age-related decline than recall memory (recalling an item on demand).

Learning

1. In verbal learning tasks, older individuals are particularly disadvantaged when time to respond is short.

2. Older individuals tend not to use encoding strategies as often or as well as younger individuals.

3. At ages beyond 65, longitudinal studies show decrements in learning abilities, even though these are less than those shown in cross-sectional studies.

Motor Performance

1. Movements of large extent at maximum speed show substantial slowing with age, due seemingly to muscular limitations. However, most movements in everyday tasks are not limited by muscular factors but by the speed of decisions required to guide and monitor movements.

2. When everyday movements can be prepared for in advance, changes with age are relatively small.

3. When opportunities to monitor and inspect signals for as long as they wish are available, older people tend to be slower but more accurate than younger ones. When such opportunities are lacking, older people tend to be less accurate than younger ones.

4. Age changes in simple sensorimotor tasks show little consistent relation to sex, education, or socioeconomic status.

5. The types of industrial and road accidents and road traffic violations that increase with age can be attributed mainly to slowness in making decisions rather than to any sensory or motor impairment.

Perception

In general, most research agrees that all five senses (vision, hearing, taste, touch, and smell) tend to decline with age. More specifically there tend to be declines on the average in the following perceptual abilities:

1. Acuity of vision.
2. Light and dark adaptation.
3. Sensitivity to glare.
4. Depth perception.
5. Color discrimination.

6. Auditory threshold sensitivity.

7. Pitch discrimination.

8. Dichotic listening (discrimination between different stimuli presented to different ears).

9. Speech reception threshold.

10. Taste sensitivity.

11. Odor sensitivity.

12. Touch sensitivity (occurs in about one-fourth of the aged, particularly in the skin of the palm and sole but not in hairy skin).

13. Vibratory sensitivity (not universal but more frequent in the lower extremities than in the upper extremities).

14. Pain and temperature sensitivity (may be impaired in a small percentage of elders).

15. Noxious stimulation.

Intellectual Abilities

Most recent research in the United States agrees on the following generalizations.

1. There are general declines in intellectual abilities past age 65, particularly in those involving speed of response of nonverbal, perceptual-manipulative skills. These declines are smaller in longitudinal studies than in cross-sectional studies but are still substantial.

2. Longitudinal studies may minimize the extent of decline because of practice effects (improvements with practice) and because of selective dropout (poorer performers tend to drop out more often).

3. People who perform relatively well when younger will also perform relatively well when older.

In summary, research in the United States has tended to agree that there tend to be numerous declines in all areas of psychological functions with age. On the other hand, most of these declines among healthy elders can be compensated for by a variety of techniques and aids such as eye glasses, hearing aids, cautious driving, and taking more time so that they need not interfere with the effective performance of most normal activities.

SOCIAL SCIENCE RESEARCH

Gerontological research in many other countries has concentrated on biomedical aspects of aging. Gerontology in the United States, by contrast, has had a heavy emphasis from its beginning on social aspects of aging. The fallacy of attributing all age differences to biological processes has long been recognized. Recently it has even been asserted that most of the problems of aging in the United States are not primarily biological problems but are primarily social and political problems resulting from "ageism" (Comfort, 1976). While the early concern with the social problems of aging has continued, there has also been a steady growth in social gerontology as science. This growth has been marked by five major review volumes. In 1948, the Social Science Research Council published *Social Adjustment in Old Age: A Research Planning Report* (Pollak), which attempted to provide a common frame of reference for social research and which emphasized the changes in social opportunity for understanding the processes of aging. In 1960 the appearance of the *Handbook of Social Gerontology* (Tibbitts) and of *Aging in Western Societies* (Burgess) documented the fact that enough research and theory had accumulated to consider social gerontology as a separate discipline, or at least a subspecialty within sociology. In 1968 *Aging and Society: An Inventory of Research Findings* (Riley and Foner) provided an encyclopedic reference on most of the important social research up to 1967. Finally in 1977, the *Handbook of Aging and the Social Sciences* (Binstock and Shanas) provided a landmark in the development of social gerontology. It makes clear that each of the social sciences has made major contributions to social gerontology and helps to clarify the main theoretical and methodological issues current in United States research. This research is so extensive that I will limit this review to three major theories and one methodological problem.

Modernization Theory

This theory could be represented by a graph that shows a rise in stable agricultural society, a fall during modernization, and then a leveling off in the security, satisfactions, and status of the aged. The baseline or zero point would be represented by animal groups in which there seem to be no instincts or inborn propensities to sustain aged parents. The usual pattern among animals is to abandon the aged of the species as soon as their ability to function has seriously declined. It is only through the development of human culture that the aged have been able to achieve any security. In most primitive hunting, fishing, and collecting societies, the security and status of the aged has remained fairly low because of the constant struggle to survive and the relative inability of the aged to contribute their share to this survival. However, as soon as the group achieves some measure of security and stability, the security and status of the aged tends to rise rapidly. The peak of the graph is reached in the stable agricultural societies, which tend to become gerontocracies, with the aged controlling access to land, food, sex, recreation, religion—indeed all the desired things in the society.

As modernization develops, the status of the aged begins to decline. Increases in longevity lead to a large "supply" of aged that exceeds the "demand" for aged persons—to put it in economic theory terms. The developing technology makes the skills of the aged obsolete. Urbanization reduces the importance of the aged's control of farmland and also increases migration and social mobility, which undermines the aged's status as head of the extended family. Growing education and the mass media undermine the aged's status as the main source of wisdom and culture. This decline in the status of the aged with modernization can be seen in the inverse correlations between various measures of modernization and the status of the aged among nations today (Palmore and Manton, 1973).

A recent development in this theory suggests that this decline is beginning to level out and may even swing back up in postindustrial societies. For example, it appears that in the United States the relative status of the aged in terms of health, income, occupation, and education has begun to rise and will be substantially higher in the year 2000 (Palmore, 1976b). This appears to be due to a leveling off of the aspects of modernization that contributed to their declining status, such as urbanization, social mobility, and increasing education. In addition, the growth of gerontology and programs for the aged probably contributes to this rise in status.

Minority Group Theory

A recurrent and controversial issue in American gerontology is the degree to which the aged are integrated in society and whether it is useful to view them as an emerging minority group. Several gerontologists have argued that minority group concepts and theory help to explain why many of the aged suffer from negative stereotyping, segregation, and discrimination and, as a result, often develop feelings of inferiority and group consciousness (Barron, 1961; Breen, 1960; Rose and Peterson, 1965; Palmore, 1978a). Others argue that the aged are different from racial and ethnic minority groups in several respects, such as not having been "born that way" (Streib, 1965).

Research has shown that elders in the United States do share three characteristics with other minority groups. First, they are subject to widespread prejudice in the form of numerous negative stereotypes, such as the belief that most elders are sick or infirm or soon will be; that they have neither sexual interests nor abilities; that most are senile; that most are depressed or irritable; that most are unable to work or be useful; that most are isolated and lonely; and that a majority are poor. The facts clearly show that all these beliefs are false (Palmore, 1977b). Second, the elders suffer from various forms of discrimination, such as mandatory retirement and other job discrimination, discrimination by lending institutions, and segregation in certain neighborhoods and institutions. Third, as a result of this prejudice and discrimination, they tend to be a deprived group in terms of income, occupation, education, and general social prestige.

On the other hand, elders in the United States are different from other minority groups in at least two ways. First, they are not born into the group. This gives them an advantage over all other minority groups in that everyone who lives long enough will move into the category of aged and thus everyone has a long-term self-interest in the status of the aged. Second, most elders have so far shown little evidence of organizing, or even of self-consciousness as a group, or of developing a subculture, as have the other minority groups. Many, if not most, elders seem ashamed of their age and are unwilling to identify themselves as aged, much less will they join advocacy groups for the aged. However, there are some signs that this may be changing. It is paradoxical that as their socioeconomic status rises (thus making them less of a deprived group), their willingness to identify with other elders and organize to overcome prejudice and discrimination seems to be rising also (thus making them more like a minority group). However, this paradox has previously been observed among blacks and is related to rising levels of expectation that outpace actual gains in status.

Disengagement versus Activity Theories

In 1961 the theory of disengagement was first introduced, along with some evidence from a cross-sectional study in Kansas City. The basic tenets of the theory are that the process of mutual withdrawal of aging persons and of society from each other is typical of most aging persons; this process is biologically and psychologically intrinsic and inevitable; and the disengagement process contributes to healthy, satisfying adjustment in old age (Cumming and Henry, 1961). In contrast, activity theory holds that the majority of normal aging persons maintain stable levels of activity and engagement; the actual amount of engagement or disengagement is more influenced by past life-styles and the culture than by any intrinsic processes; and maintaining substantial levels of physical, mental, and social activity is usually necessary for successful aging.

There has been a voluminous amount of research dealing with this controversy, but most of the methodologically sound research tends to support the activity theory: continued substantial engagement of various forms appears to be typical of at least the majority of normal aging persons; disengagement is not intrinsic or inevitable, except perhaps just before death; and maintaining activity is usually associated with more successful aging and life satisfaction. It may be that activity theory is especially applicable to the culture in which American elders were reared with its emphasis on a work ethic, on active mastery rather than passive acceptance of nature, on extroversion, and similar factors.

Age, Period, and Cohort

Since the mid-1960s, there has been growing recognition that the problem of separating out age, period, and cohort effects is a fundamental one for most of gerontology. There was early recognition that age differences found in cross-sectional research (done at one point in time) could be due more to cohort or generational differences than to aging processes. For this reason, longitudinal studies of the same group of people over time were proposed as the better way to study aging processes. However, it became apparent that longitudinal research has another problem: the differences observed over time could be due more to changes in the environment or practice effects than to aging processes. To remedy the defects of both cross-sectional and longitudinal studies, a combination of the two has been utilized, generally called cross-sequential studies. In these studies, several birth cohorts are studied longitudinally, and the range of years in each birth cohort must equal the interval(s) between measurement(s) in the study. This technique allows analysis and comparison of all three possible differences: cross-sectional (between age cohorts at one point in time), longitudinal (within the same cohort at different points in time), and time lag (between the same age groups at different points in time). From the analysis and comparison of these three kinds of differences, the three possible effects of age, period, and cohort can be inferred and estimated under certain conditions (Palmore, 1978b). The reason is that each difference reflects two of the possible effects while controlling the third: cross-sectional differences equal the sum of age and cohort effects, longitudinal differences equal the sum of age and period effects, and time-lag differences equal the sum of cohort and period effects. The third stage in such analysis is the imputation of causes (such as biological aging, social change, practice effects, or change in status) for the inferred effects based on evidence and theory from outside the model. The multiple conceptual and methodological confusions that have surrounded this problem have only recently been clarified, and there are several alternate strategies recently developed to attack this problem (Palmore, 1978b; Binstock and Shanas, 1977). American gerontologists appear to be the pioneers in this area.

INFORMATION SOURCES

There are several major information sources in the United States devoted entirely to information on aging. The three major ones are described below with their addresses.

Aging Research Information Service (Texas Department of Public Welfare, John H. Reagan Building, Austin, Texas 78701) has collected and stored about twelve thousand abstracts of research reports on aging. It has an automated system for retrieval of information from these abstracts.

Keyword Indexed Collection of Training Resources in Aging (Box 3003, Duke Medical Center, Durham, N.C. 27710) has indexed about a thousand resources for training in aging such as bibliographies, course outlines, syllabi, audiovisuals, and manuals. Another fifteen hundred resources are held for staff reference purposes.

National Clearinghouse on Aging (330 Independence Ave. SW, Washington, D.C. 20201) contains a collection of twenty-five hundred statistically oriented documents, fifteen hundred federally funded research projects, Administration on Aging discretionary grant reports, sixty periodicals, and congressional reports. The statistical collection is indexed using terms from the AoA thesaurus and is retrieved with an on-line computer system.

In the area of education in gerontology, there is now a comprehensive directory, the *National Directory of Educational Programs in Gerontology* (Sprouse, 1976). This directory lists 1,275 institutions that offer programs in gerontology in the United States and includes comprehensive information on each program.

In summary, although the United States has led most of the world in gerontological research, it has tended to lag in the practical application of gerontology to the solution of problems of aging. However, there are signs that we may be catching up, and the outlook appears promising.

REFERENCES

Barron, M., ed. 1961. *The Aging American*. New York: Crowell.

Binstock, R., and Shanas, E., eds. 1976. *Handbook of Aging and the Social Sciences*. New York: Van Nostrand.

Birren, J., and Schaie, K., eds. 1977. *Handbook of the Psychology of Aging*. New York: Van Nostrand.

Breen, L. 1960. The aging individual. In C. Tibbitts, ed., *Handbook of Social Gerontology*. Chicago: University of Chicago Press.

Brotman, H. 1977. Population projections. *Gerontologist* 17:203–209.

Burgess, E., ed. 1960. *Aging in Western Societies*. Chicago: University of Chicago Press.

Butler, R. 1969. Age-ism: another form of bigotry. *Gerontologist* 9:243–246.

Comfort, A. 1976. Age prejudice in America. *Social Policy* 7:3–8.

Cumming, E., and Henry, W. 1961. *Growing Old*. New York: Basic Books.

Finch, C., and Hayflick, L., eds. 1977. *Handbook of the Biology of Aging*. New York: Van Nostrand.

Fowles, D. 1977. *Income and Poverty among the Elderly: 1975*. Washington, D.C.: Administration on Aging, Department of Health, Education and Welfare.

Gibson, R.; Mueller, M.; and Fisher, C. 1977. Age differences in health care spending, fiscal year 1976. *Social Security Bulletin* 40:3–14.

Harris, L. 1975. *The Myth and Reality of Aging in America*. Washington, D.C.: National Council on Aging.

Office of Management and Budget. 1977. *Catalogue of Federal Domestic Assistance*. Washington, D.C.: U.S. Government Printing Office.

O'Meara, J. 1977. *Retirement: Reward or Rejection*. New York: Conference Board.

Palmore E. 1972a. Compulsory versus flexible retirement. *Gerontologist* 12:343–348.

———. 1972b. Medical care needs of the aged. *Postgraduate Medicine* 51:194-200.

———. 1975. *The Honorable Elders*. Durham, N.C.: Duke University Press.

————. 1976a. Total chance of institutionalization among the aged. *Gerontologist* 16:504–507.

————. 1976b. The future status of the aged. *Gerontologist* 16:297–302.

————. 1977a. Change in life satisfaction. *Journal of Gerontology* 32:311–316.

————. 1977b. Facts on aging. *Gerontologist* 17:315–320.

————. 1978a. Are the aged a minority group? *Journal of American Geriatrics Society*. 26:214–217.

————. 1978b. When can age, period, and cohort be separated? *Social Forces*. 57:282-295.

Palmore, E., and Manton, K. 1973. Ageism compared to racism and sexism. *Journal of Gerontology* 28:363-369.

————. 1974. Modernization and status of the aged. *Journal of Gerontology* 29:205-210.

Pollak, O. 1948. *Social Adjustment in Old Age*. New York: Social Science Research Council.

Riley, M., and Foner, A., eds. 1968. *Aging and Society: An Inventory of Research Findings*. New York: Russell Sage Foundation.

Rose, M., and Peterson, W. eds. 1965. *Older People and Their Social World*. Philadelphia: Davis.

Shanas, E., et al. 1968. *Old People in Three Industrial Societies*. New York: Atherton Press.

Sprouse, B., ed. 1976. *National Directory of Educational Programs in Gerontology*. Washington, D.C.: Administration on Aging, Department of Health, Education and Welfare.

Streib, G. 1965. Are the aged a minority group? In A. Gouldner and S. Miller, eds. *Applied Sociology*. New York: Free Press.

Tibbitts, C., ed. 1960. *Handbook of Social Gerontology*. Chicago: University of Chicago Press.

United Nations. 1976. *Demographic Yearbook*. New York: United Nations.

URUGUAY

AMERICO S. ALBERIEUX MURDOCH

A study conducive to a better understanding of aging and of the condition of the aged in the different countries is an important undertaking in view of the increased life span and its repercussion upon society. The growth of the aged population is a worldwide phenomenon resulting from technological advances and social changes that have taken place during this century. Today's society, planned and executed by those who are now the subject of study and discussion, has the obligation to find a solution to the problems posed by old age. Today's situation is not the same as at the beginning of the century; ignorance of biology and psychology has led, in the near past, to a childlike rejection of things unpleasant. Prejudices, social standards, and false beliefs have given rise to negative feelings toward old age, although not toward the individual old person (Parodi, 1977). Goethe said: ''The old man has lost one of the greatest human privileges: he is no longer judged by persons of his same condition.''

Knowledge of programs and research in gerontology in different countries will prove useful to students of old age. It will enable them to channel conceptions, establish comparisons, and derive conclusions regarding programs for local application. It will promote close relationships between gerontologists of different countries.

Uruguay is economically an underdeveloped country, but culturally, socially, and politically, it may be regarded as developed. It exhibits a large old population, high life expectancy, and low mortality, as do industrialized countries. It has a low birthrate, thus lacking the population explosion characteristic of the other Latin American countries. However, from the turn of the century until the 1930s, this low birthrate was counteracted by youthful immigration. Its advanced social legislation has enabled the retirement of a large number of inhabitants at ages when production is still feasible, thereby leading to an unbalance and overloading of production persons (Parodi, 1977).

To this may be added generational conflicts that give rise to a certain degree of social strain. Short-term solutions are required and an understanding of the development of gerontology and its future implications assumes both a national and an international interest.

DEVELOPMENT OF GERONTOLOGY

The Society of Geriatrics and Gerontology of Uruguay, founded in 1959, was the first scientific institution of its kind in Uruguay. It has carried out profitable medical and research work. It is affiliated with the International Association of Gerontology and has been represented at international and Latin American congresses. It is the founding member of the Federation of Latin American Societies of Geriatrics and Gerontology. In 1979 it attended the Third Congress of the federation in Venezuela and will be in charge of the implementation of the Fourth Congress of Latin American Societies and the First Uruguayan Congress of Gerontology in 1982.

The National Group of Private Entities, founded in 1972, studies old-age issues aiming at the search for solutions both for society and the aged. It has available a group of very efficient social workers. The Gerontologic Association, of recent foundation, promotes the discussion of scientific and social problems. The Uruguayan Society of Gerontology and Geriatrics has existed since January 1979. The Social Service Institute studies social problems. The grandparents' club holds weekly meetings and yearly parties and organizes excursions.

There is no national research project, either official or private, for the aid of aged; however, there have been attempts in this direction. In 1975 the Society of Geriatrics and Gerontology of Uruguay sponsored, within the School of Medicine of Montevideo, the establishment of a geriatric and gerontology clinic as a national requirement for the training of technicians. On the basis of this initiative a course of introduction to geriatrics-gerontology, theoretical and practical, has been established and implemented by the university hospital (Hospital de Clinicas) and sponsored by the graduate school. Important programs have been developed (Morelli, 1977).

DEMOGRAPHY

Uruguay's climate is temperate with a mean temperature of 57 to 60 degrees F; snow is rare. It is the smallest country in South America; according to the 1975 census it has a population of 2,782,000 inhabitants (1,375,000 males and 1,418,700 females). The population density is 14.7 per square kilometer, ranging from 4.5 to 22.64 in rural or urban areas. Despite this low population density, it is the highest in South America.

The demographic evolution of Uruguay is shown in table 76. The population growth starting from 1908 is low and was concomitant with a sustained immigration trend until 1930. The rate of population growth was markedly and progressively reduced, with a 0.5 figure in 1975. The old-age population rose to 7.9 percent in 1963 and 10.2 percent in 1975. The ratio of old-age population to child population was unbalanced. In 1908 there were 302,600 inhabitants 9 years and under and 26,000 aged 65 or more, with a ratio of 11.6

children per old person. In 1963 the corresponding figures were 523,000 and 200,000 with a ratio of 2.6 per old person; in 1975 this figure was less than 2 children per old person. Tables 77 and 78 show the rates of population growth and birthrates in Uruguay compared with those of other Latin American countries. This decline in birthrate has a sharp bearing upon the total population volume within the overall framework. It is due to the decline in the number of offspring per child-bearing-aged woman, the frequency of abortion, the use of oral contraceptives, and social status.

Table 76: TOTAL POPULATION AND POPULATION 65 AND OVER

Year	Total	Annual Rate of Growth (percent)	65 Years and Over	Annual Rate of Growth (percent)
1852	132,000			
1860	330,000	7.2		
1908	1,043,000	3.2	26,600	
1963	2,659,000	1.7	200,200	7.9
1975	2,782,000	0.5	286,200	10.2

Source: National Census of Population, 1975. Department of Statistic and Census. Ministry of Economy and Finances, Montevideo.

Table 77: RATES OF POPULATION GROWTH IN SELECTED LATIN AMERICAN COUNTRIES

	1920–1925	1940–1945	1965–1970
Argentina	3.17	1.67	1.56
Brazil	2.05	2.27	2.87
Colombia	3.94	2.36	3.46
Chile	1.54	1.54	2.26
Guatemala	1.11	3.36	2.89
Mexico	0.95	2.88	3.50
Uruguay	2.06	1.33	0.53
Venezuela	1.93	2.84	3.31

Source: Bulletin No. 137 of CEPAL (1973).

Table 78: BIRTHRATES IN SELECTED LATIN AMERICAN COUNTRIES, 1960–1965

Country	Birthrate
Uruguay	23.5
Argentina	23.0
Chile	35.0
Brazil	42.0
Dominican Republic	46.5
Mexico	44.5
El Salvador	48.0
Nicaragua	48.5

Source: CEPAL, *Social Changes and Policy of Social Development in Latin-America.*

The young population between the ages of 15 and 39 years, making up the labor and reproductive force of the country, which in 1903 constituted 43 percent of the total population, decreased to 37 percent in 1963 and 35 percent in 1975. Emigration, particularly of young people, increased over the last decade, but it has been somewhat restrained by the current government.

Life expectancy has been steadily rising since the beginning of the century, and according to estimates of the Office of Statistics and Census, in 1963 life expectancy at birth was 68.5 years—65.5 for males and 71.6 for females. In 1975 these figures were higher. According to the 1972 demographic yearbook of the United Nations, Uruguay has the highest life expectancy of Latin America, surpassed only by developed countries.

Death rates in Uruguay have experienced a progressive decline, despite the growing rise of aged population, and at present it is listed among the countries with the lowest mortality rates. According to the figures provided by the United Nations, the death rate per 1,000 inhabitants was 8.8. This figure would be lower were it not for the high proportion of aged population, since the child death rate has drastically decreased since 1920. For instance, in 1975, of 27,437 deaths, 15,287 were among persons aged 65 or older, accounting for 55 percent of the deaths (deaths classified by sex and age, Ministry of Public Health, Department of Statistics, 1975).

The censuses of 1908, 1963, and 1975 show that the phenomenon of population aging in Uruguay still holds true, and the difference by sexes favors females even more markedly. The economic and social consequences deriving from this trend are varied and complex; an increase in the percentage of economically inactive persons who, together with the increase of aged, cause the labor force to bear the load of this sector of the population with its ever growing needs. Tables 79 and 80 show the number of persons aged 60 and over according to sex. The tables confirm the female prevalence: the rate of yearly growth is 0.53 for the total population (0.42 for males and 0.64 for females).

Demographic changes and their relationships with old age are important. Of the 2,782,000 inhabitants of Uruguay by 1975, 1,229,718 resided in Montevideo and 1,553,000 in the interior of the country. There is a constant migratory flow from the countryside to the capital. The same trend is seen in the interior where the rural population is moving into urban centers.

These migratory trends are more marked for the aged. The attraction of large cities with their favorable educational, labor, and health care features prompt the aged to seek protection from biologic aging. According to the figures provided by the censuses of 1963 and 1975, the total population growth did not exceed 6.5 percent, with an annual rate of 0.53; the actual increase over twelve years was 168,454, comprising 65,468 men and 102,986 women. For the Montevideo county, growth was only 2 percent, due to the fact of emigration from Montevideo.

The distribution of aged population between urban centers and rural areas according to the 1963 census is as follows: Montevideo and urban centers,

Table 79: POPULATION 60 AND OVER, BY AGE AND SEX

Age	Total	Males	Females
60–69	224,600	106,700	117,000
70–79	126,300	55,400	70,900
80 and over	47,600	17,200	30,400

Source: National Census of Population, 1975. Department of Statistic and Census. Ministry of Economy and Finances, Montevideo.

Table 80: POPULATION AGE 60 AND OVER, BY AGE, MARITAL STATUS, AND SEX, 1963

	Total	Unmarried	Married	Widower or Widow	Divorced	Never Married
Both sexes	298,763	48,728	148,707	83,889	5,398	10,910
Males	139,649	20,212	92,240	18,096	2,303	6,426
Females	159,108	29,216	56,362	66,213	3,145	4,494

Source: National Census of Population, 1963. Department of Statistic and Census, Ministry of Finances, Montevideo.

93,501; rural areas, 2,569; interior of the country and urban centers, 73,398; rural areas, 27,050. The prevalence of older females in Montevideo is overwhelming: 55,124 females compared with 38,385 males.

PROBLEMS AND PROGRAMS

Health and Nutrition

The fundamental pillars of good health are directly related to the diet, housing, and education. The organization of the health system should effectively cover the entire population. Uruguay allots to health expenditures from 5.1 percent to 6.5 percent of its gross national product, one of the highest rates among the Western countries (Studies on Health Expenses, 1972).

The health status of the population is a good one, health coverage being committed to 210 institutions, including the Ministry of Health. The private sector has 168 institutions of which 112 are cooperative groups, and the remaining 56 are made up of outpatient departments and old-age homes, which have increased in number in step with the growing rate of aged population.

In Montevideo, 63.8 percent of the population have health coverage in cooperative groups, comprising 900,000 members; 11.7 percent (167,000) are provided medical service at other centers. Those with low incomes, 13.6 percent of the population, are provided for at public health centers. Those who lack any permanent system of health care comprise 16.5 percent.

According to a survey of households carried out in the city of Montevideo by the Office of Statistics and Census, the population with health problems is grouped by ages and sex according to the following figures: of the population aged 60 or more (205,700), those with consultations for health problems number 43,700 (15,700 males and 28,000 females). The rate of health consultations increases progressively with age and is as high as 21 percent among the population aged 60 and more. However, repeated consultations failed to increase with age over 60 years or more, despite the presence of chronic diseases peculiar to old age.

No data are available regarding health care levels in the interior of the country where health coverage is provided by the Ministry of Public Health and private service. The number of inhabitants without coverage is rather high. There is one physician per 500 inhabitants; by contrast, the rate in the capital is 260 per doctor (1978). According to the Medical Labor Union of Uruguay, in Uruguay therer are 5,668 physicians, in Montevideo 4,674, and in the interior of the country 994 (University Culture Foundation, 1975).

The most frequent diseases of the aged population in Uruguay are like those of other Western countries. In decreasing order, they are cardiovascular diseases; malignant tumors; disorders of the locomotor, respiratory, nervous, and digestive systems; and metabolic diseases. The motives for consultation at the Department of Geriatrics of IMPASA (a cooperative group) and the geriatrics outpatient department of the Pasteur Hospital include 48 percent for cardiovascular diseases, 14 percent for the locomotor system, and 17 percent for the nervous system. Tumors and diseases of the respiratory and urinary systems are referred to the specialized services.

Another interesting set of statistics is that of deaths classified by cause and age. According to the information provided by the Ministry of Public Health Department of Statistics (1975), the figures for deaths over age 65 are as follows: cardiovascular disease, 56.53 percent; tumors, 10.57 percent; respiratory disease, 4.97 percent; digestive disorders, 3.22 percent; urinary duct disorders, 0.86 percent; diabetes, 2.75 percent; accidents, 1.08 percent; suicides 0.51 percent; other causes, 21.32 percent. The frequency of obesity, particularly in older women, is very high and reflects the excessive caloric intake in a large sector of the population. Surveys of aged at different socioeconomic levels showed that protein intake was lower among the aged than among others. This is due to factors of limited supply as well as to modifications in the digestive tract (teeth, decrease of digestive secretions and of motor responses of the walls, absorption disturbances, and so on).

Family, Work, and Society

The family has been one of the pillars in the development of Uruguayan society. In general, if the family is intact, the old person is attached to it. However, as in other developed or developing countries, the Uruguayan family has undergone changes regarding structure and unity. Present-day Uruguayan society is changing. Industrialization, economic pressures, migra-

tion movements, changes in housing, equal rights for women, and the introduction of the conjugal family in place of the consanguineous family influence
the relations of the old person with the family and therefore with society
(Solari, 1964).

The traditional family, led and supported economically by the patriarch, is
giving way to the so-called urban family in which the roles of the members and
therefore the social status of the old person are changing. In this new type of
family, almost every member contributes his or her energy and income. These
new sociocultural trends lead to the breakdown of the old family bonds,
establishing a new organization in which every member has duties and rights.

At the thirty-third meeting of the World Health Organization, the conclusion
reached by way of sociologic survey was that the aged are a social problem
caused by the loosening of family bonds that lead to family breakdown. The
links between the old person and the family in Uruguayan society depend,
among other factors, upon health, age, education, economic status, and type of
family. While the old person preserves an acceptable state of health and
contributes to the family budget, no problems arise. But when organic
changes, economic deterioration, or death of a spouse takes place, the family
framework is disturbed, and there arise problems that often end in institutionalization or isolation within the home itself. This change of ambience,
either at home or away from it, leads to a new life, frequently against the will of
the aged individual. Then a feeling of frustration begins; the old person
realizes that his role in the family and social life has changed. He feels inferior
to others since his current position is different, and he experiences a reduction
in his physical and intellectual faculties. For a woman, the problem is not so
serious; she is able to carry on with her domestic activities and, if actual family
breakdown does not ensue, there is no maladjustment syndrome (Albrieux,
1957, 1963, 1978). Institutionalization is not so severe as for men. Hence
sociologic investigation applied to gerontology should be designed to reduce
these trends toward transformation of the system of roles and status of the aged
either within the family or society.

In Uruguay the sociologic studies applied to gerontology have been developed on the basis of data supplied by censuses and surveys, providing
conclusions deriving from questionnaires. They are macrosocial studies of
considerable value in the economic, political, and social orientation of the
nation. Variables called ''BASIC'' are used, which are those not easily
modified by the action of the subject, such as age, sex, geographic residence,
emigration, occupation, and housing. Conclusions related to the position of
old persons in the family may also be derived from surveys of such areas as
their associations and family relations.

The economic dependence of the aged on the primary family is greatly
variable and is conditioned by social class. Economic dependence is particularly marked at low social class levels. A survey undertaken by the National

Group of Private Entities (1975) shows that only 26 percent of old persons enjoy economic autonomy, a figure that is lower for females and for the very old of both sexes. These basic variables also diminish the possibility of holding a job. The same survey points out that 18 percent lack personal autonomy.

In gerontology, the importance of inquiry into internal factors operating below the surface should be mentioned—for instance, an understanding of how the old person experiences the process of aging, to what degree he regards old age as a legitimate status; to what extent his problems are understood by society; and in what manner he is identified with his age group. In the survey under consideration, females value themselves socially at a higher level than old men do; however a high percentage of the aged, men and women, fail to find recognition in old-age status. In a like manner, attention should be focused upon the knowledge of the existence of relief resources on the part of the community. A relationship was also found between social appraisal and identification with the age group. Through identification with the group, they develop a higher esteem for their aged status. This situation favors their integration into organizations for the aged: clubs, camping sites, dining halls, and cultural and manual activities. Thus 62 percent of the surveyed aged stated that they enjoy joining in activities with people of their age. This has been pointed out by Kruse and Bouzas in "Seminar of Social Promotion of the Aged." They contend that old people are primarily in need of meeting other people of their age and with similar cultural backgrounds.

The aged of Uruguay present other problems in connection with their peculiar demographic, economic, political, and social structure, such as generational conflicts. There is a competitive coexistence of at least five generational mentalities. These conflicts have come into the open in the last few years and have threatened social peace. At the beginning of the century there existed only three generations, and coexistence among them was not difficult. A high proportion of old persons preserve a high degree of psycho-physical effectiveness and are therefore active, partly as a necessity to keep up an acceptable living standard. Gerontocracy and lawful or clandestine withholding of jobs promotes intergenerational strains. On the other hand, a majority of the surveys of the aged people, when asked how present-day youth were getting along, answered that they were going wrong.

So far consideration has been given to the sector of the aged population who are more or less in close contact with society. But there is another sector residing in institutions whose relation with the outward world is more limited. The study of these so-called captive populations requires a different approach. In a survey carried out by the Social Service Institute at the Home Hospital Dr. Luis Pineiro del Campo, 564 inmates—302 males and 262 females—were considered. Of the men, 72.4 percent were unmarried; 75 percent of the total had never held a job; and the percentage of illiterates was double the average figure for the rest of the aged in Uruguay (Prat, 1974).

These studies are not accurate because in Uruguay there are limitations of a technical and financial nature that restrict studies of social gerontology at a national level. Also there are no national publications to serve as guides.

Work and the Aged

In accordance with information by the Bureau of Statistics and Census, in 1963 the economically active population aged 60 and over was 54,789 (26 percent)—46,243 men and 8,446 women, with a decreasing rate of activity with older age. These figures from official sources, however, do not correspond to the real situation (table 81). When an old man is capable of working, he usually carries on with his job; in a clandestine manner, the retired person often returns to the labor market. Also in the high and middle classes, where the cultural level is higher and health care is better, work activity is sustained until 70 years on average. Hence the 26 percent figure for economically active old people climbs up to rates over 50 percent. Thus there is an aged labor force that does not appear in the censuses. This capital should be preserved and channeled to the benefit of society. Such a trend might contribute to the decisions concerning a retirement policy (Albrieux, 1957, 1963, 1978). Surveys independent of censuses, in areas with a high prevalence of low-class people, show that 90 percent of the population receives per month less than the equivalent of forty dollars, so that in order to be able to subsist, they must supplement their income with a job. (These surveys were conducted by the Department of Statistics, Ministry of Work and Social Security in 1978). Uruguayan workers possess a high degree of efficiency which is preserved throughout many years (table 82). Stieghtz's (1956) view holds true in Uruguay: "A useful, interesting, and preferably paid activity is essential for the physical welfare of an old person."

Table 81: ECONOMIC ACTIVITY RATE BY AGE AND SEX (IN PERCENT)

Age	Total	Males	Females
12–14	8.9	12.7	5.0
15–19	44.2	61.2	27.5
20–24	66.3	90.6	42.8
25–34	68.5	96.5	45.3
35–44	67.6	97.0	39.3
45–54	62.0	92.4	32.4
55–64	42.6	70.0	16.8
65 and over	11.1	20.8	3.6

Source: National Census of Population, 1975. Department of Statistic and Census. Ministry of Economy and Finances, Montevideo.

Note: These figures are lower than those obtained by the United Nations in 1963. Demographic Year Book, Inform. No. 1.

Table 82: ECONOMICALLY ACTIVE POPULATION (PERCENT) IN SELECTED LATIN AMERICAN COUNTRIES

Uruguay	64.2	Bolivia	54.9
Argentina	63.8	Brazil	54.4
Chile	56.0	Peru	52.9

Source: R. Franco and A. Solari. *The Family—Social Studies*. Montevideo: Ed. Alcali, 1977.

Housing and Transportation

Uruguay has no houses specially built for senior people. A project of the Gerontology Foundation (1969) has been thoroughly documented, but it has not been followed through because of financial problems. Asylums, shelters, and houses for senior people are not very satisfactory, although some modifications have been made to make life easier for senior people.

Senior people of the upper and middle classes live in reasonable comfort. Heating in the winter is becoming commoner, and it is most beneficial for older persons.

Trains and urban transport companies grant discounts to retired and pensioned people. There is a high rate of traffic accidents among the aged.

Legal Protection

In Uruguay protection of the aged takes place through two mechanisms: legal and institutional. The economic risk entailed by the aged is met by the retirement allowance or pension, a right established by the constitution. There is an Institute of Social Security with offices corresponding to state employees, industrial and business workers, rural workers, and domestic service. In addition, there are independent retirement and pension offices for university graduates, banking clerks, and other occupations.

At present, the retirement allowance is given when a male worker reaches 50 years of age and has completed thirty years of work. Only twenty-five years of work are required of women. In the near future, a rise in the general retirement age to 60 years for men and 55 for women, will be enacted. For government employees, the obligatory retirement age is 70. The retirement scheme has been overgenerous and has resulted in a maladjustment and overload for active workers. Pension is the allowance granted to the family of the worker in case of death. Old-age pension is granted to persons over 60 who are destitute and without means for an income.

Institutional Protection

Institutionalization is granted to those aged with disability, whether economic, physical, or mental.

The Home Hospital Dr. Luis Pineiro del Campo houses people over 60 and destitute persons who, although not ill, require some social care. This institution has a high number of residents, far above its physical and functional capacity. It meets neither the requirements of a hospital nor of a home (Prat, 1974).

The Hospital of Ministry of Public Health provides medical care at the outpatient departments and inpatient services. There are two geriatric outpatient departments: Maciel Hospital and Pasteur Hospital. No social service is available.

Hospital de Clinicas is a university hospital. It provides medical care and some degree of social service. Private institutional protection is provided by several religious or national communities: Don Orione Home, Jewish Home, Old-age Home of Colonia Valdense, Spanish Home, British, Italian and German Home. In the interior of the country there are also some homes for the aged related to some medical care centers by the Ministry of Public Health.

SUMMARY

Uruguay, a country with good social, cultural, and political development but economic underdevelopment, has a senior population ranging from 9.8 and 11.2 percent of the total population, which is near the rates of industrialized countries. It has a low birthrate and lacks the population explosion characteristic of the other Latin-American countries. A low death rate and the immigration of young people are the determining factors of the progressive growth of the aged population. The numerical superiority of women relative to men is increasing. There is a great difference between the numbers of widowers and widows.

Aged people are concentrated in urban centers, especially the capital city. The extended family is being replaced by the conjugal and urban family, with the consequent loss of roles for the aged in the family and social isolation.

Retired and pensioned people are economically protected, but their allowance is not sufficient. This generates the economic dependence of 50 percent of senior people and forces them to seek clandestine work. Early retirement due to generous laws increases the economically inactive population, which overburdens the working class and causes generational conflicts. In general, the health, nutrition, and education of the elderly are acceptable.

Governmental institutional protection is deficient, but there are private homes that depend on national or religious institutions. Social protection is being organized. Sociological research is based on macrosocial surveys, but there already exist some studies in social gerontology, based on psychosocial factors.

Geriatric and gerontologic teaching has begun, due to the efforts of geriatric and gerontologic societies of Uruguay. Biomedical research exists, but it is isolated.

REFERENCES

Albrieux, Américo S. 1957, 1963, and 1978. Conferences on Gerontology held at the Rotary Club of Montevideo: *Longevity* (1957), *Personality after Fiftieth* (1963), and *Gerontology Today* (1978). Rotary Club, Montevideo.

Demographic Yearbook of the United Nations, 1972.

Demographic Yearbook of the United Nations, 1966.

Latin American Federation of Societies of Gerontology and Geriatrics. 1970. *Acta of Foundation*. Buenos Aires. May.

Morelli, A. 1977. *Conferences on Geriatric and Gerontology*. Vols. I-III. Montevideo: University of Uruguay Press.

Mortality Classified by Cause, Sex, and Age. 1977. Department of Statistics. Ministry of Public Health, Montevideo.

National Group of Private Entities. Conferences 1975 (unpublished).

Parodi, Hernan. 1977. *Work, Retirement and Aging*. Conferences on Geriatric and Gerontology. Montevideo: University of Uruguay Press. I: 229.

Prat, D. 1974. *Survey of Older People*. Institute of Social Service. Ministry of Work and Social Security, May. Montevideo.

Solari, Aldo. 1964. *Studies about Uruguayan Society*. I: 55-64. Montevideo.

Stieglitz, E. J. 1956. *Geriatric Medicine*. Philadelphia: Lippincott.

Studies on Health Expenses 1971. 1972. Planned Division MSB/OPS. Uruguay Basic Data. University Culture Foundation, Montevideo, pp. 171, 1976.

Survey of Homes. Demand for Medical Assistance. 1971. Department of Statistics and Census. Ministry of Economy and Finances, Montevideo. May-October.

VENEZUELA

L. FIGALLO-ESPINAL

DEMOGRAPHY

Venezuela, which lies on the north coast of South America, has an area of 350,000 square miles. According to the last census (1971) it has a population of about 12 million; approximately 500,000 are over 60 years of age.

Venezuela is a developing country, and only recently have old-age problems been noticed. Not many years ago many tropical diseases were common, and the average life expectancy was only about 47 years. Due to the sanitation campaigns carried out and to better standards of living, life expectancy has risen to 67 years. About half of the population works and supports the other half (the children and the retired).

PROGRAMS

Only half of the total population benefit from the social security scheme, which was started for workers about thirty years ago. Thus a large part of the population is unprotected from a social insurance point of view. However, regarding the care of the elderly, it is believed that protection is usually given by the family, which remains a strong nucleus and shows devotion to old relatives. Actually, among the 500,000 old persons, we believe that only about 20 percent lack any social protection. An old-age pension scheme has been introduced recently in Venezuela.

The Patronato Nacional de Ancianos e Invalidos, ("National Organization for the Elderly and the Invalid") was begun in 1949 and has been fully functioning since 1950. Since 1978 it has been the Instituto Nacional de Geriatria. It deals mainly with the old and, to a lesser extent, with invalids who are outside the established social security scheme. The patronate is an autonomous institute under the Ministry of Health. It has a central office with administrative and technical departments. A general secretary acts as a director under the supervision of a directive council. The budget assigned is small, and for several reasons the patronate now is functioning as a charitable entity. However, despite all difficulties it is doing excellent social work. The patronate deals with old people's problems in several ways.

1. Lodging the elderly in homes equipped with amenities and staffed by trained personnel. Old people live in them free of charge, although in some cases a small contribution is accepted. The homes provide shelter, a balanced diet, clothes, and amenities. Each home has a physician in charge responsible for the health of the elderly. About two thousand people live in these homes, mainly old people who are fairly healthy; a great majority are fully ambulant and have a good mental state. In case of emergency, the elderly have to be admitted to a general hospital. In different parts of the country there are homes that belong not to the patronate but to the local authority or to private organizations. The patronate gives them financial help and tries to solve any technical problems that arise, since one of its functions is to supervise those institutions. In the central office as well as in the several branches of the patronate, geriatric clinics deal with ambulatory old people seeking treatment.

2. Providing temporary allowances to the elderly, in the form of fixed pensions.

3. Offering occasional assistance—money, food, or medicine.

About fifteen thousand old persons are under the care of the patronate, which recently has started constructing modern gerontological units; five have been completed in different parts of the country. We hope that in the near future all of the patronate's plans will be finished.

DEVELOPMENT OF GERONTOLOGY

Sociedad Venezolana de Geriatria y Gerontologia ("Venezuelan Geriatric Society") was founded in 1957; it is affiliated with the International Association of Gerontology. According to the Venezuelan Medical Federation, all members of the organization must be physicians. Most of them work in homes for the elderly. The Third Latin American Congress of Gerontology, together with the First Venezuelan Congress of Geriatrics and Gerontology, was held in Caracas February 18-23, 1979.

We are optimistic regarding the future of geriatrics and gerontology in Venezuela because we believe that the problem has been faced from its beginning.

REFERENCE

Figallo-Espinal, L. 1965, "Geriatics in Venezuela." *Geront. clin.* 7:227-230.

YUGOSLAVIA

DJORDJE KOZAREVIC

The socialist Federal Republic of Yugoslavia, located in southeastern Europe on the Balkan peninsula along the Adriatic coast, is a federal state with six republics and two provinces; it is a multinational community voluntarily united on the principles of equality and mutual solidarity and on the determination to construct a socialist society. Geographically Yugoslavia belongs to the Mediterranean, to Central Europe, and to the Danubian basin, which has had an important influence on its historical, social, and economic development.

Significant interest in gerontology in Yugoslavia has been growing, especially since the mid-1960s (Medicinski Glasnik, 1966). The development of gerontology is taking place within the social system, which is a self-management one. A self-management socialist society can be described as one that is directed and whose development is determined by a group of associated producers. Self-management in Yugoslavia implies a political system in which the producers—the workers—gradually take over the management of all labor, including the management and disposition of the products of the work. The standards of humanity, justice, and democracy in every modern socioeconomic system must also be judged by the degree of organized social welfare as it concerns the health and social well-being of its elderly citizens. The whole self-management system, and especially organized social forces such as the self-managing communities of interest (for social and health protection, pensions, housing, and education, for example), organizations of united labor, families, local communities, the assemblies of sociopolitical communities, and sociopolitical and social organizations are oriented toward and guarantee the elderly high standards of health and social well-being. Other social structures (political, social, professional, and scientific organizations) must also direct part of their activities to the care of the aged and pensioned people in the community.

DEMOGRAPHY

The age structure of the population of Yugoslavia shows that of its 20,522,972 inhabitants in 1971, the age group 60 and over accounted for 12.2 percent; in 1973 the percentage in this age group was 12.6. The estimate for 1981 is 22.5 million inhabitants with 11 percent in the age group 60 and over.

In 1931 out of 13.9 million 8.2 percent were in the age group 60 and over, whereas in 1948 there were 8.7 percent, and at the 1961 census there were 10.0 percent.

Corresponding figures for those 65 and over were 6.4 percent in 1961, 7.9 percent in 1971, and 8.6 percent in 1975. In some parts of the country the population of those 65 and over was 13 to 20 percent, and it has since been increasing rapidly, especially in rural areas where the problem of aging is even more complex.

In Yugoslavia in the 1971 census, there were relatively few people in the 50–55 and 25 year age groups because of great losses during and immediately after World Wars I and II. Increased infant and general mortality, a lower birthrate, and the deaths of about 10 percent of the population (about 1.7 million inhabitants) during World War II are reflected in the composition and shape of the age structure. These facts will have considerable influence on the age structure of the population of Yugoslavia in the coming years.

At the 1971 census (table 83), there were 10,077,000 (49.1 percent) males and 10,445,690 (50.9 percent) females. In the age groups 65 and over, there were more females (8.9 percent) than males (7.0 percent). Population projections show a further increase in this difference. It has been estimated that in 1980 3.8 percent of the total will be males over 65 and 5.2 percent will be females over 65.

Table 83: STRUCTURE OF THE POPULATION BY AGE AND SEX (IN PERCENT)

Census Year	Sex	Total	Age Groups		
			0–59	60–64	65 and Over
1953	M	8,204,595	92.2	2.6	5.2
	F	8,731,978	90.0	3.3	6.7
1961	M	9,043,424	91.4	3.4	5.2
	F	9,505,867	89.0	3.9	7.1
1971	M	10,077,288	88.6	4.2	7.0
	F	10,445,690	86.5	4.6	8.9

Source: Statistical Yearbook of Yugoslavia (1976).

Until World War II, Yugoslavia was a relatively undeveloped, predominantly agrarian country with 82.6 percent rural and 17.4 percent urban population (1931 census). At the 1971 census, the population was 63.7 percent rural and 36.3 percent urban (Federal Institute of Public Health, 1975). By the 1971 census, of a total 1,614,902 inhabitants in the age group 65 and over, 793,282 (49.1 percent) belonged to the agricultural sector. The dynamic industrialization and urbanization of the country resulted in migration of younger and older people from the rural to the urban areas.

From the basic vital statistic indexes (table 84), it can be seen that the great changes occurred in the last twenty-five years, resulting in the prolongation of the average duration of life and the expectation of life, which has increased considerably in the postwar period.

Table 84: BASIC VITAL STATISTICS INDEXES

	1953	1961	1971
Live births per 1,000 inhabitants	28.4	22.7	18.2
Crude death rate per 1,000 inhabitants	12.4	9.0	8.7
Infant mortality	116.1	82.0	49.5
Average age (years)			
Male	27.7	28.6	30.2
Female	29.5	30.7	32.3
Expection of life at birth (years)			
Male	56.9	62.3	64.8
Female	59.3	62.4	69.2

Source: *Statistical Yearbook of Yugoslavia* (1976).

Since 1953 the percentage of the active population (table 85) has been proportionally decreasing while that of the supported population has been slightly increasing. In 1953 there were 7,848,857 or 46.3 percent active and 8,545,935 or 50.5 percent supported out of the total population.

Table 85: ACTIVE AND SUPPORTED POPULATION BY AGE, 1971

	Total	64 and Under	65 and Over
Agricultural			
Active	4,207,645	88.9%	11.1%
Supported	3,636,341	91.0%	9.0%
Nonagricultural			
Active	5,923,669	90.7%	9.3%
Supported	6,755,317	96.0%	4.0%

Source: *Statistical Yearbook of Yugoslavia* (1976).

The number of marriages and divorces (table 86) show a slight increase, although the rate since 1961 has been almost stable. About 60 percent of women 65 years and over were widows according to the 1961 census; 34.7 were married. Among men over 65, only 25.8 percent were widowers and 69.3 percent were married.

The number of illiterate persons among the aged is steadily decreasing. In 1953 among those 65 and over, there were 40.5 percent male and 64.9 percent female illiterates; in 1961 there were 34.1 percent male and 59.3 percent females; and in 1971 this had decreased to 29.7 percent for males and 59.3 percent for females 65 years and over.

Table 86: MARITAL STATUS

	1953	1961	1971
Marriages			
Number	167,940	168,510	184,011
Rate per 1,000 inhabitants	9.9	9.1	9.0
Divorces			
Number	16,020	21,532	21,347
Rate per 1,000 inhabitants	0.9	1.2	1.0
Widows[a]	10.4	9.0	8.1
Divorcees[a]	1.0	1.4	1.8

Source: Statistical Yearbook of Yugoslavia (1973).

a. As percentage of total population.

ROLE AND STATUS

Family life in Yugoslavia was traditionally patriarchal. All members of the family lived in the same household, and the position of each was determined by his age, his work, and the family relationship. In areas where a cooperative family system existed, the aged had a much higher status than in other parts of the country. The general closeness of the family even today has not weakened much. In such families, older persons satisfy most of their needs inside the family and are taken care of by the family until the end of life (Smolic-Krkovic, 1977; Nedeljkovic, 1971; St. Erlich, 1971).

The number of households with only one or two members has increased from 1,047,139 (26.5 percent) in 1965 to 1,568,485 (29.2 percent) in 1971; the percentage of those with three to seven members remained between 63.5 percent in 1953 and 65.5 percent in 1971, while the number of households with eight or more members decreased from 392,999 (10.0 percent) in 1953 to 283,798 (5.3 percent) in 1971.

PROBLEMS OF THE AGED

Most of the problems arise in the sphere of care (health, medical, and social) for those in the so-called pathological stage of aging—elderly people with long-term diseases and disabilities. Also important are problems in under-taking active measures to prevent or postpone the development of diseases, to rehabilitate many cases, and to ensure proper solutions for the complex problems of the elderly.

A relatively high and increasing proportion of aged persons, particularly those with chronic conditions, has been a reality in the most developed parts of Yugoslavia. Furthermore, it has been recognized as an even greater and cumulative problem in most parts of the country, especially in the developing areas (International Center of Social Gerontology, 1972).

Morbidity, Disability, and Aging

As far as the rapid changes in the state of health are concerned, long-term diseases, disability, and invalidity have reached a level of epidemiological importance, especially among the aged. This is the direct and indirect effect of many unfavorable conditions in the living and working environment in the past that have affected today's elderly population (Kozarevic, 1972).

Global aspects of the role of chronic diseases as a cause of permanent working disability are illustrated by the fact that the rate of workers pensioned due to disease is increasing. Cardiovascular, respiratory, and psychoneurotic diseases in the last decade have become the three leading causes of invalidism; they are responsible for almost half of all invalidism among the active workers. Coronary heart, cardiovascular disease, and hypertension alone amount to almost 80 percent. These diseases are much more prevalent among the aged (World Health Organization, 1976), indicating that in the future we might expect a higher proportion of disabled among those pensioned.

In the Belgrade region (population 1.2 million), out of 165,000 persons 60 years and over, 33,000 (20 percent) reported some kind of long-term disability. Among them 20,000 (12 percent of the total) were partially, 8,250 (5 percent) markedly and 5,000 (3 percent) severely disabled (Dovijanic, 1976).

Data from the Yugoslavia Cardiovascular Prospective Epidemiological Study of 11,121 males 35 to 64 years of age clearly show higher disability rates from chronic conditions in the less developed areas (32.4 per 1,000) and lower rates (19.6 per 1,000) in the more developed ones, which indicates the more complex situation for the aged in rural areas (International Center of Social Gerontology, 1972).

Chronic illnesses not only lead to disability and invalidity but also to premature aging and death; they also imply the continuous extension of long-term care, which entails increasing costs and demands on the insurance funds.

From 1971 to 1974 a special survey on medical needs and demands in the field of chronic diseases during the process of aging, based on a representative sample in three regions of Yugoslavia covering 48,000 interviewed and 4,738 examined persons, established that one-third of total population was healthy; the other two-thirds had one or more chronic conditions, out of which only half were known to health services (Kozarevic, 1977). With aging, the number of persons with chronic diseases increased. In the age group of 60 and over, 75 percent had three or more chronic diseases.

In a health examination survey of a representative sample of 1,464 adults (in the Belgrade population) completed in 1976, there was established a list of prevalence rates (table 87) for leading diseases among those 65 years of age and over.

In all groups of diseases, rates for the aged are much higher than the rates for the average adult population. This fact alone has a great influence on the rate of

Table 87: LEADING DISEASES AMONG ADULTS IN BELGRADE, 1976 (PREVALENCE RATES PER 1,000)

Diseases	Rate per 1,000			
	Total Sample (N=1,464)		65 and Over	
	MALE	FEMALE	MALE	FEMALE
Cardiovascular system	442	496	728	805
Hypertension	296	344	430	590
Myocardial infarct	22	7	53	19
Angina pectoris	42	30	60	52
Respiratory system	549	453	668	481
Chronic bronchitis	194	100	291	167
Obstructive pulmonary disease	111	66	265	143
Asthma bronchitis	26	21	53	43
Osteomuscular system	198	244	218	295
Gastrointestinal system	165	160	119	224
Urogenital system	89	117	119	95

Source: Institute of Chronic Diseases and Gerontology, Belgrade, 1977.

utilization of medical care services in the community. Rates of utilization of general medical and specialist services were also an average of 50 percent higher for aged and pensioned persons than for the middle aged.

Without neglecting acute conditions, which are even higher among the aged, long-term disability and pathological aging are the most vital concerns in organizing and operating services for the aged in Yugoslavia. Also, the high prevalence of risk factors—precursors of leading chronic diseases hypertension, sedentary activity, smoking, hypercholesteremia, and obesity, hyperglycemia—among the middle aged indicates that gerontology in Yugoslavia will have to cope with a new situation in the near future; these factors are also increasing rapidly and are highly associated with the higher incidence of the most important cardiovascular and other long-term diseases later in life (Kozarevic et al., 1976).

Mortality

Age-specific death rates by sex per 1,000 for those 65 and over are presented for Yugoslavia in 1965, 1970, and 1974 in table 88. The rates for males are higher than for females and also higher in older age groups, especially for those in the age group 80–84. There was a slight tendency toward a decrease in the period 1965–1974, which together with the decrease of infant mortality rates, is reflected in the lower crude death rates in 1974 in comparison with the 1965 rates.

There have been great changes in the mortality structure and leading causes of death in Yugoslavia in the last twenty years. Chronic degenerative, non-

Table 88: AGE- AND SEX-SPECIFIC DEATH RATES (PER 1,000 POPULATION)

Age Groups	Sex	1965	1970	1974
60–64	M	26.7	24.9	23.1
	F	19.5	15.1	13.3
70–74	M	62.0	65.3	57.8
	F	51.7	47.8	40.7
80–84	M	144.4	151.2	146.3
	F	123.8	127.5	125.9
Crude death rate (all ages)	M	11.7	9.5	9.0
	F	11.1	8.4	7.9

Source: *Statistical Yearbook of Yugoslavia* (1976).

infectious diseases (cardiovascular disease, malignant neoplasms, and injuries) are the leading causes of death in Yugoslavia (table 89). Of the total number of deaths, cardiovascular disease accounts for 39.5 percent; in the older age group the rate is much higher. Specific death rates for cerebrovascular disease in the age group 65–69 were 427 (males) and 364 (females) per 100,000; in the age group 75–79, the rates were three times higher. For stomach cancer in 1974, specific death rates in the age group 65–69 were 153 (males) and 65 (females); in the age group 75–79, the rates were 256 for males and 131 for females. In all age groups rates were higher for males than for females and are still increasing.

Table 89: LEADING CAUSES OF DEATH (RATE PER 100,000 POPULATION)

	1970			1974		
	Rate	Number	Percent	Rate	Number	Percent
All causes	892	181,842	100	840	177,691	100
Cardiovascular	287	58,503	32.0	337	70,151	39.5
Malignant neoplasms	98	20,030	11.0	109	23,083	13.0
Accidents	64	12,985	7.1	60	12,751	7.2

Source: *Statistical Yearbook of Yugoslavia* (1976).

The total number and rate of suicides, as well as the number of suicides among those 50 years and older as a percentage of the total, have not changed in the last twenty years.

Although mortality cannot reflect the pathology of the aged exactly, it is of interest to stress the fact of rapid change in structural mortality, especially among the aged, which has occurred in the last twenty years in Yugoslavia. Of course, there is still a great difference in mortality and morbidity between the most developed and developing areas in Yugoslavia. General morbidity rates for the prevailing chronic noninfectious diseases are much higher in the northwest than in the less developed southern and eastern areas, where infectious and parasitic diseases are much more frequent.

In conclusion, in view of the present epidemiological situation in Yugoslavia, chronic diseases and disability and problems connected with these situations are expected to play a major role in the care for the elderly. The trend is expected to continue with vast increases in the incidence of cardiovascular diseases and also disorders of the respiratory system.

These forecasts have significance for planning and organizing more efficient and more economical care for the aged. At least two types of activities seem necessary: planning of comprehensive and efficient care for the elderly, especially those affected by diseases, and initiation of long-term programs in active preventive work for combating risk factors, particularly in the process of aging, with the goal of improving the quality of life for the aged and to postpone the onset of disability as long as possible.

PROGRAMS

General Principles

Care for the aged in Yugoslavia is an integral part of the community's general concern for man. Within the framework of the freedom, rights, duties, and responsibilities of citizens, the 1974 constitution and the constitutions of the socialist republics and socialist autonomous provinces proclaim the following:

Everyone shall be entitled to health care. Cases in which uninsured citizens are entitled to health care using social resources shall be spelled out by state. [Article 186]

Veterans, disabled veterans and survivers of fallen veterans shall be guaranteed rights which ensure their social security as well as special rights as spelled out by statute. Disabled veterans shall be entitled to vocational rehabilitation, disability benefits, and other forms of care. [Article 187]

The family shall enjoy social protection. . . .Parents shall have the right and duty to raise and educate their children. Children shall be bound to care for their parents in need of assistance. [Article 190]

The right to workers to social security shall be ensured through obligatory insurance based on the principles of reciprocity and solidarity and past labor, in self-managing communities of interest, on the basis of contributions collected from workers' personal incomes and contributions collected from the income of organizations of associated labor. . . .On the basis of this insurance, the workers shall have . . .benefits in the case of diminution or loss of working capacity, unemployment and old age, and other social security benefits, and for their dependents—the right to health care, survivors' pensions, and other social security benefits. Social security benefits for working people and citizens who are not covered by the compulsory social insurance scheme shall be regulated by statute on the principles of reciprocity and solidarity. [Article 163]

The care of the aged is not separated from other social structures in any form and is put into practice by social institutions of all kinds and through activities of sociopolitical communities.

The basis of health and pension insurance in Yugoslavia is individual contributions made during the working years and specific insurance payments. Social security funds, which are grouped in the various self-management organizations, are used for payment of sick leave days, invalidity pension, family insurance, help and nursing of other persons, and similar reasons.

Men are entitled to old-age pensions at the age of 60 and women at 55 if they have been insured for twenty years. Men with forty years of insurance coverage and women with thirty-five years of coverage are entitled to insurance regardless of age.

If an enterprise is particularly profitable, the workers may have greater salaries and thus greater pensions in old age or during sick leave or better invalidity pension.

Health care for farmers is provided by health insurance plans for all farmers and their dependents and is based on the process of self-management decisions for a given region. In SR Serbia a free medical care system was introduced in 1970 for all people 65 and older, regardless of whether they were previously insured.

Planning Comprehensive Care

Some social principles have considerable influence on the practice of gerontology in Yugoslavia, especially in health care. They emphasize that every elderly citizen must be under systematic and organized health supervision in the care of the so-called health homes (basic district medical centers), particularly their visiting nurse services, and that every elderly must be hospitalized, treated, and rehabilitated in a similar social milieu to the one in which he lives and to which he will subsequently return after his treatment and rehabilitation. The basic thesis of this conception has been developed only recently. It springs from the experience and development of the social attitudes that point out the enormous significance of the human aspects of care for elderly patients.

The establishment of so-called self-management communities of interest (which are the form of social organization where the specified interests of consumers and those who provide services meet, create policy, coordinate, make priorities, and handle other details) in the field of health, social welfare, and other fields of importance for the aged already have shown a positive influence on the care provided to older citizens.

Determination of the state of health and major health problems among the elderly has great importance. It is especially useful to classify those who are healthy, those with disease who can walk unaided, those who need assistance to get around, and those who are totally bed-ridden.

Health services for old people should be comprehensive, coordinated, and continuous in order to meet all known needs of the old person and his family. This means that in each situation we want to preserve, and we hope to improve, the health situation of the elderly, trying to postpone the onset or further complications of disease and disability (World Health Organization, 1974b; U.S. Department of Health, Education and Welfare). Thus, undertaking preventive measures, early detection of disease, ambulatory care, screening for hospitalization, rehabilitation, long-term care, home care, and similar programs are of great importance (Smolic-Krkovic, 1974; World Health Organization Report, 1974, 1977).

The application of epidemiological methods to gerontological work in the community is the basis for an organized approach to care for the elderly (Leavell and Clark, 1958). No separate gerontological dispensaries are suggested in our setting. Comprehensive, coordinated, and continuous care for the elderly is recognized within the care for other adults in general medicine dispensaries.

Home care is an important part of long-term care for the aged in Yugoslavia. At the First Yugoslav Congress of Gerontology in December 1977, a special symposium summarized twenty years of experience in organized home and long-term care for the elderly.

The Epidemiologic-Ecologic Concept in Planning

The contemporary epidemiologic-ecologic concept of determining the results of the host-agent-environment interaction is probably a good possibility for planning and organizing a comprehensive approach to health care in general, and nursing care for the elderly in particular. Instead of concentrating primarily on aetiological studies, we need to focus more broadly on ecological studies and work that, while not denying the importance of specific aetiological agents, acknowledges the importance of the human host as psychobiological respondents to the incursions of noxious stimuli, and the environment as a social as well as a physical and biological medium in which interactions between agent and host take place. According to this concept, the progress of a disease has a time dimension, and its end point is death, disability, or cure. Epidemiological research consists of an analysis of the system to determine how all of its points fit together and what the contributions are of the three groups of factors in inducing the development of diseased or healthy states in particular population groups.

Based on such an epidemiological approach, it is possible to work out steps in planning care for both individuals and groups by transforming the broad concept of comprehensive care into specific measures of prevention and nursing care for the elderly. This involves the formulation of precise measures at each of the so-called five levels of comprehensive care or measures of primary and secondary prevention (Kozarevic, 1973).

Accepting this approach, we must bear in mind that there are many biologically determined universals that vary relatively little from one part of the world to another but that there are many environmentally influenced specifics that vary considerably from one locality to another. Such epidemiologic-ecologic concepts have already been accepted for application by the World Health Organization and many national planning authorities. This concept also enables planning at the community, local, regional, state, and other levels, as well as proper evaluation of the quantity and quality of work introduced to improve the physical, mental, and social health of the aged at all levels (Kozarevic, 1975). A similar concept has been applied in our own planning work in the field of chronic diseases and gerontology.

The Need for Preventive Gerontology

Achievements in epidemiological research and modern gerontology have made it possible to apply practical measures of community health care in the process of aging and for the aged. Taking into account the fact that, among the aged, clinical manifestations of the arteriosclerotic process upon the cardiovascular system (primarily coronary, cerebrovascular, and other diseases) are highly prevalent, it is necessary to undertake proper measures in promoting an organized risk-factors control in the process of aging as a basic concept in improving preventive gerontological activities.

Among the elderly in Yugoslavia, the proportion of persons in the group of the so-called pathological aging is increasing. This prevailing pattern of ill health clearly differs from that of the past. Therefore instead of a passive health service (perhaps appropriate in the past), organized community preventive health work in suppressing chronic long-term diseases, especially clinical manifestations of the arteriosclerotic process and measures against environmentally influenced risk factors (such as hypertension, smoking, hypercholesteremia, obesity, and physical inactivity), are imperative not only in the modern approach to improving health but also in effective and better preventive work in gerontology (Svanbor, 1976; Gudman, 1974).

Since chronic diseases, conditions, and disabilities are prevalent among the elderly and since a number of epidemiological and other studies all over the world have already identified many of the main risk factors contributing to the onset and high incidence of those diseases, it is both realistic and possible to implement practical measures in programming prevention for the better health of old people by controlling these factors and undertaking all possible health care measures much earlier in life (First World Conference, 1977). This is actually the basis of the concept of active preventive work in gerontology, which is multidisciplinary, highly complex, and multidimensional in its practical approach (Neugarten and Havighurst, 1976; Office of Health Economics, 1964; Ferguson-Anderson, 1976).

Socioeconomic development has led to the replacement of epidemics of infectious diseases by mass degenerative disease, mostly atherosclerotic, cardiovascular, and other diseases. More specifically, epidemics of these diseases and working, recreational, and personal disabilities in the industrialized countries are particularly due to the evolution of nutrition and smoking habits, aided probably by the concomitant widespread emergence of sedentary living habits and also possibly by personality and behavior patterns that have become common in modern industrial societies (Stamler, 1976).

If this concept is correct, then prevention must be related to the detection and control of the most important factors operating in the process of aging and resulting in a higher proportion of those with disease and disabilities among the aged. In order to achieve this, especially with the purpose of preventive gerontology, identification of the main and new factors operating and affecting the aged in given ecologic systems should also be undertaken.

INFORMATION SOURCES

In preparing basic elements for the application of effective solutions and for planning purposes in such complex problems as improving the health and social well-being of the elderly, a considerable amount of epidemiological, biomedical, psychological, social, economic, and other research work has been completed, and further research is in progress. During this work, important advances in the practice of gerontology and training of personnel have been made. Detailed information about this work in Yugoslavia can be obtained from:

- Institute of Gerontology-Medical School, Ljubljana, SR Slovenia: Prof. dr Bojan Accetto, Director of the Institute and Gerontological Association of SR Slovenia or dr Marija Zmidarsic.
- Department of Internal Medicine-Medical School, Ljubljana, SR Slovenia: Professor dr Ivan Matko.
- Interdisciplinary Study in Social Work—Chair of Gerontology, University of Zagreb, SR Croatia: Professor dr Nada Smolic-Krkovic.
- Gerontological Association of SR Croatia, Zagreb: Professor dr Miro Mihovilovic and dr Svetozar Livada.
- Institute for Occupational Health, Yugoslav Academy of Sciences, Zagreb, SR Croatia: Professor dr Marko Saric and Professor dr Milorad Mimica.
- Thalasotherapia, Opatija, SR Croatia: Professor dr Cedomil Plavsic.
- Institute of Public Health of SR Croatia, Zagreb: Professor dr Zivko Kulcar and School of Public Health, University of Zagreb—Professor Jaksic.

- Institute of Public Health, City of Zagreb, SR Croatia: director dr Berislav Defilipis and dr Ivan Vodopija.
- Geriatric Unit, City Hospital Medical School Belgrade: doc dr Petar Korlija and collaborators.
- Institute of Social Policy of SR Serbia, Belgrade: director dr sci. Milosav Milosavijevic, Petar Manojlovic, secretary general.
- Gerontological Association of SR Serbia: dr sci. Miroslav Zivkovic.
- School of Political Science, University of Belgrade: Professor dr Iv Nedeljkovic.
- Institute of Mental Health, Medical School, Belgrade: Professor dr Dusan Petrovic.
- Belgrade Medical School, University of Belgrade: Professor dr Bozidar Djordjevic; Professor dr Slobodan Krajinovic; Professor dr Vladan Josipovic; Professor dr Srecko Nedeljkovic and collaborators in cardiology and epidemiology research; Professor dr Borislav Bozovic and collaborators in endocrinology; Professor dr Bozidar Simic, nutrition: Professor dr Radomir Geric; Professor dr Predrag Micovic, gerontology and public health; Professor dr Najdanovic, cardiology and field surveys; Professor dr Z. Conjic, rehabilitation; Professor dr Stanoje Stefanovic; Professor dr Miroslav Kovacevic; doc. dr Ranko Stefanovic, metabolism, hematology, cardiology, and long-term care.
- Institute of Evaluation of Working Capacity of SR Serbia: director doc. dr Svetozar Nagulic.
- Secretariat of Health and Social Policy of Serbia and the Institute of Public Health of SR Serbia: Prim. dr Sumenkovic; prim dr. Aleksandar Nikolic; prim. dr Zoran Cucic; prim. dr Borislav Antic; doc. dr Velibor Tomic; prim. dr Dragan Urosevic.
- Center for Multidisciplinary Studies, University of Belgrade: prof. dr Zvonko Damjanovic; prof. dr Vladimir Glisin; dr Ljubomir Radanovic.
- Self-management Community of Interests in Health Care, Belgrade; prim. dr Marko Jovanovic; dr med. sci prim. Bozidar Micic.
- Institute of Chronic Diseases and Gerontology, Department of Gerontology and Home Care: dr Zarko Vukovic; dr Nikola Vojvodic; dr Zivorad Racic.
- Institute of Public Health of Socialist Province Vojvodina, Novi Sad: prof. dr Djordje Jakovljevic; prof. dr Svetislav Trifunovic; prim. dr Vera Mihajlovic.
- Medical School University of Pristina, SA Kosovo: prof. dr med. sci. Svetomir Stozinic; doc. dr sci. I. Kocynoj and their collaborators.
- Department of Sociology, University of Skopje, SR Macedonia: prof. dr Sinadinovski and collaborators.
- Institute of Public Health of SR Bosnia and Herzegovina, Sarajevo: doc. dr. med. sci. Tomislav Hrabac; dr. med. sci. Hasan Kapetanovic; prim. dr Adila Filipovic.
- Medical Center Titograd, SR Montenegro: director prim. dr Bozidar Raspopovic; prim. dr Bozina Culafic; prim. dr Ljubomir Ulicevic.

RESEARCH

Most of the institutions and experts dealing with gerontological problems in Yugoslavia, particularly in specialized institutions, are concerned with the aspects of aging connected with activities and with the field of practice, research, and training personnel.

The Institute of Gerontology, Medical School, in Ljubljana; the Geriatric Unit, City Hospital Medical School, Belgrade; the Interfaculty Study in Social Work, Chair of Gerontology, University of Zagreb; and many other public health, medical, and social institutions throughout the country conduct research work as well as postgraduate training in gerontology. In Ljubljana, a regular four-semester postgraduate course in gerontology is already in its fifth year.

The Institute of Chronic Diseases and Gerontology, Belgrade, Yugoslavia, in close cooperation with the above-mentioned institutions and especially with public health institutes and experts in Yugoslavia undertaking the main responsibilities in gerontology and chronic diseases, does a considerable amount of work in epidemiology and mass field surveys on chronic diseases and other sociomedical problems in the process of aging and among the aged. The institute has developed from the former Department of Chronic Diseases, which was an integral part of the Federal Institute of Public Health, Belgrade. Therefore the concepts of contemporary public health work in the field of chronic diseases and gerontology have been initiated with the aim of putting them into the practice.

The institute is concerned with aspects of public health and improvement of health care in the sphere of chronic diseases, such as cardiovascular—particularly coronary heart disease and hypertension—chronic respiratory, and gastrointestinal diseases, diabetes, and others in the process of aging and for the aged.

The institute is also concerned with other issues of importance in the investigation of the health of the population as well as the promotion of health care in general. The institute therefore studies both the distribution and the trends of major chronic diseases. The institute is engaged in the determination of the magnitude of the problem and in the solving of priority tasks in chronic diseases, with special reference to the investigation of the epidemiology of the major chronic diseases. In this connection the institute is concerned with priority problems related to the promotion of health care. Among various health institutions, cooperation and work with physicians in general practice from all republic, regional, and local institutes of public health is of the greatest importance.

The institute conducts scientific, clinico-epidemiological projects in a defined population with regard to the major chronic diseases, aging, and gerontology. Some of the areas are:

- Cardiovascular, especially hypertension, and coronary heart diseases. The prevalence and incidence of coronary heart disease and hypertension in newly industrialized populations in Yugoslaiva is a prospective clinico-epidemiological study of

11,121 males 35 to 62 years of age at entry. It started in 1964 and is still in progress.

- Chronic respiratory diseases, especially chronic bronchitis, emphysema, and others. The etiologic and risk factors in respiratory diseases is a study of 10,000 males 35 to 70 years of age. It started in 1970 and is still in progress.
- Epidemiology of Essential Hypertension Among Varous Ethnic Groups in Yugoslavia - study of 9,600 males and females 30 to 59 years of age in seven locations in Yugoslavia.
- The consequences of war on the status of health and the economic and social position of war veterans is a cross-sectional study of 12,000 war veterans in nineteen locations in Yugoslavia.
- Chronic gastrointestinal, diabetes, and other mass chronic diseases in various population groups are under study.

In the sphere of studies concerned with comprehensive gerontological work and determination of the health of the population, the institute is working in these areas:

- Identifying the state of health of the population and trends in major diseases in the light of the interdependence of the state of health, specific features of individual demographic structures, and population movements, as well as rapid urbanization and industrialization.
- Keeping track of current issues concerned with the health care to be provided to individual population groups, especially the old and the farming group and the interrelation of those issues with chronic diseases.
- Identifying problems of chronic diseases with regard to the utilization of health care and health economics, based on the results of special investigations;
- Preparing materials and papers on individual problems concerning the quality of health care in the sphere of chronic diseases and gerontology with special reference to the public health aspects of morbidity and mortality.

In close cooperation with universities, medical schools, and other institutions at federal, republic, regional, and local levels, especially public health and medical institutions, the institute is extending its activities in the field of public health, training, and research for the advancement of health care for adults and the aged. In collaboration with the World Health Organization, gerontological and other associations, international scientific and technical organizations and institutions, and universities, the institute is involved in various activities in the field of investigation of major aspects of specified chronic diseases, as well as in work of great importance for the improvement of health care. To carry out these activities, the institute is making efforts to ensure the continuity of analytical and planning work, technical and scientific health and medical work, as well as the training of personnel for better public health practice in the field of chronic diseases and gerontology.

REFERENCES

Basis for Policy in Health Protection in Beograd - Executive Council-Assembly of the City of Beograd and Executive Board of The Self-managing Association of Interest in Health Insurance-Beograd, Beograd (1976).

Dovijanic, P. 1976. *The present day organization of comprehensive health care of the elderly in large urban centres, with particular reference to the city of Beograd.* Beograd: EURAG. (1976).

Ferguson-Anderson, W. 1976. *Practical management of the elderly.* Oxford: Blackwell Scientific Publication, Ltd.

First World Conference. 1977. Aging—A challenge to science and social policy. Vichy.

International Center of Social Gerontology. 1972. *Elderly people living in Europe.* Paris: The Center.

Kozarevic, Dj. 1972. Disability and programming preventive measures in the process of aging. Paper presented at the Ninth International Congress of Gerontology, Symposium of Social Sciences, devoted to Occupational Aging and Working Capacity. Kiev.

———. 1973. *Recruitment and training of personnel—Applied gerontology.* Oslo.

———. 1975. Planning and organization of medical services for old people. Paper presented at the Tenth International Congress of Gerontology, Jerusalem.

———. 1977. *Chronic diseases, aging and long term care in Yugoslavia—Problems and position.* Uppsala: Working Group on the Organization and Operation of Long Term Care Services.

Kozarevic, Dj.; Pirc, B.; Racic, Z.; Dawber, Th.; Gordon, T.; and Zukel, W. 1976. The Yugoslavia cardiovascular disease study—II. Factors in the incidence of coronary heart disease. *American Journal of Epidemiology* 104.

Leavell, H. R., and Clark, E. G. 1958. *Preventive medicine for the doctor in his community.* 2d ed. New York: McGraw-Hill.

Medicinski Glasnik - *Gerontologija, Savez Lekarskih drustava SFRJ, No 1-2,* Beograd (1966).

Nedeljkovic, I. 1971. *Old people in Yugoslavia.* Belgrade:

Neugarten, B., and Havighurst, R. 1976. *Social policy, social ethics and the aging society.* Chicago.

New frontiers in health. 1964. London: Office of Health Economics.

Smolic-Krkovic, N. 1974. *Gerontologija.* Zagreb:

———. 1977. "Aging, Bureaucracy and the Family," in Shanas, E., and Sussman, M., eds. *Family Bureaucracy and the Elderly.* Durham, N.C.: Duke University Press.

Stamler, J. 1976. Sudden coronary death—Approaches to its prevention. *Medical Clinics of North America* 60.

Svanbor, A. 1976. *Trends in Health Protection of the Elderly,* Working Group on Nursing Aspects in the Care of the Elderly, W. Berlin (1976).

The Public Health Service in Yugoslavia. The Federal Institute of Public Health. Beograd (1975).

V. St. Erlich. 1971. *Jugoslovenska proodica u transformaciji.* Zagreb.

White, Kerr, L. 1974. Contemporary epidemiology. *International Journal of Epidemiology* 3.

U.S. Department of Health, Education and Welfare. Public Health Service. *Working with older people: A guide to practice.*

World Health Organization. 1974a. *Report of planning meeting on a medium-term programme in nursing/midwifery in Europe.* Kiel: WHO.

————. 1974b. *Planning and organization of geriatric services.*

————. 1976. *Summary on working group on nursing aspects in the care of the elderly.* West Berlin: WHO.

————. 1977. *Report of the working group on the organization and operation of long-term care services.* Uppsala: WHO.

APPENDIX 1

INTERNATIONAL DIRECTORY OF ORGANIZATIONS CONCERNED WITH AGING

This list of the names and addresses of the major international, regional, and national organizations concerned with aging is derived from the United Nations *International Directory of Organizations Concerned with the Aging* (1977). The organizations are listed in alphabetical order by continent and then by country.

INTERNATIONAL

International Association of Gerontology
Weizmann Institute of Science
P.O. Box 26
Rehovot, Israel

International Center for Social Gerontology, Inc.
425 13th Street, N.W.
Suite 350
Washington, D.C. 20004, United States

International Center of Social Gerontology
Avenue Molière 195
1060 Brussels, Belgium

International Federation on Aging
1909 K Street, N.W.
Suite 690
Washington, D.C. 20049, United States

International Organization for Advancement of Longevity Research
4408 Medical Parkway
Austin, Texas 78756, United States

International Senior Citizens Association
11753 Wilshire Boulevard
Los Angeles, California 90025, United States

International Social Security Association
Case Postale 1
CH-1211 Geneva 22, Switzerland

REGIONAL

Conseil de l'Europe (Council of Europe)
67006 Strasbourg, France

European Federation for the Welfare of the Elderly (EURAG)
Moserhofgasse 47
A-8010 Graz, Austria

Nordisk Gerontologisk Forening (Scandinavian Federation for Gerontology)
Department of Anatomy
University of Aarhus
DK-8000 Aarhus C, Denmark

AFRICA

South African National Council for the Aged
P.O. Box 2335
Cape Town 8000, South Africa

ASIA

Bangladesh

Bangladesh Association for the Aged/Institute of Geriatric Medicine
78, Dhanmandi Residential Area
Road No. 5
Dacca, Bangladesh

Israel

Israel Gerontological Society
P.O. Box 11243
Tel Aviv, Israel

Japan

Gerontological Research Association of West Japan
3 Nakamichi 1-Chome
Higashinari-ku
Osaka 537, Japan

Japan Gerontological Society
Department of Geriatrics
Faculty of Medicine

University of Tokyo
7-3-1 Hongo, Bunkyo-ku
Tokyo, 113, Japan

EUROPE

Belgium

Le troisième âge
6 rue du Méridien
1030 Brussels, Belgium

Czechoslovakia

Czechoslovak Gerontological Society
Third Medical Clinic
Unemocnice 1, Prague 2, Czechoslovakia

Denmark

Dansk Gerontologisk Selskab (Danish Gerontological Society)
Langtidsmedicinsk afd.
Centralsysgehuset
DK-4700 Naestred, Denmark

Finland

Societas Gerontologica Fennica
Institute of Physiology
University of Helsinki
Siltavuorenpenger 20 A
Helsinki 17, Finland

France

Fondation nationale de gérontologie
40 rue Mirabeau
75016 Paris, France

German Democratic Republic

Gesellschaft für Gerontologie der DDR
GDR-104 Berlin, Hermann-Matern-Strasse 13 a
Medizinische Poliklinik (Charité), German Democratic Republic

Germany, Federal Republic of

Deutsches Zentrum für Altersfragen e.V.
Rankestrasse 17
1 Berlin 30, Federal Republic of Germany

Greece

Hellenic Association of Gerontology
137, Kifissias Avenue
Athens 606, Greece

Hungary

Hungarian Gerontological Association
1428 Budapest Pf. 45
Budapest, VIII. Somogyi Béla u. 33, Hungary

Ireland

Irish Gerontological Society
Department of Social Medicine
Trinity College
Dublin 2, Ireland

Netherlands

Nederlandse Federatie voor Bejaardenbeleid (Netherlands Federation for Old People's
   Welfare)
Eisenhowerlaan 114
The Hague, The Netherlands

Netherlands Society of Gerontology
Verlengde Groenestraat 75
Nijmegen, The Netherlands

Norway

Norsk Geriatrisk Forening (Norwegian Geriatric Society)
Okern Alders-og sykehjem
Okernvn 151, Oslo 5, Norway

Norsk Gerontologisk Institutt (Norwegian Institute of Gerontology)
Oscarsgt. 36
Oslo 2, Norway

Poland

Polish Medical Association—Geriatrics Section
00-658 Warszawa
ul, Iwowska 4 m.3, Poland

Rumania

National Institute of Gerontology and Geriatrics
9, Minastirea Caldarusani Street
Bucharest 8, Rumania

Sweden

Swedish Society of Gerontology
Vasa Sjukhus Klinik I
411 33 Göteborg, Sweden

Switzerland

Schweizerische Gesellschaft für Gerontologie (Société Suisse de Gérontologie)
Inselspital, CH-3010 Berne, Switzerland

United Kingdom

Age Concern England (National Old People's Welfare Council)
Bernard Sunley House
60 Pitcairn Road
Mitcham
Surrey CR4 3LL, England

British Council for Ageing
c/o National Corporation for the Care of Old People
Nuffield Lodge
Regent's Park
London NW1 4RS, England

British Geriatrics Society
c/o Bernard Sunley House
60 Pitcairn Road
Mitcham
Surrey CR4 3LL, England

British Society of Social and Behavioral Gerontology
c/o Medical Sociology Research Centre
Park Buildings, Park Street
Swansea SA1 3DJ
Wales, United Kingdom

National Corporation for the Care of Old People (NCCOP)
Nuffield Lodge
Regent's Park
London NW1 4RS, England

Union of Soviet Socialist Republics

Institute of Gerontology of the Academy of Medical Sciences of the U.S.S.R.
Vyshgorodskaya St. 67
252655 Kiev—114, U.S.S.R.

LATIN AMERICA

Brazil

Associacão Brasileira de Gerontologia
Rua Candido Mendes 271
Rio de Janeiro, Brazil

Chile

Sociedad Chilena de Gerontología
Avenida Bulnes 377
Santiago, Chile

Peru

Primer Congreso Nacional de Jubilados, Retirados, Cesantes y Pensionistas
P.O. Box 246
Arequipa, Peru

Uruguay

Agrupación Nacional de Entidades Privadas Pro Bienester Social del Anciano
  (ANEPA)
Plaza Independencia 838, piso 2, oficina 9
Montevideo, Uruguay

NORTH AMERICA

Canada

Canadian Association on Gerontology
c/o Maimonides Hospital and Home for the Aged
5795 Caldwell Avenue
Côte St. Luc
Montreal, P.Q. H4W 1W3, Canada

United States of America

Federal Council on the Aging
330 Independence Avenue, S.W.
Washington, D.C. 20201, United States

Gerontological Society
Suite 520, One Dupont Circle
Washington, D.C. 20036, United States

National Council on the Aging, Inc. (NCOA)
1828 L Street, N.W.
Washington, D.C. 20036, United States

National Geriatrics Society
212 West Wisconsin Avenue
Milwaukee, Wisconsin 53203, United States

National Institute on Aging
Department of Health, Education and Welfare
Bethesda, Maryland 20014, United States

OCEANIA

Australia

Australian Association of Gerontology
c/o Science Centre
35 Clarence Street
Sydney, N.S.W. 2000, Australia

Australian Council on the Ageing
P.O. Box 1817Q, G.P.O.
Melbourne, Australia

New Zealand

New Zealand Society for the Study of Aging
P.O. Box 5546, Wellesley Street
Auckland 1, New Zealand

APPENDIX 2

INTERNATIONAL AND REGIONAL
ORGANIZATIONS ON AGING
DAVID A. HALL and ANDRUS VIIDIK

There are several different types of organizations on the international scene that concern themselves with aging. Some are primarily devoted to charity among the elderly, others to promoting the cause of the aged, influencing legislators, or disseminating and circulating information. The only truly international organization in the scientific field is the International Association of Gerontology. This appendix will deal mainly with this organization, which is based on the various national scientific societies. Some attention will also be paid to its European sections, since the need for cooperation among small national units is pronounced. As an example, the European Biological Section will be discussed in some detail (the Clinical Medicine and Social Research sections function similarly). Finally the Scandinavian Federation for Gerontology will be presented; it seems that even Europe is too big or too heterogeneous for close cooperation; a smaller regional organization is needed as a coordinating body.

INTERNATIONAL ASSOCIATION OF GERONTOLOGY

Aims

Article III of the bylaws of the International Association of Gerontology, revised in 1960 and ratified by all the constituent national societies, cites the association's purposes:

a) To promote gerontological research in biologic, medical and social fields carried out by gerontologic associations, societies or groups, by all possible means and in particular to promote cooperation amongst the members of these societies, associations or groups;
b) To promote the training of highly qualified professional personnel in the fields of ageing; and
c) To protect the interests of the gerontologic societies, associations or groups in all questions pertaining to foreign or international matters (for instance, by applying to organizations such as U.N.O., U.N.E.S.C.O., C.I.O.M.S., W.H.O., B.I.T., or to the government of any country).

History

The International Association of Gerontology was founded on July 10, 1950, at a meeting convened at Liège, Belgium. The organizing committee for the meeting was chaired by Professor L. Brull, who was subsequently elected the first president of the association, but much of the responsibility for the organization of international age research must be attributed to Dr. V. Korenchevsky. Dr. Korenchevsky, not content with founding the British Ageing Club, the forerunner of the present British Society for Research on Ageing, set himself the task of acting as a missionary for gerontology, traveling throughout the world and encouraging workers in many countries to found their own national gerontological societies. It was at his suggestion in 1949 that Professor Brull called ninety-seven representatives from fifteen countries to Liège to take part in the first Congress on Ageing. The governing body elected at that meeting consisted of one representative from each national society rather than from each nation. Thus there were two British, two French, and two American members; other countries contributed only one member each. This arrangement has been maintained, an extra member being added to the council as each new society has applied for membership in the association and has been elected. The format of the association was determined at this first meeting as a federation of national gerontological societies with more than ten members. There are no individual members.

At this meeting it was decided that the congresses organized by the association should take place every three years, although in the first instance, the United States' representatives were in a position to invite the association to St. Louis in the following year, 1951. It was also decided that the president elected at each congress should hold office for a three-year period and be succeeded by the vice-president, or as later designated, president elect. The secretariat, consisting of an elected secretary and a treasurer, would be of the same nationality as the president and would hold office for the same three-year period. These rules have been retained with little alteration during the twenty-eight years since their original pronouncement (they were ratified in 1960 at the San Francisco Congress).

The locations of the eleven congresses and the names of the presidents follow:

1.	Liège, Belgium	Professor L. Brull	1950
2.	St. Louis, United States	Professor E. V. Cowdry	1951
3.	London, Great Britain	Dr. J. H. Sheldon	1954
4.	Merano, Italy	Professor E. Greppi	1957
5.	San Francisco, United States	L. Kuplan	1960
6.	Copenhagen, Denmark	Professor T. Geill	1963
7.	Vienna, Austria	Dr. W. Doberauer	1966

8. Washington, D.C., United States	Dr. H. W. Shock	1969
9. Kiev, U.S.S.R.	Professor D. Chebotarev	1972
10. Jerusalem, Israel	Dr. D. Danon	1975
11. Tokyo, Japan	M. Murakami	1978

The Functions of the Council

As laid down in the bylaws of the association (1960 revision), the council constitutes the governing body of the association with full powers to act on the association's behalf. It determines the place and date for each international congress, thus delegating the choice of president elect and hence, at a later stage, president, to each successive host country. Between meetings, the activities of the council are delegated to the chairmen of the regional executive research committees and, through them to the officers of the regional research committees of the individual sections.

The president, or the chairman of the congress organizing comittee, becomes the chairman of the regional executive committee in the area in which he or she resides.

For the period 1975–1978 the officers of the International Association are:

President	David Danon
Secretary-general	Samuel J. Leibovich
Treasurer	Gershon Dror
Chairman of the European Executive Committee	Simon Bergman
Chairman of the American Executive Committee	Harold Brody

In addition to the chairmen, the two executive committees consist of the following:

European

J. Schouten	Chairman	Clinical Section
E. Beregi	Secretary	Clinical Section
J. Hellander	Chairman	Social Research Section
M. Asiel	Secretary	Social Research Section
A. Viidik	Chairman	Biological Section
D. A. Hall	Honorary chairman	Biological Section
U. J. Schmidt	Secretary	Biological Section

American

Secretary of Executive Committee,
  G. L. Maddox
E. Pfeiffer   Clinical Medicine
R. C. Edelman   Biology
M. M. Clark   Social and Behavioral Sciences
J. Kaplan   Applied Social Welfare

American Geriatric Society   E. W. Busse
  Representative
Canadian Representative   G. A. McDonnell

EUROPEAN BIOLOGICAL SECTION

Role in the International Association

At the Seventh International Congress of Gerontology in 1960, it was decided to found two major geographical executive committees to organize the activities of the international association: one in Europe and one on the North American continent. The membership of these committees would be composed of the officers of various sections devised to cover the different aspects of age research. In America, four such sections were founded, dealing especially with the biological, clinical, behavioral, and sociological fields. In Europe the last two topics have been covered by one section, thus giving a total of three.

In its role as a member of the European Executive Committee, the Biological Section sends one or more of its officers to the working parties set up every three years to assist in the organization of the triennial international congresses.

Function of the Section

The Biological Section, founded in 1960 with Professor F. Verzár of Basel and Professor F. Bourliére of Paris as chairman and secretary respectively, has sponsored triennial symposia on basic research in gerontology. Five have been organized, in 1964 in Basel, Switzerland, by Professor F. Verzár; in 1967 in Liblice, Czechoslovakia, by Dr. Z. Deyl; in 1970 in Leeds, England, by Dr. D. A. Hall; in 1973 in Varberg, Sweden, by Professor A. Viidik; and 1976 in Weimar, German Democratic Republic, by Professor G. Bruschke. The sixth symposium was arranged by Professor D. Platt in the German Federal Republic in 1979. (Two meetings that might be regarded as forerunners of the series were held in Basel in 1957 and Paris in 1960 at the invitation of Professors Verzár and Bourliére respectively, but since the organization of the Biological Section had not been settled by then, they are not included in the numbered series of symposia.)

Each symposium has been organized by the gerontological society of the host country. Of the 150 participants who have on average attended, between 12 and 20 percent have been nationals of countries other than the host. Participants from the rest of the world have always been welcome, and one or two of the keynote lectures have been presented by workers from the United States.

Membership, as in the case of the international association, is on a national basis, and the control of the section lies in the hands of the representatives from each national society who meet during each triennial symposium. The following countries are represented: Belgium, Bulgaria, Czechoslovakia, Denmark, Finland, France, Great Britain, Hungary, Italy, Netherlands, Norway, Rumania, the Soviet Union, Sweden, and Switzerland; in addition, workers from Canada, the Republic of Ireland, India, Israel, the Peoples' Republic of Korea, Poland, and the United States have attended some of the symposia.

To maintain continuity in an organization, the membership of which only meets once every three years, the officers have tended to hold their posts for appreciable periods. Professor Verzár held the post of chairman for six years from 1960 to 1966, Dr. Hall from 1966 to 1976, and Professor Viidik from 1976 to the present. In 1976 Dr. Hall was elected to a newly instituted office of honorary chairman. The secretaries of the section have been Professor Bourliére, Professor E. Guman, Dr. H. P. von Hahn, Dr. P. B. Gahan, Professor A. Viidik, and, since 1976, Dr. U. J. Schmidt.

During the periods between symposia, the identity of the section is maintained by the officers who keep in touch with the constituent societies by post and, where possible, by travel to meetings of the national societies, especially those identified as having international involvement. The cost of this work has been borne either by individual societies or by the use of any surplus from the funds raised by each host society for the triennial symposia. The section has no funds of its own, a fact that has made it difficult to expand its functions.

SCANDINAVIAN FEDERATION FOR GERONTOLOGY

From June 3–6, 1973, the first Scandinavian Gerontological Congress was held in Aarhus, initiated and chaired by Dr. Jörgen Scherwin. One of the topics at the meeting was the present state of gerontology in biology, clinical medicine, and social and behavioral sciences, with reports from Denmark, Finland, Iceland, and Norway. It was found that the problems with establishing research and teaching curricula were similar in these countries, although some had progressed more than others in establishing academic gerontology. An informal group worked on the proposal to establish a Scandinavian federation. A year later, the nine gerontological and geriatric societies in the five Scandinavian countries had ratified the bylaws of the federation, and at the second Scandinavian Gerontological Congress, which was held in Göteborg, Sweden, May 4–7, 1975, the federation held its first general assembly.

The aim of the federation is to be a coordinating and advisory board for the gerontological and geriatric (including long-term medical care) societies in Denmark, Finland, Iceland, Norway, and Sweden. Its purpose is to support, coordinate, and develop gerontological and clinical geriatric research and teaching. It functions according to the principles of the International Association of Gerontology and in cooperation with its European Section. It sponsors Scandinavian conferences of gerontology (biannually) and promotes dissemination of scientific information.

Chairman of the federation since its start in 1974 has been Professor A. Svanborg. Its secretary is A. Viidik. Representatives for the national societies are from Denmark, A. Viidik and J. Worm; from Finland, A. Kahanpää and L. Sourander; from Iceland, A. Gislason and T. Halldorsson; from Norway, A. C. Julsrud and Sol Seim; and from Sweden, A. Svanborg and S. M. Samuelson.

The activities have increased through the years. The federation now circulates a newsletter (NGF-aktuellt) four times a year to all the members of the Scandinavian national societies. The next congress was held in Oslo in 1979.

APPENDIX 3

THE INTERNATIONAL DEVELOPMENT OF ACADEMIC GERONTOLOGY

DONALD O. COWGILL and ROSEMARY A. ORGREN

I have been asked to give an international perspective on promoting the growth of gerontology in higher education. No doubt I drew this assignment because of my prior work on aging in various societies (Cowgill and Holmes, 1972; Cowgill, 1974). However, close examination of those earlier works will reveal practically nothing about the development of gerontology as a discipline or about gerontology in higher education. They have all been concerned with the phenomenon of aging as a socio-cultural process, the condition of older people within specific social settings or with the theory of the interrelationships between general social structure and the status and condition of older people. The works themselves may be considered a part of the growing corpus of gerontology, but gerontology as a system of thought and a discipline has not usually been part of the subject matter which has been treated in them. However, as I came to contemplate the assignment it posed a challenge because it appeared very probable that the development of gerontology as a self-conscious discipline was interlinked with the other types of developments with which I had been concerned and it seemed that the study of this development could possibly prove to be just an extension of the work in which I had already been involved. In other words, the development of gerontology is probably an intellectual reaction to some of the demographic and social conditions which have been the subject matter of my earlier study and writing.

Therefore, this paper is devoted to the examination of the emergence of gerontology as a system of thought, and its varying stages of development in relation to the types of societies and social conditions in which it has happened. A more direct statement of the theory, which is being presented, is that gerontology as an intellectual corpus and scientific discipline emerges only in certain social and historical contexts and its development is conditioned by further social and historical changes. More concretely we may posit that societies which have small proportions of their populations in advanced ages and whose institutions have evolved in such a way as to absorb and care for the needs of such older people, as they have will not develop a self-conscious analysis of old age and will not be concerned with the problems and conditions of aging.

Source: Reprinted by permission from H. Sterns (Ed.), *Promoting the Growth of Gerontology in Higher Education*. Belmont, California: Wadsworth, 1979.

On the other hand we may posit that with increasing numbers and proportions of older people in modernizing societies and with the concomitant institutional changes attendant upon modernization which render traditional institutional forms either obsolete or inadequate for the management of problems of aging there will be a development of study, analysis and teaching about aging, i.e., the study of gerontology will emerge.

No doubt the best way of testing this proposition, from a methodological point of view, would be longitudinal, historical studies in specific societies in which such development has occurred. Little systematic work of this kind has yet been done. Therefore I am thrown back upon a cross-sectional or cross-cultural approach. I am well aware of the dangers of such a methodology and I shall try to be sensitive to the points at which such a methodology might tend to mislead us.

For some twenty societies I have hurriedly assembled information on the volume and types of research being conducted, the number of academic specialists devoting major attention to some aspect of gerontology, the number and kind of courses being taught, whether there are institutes or centers devoting themselves primarily to gerontology, whether there are national associations or professional organizations of gerontology, whether there are professional journals in the area, and to some extent the nature of the sponsorship of both research and teaching in those societies. On the basis of this information I wish tentatively to suggest that there appear to be about five different stages of development of academic gerontology which are closely associated with different levels of demographic and social modernization.

The first stage is that in which there is no gerontology of any form—no research, no teaching, and usually no specialized service programs. Without exception these are societies which we now label as developing societies, in which demographic aging has not yet occurred to any measurable degree and in which older persons are cared for and integrated into familial and kinship institutions which have traditionally operated to manage this social function. Indeed in none of the countries which showed no sign of gerontological development was there more than three percent of the population 65 and over. In many of the societies in this stage of development, modernization has had the demographic effect of "younging" their populations and of increasing the emphasis upon youth, rather than developing any emphasis on aging. One of my informants illustrates this by the statement, "The present concerns of this country are with youth and economic dependency of the young rather than of the aged." Thus in these societies it is not merely that the aged have not yet been defined as a social problem, it is more that the present social problems are overwhelmingly concerned with youth. Therefore we cannot expect much intellectual attention to be given to older people, and we cannot expect much programmatic response or innovation in the direction of aging. Some of the sample countries in this stage of development included: Brazil, Peru, Iran, Jordan, Nigeria and American Samoa.

However, in several other countries with no greater demographic aging, there are indications of some beginning interest in research relative to aging. In each case this is either a transplanted interest stimulated by contact with gerontology elsewhere or a response to some specific problem. For example, in Thailand a former student of mine is planning to study the inmates of several of their old folks residential homes. In Egypt, there has been a study of widows and some attention to poverty, including poverty among the aged. In Taiwan a survey of old people in institutions for the aged is currently being completed and some attention is being given to the problems of differential service (not to say discrimination) as between mainlanders and native Taiwanese in services for the aged, including institutionalization. A recent migrant to Kuwait is a demographer with a considerable interest in and commitment to gerontology. Thus research interests and expertise are being diffused from developed areas to less developed ones. And it is evident that many of the limited services available to the elderly in these societies are also imitative responses of western patterns. Certainly this is the case in Kenya where Cox and Mberia (1977) report on an old folks home established by missionaries.

Another observation about the kind of research which is either under way or being planned in the societies in this stage of development is that most of it is either demographic or sociological in nature. This appears to be a case in which our cross-sectional method provides a kind of observation which would not be expected in longitudinal study of more advanced development in gerontology. In Europe and the United States, for example, biological and medical research in aging preceded socio-logical and psychological research by several decades. However, currently developing countries, now beginning to face some social problems related to age, seem to be leaving the basic research on biological and medical aging to the more advanced societies and they are devoting their research attention to the demographic and socio-logical problems specific to their societies.

The third stage of gerontological development is to be found in such places as Australia and Japan where we certainly have both bio-medical and sociological research under way. Furthermore, much of this research is taking place within organized structures, the results are being published in formal journals, and the researchers are affiliated with formal professional associations. There are still no formal courses in aging or gerontology and few if any faculty describe themselves as gerontologists. It is interesting and probably significant that in both of these societies about eight percent of the population is 65 or over and in both the proportion is increasing quite rapidly. Some of the research interest is undoubtedly anticipatory response.

The fourth stage of development is represented by societies which have developed a full range of academic programs in gerontology, including not only research institutes, associations and journals, but have added formal teaching and faculty who are self-consciously associating themselves with the field of gerontology both for research and for instructional identification. This seems to have happened in many of the countries of Europe such as Sweden, Norway, Austria, West Germany, Holland and France all of which have populations with 14 or 15 percent 65 and over. However there appear to be a couple of cases of countries where similar developments have happened at an earlier stage of demographic development. One of these is Israel, but in this case we know that a large proportion of the population are migrants from Europe who have carried their skills and interests with them and have developed programs very much upon the European model. The other case is Canada with only eight percent of its population 65 and over, and here we appear to see the development of gerontology paralleling that in its neighbor to the South and interacting very intimately with programs and develop-ments within the United States.

In not many parts of the world has the national government formally sponsored gerontological research and training. This appears to be the fifth stage of gerontological growth. The entry of the national government into this role has been painful and unsteady here in the United States.

If these stages represent a fair approximation to the order of development of gerontology in general there are also some subordinate principles which seem worthy of enunciation. One of these is the sequence of institutional response to demographic aging which is also reflected in research interests. The earliest area of concern appears to be with sheer economic security, with the means of survival. Thus we find the establishment of almshouses, old folks homes, social security and pension schemes and this is shortly reflected in research aimed at finding ways to accomplish the ends better or at least more cheaply. So we have studies such as Charles Booth's (1894) classic study of *The Aged Poor* in England in the 1890's and a parallel concern with poverty among the aged in Egypt today. When we get past the concern for sheer survival it appears that the next general interest is in health but even here there is a sequence in which the first line of attention is an extension of curative medicine; the doctors and hospitals continue to apply the views and skills appropriate to younger populations, the effort to cure people of acute and reversible conditions. It takes a considerable period of time for our institutions to adjust themselves to the reality of a changed population and to come to the realization that health care in an aged population must stress preventive maintenance and treatment of chronic conditions. Beverfelt reports that medical schools in Norway provide for specialization in geriatrics, but that there is nothing on aging in the training of other specialists. Still later comes the acknowledgment that old people are total human beings with all of the psychological and sociological needs of any persons. The adaptation of our mass urban institutions to this need is a continuing challenge. No one has succeeded very well in this effort as yet.

A second subordinate sequence has to do with the emphasis and interpretation of research—what we research and how it is interpreted. In the early stages, as we become conscious of the reality of an aging population and of the evident needs of these people, our research tends to concentrate on problematic aspects of aging. Part of the reason for this is that often researchers concentrate upon captive audiences in clinics and in hospitals. But another part of the reason is that the motivation for the research is frequently to convince decision makers that something needs to be done about perceived problems. Therefore there is an effort to count problem cases and a tendency to exaggerate the seriousess of the problem. Much of the research here in the United States prior to about 1960 was of this kind and it tended to reinforce the stereotype of old age as a period of decline, weakness, senility, poor health, and poverty. It takes some time for science to escape from the intellectual confinement of its clinical and hospital cases and from the stereotype which they build and reinforce, to undertake the more difficult and costly research of looking at normal representative people who often don't stand still and wait to be studied, and especially to study these live and lively people over a long enough period of time to see the real consequences of aging. Gerontology in the more advanced areas of the world is just now attempting to readjust both its method and its interpretation to these imperatives. Ageism is still rampant and the stereotypes are still abundant even among gerontologists, many of whom are attempting to escape these intellectual shackles. The reason for these vestiges in the literature is not merely inertia, biased samples and cross-sectional research designs. Many continue to feel the need for the ''poor old dear'' approach as a means of tugging at the heart strings in justifying appeals for money for services and research. How do we justify our appeals for funds to the bureaucrats, to Congress, or even to Maggie Kuhn, except in terms of serious and prevalent problems to be solved? Most of us don't find the Louis Harris (1974) survey which showed most old people as reasonably happy, healthy, comfortable and active people very helpful in promoting programs or grants. In this stage of development the appeals must be much more sophisticated and precise. No longer can we ascribe to the old in general a prevalent failing to which our particular project will supply the ultimate answer. Now we must say with precision where the problem is, how extensive it is, and probably we must put forward a more convincing argument that our project will have any significant impact upon the target population.

In conclusion, it appears that the development of academic gerontology does occur in response to demographic and institutional changes in society. There are reasonably regular stages of its development, beginning with individually initiated scattered research, gradually maturing into organized activities in institutes and professional associations, ultimately culminating in a full range of research and teaching. Biological and medical research seems to have preceded social and psychological research in the developed parts of the world, but in the developing areas this sequence is not as clear. In most places early concerns are with sheer economic survival, then with the availability and practice of curative medicine, followed by attention to health maintenance programs, and ultimately by a realization that older people must be treated in all institutional settings as whole persons. In early stages our research tends to concentrate upon problematic aspects of aging and only later, with more representative samples and longitudinal designs, do we arrive at a more balanced and sanguine view of the aging process. Needless to say we in the United States have not yet fully arrived in this latter projected stage and it remains to be seen whether the developing societies must pass through all of the painful stages of development which the more advanced societies have undergone.

REFERENCES

Beverfelt, E. 1973. Training within gerontology: Needs and organization. In *Recruitment and training of personnel*. Paris: International Center of Social Gerontology.

Cowgill, Donald O. 1974. Aging and modernization: A revision of the theory. In Jaber Gubrium, *Late Life*. Springfield, Ill.: Charles C. Thomas, Publisher.

Cowgill, Donald O., and Holmes, Lowell D. 1972. *Aging and Modernization*. New York: Appleton-Century-Crofts.

Cox, Frances M., and Mberia, Ndung'u. 1977. *Aging in a changing village society: A Kenyan experience*. Washington, D.C.: International Federation on Aging.

Harris, Louis and Associates, Inc. 1975. *The myth and reality of aging in America*. Washington, D.C.: National Council on the Aging.

INDEX

LIST OF
CONTRIBUTORS

A. Amann, University Assistant Magister
Lehrkanzel fur Soziologie
A-1080-Wein
Aeserstrasse 33
Vienna, Austria

Ana Aslan, Professor and Director
Institutul de Geriatrie
Str. Minastirea Caldarusani, 9
Casuta Postala 1004
Bucuresti, Rumania

Edit Beregi, C.M.Sc., D.M.Sc.
President, Hungarian Gerontological Association
Director, Research Department of Gerontology
Semmelweis Medical School
1428 Budapest, Postafiok 45, Hungary

Shimon Bergman, ACSW
School of Social Work, University of Tel Aviv
Brookdale Institute of Gerontology and Adult Human Development
P.O. Box 13087
Givat Ram, Jerusalem, Israel

Eva Beverfelt
Norwegian Gerontological Institute
Oscarsgate 36
Oslo 2, Norway

W. R. Bytheway, Ph.D.
Honourable Secretary, British Society of Social and Behavioral Gerontology
Medical Sociology Research Center
University College Swansea
University of Wales
Park Buildings, Park Street
Swansea SA1 3DJ, South Wales, United Kingdom

Dmitri F. Chebotarev, Professor, Dr. Med. Sc.
Director, Institute of Gerontology of the Academy of Medical Sciences
Vyshgorodskaya St., 67
252655 Kiev—114, U.S.S.R.

S. P. Cilliers, Professor
Department of Sociology
University of Stellenbosch
Stellenbosch, South Africa

Donald O. Cowgill, Ph.D.
Professor of Sociology and Rural Sociology
Director, Joint Centers for Aging Studies
University of Missouri
Columbia, Missouri 65201

David Danon, M.D.
President, International Association of Gerontology
Head, Section of Biological Ultrastructure
Weitzmann Institute of Science
P.O. Box 26
Rehovot, Israel

B. Doberauer, Oberarzt Doctor
Osterreichische Gesellschaft für Geriatrie
A-1140 Wien XIV
Hotteldorferstrasse 188
Vienna, Austria

W. Doberauer, Oberarzt Doctor
Osterreichische Gesellschaft für Geriatrie
A-1140 Wien XIV
Hotteldorferstrasse 188
Vienna, Austria

Lucjan Dobrowolski, Professor, Dr.
President, Geriatrics Section, Polish Medical Association
Lwowska 4 m 3
Warsaw 00-658, Poland

S. Eitner, Professor, Dr., Sc. Med.
Forshungsprojeckt Gerontologie der DDR
Hermann-Matern-Str. 13a
104 Berlin, German Democractic Republic

L. Figallo-Espinal, Dr.
Colegio de Medicos del Distrito Federal
Caracas, Venezuela

John F. Fleetwood, Dr.
Secretary, Irish Gerontological Society
11 Proby Square
Blackrock, Dublin, Ireland

Aurelia Florea, Dr. ssa.
Istituto per gli Studi di Servizio Sociale
Via Arno 2
Rome 00198, Italy

Anne Fontaine, Documentaliste
Fondation National de Gérontologie
49 rue Mirabeau
75116 Paris, France

Bent Frijs-Madsen, M.D.
Secretary, Danish Gerontological Society
Department of Geriatric Medicine
Gentralsygehuset
4700 Naestved, Denmark

José Froimovich, M.D., President
Sociedad Chilena de Gerontologia
Avenida Bulnes 377, Departmento 605
Santiago, Chile

Barbara Fülgraff, Ph.D.
Professor of Sociology and Adult Education
University of Oldenburg
Ammerlander Heerstr. 67-99
2900 Oldenburg, West Germany

Bernard Grad, Associate Professor
Department of Psychiatry
McGill University
Montreal, Quebec, Canada

David A. Hall, M.D.
Senior Lecturer in Biochemistry
Department of Medicine
University of Leeds
Leeds, LS1 3EX, United Kingdom

J. Hoerl, University Assistant Magister
Lehrkanzel fur Soziologie
A-1080-Wein
Aeserstrasse 33
Vienna, Austria

J. A. Huet, Professor and Président
Centre d'Etudes et de Recherches Gérontologiques
1, Place Iena
75016 Paris, France

Jean-Pierre Junod, M.D.
Medecin-Directeur, Hospital de Gériatrie
1226 Thonex
Geneve, Switzerland

I. Kalbe, Dr. rer. nat.
Forchungsprojeckt Gerontologie der DDR
Herman-Mattern-Str. 13a
104 Berlin, German Democractic Republic

Djordje Kozarevic, M.D., M.P.H.
Director, Institute of Chronic Diseases and Gerontology
11000 Belgrade
Slobodana Penezice Krcuna 35, Yugoslavia

E. G. Loten, M.B., Ch.B., F.R.A.C.P.
President, New Zealand Society for the Study of Aging
P.O. Box 5546, Wellesley Street
Auckland 1, New Zealand

Daisaku Maeda
Chief, Social Welfare Section
Tokyo Metropolitan Institute of Gerontology
35-2 Sakaecho, Itabashiku
Tokyo 173, Japan

G. Majce, University Assistant Magister
Lehrakanzel fur Soziologie
A-1080-Wein
Aeserstrasse 33
Vienna, Austria

Americo S. Alberieux Murdoch, M.D.
Hon. President, Sociedad de Geriatria y Gerontologia del Uruguay
Duvinioso Terra 1567, AP 402
Montevideo, Uruguay

Rosemary A. Orgren
Educational Gerontologist
Joint Centers for Aging Studies
University of Missouri
Columbia, Missouri 65201

Erdman Palmore, Ph.D.
Professor of Medical Sociology
Senior Fellow, Duke University Center for the Study of Aging and Human Development
Box 3003, Duke Medical Center
Durham, North Carolina 27710, United States

Manuel Payno, Dr.
Academia Mexicano de Gerontologia
Pitagoras 617
Narvarte, Mexico, D.F.

H. Richter, Dipl. rer. pol.
Forshungsprojeckt Gerontologie der DDR
Hermann-Matern-Str. 13a
104 Berlin, German Democratic Republic

Gilbert Rosenberg, M.D., F.R.C.P. (C)
Professor, University of Calgary, and Director, Fanning Extended Care Center
722 Sixteenth Ave., N.E.
Calgary, Alberta T2E 6V7, Canada

Nina N. Sachuk, Dr. Med. Sc.
Institute of Gerontology, AMS
Vyshgorodskaya St. 67
252655 Kiev-114, U.S.S.R.

U. J. Schmidt, OA Doz, Dr., Sc., Med., Secretary
International Association of Gerontology
Medizinische Poliklinik der Bereiches Medzin der Humboldt-Universitat
Hermann-Matern-Strasse 13a
104 Berlin, German Democractic Republic

P. H. Schulz, Professor, Dr.
Forshungsprojeckt Gerontologie der DDR
Hermann-Matern-Strasse 13a
104 Berlin, German Democractic Republic

Leif Sourander, M.D.
President of Societas Gerontologica Fennica
Assistant Professor of Geriatric Medicine
University of Turku
City Hospital
20700 Turku 70, Finland

Andrus Viidik, M.D., Ph.D.
President, Danish Gerontological Society
Professor of Anatomy
Department of Connective Tissue Biology
Institute of Anatomy
University of Aarhus
DK-8000, Aarhus C., Denmark

R. J. van Zonneveld, Dr.
Secretary-Treasurer, Netherlands Society for Gerontology
Director, Bureau Council of Health Research, TNO
Juliana van Stolberglaan 148
Postbus 297, den Haag, 2076, Netherlands

John Zarras
Lecturer, University of Athens
Executive Committee of Helennic Association of Gerontology
8 Pittakou Street
Athens 119, Greece

ABOUT THE EDITOR

Erdman Palmore is Senior Fellow at the Duke Center for the Study of Aging and Human Development, and Professor of Medical Sociology at the Duke University Medical School in Durham, North Carolina. His previous books include *Honorable Elders, Normal Aging,* and *Prediction of Life Span.*